1987.

For Elizabeth and the boys

Epilepsy

EDITED BY

Anthony Hopkins

Department of Neurological Sciences,
St Bartholomew's Hospital, London

London
CHAPMAN AND HALL

First published in 1987
by Chapman and Hall Ltd
11 New Fetter Lane, London EC4P 4EE

© 1987 Chapman and Hall

Printed in Great Britain
at the University Press, Cambridge

ISBN 0 412 26520 6

British Library Cataloguing in Publication Data

Epilepsy.
  1. Epilepsy
  I. Hopkins, Anthony
  616.8'53   RC372

ISBN 0-412-26520-6

Contents

Contributors

Thomas L. Babb, Department of Neurology, Reed Neurological Research Institute, Brain Research Institute, University of California School of Medicine, Los Angeles, California, USA.

Colin D. Binnie, The Maudsley Hospital, Denmark Hill, London, UK.

W. Jann Brown, Department of Pathology/Neuropathology, Reed Neurological Research Institute, Brain Research Institute, University of California School of Medicine, Los Angeles, California, USA.

Stephen W. Brown, The David Lewis Centre for Epilepsy, Cheshire, UK

Sarah Bundey, The Infant Development Unit, Birmingham Maternity Hospital, Queen Elizabeth Medical Centre, Edgbaston, Birmingham, UK.

Antonio V. Delgado-Escueta, Comprehensive Epilepsy Program, Department of Neurology, Reed Neurological Research Center, UCLA Center for the Health Sciences, and VA Southwest Regional Epilepsy Center, Neurology and Research Services, West Los Angeles VA Medical Center (Wadsworth), Los Angeles, California, USA.

Fritz E. Dreifuss, University of Virginia Medical Center, Charlottesville, Virginia, USA.

Peter Fenwick, Institute of Psychiatry, de Crespigny Park, Denmark Hill, London, UK.

Andrea Garman, Department of Neurological Sciences, St Bartholomew's Hospital, West Smithfield, London, UK.

Peter K. P. Harvey, Department of Neurology, Royal Free Hospital, Pond Street, London, UK.

Anthony Hopkins, Department of Neurological Sciences, St Bartholomew's Hospital, West Smithfield, London, UK.

John G. R. Jefferys, Sobell Department of Neurophysiology, Institute of Neurology, Queen Square, and Department of Physiology and Biophysics, St Mary's Hospital Medical School, London, UK.

Bryan Jennett, Department of Neurosurgery, Institute of Neurological Sciences, University of Glasgow, Glasgow, UK.

S. Roy Meadow, Department of Paediatrics and Child Health, St James's University Hospital, Leeds, UK.

Niall V. O'Donohoe, Department of Paediatrics, National Children's Hospital and Trinity College, Dublin, Eire.

Richard Roberts, University Department of Medicine, Ninewells Hospital and Medical School, Dundee, UK.

Ernst A. Rodin, Epilepsy Center of Michigan, 3800 Woodward – Seventh Floor, Detroit, Michigan, USA.

Danuta Rosciszewska, Department of Neurology, Silesian Medical Academy, 41-800 Zabrze, 3-go Maja 15, Poland.

Graham Scambler, Academic Department of Psychiatry, Middlesex Hospital Medical School, London, UK.

Simon Shorvon, Institute of Neurology and National Hospital for Nervous Diseases, Queen Square, London, and the National Hospital–Chalfont Centre for Epilepsy, Buckinghamshire, UK.

Barbara E. Swartz, Department of Neurology, Reed Neurological Research Center, UCLA Center for the Health Sciences, and VA Southwest Regional Epilepsy Center, Neurology and Research Services, West Los Angeles VA Medical Center (Wadsworth), Los Angeles, California, USA.

Sheila J. Wallace, Department of Paediatric Neurology, University Hospital of Wales, Cardiff, UK.

Preface

There has been renewed interest in the scientific and sociological aspects of epilepsy in the last fifteen years, reflected in a mass of scientific and popular communications. There are a number of monographs about aspects of epilepsy on the market, but some, though excellent, concentrate on one particular aspect such as anticonvulsant medication, and others are no more than a collection of manuscripts reflecting the disparate interests of contributors and editor. None seem to provide a coherent guide to epilepsy to the resident training in neurology, to the practising 'general' neurologist, or to one whose special expertise lies in other fields. I hope this book meets these needs. It is difficult to impose an architecture on a field as wide as epilepsy, but I hope that my co-authors and I succeed in leading the reader from the epidemiology of epilepsy, through the biophysical principles, to the clinical aspects of the different epileptic syndromes and their investigation and treatment. Psychiatric, sociological and legal aspects are considered towards the end of the book.

I am grateful to all my colleagues for the prompt submission of their chapters, and for contributing their experience to this book. My secretary, Mrs Joyce Bennett, provided splendid help and support and I am also grateful to Dr Peter Altman and Miss Sharon Duckworth of Chapman and Hall for their help and skill up to publication.

Anthony Hopkins,
February, 1987

CHAPTER ONE

Definitions and Epidemiology of Epilepsy

Anthony Hopkins

All epidemiology is bedevilled by problems of definition of the disease and of the population base under study, and of case ascertainment, but the epidemiology of epilepsy is more complex than that of most other neurological illnesses. In the case of cerebrovascular disease, for example, an illness which like epilepsy ranks high in neurological importance, the vast majority of cases occur in older age groups, are related to atherosclerosis, and the events under study are reasonably clearly defined. Epileptic seizures occur at any age, are of many different types, arise as a result of many different pathologies, have a variable genetic basis, may be precipitated by environmental events, and may start, or stop for no clearly defined reason. Older physicians used to state, with some justification, that epilepsy was a symptom. This immediately raises the problem that analysis of symptoms is hardly an adequate basis for the understanding of pathophysiological events. If epilepsy is a symptom, like breathlessness, who now would attempt to write '*A textbook of dyspsnoea*'? However, as 'epilepsy' is the present and best framework within which neurological medicine operates, it is of crucial importance to define the operational terms.

1.1 AN EPILEPTIC SEIZURE

An *epileptic seizure* may be defined as a *paroxysmal discharge of cerebral neurones sufficient to cause clinically detectable events that are apparent either to the subject or to an observer*. Each of the adjectives or nouns in this sentence is of importance. '*Paroxysmal discharge*' is more fully analysed in Chapter 2 but its purpose in this definition is to exclude clinical events such as a transient hemiparesis caused by depression of neuronal inactivity resulting from, for example, migraine, or ischaemia due to vascular occlusion. The word '*cerebral*' excludes the activity of spinal neurones resulting in spinal myoclonus, stretch-induced clonus or flexor spasm in paraplegia.

Events resulting from a paroxysmal neuronal discharge may be apparent only to the subject, as in some distorted perception resulting from a seizure beginning in the mesial temporal lobe, or, less commonly, in the somatosensory area. Alternatively events may be apparent only to the observer – for example, a generalized tonic-clonic seizure arising during sleep. More commonly, however, the epileptic event is detected by both subject and observer.

The modifiers *'clinically detectable'* to the word *'events'* are present in the definition so that an epileptiform discharge in the electroencephalogram (EEG) (p. 169) without clinical concomitants, is not called a seizure. There are, however, difficulties here, as sophisticated analysis of performance during psychological tests have shown that cognitive function is impaired during the 3 Hz activity associated with absence seizures, even though there is no 'clinically detectable' event at this time, as judged by bedside assessment [1]. A parallel disturbance of cognitive function, as judged by impaired performance on video games, has been shown during subclinical discharges arising in the temporal lobe [2]. These studies have raised a problem of definition – just how much impairment of function warrants an event being called a seizure. For operational purposes, however, the definition continues to require a 'clinically detectable event'.

The adjective *'epileptic'* itself causes difficulties in epidemiological study. Febrile convulsions, for example, are included in the proposed International Classification of the Epilepsies (Chapter 3). However, numerous studies (reviewed by Wallace in Chapter 15) have shown firstly that a febrile convulsion is an incident arising in the childhood of up to 5% of perfectly healthy children, and secondly that febrile convulsions are not followed by later epilepsy except in certain clearly defined circumstances. The consensus view is that febrile convulsions, although undoubtedly associated with a paroxysmal discharge of cerebral neurones, should not be regarded as 'epileptic'.

The same caveat applies to anoxic seizures. A period of cerebral hypoperfusion resulting from cardiac or vasovagal syncope may terminate in anoxic convulsions, but the EEG changes preceding and during these are quite different from those of epilepsy [3].

There is no great intellectual difficulty in distinguishing anoxic seizures or febrile convulsions from epilepsy, but a much greater problem arises in so-called isolated seizures.

It used to be thought that isolated seizures were quite common, and did not herald the onset of epilepsy. As, however, anyone suffering from recurrent epileptic seizures must at some stage have had his first of many it is not possible to say of any individual that his first seizure is not epileptic. Indeed, the epidemiological studies of first seizures reviewed on p. 152 show that 30–70% of first seizures are followed by others within a few years. Take the example of a man who has a single seizure at the age of 20, and is seen at the age of 30, having had no others. It might seem reasonable to say that this man had once had an epileptic seizure, but not that he was 'an epileptic'. What if he then has a second seizure at the age of 40? Does he then become 'an epileptic' after this interval of 20 years, or was he an undiagnosed epileptic the whole time?

1.2 EPILEPSY

Some of the difficulties recorded above can be avoided by an operational definition of epilepsy in the following terms: *epilepsy is a condition in which more than one non-febrile seizure of any type has occurred at any time*. This is distinctly different from the definition given in the *WHO Dictionary of Epilepsy*: 'a chronic brain disorder of various aetiologies characterized by recurrent seizures due to excessive discharge of cerebral neurones. Single or occasional epileptic seizures as well as those occasioning during an acute illness should not be classified as epilepsy'. It is quite true that some patients have only occasional seizures [4] but that seems insufficient grounds to exclude them from a diagnosis of epilepsy.

Once again, however, the proposed definition raises a difficulty. As will be seen on p. 11, the ratio between the incidence and prevalence rates indicates, and long term follow-up studies confirm (p. 12) that epileptic seizures often cease. Take the example of a girl who had many seizures in adolescence, but then none after the age of 21. When does she stop suffering from epilepsy – after an interval of five years free from seizures, or ten – or should she be regarded throughout her life as 'an epileptic'? Leaving aside the use of the term 'epileptic', which some find perjorative, it would seem best to record this patient as being 'in remission for *x* years' as undoubtedly she is at greater risk from recurrent seizures in later life than some one who has never had a single seizure.

1.3 PROVOKED SEIZURES

There is another aspect upon which an epidemiologist has to make up his mind. Many authors of studies of first seizures or epilepsy (e.g. [5]) exclude what they call *provoked seizures*, in relation to intoxication with alcohol, or as an unwanted effect of some other drug such as a tricyclic antidepressant, or in relation to withdrawal from alcohol or barbiturates. While there is little doubt that seizures may be provoked by such circumstances, epidemiological studies usually fail to state specifically their criteria for exclusion. How many drinks do you have to take before you can fairly attribute your seizure to alcohol?

1.4 SEIZURE THRESHOLD

The concept of a '*seizure threshold*' is helpful in resolving some of these semantic difficulties. Anyone can have an epileptic seizure, but the majority of the population never do. Those with low thresholds have a greater tendency to seizures. In those with low thresholds, a variety of stimuli throughout life may be sufficient to trigger a seizure.

This, then, is the touchstone of the epidemiology of epilepsy. What is it that leads some people to have seizures after a head injury, while others with an identical head injury do not? What is the *pattern of susceptibility* to epilepsy in the population? Unfortunately there is no methodology yet devized for surveying the population's propensity to seizures. All an epidemiologist can do is to survey the results of that propensity – the seizures themselves.

To summarize so far, an epidemiologist working on epilepsy has to decide exactly what constitutes a seizure, whether to include febrile, anoxic, isolated, first or rarely recurrent seizures, seizures in remission, and provoked seizures. He or she has to remember that the seizures are only markers of a widely distributed and varying propensity to seizures, and the variation in epileptic threshold, so far unmeasurable, determines whether or not a subject will have a seizure in response to some insult such as a head injury or stroke.

1.5 THE POPULATION UNDER STUDY

Many earlier studies on the epidemiology of epilepsy were based upon the population attending neurologists, and sometimes clinics specializing in epilepsy. The prognosis of such selected patients (e.g. [6]) is, it is now known, much more unfavourable than that of the population with epilepsy as a whole. In the last 20 years, however, a number of studies have been done based upon the population 'as it really is' in the community. Pioneers of this approach included Kurland in Minnesota [7], Crombie [8], Pond [9] and Brewis [10] and their various colleagues in England, Gudmundsson [11] in Iceland, and Zielinski [12] in Poland. One of the fullest studies of the 1970s was that of Hauser and Kurland [13]. Their population base was the people of Olmsted County, Minnesota, a moderately stable rural and professional population of about 55 000, where primary medical care was and is undertaken by the sophisticated medical facilities of the Mayo Clinic. Many of the subsequent writings on the epidemiology of epilepsy draw heavily upon this material. Later studies based upon English primary care practice are those of Hopkins and Scambler [14] and Goodridge and Shorvon [15].

1.6 ASCERTAINMENT OF CASES

Many people with epilepsy are reluctant to disclose their condition (Chapter 17). Some patients with undoubted seizures therefore probably do not seek medical advice, and do not come under medical care [12]. Indeed personal experience shows that, when talking about eligibility to hold a driving licence (Chapter 20), many patients remark that they wish they had never been to the doctor about their seizure(s). However, a proportion of those with seizures that, to a neurologist, is surprisingly large – 80% – do not suspect the diagnosis of epilepsy before consulting their doctor [14]. If medical records are complete, which is, unfortunately, unlikely for administrative reasons even in the UK with a constant patient-linked record system, then it is unlikely that many patients with epilepsy are overlooked in a competent survey. However, surveys which rely upon the records of a population of which members have been to a number of different doctors and clinics may seriously underestimate the lifetime incidence (p. 7) of epilepsy. Even door-step surveys, with carefully constructed questionnaires, may fail as patients known to have epilepsy have been shown to be very likely to deny it [16].

1.7 PROBLEMS WITH THE DIAGNOSIS OF AN EPILEPTIC SEIZURE

These are considered on p. 157. In epidemiological terms, in the absence of the histological proof that allows one to write, for example, with greater certainty about the epidemiology of cancer of the breast, most surveys imply that the diagnosis of epilepsy is made on clinical grounds by a neurological specialist. It is likely that most surveys are contaminated by some anoxic seizures, simulated seizures and ischaemic events.

In practical terms, apart from the operational definitions of epileptic seizure and epilepsy, the forgoing paragraphs are not of great concern to any except those who are writing specifically about their epidemiological techniques. It is of no great interest to know that the prevalence of epilepsy is 8 per 1000 in Poland and 5 per 1000 in the UK, for example. What is important is the use of epidemiology to define, for example:

(1) populations at risk so that methods of prevention can be considered;
(2) populations that require specific investigation and treatment, so that appropriate facilities can be provided;
(3) populations that require special care, for example in special schools or caring institutions, so that appropriate budgets can be allocated.

1.8 INCIDENCE OF EPILEPSY AT DIFFERENT AGES

The age-specific incidence rates from the Rochester study [13] are shown in Fig 1.1. The high incidence in early childhood reflects particularly the high incidence of seizures occurring in the first year of life ([17, 18] and Chapter 16). Figure 1.1 shows more or less steady age-specific incidence through maturity and middle life of about 20–40 cases per 100 000 per year. There is no particular 'peak' reflecting 'epilepsy of late onset' as traditionally described, until the last decades, when epilepsy in association with atrophy and vascular disease (p. 119) adds to the figures. Two studies show either a prominent increase in the number of cases in the last decades of life [13], or a high incidence of epilepsy in those over the age of sixty – 77 per 100 000 [18b].

Juul-Jensen and Foldspang [19] report similar figures in middle life based upon their survey of nearly 250 000 people in Greater Aarhus, Denmark, but these writers did not find an increased incidence after the age of 50.

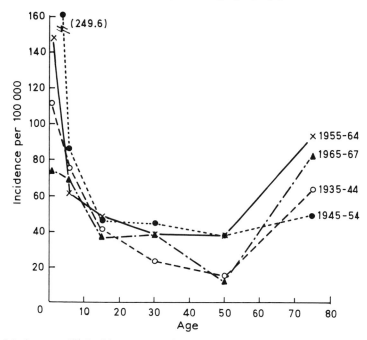

Figure 1.1 Age-specific incidence rates of epilepsy first diagnosed at different intervals in Rochester, Minnesota, 1935–1967. (Reproduced with kind permission from Hauser and Kurland [13].)

1.9　CUMULATIVE INCIDENCE OF EPILEPSY

This concept in relation to epilepsy was first introduced by Crombie and colleagues [8]. They wrote:

> 'From the annual rates of occurrence of first fits per 1000 patients alive, by sex and age groups . . . it is possible to make an estimate of the number of persons in a community who are likely to have a fit of some sort during their life time.' Their calculations are not clear, but they estimated that 'just over 4% of all persons are likely to have a fit at some time during their life . . .' and (later) '. . . 32 persons per 1000 may be expected to have had a chance of being classed as a chronic epileptic . . .'

The concept of cumulative incidence has been furthered by longitudinal follow-up of a national population sample including all children born in one week in March, 1958 in the United Kingdom. The cumulative incidence of epilepsy was 4.1 cases per 1000 (0.41%) by the age of 11 (64 cases in 15 496 children) [20]. Preliminary date from a further follow up of this cohort suggest that the cumulative incidence is 0.6% by the age of 16 and 1.0% by the age of 23 [21].

Hauser and Kurland [13], combining the incidence rates for isolated

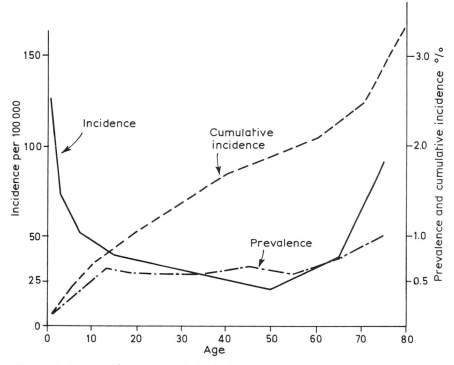

Figure 1.2 Age-specific rate, cumulative incidence rate and prevalence rate of epilepsy. Data from Rochester, Minnesota, 1935–1974. (Reproduced with kind permission from Hauser *et al.* [20]).

seizures with those for epilepsy, calculated that 5.9% of the total population of the community may be expected to experience at least one non-febrile seizure in their lifetime. The Minnesota experience for recurrent seizures is illustrated in Fig. 1.2 [22]. The lifetime incidence of ever having been epileptic is 3.2%; the Danish experience gives a figure of 2.44% [19].

These high figures have received direct support from observations by Goodridge and Shorvon [15, 23]. They inspected 6000 records of one general practice. In the UK system of health care, if a patient relocates, his health record is sent, at least in theory, to his new primary care physician. Goodridge and Shorvon found 122 patients had had at least one non-febrile seizure, giving a lifetime incidence of 2.03%. Recurrent seizures (at least two non-febrile seizures) had affected 1.67% at some time. Clearly, many of this population were in youth or middle age, and as some of the records were incomplete, the lifetime incidence will be even more than this, supporting the estimated American and Danish figures quoted above.

This concept of cumulative incidence makes a nonsense of the sort of statement often heard in legal hearings after cranial trauma, when it may be said that the risk of post-traumatic epilepsy is 3%, without any recognition of the fact that the population as a whole carries a lifetime risk of this order.

1.10   PREVALENCE OF EPILEPSY

Figures quoted for the prevalence of epilepsy can again be remarkably uninformative, unless the population is defined scrupulously. The principal difficulty is deciding how long a remission should be allowed before a patient is excluded from 'being epileptic'. One criterion that has been used (e.g. [14, 15]) is that a subject is included if a seizure of any type has occurred within the last two years. Such studies give prevalence rates of around 3–6 per 1000 (0.3–0.6%).

The prevalence of epilepsy at different ages is a reflection of the balance between the ages at onset, and the duration of illness before remission (or, in a few cases, death). The Rochester experience is illustrated in Fig. 1.2, which shows a more or less constant prevalence through the middle years of life, of about 0.68%, being lower in children and increasing with advancing age.

1.11   THE PREVALENCE OF SEVERE EPILEPSY REQUIRING RESIDENTIAL CARE

This figure is obviously of importance to health care planners. The Commission for the Control of Epilepsy and its Consequences [24] suggested a prevalence of 0.36 such cases per 1000. In the UK it has been estimated that there are about 3100 patients with epilepsy in residential care [25]. This gives a rate of about 0.06 per 1000. This six-fold difference may reflect no more than different availability of residential places.

There may well be a pool of patients in the community who might have a better quality of life in residential care. Conversely, many of the patients in caring institutions are there not because of their epilepsy, which may well be a relatively minor problem, but on account of associated mental or physical handicap.

1.12   INCIDENCE AND PREVALENCE OF DIFFERENT SEIZURE TYPES

This is again age-dependent. Salaam seizures, for example, are seizures only seen in infancy. Typical absences, although a reflection of primary generalized epilepsy which may continue through life, are rare outside childhood and adolescence.

Figure 1.3 reflects, schematically, the examples of the cumulative incidence and prevalence rates for typical absences and for partial seizures with secondary generalization based upon the data of Juul-Jensen and Foldspang [19]. The continuing climb of the cumulative incidence curve for partial

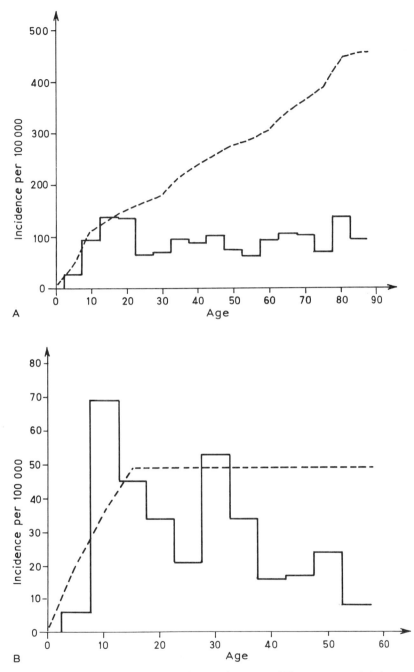

Figure 1.3 Cumulative incidence, and prevalence at different ages of (A) partial epilepsy with secondary generalization and (B) typical absences. Data from Juul-Jensen and Foldspang [19] reproduced with kind permission.

seizures with secondary generalization (A) reflects the incremental influence through life of neurological events resulting in epilepsy. The flat prevalence line, in contrast, indicates that for roughly every new case of epilepsy that begins, another enters a long term remission. For typical absences (B) the flattening of the cumulative incidence curve indicates that virtually no cases have their first such seizure after the end of the second decade.

There are few reliable studies on the incidence and prevalence of different seizure types in the community, as clearly hospital investigation is often necessary to classify the seizures accurately. Table 1.1 shows the incidence of different types of seizures in the Danish [19] and Rochester [13] surveys, but in each of these surveys each patient was allocated to one seizure type only, whereas, of course, it is common for patients to experience more than one type – most commonly a mixture of partial and secondarily generalized seizures. The prevalence of different types of seizure in the community was reported by Hopkins and Scambler [14] for a population aged over 16 who had had more than one non-febrile seizure of any type with at least one seizure in the last two years, and/or were continuing on anticonvulsants for seizures in the past. Their findings are shown in Table 1.2. In addition to the 56% who had

Table 1.1   Incidence of different types of seizure (%)

	Danish study [19]	Rochester, USA [13]
Primary generalized tonic-clonic	36.0 ⎫ 56.3	35.0
Partial with secondary generalization	20.3 ⎭	
Partial elementary	6.5 ⎫ 31.7	53.0
Partial complex	25.2 ⎭	
Typical absences	5.4	8.2
Other	6.6	3.7
	$n=1505$	$n=451$

The data in the Danish study are recalculated from Table 1 of [19], after omission of isolated and provoked seizures. The data in the Rochester study are recalculated from Table V-7 of [13].

Table 1.2   Prevalence of different types of seizure in the community (%)

Seizures experienced	Typical absences	Partial seizure	Tonic-clonic	Seizure of any type
In past two months	2	37	26	50
In past two years	2	45	47	69
At any time	7	56	95	100

In addition to the 56% who had experienced a partial seizure at some time. there was clear clinical or EEG evidence of partial onset to generalized seizures in a further 12%. $n=94$. From Hopkins and Scambler [14].

experienced a partial seizure at some time, there was clear clinical or EEG evidence of partial onset to generalized seizures in a further 12%.

1.13 THE INFLUENCE OF SEX

Most epidemiologists record a slight excess of males with epilepsy – e.g. 1.1:1 [12]; 1.4:1 [19]. Studies of seizures in early childhood have shown a differential effect of seizures upon the brains of infant boys and girls at different maturational ages (see Chapter 15). It has always been said that a proportion of the excess of males with epilepsy is accounted for by their different occupational and social exposure to epileptogenic insults such as cranial trauma and alcohol; however studies in less developed societies, for example in Colombia [26], in which trauma and abuse of alcohol might be thought to be higher in males show a greater prevalence in females (M:F=0.67).

1.14 SOCIAL CLASS AND RACE

There was no significant difference in the prevalence rates of epilepsy in different social classes in Colombia in the study just quoted [26], but, in the more developed USA, a study by Shamansky and Glaser [27] found a much higher risk of childhood epilepsy for black children than for white. The cumulative risk per 1000 to age 15 was 19.63 for black boys, 19.51 for black girls, 9.53 for white boys, and 9.10 for white girls. After controlling for age and race, Shamansky and Glaser [27] found an excess incidence of epilepsy in areas in which resided those of lower socio-economic groups. Other studies under way (Hauser, personal communication) confirm the high risk of epilepsy in young, poor blacks. Such findings are of importance as they imply that at least part of the burden of the incidence of epilepsy can be solved by preventive methods to improve social health.

1.15 THE PROGNOSIS OF PATIENTS WITH EPILEPSY

Chapter 11 analyses in depth the different factors that predict prognosis for different types of seizure at different ages. In this section is given an overview of the prognosis of epilepsy in the community.

Studies separated by more than 60 years [6, 28] suggested that only about one-third of those with epilepsy could hope to achieve a worthwhile long term remission of seizures. It is now realized that this is an artefact of patient selection, both these and similar reports emanating from units specializing in epilepsy, and thereby attracting patients refractory to treatment. The first hint that this was unduly pessimistic came from the works of Crombie and colleagues [8] in primary care practice in the UK. They divided their calculated cumulative incidence by the prevalence of active epilepsy, and estimated that there was only one chance in eight of a first fit being repeated at intervals and requiring continuous treatment.

A definitive paper was published by Annegers, Hauser and Elveback based upon the Rochester, Minnesota study, in 1979 [29]. Their principal findings are reproduced in Fig. 1.4. The point to note from Fig. 1.4 and its legend is that a large number of patients (42%) enter a remission that will last for at least five years within one year of diagnosis. Furthermore, as the narrow gap between the top two curves show, relapses once a long remission has been achieved are unusual. Similar shaped remission curves have been reported by Goodridge and Shorvon [30] and Elwes and colleagues [31], the last being a prospective survey.

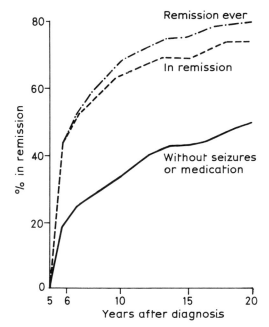

Figure 1.4 Remission of seizures. *Top curve*: probability of completing a period of five consecutive years without seizures. For example, six years after diagnosis 42% of subjects have been seizure-free for five years. *Middle curve*: the probability of being in remission for at least the past five years. The difference between the top and middle curves is due to relapse after achievement of a five-year remission. For example, at 20 years after diagnosis 70% are currently free from seizures, and have been for five years, and a further 6% have had at least one seizure-free period of at least five years' duration, but have subsequently relapsed. *Lowest curve*: the probability of being free of seizures for at least five years whilst not taking anticonvulsant drugs.

In summary, 20 years after diagnosis 50% have been free from seizures without anticonvulsants for at least five years. A further 20% continue to take anticonvulsant medication and have also been free of seizures for at least five years. Seizures continue, in spite of medication, in 30%. (Reproduced with kind permission from Annegers *et al.* [25].)

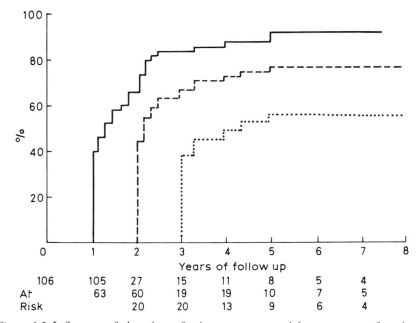

Figure 1.5 Influence of duration of seizures on actuarial percentage of patients completely free of seizures for one year. The top curve represents all patients from start of treatment, the middle curve patients with seizures in the first year of follow-up, and the bottom curve patients with seizures for the first two years of follow-up. Reproduced with kind permission from Elwes *et al.* [27].

Annegers and colleagues [29], Elwes and colleagues [31] and subsequently Shorvon [32] note the interesting point that the shape of the remission curves indicates that the chances of achieving a remission fall rapidly if a remission has not been achieved in the first one or two years. Figure 1.5 shows the reduced chance of achieving a remission lasting one year in the second year after onset if the seizures have already lasted one year, and the even lesser chance of achieving a remission in the third year if the seizures have already lasted for two. This, and the interesting observation by this group that intervals between the second and third seizures are shorter than between the first and second has led to a resurrection of the view, originally proposed by Gowers [33] that epilepsy may tend to escalate in the early weeks. He wrote: 'Each attack facilitates the occurrence of another, by increasing the instability of the nerve elements.' It has also been suggested [31, 32, 34] that early treatment with anticonvulsants may actually alter the natural history of epilepsy – that is to say, if seizures are allowed to continue in the early stages, then subsequent control may be more difficult. The alternative, of course, is that those seizures which are difficult to control at first remain difficult to control. The distinction between these two possibilities could only be made by a large scale randomized controlled trial of anticonvulsants against placebo.

1.16   THE MORTALITY OF EPILEPSY

Death certification of those who die having suffered from epilepsy is likely to be unreliable in any country. If epilepsy had been due to, for example, a cerebral tumour, then it is probable that the tumour would take precedence on certification. Conversely others who die from an unrelated cause, such as myocardial infarction, may have epilepsy entered on their certificates as a confounding factor. These problems have been discussed by Hauser and colleagues [13, 35], Zielinski [36] and Chandra *et al.* [37]. Hauser and Kurland [13] preferred to rely upon *survival* of those with epilepsy, as giving the best measure of excess mortality. They compared survival for up to 23 years after diagnosis in 516 patients with epilepsy matched to Minnesota controls of the same age and sex. Five years after diagnosis, the ratio of epileptic survivors to controls was 95%, at 10 years 90% and at 15 years 89%. Most of the excess mortality therefore shows in the early years after diagnosis. As might be expected, survival was much less in those patients with a cause assigned to their epilepsy, the figures, matched against controls being 69%, 58% and 53% at 5, 10 and 15 years. Hauser and Kurland point out that since the survival ratio of all cases is not far from 100%, a reduction in a few percentage points appears minor when expressed in these terms, but the mortality ratio, as its base is close to zero, may be doubled or tripled by the same difference. The mortality ratio at five years, for example was 252 if no cause was allocated for the epilepsy and 336 if a cause was suspected.

Hauser *et al.* [35] returned to the subject of excess mortality in 1980, noting that the standardized mortality ratio (SMR) was highest in the first ten years after diagnosis (SMR was 3.8 in the first year after diagnosis, falling to 2.0 five to nine years after diagnosis). An unexplained point is that even patients in remission have an increased mortality, suggesting that factors other than seizure occurrence influence mortality, although there seemed to be no cause of death unique to the study group. Subjects with partial complex seizures without a demonstrated cause, and subjects with absence seizures, did not have an increased mortality.

An alternative epidemiological approach has come from forensic pathology. Leestma and his colleagues [38] report on the incidence of sudden unexpected death associated with seizures. During one year in which a special effort was made, in Cook County, Illinois, to identify all sudden deaths occurring in those with epilepsy, 50 cases were identified. Assuming a prevalence of epilepsy of 0.5% in the Cook County population, the authors calculated an annual incidence of sudden death amongst those with epilepsy of one per 525 cases. Although some epileptics undoubtedly die through road traffic accidents and drowning, the authors stressed that these were 'extra' deaths, without anatomical evidence of any cause. They suggest that a fatal arrhythmia is induced by the seizure discharge spreading into the neurovegetative system. Certainly there is evidence that cardiac arrhythmias can occur during clinical and experimental seizures (see [38] for references). It could, however, be argued that the cumulative incidence rather than the prevalence of epilepsy should have been employed in the calculations of Leestma *et al*. [38], and, if this is done, the excess mortality disappears.

Another cause of excess mortality in those with epilepsy is suicide. Unfavourable life events, such as redundancy, and a break down in personal relationships due to epilepsy may precipitate depressive illness. Unfortunately, anticonvulsant drugs provided a readily available means of self-destruction. The suicide rate amongst those with epilepsy is five or six times the rate of the population at large, and the attempted (para-) suicide rate is probably even higher, though statistics cannot be reliable [39].

ACKNOWLEDGEMENT

I am grateful to Dr W. Allen Hauser for helpful discussion.

REFERENCES

1. Schwab, R. S. (1939) A method of measuring consciousness in petit mal epilepsy. *J. Nerv. Ment. Dis.* **89**, 690–6.
2. Aarts, J. H. P., Binnie, C. D., Smit, A. M. and Wilkins, A. J. (1984) Selective cognitive impairment during focal and generalized epileptiform activity. *Brain*, **107**, 293–308.
3. Gastaut, H. and Fischer Williams, M. (1957) Electroencephalographic study of syncope. Its differentiation from epilepsy. *Lancet*, **ii**, 1018–25.
4. Janz, D. (1969) *Die Epilepsien*. Thieme, Stuttgart.
5. Hauser, W. A., Anderson, V. E., Loewenson, R. B. and McRoberts, S. M. (1982) Seizure recurrence after a first unprovoked seizure. *N. Eng. J. Med.*, **307**, 522–8.
6. Rodin, E. A. (1968) *The Prognosis of Patients with Epilepsy*, Charles C. Thomas, Springfield, Ill.
7. Kurland, L. T. (1959) The incidence and prevalence of conclusive disorders in a small urban community. *Epilepsia*, **1**, 143–61.
8. Crombie, D. L., Cross, K. W., Fry, J. *et al.* (1960) A survey of the epilepsies in general practice: a report by the Research Committee of the College of General Practitioners. *Br. Med. J.*, **2**, 416–22.
9. Pond, D. A., Bidwell, B. H. and Stein, L. (1960) A survey of epilepsy in fourteen general practices. I. Demographic and medical data. *Psychiatr. Neurol. Neurochirurg.*, **63**, 217–36.
10. Brewis, M., Poskanzer, D. C., Rolland, C., *et al.* (1966) Neurological disease in an English city. *Acta Neurol. Scand.*, **42** (Suppl. 24), 9–89.
11. Gudmundsson, G. (1966) Epilepsy in Iceland: a clinical and epidemiological investigation. *Acta Neurol. Scand.*, **43** (Suppl. 25), 1–124.
12. Zielinski, J. J. (1976) People with epilepsy who do not consult physicians, in *Epileptology* (Ed. D. Janz), George Thieme, Stuttgart, pp. 18–23.
13. Hauser, W. A. and Kurland, L. T. (1975) The epidemiology of epilepsy in Rochester, Minnesota, 1935 through 1967. *Epilepsia*, **16**, 1–66.

14. Hopkins, A. and Scambler, G. (1977) How doctors deal with epilepsy. *Lancet*, **i**, 183–6.
15. Goodridge, D. M. G. and Shorvon, S. (1983) Epileptic seizures in a population of 6000. I Demography, diagnosis and classification, and role of the hospital services. *Br. Med. J.*, **287**, 641–4.
16. Beran, R. G., Michelazzi, J. *et al.* (1985) False negative response rate in epidemiologic studies to define prevalence rates of epilepsy. *Neuroepidemiology*, **4**, 82–5.
17. Goldberg, H. J. (1983) Neonatal convulsions – a 10 year review. *Arch. Dis. Child.*, **58**, 966–8.
18. Chevrie, J. J. and Aicardi, J. (1977) Convulsive disorders in the first year of life: etiologic factors. *Epilepsia*, **18**, 489–98.
18b. Luhdorf, K., Jensen, L. K. and Plesner, A. M. (1986) Epilepsy in the elderly: incidence, social function and disability. *Epilepsia*, **27**, 135–41.
19. Juul-Jensen, P. and Foldspang, A. (1983) Natural history of epileptic seizures. *Epilepsia*, **24**, 297–312.
20. Ross, E. M., Peckham, C. S., West, P. B. *et al.* (1980) Epilepsy in childhood: findings from the National Child Development Study. *Br. Med. J.*, **1**, 207–10.
21. Kurtz, Z., Tookey, P. and Ross, E. M. (1986) *The epidemiology of epilepsy in childhood*. John Wiley & Sons, in press.
22. Hauser, W. A., Annegers, J. F. and Anderson, V. E. (1983) Epidemiology and the genetics of epilepsy, in *Epilepsy* (eds A. A. Ward, J. K. Penry *et al.*), Raven Press, New York.
23. Goodridge, D. M. G. and Shorvon, S. D. (1983) Correction. *Br. Med. J.*, **287**, 1020.
24. *Commission for the Control of Epilepsy and its Consequences* (1978) United States Department of Health, Education and Welfare publication of National Institute of Health 78–276, Washington DC.
25. *Epilepsy in Society* (1971) Office of Health Economics, London.
26. Gomez, J. G., Arciniegas, E. and Torres, J. (1978) Prevalence of epilepsy in Bogota, Columbia. *Neurology*, **28**, 90–4.
27. Shamansky, S. L., Glaser, G. H. (1979) Socioeconomic characteristics of seizure disorders. *Epilepsia*, **20**, 457–74.
28. Turner, W. A. (1907) *Epilepsy – a study of the idiopathic disease*. Macmillan, London.
29. Annegers, J. F., Hauser, W. A. and Elveback, L. R. (1979) Remission of seizures and relapse in patients with epilepsy. *Epilepsia*, **20**, 729–37.
30. Goodridge, D. M. G. and Shorvon, S. D. (1983) Epileptic seizures in a population of 6000. II Treatment and prognosis. *Br. Med. J.*, **287**, 645–7.
31. Elwes, R. D. G., Johnson, A. L., Shorvon, S. D. *et al.* (1984) The prognosis for seizure control in newly diagnosed epilepsy. *N. Engl. J. Med.*, **311**, 944–7.
32. Shorvon, S. D. (1984) The temporal aspects of prognosis of epilepsy. *J. Neurol. Neurosurg. Psychiat.*, **47**, 1157–65.
33. Gowers, W. R. (1964) *Epilepsy and other Chronic Convulsive Diseases: their causes, symptoms and treatment*. Dover Publications, New York. Originally published (1885) by William Ward.
34. Reynolds, E. H., Elwes, R. D. C. and Shorvon, S. D. (1983) Why does epilepsy become intractable? Prevention of chronic epilepsy. *Lancet*, **ii**, 952–4.
35. Hauser, W. A., Annegers, J. F. and Elveback, L. R. (1980) Mortality in patients with epilepsy. *Epilepsia*, **21**, 399–412.

36. Zielinski, J. J. (1974) Epilepsy and mortality rates and cause of death. *Epilepsia*, **15**, 191–9.
37. Chandra, V., Bharucha, N. E. and Schoenberg, B. S. (1983) Deaths related to epilepsy in the United States. *Neuroepidemiology*, **2**, 148–55.
38. Leestma, J. E., Kalelkar, M. B., Teas, S. S. *et al.* (1984) Sudden unexpected death associated with seizures. *Epilepsia*, **25**, 84–8.
39. Mackay, A. (1979) Self poisoning – a complication of epilepsy. *Br. J. Psychiatr.*, **134**, 277–82.

CHAPTER TWO

The Biology of Epilepsy

John G. R. Jefferys and Richard Roberts

In this chapter we plan to illustrate the impact of advances in research in the basic neurosciences on our understanding of the mechanisms of the epilepsies, and on the ways in which the study of the epilepsies probe neural function. More detailed reviews of many of the specific issues we will address are scattered through the several good multiauthor books on experimental epilepsies which have been published recently [1–3] (reviewed in [4]). We have tried to provide in this chapter a concise, balanced overview of experimental epilepsy and its clinical context.

The epilepsies are not simply due to an imbalance of excitation over inhibition (p. 43 and review in [5]).Certainly the experimental disruption of inhibition does cause seizures in many acute models, and in at least some chronic models, and we will discuss the role of inhibition in some detail (p. 43). However, a simple increase in discharge frequency is not epilepsy; other factors must be present to synchronize the neural discharge in order to generate the electroencephalographic (EEG) and behavioural signs of the epilepsies. Thus synchronization is a crucial issue, and can arise from a variety of mechanisms (p. 28). In the extreme case one could, in principle, cause seizures without changing the total inhibitory or excitatory input to a population of neurones simply by reorganizing their connections to increase synchrony (p. 47). We believe that the analysis of the microcircuitry of epileptic foci will add a major new perspective to the basic mechanisms of the epilepsies. The great variety of experimental and clinical epilepsies argues against any single unified mechanism of epilepsy. Rather we should expect that the functional balance of the neurones of the mammalian brain can be disrupted in many different ways. By understanding the different ways in which epilepsies arise, we can expect to learn about the functional organization of the normal brain.

We will start with the major advances in our understanding of the cellular physiology of acute focal epileptic discharges, which have resulted largely from the use of the brain slice preparation. We will then consider how chronic experimental models can help bridge the gap between such acute work and clinical partial seizures and their behavioural, physiological and histopathological consequences. Subsequently we will consider the generalization of partial seizures and the mechanisms of primary generalized seizures. Finally we will briefly review the use of experimental models in the development of anticonvulsant drugs.

2.1　MECHANISMS OF PARTIAL (FOCAL) SEIZURES

2.1.1　The interictal spike produced by acute convulsants

The epileptic event arguably understood in greatest detail is the interictal 'spike' produced by acute convulsants applied to neocortex, hippocampus and other brain structures. The essential cellular events in strychnine foci in the neocortex were described as long ago as 1959, and in penicillin foci in the hippocampus one to two years later [6–10] (reviewed in [11, 12]). In both these situations, neurones exposed to the convulsant discharged with brief, rapid bursts of action potentials. Intracellular recordings from these neurones (using the then newly-developed glass microelectrodes) revealed that the epileptic bursts arose from abrupt, large depolarizations from the resting membrane potential, which were called 'paroxysmal depolarization shifts' (PDSs) (Fig. 2.1). The PDS is a common feature of neurones in a wide range of experimental and clinical epileptic foci, and therefore is a central issue in any fundamental analysis of the epilepsies.

The mechanism of the PDS has been controversial for many years (see the 1969 reviews by Ajmone-Marsan and by Prince [11, 12]). Major issues included whether the epileptic abnormality resided in either individual ('epileptic') neurones, presynaptic terminals ('giant excitatory postsynaptic potentials – EPSP') neuronal populations ('epileptic aggregates' [13]), tissue metabolism, or the control of extracellular ions. These ideas have all had their proponents. However, they are not mutually exclusive (c.f. much of the early literature), as we will see in the specific examples below. The mammalian brain slice, maintained *in vitro*, has had a central role in resolving many of the arguments about the generation of the PDS induced by acute convulsants. We will describe this preparation briefly before discussing its application to the PDS.

(a)　The brain slice

Warburg [14] showed in 1930 that slices of brain can survive for many hours *in vitro*, given the necessary ions, glucose and oxygen. In general they need to be cut a few hundred (*c.* 400) microns thick to strike a balance between preserving neuronal structure and adequately oxygenating the centres of the slices. Physiologists were slow to exploit the preparation [14a, 15, 16] but certainly made up for lost time over the last few years! The slice preparation has many advantages for the analysis of central neuronal membrane properties and microcircuitry. These include: (1) mechanical stability, for better and easier intracellular recordings; (2) control over the extracellular fluid for the application of drugs and for manipulation of extracellular ions; and

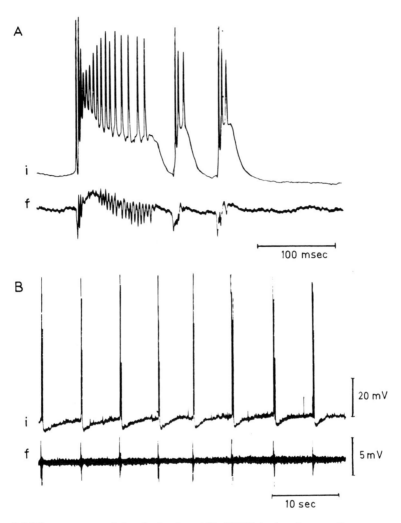

Figure 2.1 The paroxysmal depolarization shift (PDS) is the abnormality most consistently found in intracellular recordings from epileptic tissue. It consists of a massive membrane depolarization which triggers a train of action potentials, possibly followed by one or more afterdischarges (Ai). Neurones in epileptic tissue are abnormally synchronous, as revealed by the simultaneous extracellular field potential recording (Af). These data are from experiments in which hippocampal slices were incubated in picrotoxin which results in frequent and rather regular PDS's (Bi, Bf). The slower timebase (B) reveals that each PDS terminates in an after-hyperpolarization. Reproduced by permission from Miles, Wong and Traub (1984), *Neuroscience*, **12**, 1191–1200. © IBRO.

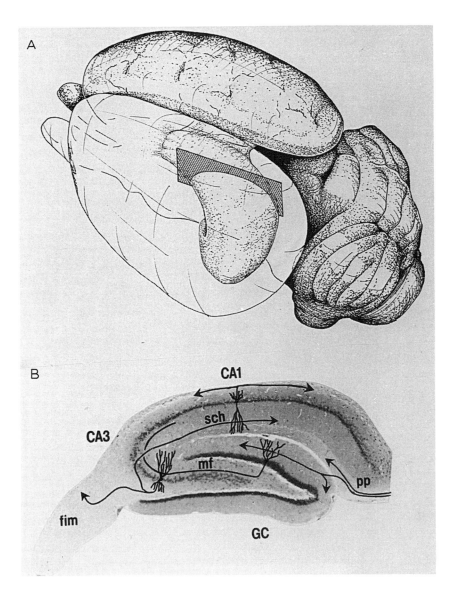

A

B

CA1

CA3

sch

mf

pp

fim

GC

(3) visualization of the tissue structure, for positioning electrodes, for local application of drugs, and for making lesions in pathways. These features have made it possible to perform biophysical analyses on mammalian brain, which previously had only been possible on invertebrate and other 'simple' preparations. As a result, the slice preparation has had a pivotal role in determining the fundamental mechanisms of acute convulsant drugs, and may be expected to have a similar role in studies of the chronic experimental epilepsies (p. 41).

(b) Inhibition and the acute PDS

We now know a great deal about the cellular mechanisms responsible for the PDS induced by blocking inhibition in rodent hippocampus (Figs 2.1 and 2.2 [6, 17, 18]). It does not matter how inhibition is disrupted. Epileptic discharges occur with (1) antagonists to the inhibitory transmitter, γ-aminobutyric acid (GABA) (e.g. picrotoxin and bicuculline [5]), (2) penicillin, which certainly blocks both inhibitory postsynaptic potentials (IPSPs) and responses to exogenous GABA [19, 20], perhaps by blocking the chloride ionophore (g_{Cl^-}) opened by GABA [5]; (3) alterations in the Cl^- gradient across the neuronal membrane, either by replacing extracellular Cl^- with larger, impermeant, monovalent anions [21, 22], or by the action of ammonium ions, which appear to prevent the extrusion of Cl^- ions from neurones [23]. Epileptic activity also can be induced by treatments which impair the synthesis or release of GABA, e.g. hyperbaric O_2 [24], thiosemicarbazide [25], and 3-mercaptopropionic acid [26]. Whether or not disruption of inhibition is involved widely in clinical or chronic experimental epilepsies is another question (pp. 43–47). However, experiments using acute blockade of inhibition have provided many important insights into basic epileptic mechanisms (pp. 24–32).

Figure 2.2 The rat hippocampus has had a central role in recent work on experimental epilepsy. In the rat it forms a relatively large part of the brain. It lies beneath the neocortex, extending from the dorsal midline laterally and ventrally as shown in the drawing (A). It has a remarkably consistent cross-section along its whole length (B). The principal (excitatory) neurones are shown schematically on a cresyl violet-stained paraffin section (B): the granule cells of the dentate area (GC) and the pyramidal cells which have been subdivided into types CA1–4 (CA=Cornu ammonis), of which CA1 and CA3 are most relevant to the present discussion. The hippocampus contains a sequence of excitatory relays: from the entorhinal cortex (which joins the caudal end of the hippocampus)→perforant path (pp)→granule cells→mossy fibres (mf)→CA3→Schaffer collaterals (Sch)→CA1→subiculum. The fimbria-fornix system (fim) contains axons (many from CA3) which project to the contralateral hippocampus and which make connections with rostral structures such as the septum. Special thanks are due to Dr I. P. Johnson for drawing a dissection by the author.

(c) Hippocampal slices and the PDS

The pacemaker for spontaneous synchronous epileptic bursts in the hippocampus such as those induced by penicillin resides in the pyramidal cells of
regions CA2 and CA3 of the hippocampus. These cells have been implicated
by several lines of evidence, by using dual or multichannel extracellular
recording (e.g. [20, 27]; Fig. 2.3), by cutting connections in the slices [20, 28],
and by local application of epileptogenic agents to specific regions in the slices
[29]. These experiments revealed that, while penicillin, picrotoxin, etc., block
inhibition in all regions of the slice, spontaneous bursts would only arise in
CA2 or CA3. They generally started close to the border with CA1 and then
spread into both CA1 and the remainder of CA3. However, most or all of CA3
(and not CA1 or dentate gyrus) could sustain spontaneous epileptic bursts,
even when isolated as small tissue prisms containing as few as 1000 pyramidal
neurones [28]. Two features of CA2/CA3 neurones have proved especially
interesting: their membrane properties and their synaptic connectivity (p. 29).

(i) Intrinsic neuronal properties

Some of the earliest intracellular recordings from CA3 pyramidal cells *in vitro*
showed that these cells possessed intrinsic burst generators (Fig. 2.4). Their

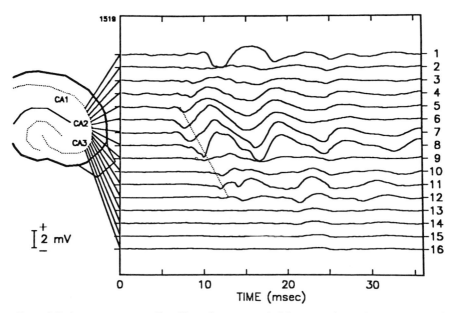

Figure 2.3 A spontaneous epileptiform burst recorded from a guinea-pig hippocampal
slice, bathed in picrotoxin, using an array of 16×61 μm diameter metal electrodes. The
burst starts in the region of CA2 or CA3 and propagates along the pyramidal cell layer
at about 0.13 m/s. Reprinted by permission from [27] © 1987 IBRO.

membranes contained mechanisms which could cause prolonged, self-sustained depolarizations, which in turn would trigger bursts of fast action potentials. These intrinsic mechanisms consist of several voltage-dependent ion channels in addition to the Na^+ and K^+ channels of the classic (fast) action potential (see Table 2.1; Fig. 2.4). The most important of these for the intrinsic burst discharge is the voltage-dependent Ca^{2+} channel (current 'I_{Ca}') which is responsible for the slow Ca^{2+} spikes recorded after fast Na^+ spikes (current I_{Na}) have been blocked, e.g. by tetrodotoxin (TTX), or by inactivation during a burst discharge (Fig. 2.4) [30–32]. These Ca^{2+} channels appear to be concentrated on the dendrites of many neurones in the mammalian brain, while the Na^+ channels responsible for the fast action potential appear to be concentrated in or near the cell body and axon [33–35]. The normal role of these dendritic Ca^{2+} channels is not entirely clear, though they may be important in integrating the synaptic inputs to long dendritic trees.

Neurones possess a variety of mechanisms to oppose sustained Ca^{2+}-dependent depolarizations. In part they are needed to control the build up of excitation (and seizures?). However, equally important is the role of free intracellular Ca^{2+} in many aspects of normal cellular and neuronal function; if intracellular Ca^{2+} increases too much it may destroy the cell (p. 54, [36, 37]). The protective (hyperpolarizing) mechanisms include K^+ channels opened by membrane depolarization (I_A, I_m, I_K) or by increased intracellular Ca^{2+} (I_c) (see Fig. 2.4 and [38] for a concise summary). These currents (notably I_m and I_c) are responsible for the hyperpolarizations recorded after bursts of action potentials, and contribute to the termination of many types of epileptic burst discharges (Fig. 2.4; e.g. [32, 39, 40]).

Computer models have been constructed which incorporate the channels described above with other experimental data, and provide a quantitatively reasonable account of the burst discharges in CA3 pyramidal cells ([41]; Fig. 2.4). The model succeeded in predicting the existence of two features of CA3 pyramidal cells, namely a voltage-dependent inactivation of K^+ currents and the partial inactivation of Ca^{2+} currents by Ca^{2+} ions [41]. The development of a realistic computer model of the individual neurone was an essential step towards understanding the roles of the assemblies of neurones in the epileptic focus (p. 29).

Spontaneous, 'pacemaker' activity has been attributed to the interactions between the membrane currents responsible for intrinsic bursts (i.e. the voltage-dependent Na^+ and Ca^{2+} channels and the Ca^{2+}-dependent K^+ channel) in a wide range of cells in many species (from molluscs to man) [42]. In mammalian hippocampal pyramidal cells or spinal motorneurones, spontaneous 'epileptic' bursting can be induced by disrupting the balance between these ionic conductances, for instance by the use of agents such as tetraethylammonium (TEA) or 4-aminopyridine, which block K^+ currents I_c or I_A, or by Ba^{2+} (c. 1 mM) which not only blocks K^+ currents (I_m and I_c), but also adds to the inward current during the Ca^{2+} spike [30, 40, 43–46].

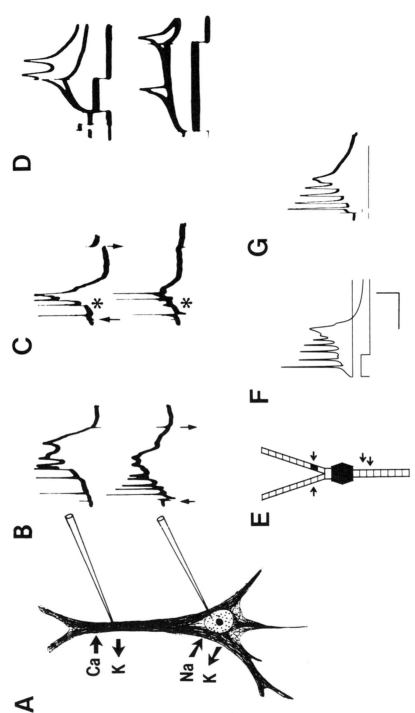

Table 2.1 Hippocampal currents (see ref. 38)

Ion	Current	Blocker	Comment
Na^{1+}	I_{Na} transient	tetrodotoxin	fast action potentials
	I_{Na} sustained	tetrodotoxin	?
Ca^{2+}	$I_{Ca(1)}$ sustained	Cd^{2+}, Mn^{2+}	high threshold Ca spike
	$I_{Ca(2)}$ transient	Cd^{2+}	low threshold depolarization
K^{1+}	I_K	Tetra-ethylammonium (TEA)	slow
	I_A	4-aminopyridine	transient
	I_m	Acetylcholine Ba^{2+}	
	I_c	TEA	Ca^{2+}-activated, fast
	I_{AHP}	Acetylcholine Noradrenaline Histamine Serotonin	Ca^{2+}-activated, non-voltage-dependent after hyper-polarization, limits burst discharges
	I_Q	Cs^{2+} (external)	activated by (and limits) hyper-polarization

Can malfunctions in the channels responsible for intrinsic burst discharges be responsible for epilepsies not caused by drugs or toxins? Work on mammalian motorneurones suggests that damage to the axons of these cells can induce abnormal dendritic action potentials (the 'chromatolytic reaction' [47, 48]); whether similar changes occur in the brain during epilepsy remains to be seen. Mutants of the fruit fly *Drosophila* exist which lack I_c, and can be

Figure 2.4 Neurones contain voltage-dependent ion conductances in their membranes. (A) The Na^+ and K^+ channels responsible for the 'classical' fast action potential tend to be concentrated in the neuronal soma, initial segment and axon, while the slower voltage dependent Ca^{2+} channel is believed to be concentrated in the dendrites. (B) Simultaneous intracellular recordings believed to be from one pyramidal neurone's soma and dendrites show how bursts evoked by current injection can spread from soma to dendrites and (C) from dendrites to soma. Note the longer and more prolonged slow (Ca^{2+}) action potentials in the dendritic recordings (B, C), and the rather poor transmission of fast (Na^+) spikes between the two sites (C*). (D) Blocking Na^+ action potentials with tetrodotoxin reveals the slower Ca^{2+} spikes in dendritic (upper trace) and somatic recordings from different neurones. (E) The ion conductances known to exist in hippocampal CA3 pyramidal cells are incorporated into multicompartmental computer models which produce a simulated burst discharge (F) which closely resembles those recorded experimentally (G). Vertical calibration (F): 20 mV in B–G; Horizontal calibration (F): 100 ms in B,C; 40 ms in D,G; 25 ms in F. (A) Reproduced from Ramon y Cajal (1911), Histologie du Systeme Nerveux. B–D redrawn from [34], with special thanks to D. A. Prince for an original print. E–G reprinted by permission from [62] © 1982 AAAS.

identified by motor disorders, such as vigorous leg-shaking in the mutant *Hyperkinetic* strain [49]. It is impossible to tell whether this motor disorder corresponds to epilepsy in higher species. To date, there is no evidence that such a dramatic loss of a specific channel occurs in any chronic mammalian or clinical epilepsy. However, it is quite likely that ion channels may be modified by abnormalities in transmitter systems which normally modulate them. It is known that acetylcholine (ACh) blocks I_m, the muscarinic K^+ channel, and that noradrenaline (NA) (norepinephrine), serotonin, acetylcholine and histamine (HA) depress I_{AHP}, the Ca^{2+}-dependent K^+ channel [38, 50–52]. Therefore, in principle, it is possible that disruption (e.g. of dopamine (DA)) or hypertrophy/upregulation (e.g. of ACh, NA, HA) of transmitter systems may be involved in clinical or chronic experimental epilepsies. It is particularly interesting that in the totterer mutant mouse, which has simple partial motor seizures and absence seizures, there is a massive proliferation of the noradrenergic projection from the locus coeruleus (p. 61). Intrinsic burst mechanisms may also be important in focal epilepsies, such as the alumina model, not because of any abnormality in the channels present, but rather because of a closer coupling of dendritic and somatic regions as a result of the shortening of dendrites, and the loss of dendritic spines [53, 54] (p. 52 and Fig. 2.9).

2.1.2 Synchronization of hippocampal neurones

A bursting discharge pattern in individual neurones does not constitute epileptic activity. The discharges of many neurones need to become synchronized to generate the EEG and other features characteristic of the epilepsies. The diversity of ion channels described in the preceding paragraphs certainly can explain how individual cells generate bursts of action potentials, but they cannot by themselves explain synchronization. Clearly some form of communication must occur between the neurones. The mechanisms of synchronization have been explored in detail for penicillin-type epileptogenesis in the hippocampus, where the synaptic connectivity has proved of prime importance in synchronizing the epileptic bursts (p. 29), but where non-synaptic mechanisms have been shown to be involved in the fine structure within the bursts (p. 35).

The idea that epileptic discharges are synchronized by some highly divergent pacemaker structure (as was the basis of the centroencephalic theory, p. 60) does not explain the origins of the synchrony; it simply changes its location.

(a) Synaptic mechanisms
Many schemes of synaptic connections can be conceived which would cause the synchronization of neuronal discharges. In principle these can rely on either inhibitory interneurones or on excitatory connections to cause syn-

chrony. The ways in which inhibition can synchronize neurones have been explored in the context of thalamocortical interactions [55] and generalized epilepsies [56] (p. 60). In the case of the hippocampus, there is no evidence to implicate inhibitory mechanisms in neuronal synchronization. Certainly when inhibition is blocked, e.g. by penicillin or picrotoxin, it cannot synchronize the epileptic activity that results. On the other hand, there is evidence of recurrent excitatory connections between some hippocampal pyramidal cells.

(i)   Recurrent excitation in the hippocampus
Early evidence of recurrent excitatory connections between CA3 pyramidal cells in the hippocampus came from experiments in which the major fibre tract to CA3 was cut. Once the afferents had degenerated, this tract should contain only the efferent CA3 pyramidal cell axons, so that stimulating it should have produced a purely antidromic activation of CA3 pyramidal cells. However, in addition to antidromic action potentials and recurrent inhibitory potentials, there also were found EPSPs, which were interpreted as being due to recurrent exitatory pathways [57–59]. These kinds of experiments do present some difficulties, for example, the risk of reactive synaptogenesis (sprouting), and the lack of topographic information. More direct evidence for the existence of monosynaptic excitatory connections between the pyramidal cells in CA2/CA3 comes from simultaneous intracellular recordings from pairs of these neurones [60, 61]. These experiments are really only feasible in the slice preparation, where intracellular recording is considerably easier than in the intact animal; even so, such recordings are technically difficult. These multiple intracellular recordings provide unambiguous evidence that excitatory connections do exist between the pyramidal cells, but they are sparse, being found in only about 1.5% of the pairs of recordings.

It is not immediately obvious that such a low incidence of recurrent excitatory connections would be sufficient to synchronize the pyramidal cells in a hippocampal slice. In order to test this quantitatively, Traub and Wong [62]; Fig. 2.5) made computer simulations of arrays of 100 individual model bursting neurones (p. 25 and Fig. 2.4), connected randomly with a realistically low percentage of excitatory interconnections. Subsequently the simulations have been enlarged tenfold [63] in order to approximate the numbers of neurones present in tissue prisms which actually generate epileptic discharges when exposed to picrotoxin [28]. The model revealed that stimulating about four neurones in the array could trigger a wave of excitation which recruited the whole population into the epileptic discharge. Experimentally, stimulating single neurones by intracellular current injection can reset the rhythm of spontaneous picrotoxin bursts in segments of CA3 maintained *in vitro* [28].

Detailed exploration of the computer model has shown that the excitatory interconnections must meet two conditions if they are to synchronize the population of hippocampal pyramidal cells. First, they must be divergent –

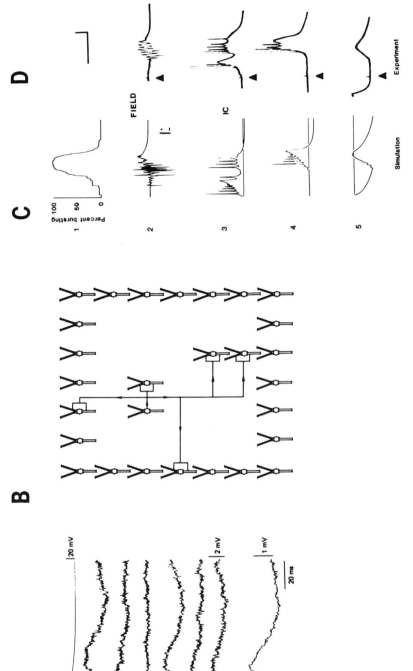

that is each neurone must connect to an average of at least two others. Secondly, they must be sufficiently powerful – that is to say, capable of exciting the postsynaptic cell to spike thresholds. The experimental exploration of these recurrent excitatory connections between the CA3 pyramidal cells is still underway. Their divergence has not yet been demonstrated explicitly, though from the profuse axonal ramifications seen in CA3 pyramidal cells filled with horseradish peroxidase (HRP) [64] it would be most surprising if this were not the case. It does appear that these synapses are powerful. Individual synapses produced depolarizations of 1–2 mV in postsynaptic neurones at resting potentials of about 70 mV, whereas unitary EPSPs in the mammalian nervous system commonly are of the order of 0.1 mV. These EPSPs summated up to 4 mV for trains of three to five presynaptic action potentials [61]. When inhibition was progressively abolished by incubating slices in low doses of picrotoxin ($\sim 10^{-6}$ M), excitatory connections between pairs of neurones became progressively more common. These additional connections appeared to be multisynaptic, from their shape, variable latency and failure rate [65]. Thus it appears that the spread of excitation through the network of excitatory connections between CA2/CA3 pyramidal cells is normally held in check by inhibition, allowing the excitatory connections to perform their normal function, which presumably is not the generation of epileptic discharges!

(ii)   The role of the N-methyl D-aspartate (NMDA) receptor
Excitatory transmission in many parts of the mammalian brain, including the hippocampus, uses excitatory amino acids, particularly glutamate. Recent progress in the pharmacology of this system [66, 67] may be important in the development of novel anticonvulsants, which ideally should block epileptic activity whilst leaving normal synaptic transmission intact [68]. It turns out that there are at least three distinct glutamate receptors which are named after their preferential agonists: the NMDA receptor (or A1 according to [67]), which we will discuss in this section; the quisqualate receptor (A2); and the

---

Figure 2.5 Recurrent excitatory connections occur between CA3 pyramidal neurones, and can synchronize epileptic bursts. (A) Simultaneous intracellular recordings from two CA3 pyramidal neurones in a guinea pig brain slice reveal that an action potential in cell 1 can trigger an EPSP in cell 2. The six successive sweeps shown for cell 2 produced one 'failure'. The lowest trace in A is the average unitary EPSP. (B) The role of these rather sparse excitatory interconnections can be assessed by computer modelling of networks of neurones of the type illustrated in Figure 2.4. (C) Such computer modelling shows that activity in a small subset of these neurones can recruit the whole population if they are randomly interconnected with a probability of 1–5% (C1); patterns of activity in the simulated (C3–5) and real (D3–5) neurones are remarkably similar. The differences between the simulated and real fields (C2 vs D2) are attributable to non-synaptic synchronization. (A) reprinted by permission from the Journal of Physiology [61]. © 1986 The Physiological Society; (B–D) reprinted from Science [62] © 1982 AAAS.

kainate receptor (A3), which has excito-toxic properties which may be relevant to the pathology of the epilepsies (p. 53).

The NMDA receptor has attracted much attention, partly because of the existence of unusually effective antagonists, such as D-2-amino-5-phosphonovaleric acid (APV), and partly because of its unusual properties (reviewed in [69]). The effects of the NMDA receptor are difficult to detect at normal resting potentials, and in the presence of normal levels of Mg^{2+}. They are greatly enhanced by depolarizing neuronal membranes, or by incubating neocortical or hippocampal slices in low Mg^{2+} solutions, indeed the latter treatment induces epileptiform responses in these slices [70, 71]. It is not clear whether such low levels of Mg^{2+} ever occur *in vivo*; however, the NMDA system is further linked to seizures by several observations under normal Mg^{2+}. APV and related compounds are anticonvulsants for several experimental epilepsies, both *in vivo* and *in vitro* [68, 70, 72]. The role for NMDA in epileptogenesis may be in amplifying the excitatory synaptic drive provided by other synaptic inputs, for example of the recurrent excitatory collateral network of the hippocampal CA3 region. In fact the anticonvulsant action of APV on slices, in models such as the acute action of picrotoxin [70], or the chronic effects of kainic acid [72], was on the later components of the epileptic response rather than on the onset of the discharges. The relatively subtle effects of this system suggest that APV and related compounds have a potential clinical use both as anticonvulsants and as protective agents against neuronal death (p. 53), although this may be complicated by their ability to disrupt learning [73].

(iii)   Convulsants which do not block inhibition
The epileptic synchronization of hippocampal neurones has been explored in most detail for convulsants whose primary action is to block synaptic inhibition (p. 23). This certainly is not the basic mechanism of all convulsants. On p. 25 we described several convulsants which affect intrinsic membrane properties, particularly currents carried by K^+. 4-Aminopyridine (4-AP) clearly acts as a topical convulsant [74] and at a biophysical level, it blocks outward K^+ currents (see the references in [45]).

Incubating hippocampal slices in 4-AP induces spontaneous, synchronous epileptiform discharges, which start in the CA2/CA3 region and subsequently propagate into the CA1 region [45]. Some of these epileptiform discharges resemble those seen under penicillin, but others differ, for example in their slow rates of propagation – about 0.01 m/s compared to 0.1 m/s for penicillin discharges [62], and in their resistance to glutamate antagonists and low extracellular Ca^{2+} ($[Ca^{2+}]_o$) [45]. The latter observations suggest that non-synaptic mechanisms have a role in the 4-AP discharges (p. 33).

Hippocampal slices exposed to 4-AP, or to elevated extracellular K^+ ($[K^+]_o$) (6.5–10 mM) also differed from penicillin (or picrotoxin) in the presence of frequent spontaneous IPSPs in hippocampal pyramidal cells, confirming the preservation of synaptic inhibition ([75]; c.f. 4-AP on olfactory cortex [46]). These intracellular recordings revealed PDSs which resembled those found under penicillin (p. 20), except that they were often preceded by an IPSP. Such IPSP – PDS sequences have been described before, in the 'intermediate zone' around a penicillin focus in the cat hippocampus *in vivo* [76] (and in a computer model, [77]. Here this sequence resulted from the interaction between a central zone where inhibition had been blocked, and surrounding regions where it had not. The data from 4-AP or increased $[K^+]_o$ on slices shows that such interactions can also occur within a focus.

At the very least, these studies demonstrate clearly that the disruption of inhibition is not essential for epileptic activity. Furthermore, they illustrate the need to extend the theoretical and experimental analysis of hippocampal microcircuitry, which was developed largely to model the penicillin discharge (p. 29), to include inhibitory connections. This is a point to which we will return when considering chronic experimental foci, and the limited data available from human tissue (p. 46); we believe that the interplay between excitation and inhibition in the epileptic focus will prove to be a central issue in the basic mechanisms of the epilepsies.

(b)   Non-synaptic mechanisms of synchronization

Synaptic interactions are clearly essential for synchronizing neurones during penicillin-type bursts in the hippocampus. However, other mechanisms are involved in the synchronization of neuronal discharges in this structure and elsewhere. This is most dramatically illustrated by epileptiform activity induced in slices of hippocampus by incubation in solutions containing fairly low (<0.5 mM) concentrations of $[Ca^{2+}]_o$. These solutions block synaptic transmission and depress Ca^{2+} currents, so that the kinds of mechanism described in the previous paragraphs could not be involved here. The phenomenon of low Ca^{2+} field bursts was first described explicitly almost simultaneously by several laboratories [78–80] (Fig. 2.6), though earlier reports did contain evidence of their existence [81]. Incubating a hippocampal slice in a solution containing 0.2 mM Ca^{2+} and 4.0 mM Mg^{2+} typically blocks synaptic transmission after a few minutes; after a further several tens of minutes the slices start to generate spontaneous synchronous discharges (Fig. 2.6). Unlike the penicillin bursts, these low Ca^{2+} field bursts occur most easily in the CA1 region of the slice, though they can be induced in the other regions [82, 82a]. Several diseases, and some kinds of therapy, can deplete ionized $[Ca^{2+}]_o$ and also cause seizures, so it is tempting to speculate that the mechanisms of the low Ca^{2+} field burst have direct clinical relevance. What kinds of mechanism might be at work in this phenomenon? Three possibilities present themselves: electrotonic junctions (electric synapses), ephaptic interactions, and fluctuations in extracellular ion concentrations.

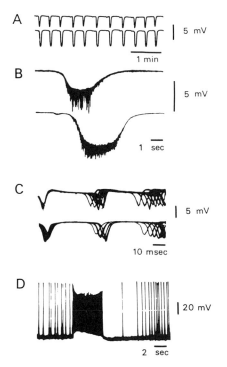

Figure 2.6 Non-synaptic synchronization of neuronal discharges is demonstrated most dramatically in the spontaneous bursts recorded from CA1 in rat hippocampal slices (Fig. 2.2) incubated in low Ca^{2+} solutions. Extracellular recordings from two electrodes in CA1 (A–C) reveal the rhythm (A) and synchrony of the bursts (A,B; electrodes 1 mm apart) and of the discharges within the bursts (C; electrodes 0.5 mm apart). An intracellular recording of one 'field burst' reveals a rapid train of action potentials on a depolarization shift. Reprinted by permission from Nature [78] © 1982 Macmillan Journals Ltd.

(i)   Electrotonic junctions (electric synapses)
Electronic junctions are structures where two cells are joined at specific sites ('gap junctions' under the electron microscope). These junctions provide low resistance connections between the cells, which can allow quite large tracer molecules to pass (up to molecular weights of the order of 1000 daltons). Contrary to earlier doubts, electrotonic junctions are now known to exist at many sites in the mammalian brain (in the hippocampus, neocortex, hypothalamus, substantia nigra, inferior olive, and elsewhere; references and reviews in [83, 84]). The evidence for the presence of such junctions in mammals comes from a variety of techniques (electrophysiological, anatomical and ultrastructural; reviewed by Dudek *et al.* [83]). However, simulations based on the measurements on the hippocampus [85] suggest that electrotonic junctions are not important in the synchronization of epileptic discharges, essentially because of the evidence from intracellular dye injection that these

junctions join neurones in small, closed clusters of only two to seven neighbouring cells, rather than the open syncytium which would be required to synchronize the population of neurones.

(ii)   Ephaptic interactions (electric field effects)
Ephaptic interactions occur when the electric currents generated in the extracellular space by the activity of one set of neurones modify the excitability of another set directly (i.e. not through specialised contacts such as gap junctions). In general the extracellular currents generated by neurones are too weak to alter the membrane potentials and excitability of neighbouring neurones, but occasionally special physical conditions do allow this to happen. This can arise when individual neuronal elements come sufficiently close together, perhaps aided by an unusually high extracellular resistivity which would tend to increase extracellular voltage gradients and intracellular currents through the recipient neurones, as originally described for peripheral nerve in about 1940 ([86] and references in [87]), and more recently for the teleost Mauthner cell and the mammalian cerebellar Purkinje cell (reviewed in [88]).

A rather different kind of electrical interaction occurs in tightly laminated cortical structures, such as the hippocampus. Here the geometry of the principal neurones causes the extracellular currents generated by their synchronous activity to sum in the axis perpendicular to the cell layers, resulting in large current densities, and field potentials (Fig. 2.7). This is not a new idea [17], but experiments to test this *in vivo* had proved contradictory. In the hippocampal slice *in vitro* the applied currents can be better controlled, revealing that neurones are sensitive to exogenous electric fields of the order of 4 mV/mm [89], well within the range of field potentials generated by the tissue.

Population spikes recorded during low Ca^{2+} field bursts are much larger than the exogenous electric fields which modulated neuronal excitability. The importance of electric field interactions in synchronizing low Ca^{2+} field bursts is shown directly by recording the 'transmembrane potentials' during the bursts. These recordings measure the intracellular potential with respect to a local extracellular electrode, rather than to a distant reference electrode. The conventional intracellular recording will be misleading when the potential just outside the membrane differs greatly from the distant reference. During the low Ca^{2+} field bursts, conventional intracellular recordings revealed that action potentials started either abruptly from the depolarizing plateau, or from a negative inflection (Fig. 2.7). When these intracellular recordings were subtracted from neighbouring extracellular recordings, a net transmembrane depolarization was revealed preceding the action potentials (Fig. 2.7; [79, 87]). These transmembrane depolarizations represent the cellular expression of the 'population ephaptic', or 'electric field' interaction.

Computer modelling suggests that electric field interactions become signifi-

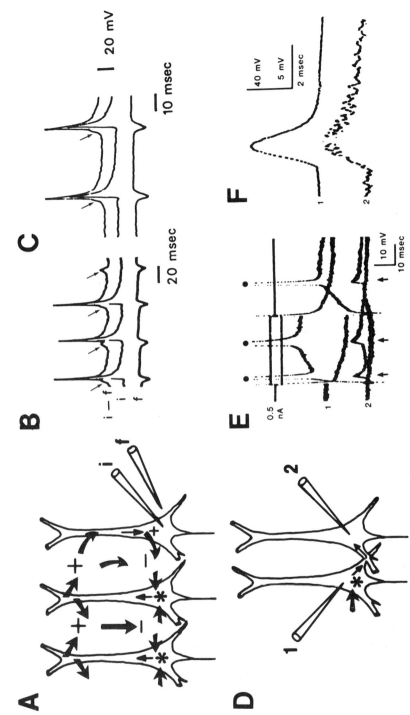

cant when the neurones are sufficiently excitable [85, 90]. This appears to be the case during incubation in low Ca^{2+} solutions, which cause a slow progressive depolarization [78], and also during the paroxysmal depolarizing shifts induced by penicillin and picrotoxin. Thus field interactions tend to organize rapid, but asynchronous, trains of action potentials into population spikes, synchronized on a 1 ms time scale. This causes the field potential to generate regular, soma-negative spikes which have the appearance of a comb (Figs 2.1 and 2.6), the 'ringing' field potential characteristic of epileptic discharges.

(iii) Extracellular ions

Neuronal activity generally involves the movement of ions across membranes, and can significantly alter the ionic composition of the extracellular fluid. In turn, the ionic composition of the extracellular fluid is crucially important to neuronal function. Particularly significant are the increased $[K^+]_o$ and decreased $[Ca^{2+}]_o$ which often result from neuronal activity (Fig. 2.4). Both these changes tend to make neurones more excitable, and thus provide a mechanism for neuronal synchronization. There has long been speculation that changes in the extracellular ion concentrations could precipitate seizures (reviewed in [17, 91]). The development of the ion selective microelectrode has allowed these speculations to be tested experimentally, and so far has failed to demonstrate that changes in ion concentration are responsible for the initiation of seizures.

Potassium is the ion which has most often been implicated in epilepsy. Measurements of ^{42}K efflux from neocortex during acute experimental seizures suggested an hypothesis in which $[K^+]_o$ and increased excitability were linked in a regenerative feedback cycle. When $[K^+]_o$ or firing rate reached a critical level, the cycle reached a threshold and would drive the

Figure 2.7 Two types of non-synaptic synchronization: ephaptic or field interactions (A–C) and electronic interactions (D–F). (A) Ephaptic interaction can occur in laminar structures, such as the hippocampus, when the currents (arrows) generated by the activity of some of the neurones (*) cause a negative field outside the neuronal cell bodies, and an outward (depolarizing) membrane current at the cell bodies of passive neurones. This results in a net transmembrane depolarization as revealed when extracellular field recordings (f) are subtracted from near-by, simultaneous intracellular recordings (i). (B,C) The transmembrane depolarization is marked by arrows. (D) Electrotonic interactions are mediated by specialized 'gap' junctions between pairs of neurones, which provide electrical continuity (albeit of high resistance). One means of demonstrating this is by intracellular recordings made simultaneously from pairs of neurones (1,2) taking care to avoid penetrating the same neurone twice (in contrast with the experiments in Figure 2.4 B,C). When a pair of neurones is joined by an electrotonic junction, potential changes induced by injecting current into cell 1 are recorded in an attenuated form from cell 2 (slow potentials E; action potentials F; different calibrations for the two traces). B, C redrawn from [87], © 1984 The Physiological Society; E,F reprinted with permission from MacVicar and Dudek, *Science*, **213**, 782–85, © 1981 AAAS.

neurones to a paroxysmal discharge. Eventually the depolarization would cause 'cathodal block', stopping the seizure [92]. The ion selective electrode eventually revealed that $[K^+]_o$ did accumulate during seizures, with the greatest concentrations at cell body layers. However, the increased $[K^+]_o$ generally occurred after electrical seizures had started, not before, and thus could not have initiated them [93–96]. During seizures $[K^+]_o$ rises from its normal 3 mM to a ceiling activity of around 10 mM (c.f. spreading depression, which is propagated by $[K^+]_o$ which reaches 80 mM, e.g. [95]). This physiological ceiling to $[K^+]_o$ (c. 10 mM) is not sufficient to block neuronal activity, and thus could not abort epileptic bursts directly (see [92]), though it could conceivably do so indirectly by activating electrogenic ion pumps [93]. There have been suggestions that pathological changes associated with chronic focal epilepsies could disrupt ionic regulation, but recent experimental evidence suggests that this probably is not the case (p. 51).

Calcium levels in the extracellular space ($[Ca^{2+}]_o$), unlike those of K^+, could change before the onset of electrical seizures induced by systemic pentylenetetrazol (PTZ) [93]. This raised the prospect that the level of $[Ca^{2+}]_o$ was related to the mechanisms which trigger the seizure. However, there was no obvious relation between the precise $[Ca^{2+}]_o$ and the seizure onset [93, 96] and it seems likely that the drop in $[Ca^{2+}]_o$ did not directly trigger the epileptic discharges, but rather reflected prodromal neuronal events, such as increased activity in excitatory synaptic circuits, and dendritic Ca^{2+} spikes.

The fluctuations in $[Ca^{2+}]_o$ have provided insights into epileptic mechanisms. The spatial pattern of the changes in $[Ca^{2+}]_o$ induced by electrical stimulation or by ionophoresis of amino acids was altered in the chronic epileptic foci induced by cobalt or by kindling ([97, 98], and compare [96]). In both cases there appears to be a greater entry of Ca^{2+} into the apical dendrites of cortical pyramidal cells, suggesting that these dendrites were more prone to Ca^{2+} spikes, or that there was a proliferation of synaptic activity or connections in this region.

Drops in $[Ca^{2+}]_o$ and rises in $[K^+]_o$ have been described in many experimental epilepsies [93, 96, 97, 99], and could have functional implications even if they do not actually trigger seizures. These changes can be very large; for example $[Ca^{2+}]_o$ fell from about 1.5 mM to 0.1–0.2 mM in the photosensitive baboon, while $[K^+]_o$ generally increased to 10–12 mM. Thus spontaneous epileptic activity could induce the kinds of conditions used experimentally in slices to produce the non-synaptic spreading excitation of 'low Ca^{2+} field bursts' (p. 33). This means that non-synaptic mechanisms such as ephaptic or field interactions may play a significant role in the development and form of epileptic discharges. The release of K^+ at cell bodies, coupled with the spatial buffering of K^+ by glia, can induce marked changes in the extracellular space during epileptic discharges [107, 169], which would further exacerbate non-synaptic synchronization.

2.1.3 Neocortex

(a) **Neocortical slices**

The theories on the cellular basis of epileptic discharges which we have described above were largely based on work using the hippocampal slice preparation. The neocortex is more difficult to analyse experimentally, but the available data do suggest that the principles developed for hippocampal epileptic activity also apply in the neocortex. Mid-cortical layers (IV and upper V) have been implicated in the initiation of synchronous epileptic bursts by several kinds of experiment (e.g. using local applications of convulsant, or chemical excitant; current source density analysis; or $[Ca^{2+}]_o$ measurements [98, 100–102]). The same layers contain a small population of neurones which, unusually in the neocortex, have intrinsic bursting properties [100, 102a]. These neurones are candidates for the pacemaker role performed by the CA2/CA3 pyramidal cells of the hippocampus. It remains to be seen whether the intrinsic-burst neurones of cortical layers IV and V are connected by an excitatory network, but it does seem likely that the theoretical framework developed for hippocampal epileptogenesis will also apply to the neocortex.

(b) **Neocortex and thalamus**

Studies of neocortical seizures *in vivo* have emphasized the importance of the thalamus in epileptogenesis. This is particularly true in the case of the penicillin model of generalized seizures, which depends on the functioning of both cortex and thalamus (p. 61). The thalamus certainly has the ion channels needed for pacemaker neurones [103]. Whether it has the mechanisms for synchronization is less clear. There are no reports on the presence or extent of excitatory connections between thalamic neurones, though they cannot yet be excluded in view of the small degree of connectivity needed to synchronize the hippocampus. Recurrent inhibition certainly is present, and has been implicated in the synchronization of the neocortical EEG [55, 104].

(c) **Terminal hyperexcitability**

Studies of focal penicillin epilepsy *in vivo* during the 1970s implicated abnormal repetitive firing of the terminals of thalamocortical axons [105]. There is no detailed model of how this would lead to the synchronization of the cortical discharge. Presynaptic bursts of action potentials would increase postsynaptic responses. Depending on the divergence of the neurones involved, this could conceivably increase cortical synchronization directly. Alternatively, the antidromic conduction of ectopic bursts could drive recurrent inhibitory circuits of the thalamus, which would synchronize the thalamic neurones, and eventually their cortical targets (p. 28).

Penicillin does affect terminal excitability directly, at least in the rat phrenic nerve – hemidiaphragm preparation [106]. Here it was possible to exclude alternative explanations such as presynaptic effects of released transmitter, ion fluxes or postsynaptic currents. However, in the brain it is more difficult to exclude secondary effects of seizure activity, for example, due to ion fluxes increasing $[K^+]_o$ or decreasing $[Ca^{2+}]_o$, both of which could easily induce repetitive firing (pp. 33, 37). Therefore it remains a possibility that ectopic bursts in thalamocortical axons arise as a consequence of seizures initiated by other mechanisms such as those described above.

2.1.4   Termination of epileptic bursts

The massive depolarization and discharge of the epileptic burst triggers many mechanisms which tend to stabilize neurones. It is specific mechanisms rather than exhaustion of the energy balance of the cells that limits epileptic bursts. We have described several of these mechanisms above. The most obvious include the various K^+ currents (p. 27), synaptic inhibition where it is preserved (p. 32), and electrogenic ion pumps triggered by the accumulation of $[K^+]_o$ [93]. Other transmitter systems can become involved, for example, opioid peptides and amines (p. 55), especially in the intact animal. Some or all of these are likely to be involved in most epilepsies, so that dissecting out their individual contributions probably will not be very easy.

On the whole, slice models generate activity which resembles the interictal spike of the epileptic EEG, that is, the brief (tens to hundreds of milliseconds) epileptic events which do not generalize, and which usually are not associated with any discernable motor component. They usually do not resemble a clinical seizure in which the epileptic discharges last much longer, and may generalize to cause obvious motor signs. Even the repetitive bursts seen in hippocampal slices under picrotoxin (Fig. 2.1 and p. 23) or from the tetanus toxin focus (Fig. 2.8 and p. 44) were much briefer than those of a full seizure. In a few experiments under the extreme conditions of the low Ca^{2+} field bursts, discharges could persist for 25 s or more [87], presumably because both inhibition and the K^+ current I_c were blocked. It is likely that a full seizure in the intact animal arises from the propagation of epileptic activity through the brain, with re-excitation of neurones after they have recovered from their protective refractory periods. As will be clear from our discussion of the generalization of focal seizures (p. 57), this greatly complicates the analysis of basic mechanisms.

2.2   CHRONIC EXPERIMENTAL PARTIAL SEIZURES

Acute experiments such as those on the slice preparation described above have revealed much about the cellular basis of the PDS and the epileptic discharge. These kinds of experiment are well-suited to the membrane or cell levels of analysis, but unfortunately they are limited as models of clinical epilepsies. They do not model clinical ictus; they provide very limited information on the propagation and generalization of seizures; they do not exhibit the more or less prolonged periods of relatively normal activity interposed between the periods of epileptic activity; and they cannot exhibit the disturbances of behaviour associated with some epilepsies such as complex partial seizures (or temporal lobe epilepsy). Chronic experimental epilepsies provide an intermediate step between the acute models and the clinical epilepsies, and are currently providing insights into the basic mechanisms which may be involved in man.

2.2.1 Cellular mechanisms in chronic epilepsies

The most obvious abnormality found when recording from neurones in chronic foci is the organization of their discharges into rapid bursts, similar to those seen with acute convulsants. For instance, extracellular unit recordings from the alumina focus [54, 108] in the monkey reveal interspike intervals of less than 5 ms during the epileptic bursts, much shorter than the interspike intervals recorded in normal cortex [54]. Similar discharge patterns have been recorded in other experimental models [99] and in human epileptic foci [109, 110]. Intracellular recordings of chronic foci *in vivo* in some cases have revealed events similar to the PDS of acute models (e.g. the cobalt focus [99]), and in others have failed to do so (e.g. the alumina focus [111]). Experience with acute models suggests that the slice preparation maintained *in vitro* has distinct advantages in the study of the cellular basis of epileptogenesis. Therefore it is likely that the slice preparation will occupy a pivotal role in exploring cellular mechanisms in chronic animal models. A start has been made with the tetanus toxin [112] and kainic acid lesion models [113–116] in the hippocampus, the amygdala kindling model in the pyriform cortex [125] and the alumina [117], and freeze lesions [118] in the neocortex.

Injecting a rat's hippocampus with a small dose of tetanus toxin induces chronically-recurring generalized seizures [119, 120]. Acute experiments suggested that the toxin blocks the release of GABA [121, 122]. It is possible to maintain the chronic focus *in vitro* in hippocampal slices prepared from these epileptic rats 3–35 days after injection [112]. These slices generate spontaneous synchronized epileptic discharges, which correspond to PDSs in most of the pyramidal cells recorded intracellularly (Fig. 2.8). The synchronous epileptic field (extracellular) potential or 'population bursts' start in the CA3 region and subsequently invade CA1, resembling the acute penicillin/picrotoxin epileptic discharges in this respect. However, intracellular recordings from the chronic focus reveal, in addition to the PDS, smaller, spontaneous depolarizations not associated with population bursts ([112], Fig. 2.8). These smaller depolarizations are quite distinct from the PDS; certainly the one cannot be transformed into the other by artifically depolarizing the neurones. They are abnormal, being larger and slower than the spontaneous EPSPs normally found in these cells (<1–4 mV; [61]). These data suggest that subsets of the pyramidal cells are recruited into the beginnings of epileptic discharges, much as they would be during the acute, complete block of

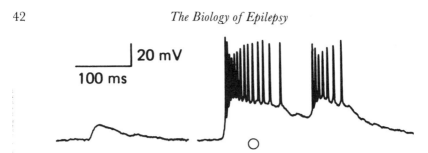

Figure 2.8 Intracellular recordings taken from a chronic epileptic focus. Hippocampal slices were prepared from a rat made epileptic 2 weeks earlier by an intrahippocampal injection of tetanus toxin. CA3 pyramidal neurones generated all or none PDS's which were synchronous with field burst discharges (○) and also partial abnormal depolarizations, which were not associated with a field potential (left). Reprinted by permission from [112] © 1986 The Physiological Society.

inhibition by picrotoxin, but that the spread of excitation through the syncytium of excitatory connections is often aborted, causing the partial depolarizations. Similar small depolarizations have been described recently during the development of picrotoxin discharges, but unlike those recorded in the tetanus toxin focus, they do not coexist with the full epileptic PDS [65]. The mechanism which aborts the propagation of excitation, which may be residual GABAergic or another inhibitory transmission, may explain why these chronically epileptic rats have intermittent seizures rather than status.

Variable or partial epileptic depolarizations, as opposed to the 'all or none' PDS, may be a general feature of chronic and clinical epileptic foci. The depolarizations found in rat cobalt foci have a very variable form when compared to those induced by penicillin for example, and occur only in a subset of cortical neurones [99]. Spontaneous, rhythmic, synchronous post-synaptic potentials, and not PDSs, have been described in one report on cortical slices from human epileptics [123] (p. 47). Graded, not 'all or none', epileptic depolarizations are evoked by stimulation of tissue slices prepared from the rat hippocampus lesioned with kainic acid [113–116] and from the alumina-treated monkey neocortex [117].

Kainic acid causes seizures acutely, presumably by activating glutamate A3 receptors [67]. It also causes lesions, which are specific for CA3 and CA4 pyramidal cells in the hippocampus (Fig. 2.2). If the dose is low enough, rats recover from their initial period of 'acute' seizures, which last 1–2 days, some days to weeks before the onset of chronically recurring seizures which persist for about one month [124]. Intracellular recordings from slices from these rats reveal a loss of inhibition (IPSPs) in the CA1 region of the hippocampi, perhaps accompanied by a disruption of intrinsic hyperpolarizing (K^+) conductances [113–115]. On the other hand, extracellular recordings and anatomical studies of the dentate granule cells implicate the sprouting of new, recurrent, excitatory connections [116] (p. 47). It is possible that both types of change occurred at both sites, but the techniques used in these respective studies did not provide the necessary data.

Repeated stimulation of certain brain structures, particularly those in the limbic system, causes an epileptic model known as 'kindling' (pp. 45 and 50). Coronal slices of pyriform cortex from amygdalar kindled animals have recently been shown to retain epileptic properties, in that their responses to stimulation are greatly prolonged compared with control slices [125]. We expect that an explanation of the differences between these epileptic and control slices would go a long way towards unravelling the phenomenon of kindling.

The analysis of cellular mechanisms in chronic foci is at an early stage of development. Clearly many different aspects of neuronal function may prove relevant to chronic epileptogenesis. For instance, abnormal dendritic properties may be important in the neocortical cobalt focus where, abnormally, partial spikes were recorded *in vivo* [99]. Other chronic epileptogenic agents, such as cholera toxin, probably affect intrinsic neuronal properties rather than synaptic properties or connectivity [126, 127] (and Jefferys, personal observation).

2.2.2 The role of inhibition in epilepsy

A major part of the microcircuitry of many brain regions appears to be devoted to containing excitation. These inhibitory circuits are now being charted in considerable detail using modern techniques [127a]. However, speculation that a loss of inhibition is responsible for clinical seizures has a much longer history (see [128] for an early version of this argument, and [5] for a more recent review). As we have already seen, blocking inhibition certainly elicits epileptic activity (p. 23). However, this does not necessarily mean that a loss of inhibition is the primary cause of chronic or clinical epilepsies. Indeed it is quite conceivable that inhibition could synchronize epileptic discharges [55, 104]; the wiring diagram, or microcircuitry of the epileptic tissue is crucial. Furthermore, the fact that many anti-epileptic drugs enhance GABA-mediated inhibition (reviewed in [5]) does not necessarily mean that the treatment reverses the initial cause; it simply means that the seizures can be damped down by increasing inhibition. More direct evidence is needed before we can conclude that inhibition is disrupted in chronic epilepsies.

(a) Loss of inhibition in chronic foci

In practice it has proved rather difficult, in most cases, to obtain compelling evidence of the loss of inhibition in chronic epileptic foci. Ideally the assessment of inhibition should be physiological, by finding out whether or not neurones can be effectively inhibited from firing. Unfortunately, it is often difficult to make suitable recordings. If there is an actual loss of inhibitory neurones, this should be detectable anatomically or neurochemically.

Antibodies to the (fixed) transmitter, GABA, or to its synthetic enzyme, glutamic acid decarboxylase (GAD), can be used to identify GABAergic neurones and synapses. However, such methods do have limitations. If they fail to reveal any changes in the GABA system, it still may be functionally disrupted (as is likely to be the case with the tetanus toxin model [129]). Conversely, the demonstration of a partial loss of GABAergic neurones does not necessarily explain the development of an epileptic focus. It might do so if this were the only change, but in real chronic models there are likely to be many other concurrent changes, so that ultimately the analysis needs to address the functional microcircuitry of the epileptic tissue.

(i)   Chronic tetanus toxin foci

Perhaps the best case for the disruption of inhibition causing chronic seizures comes from the epileptic syndrome induced by injecting a small dose of tetanus toxin into any of several sites in the brain (p. 41, [120]). The toxin blocks the release of GABA from brain slices [121, 122]. Tetanus toxin does disrupt the function of synapses using transmitters other than GABA in other parts of the nervous system (spinal cord [130], neuromuscular junction [129, 131]), so that further studies of the specificity of release from the chronic focus are needed. However, the lack of IPSPs in electrophysiological recordings from hippocampal slices prepared from rats injected some days to weeks previously, does confirm the persistent disruption of inhibition in this model [112].

(ii)   Chronic kainic acid foci

Physiological experiments on hippocampal slices have also shown that inhibition is disrupted in the CA1 region in rats where lesions had previously been made in the CA3 region with kainic acid [113–115]. Other factors, such as the sprouting of new excitatory connections also may be involved in the epileptic activity in these rats (p. 48). From the data available, it is difficult to pinpoint the way in which inhibition is disrupted by these lesions, though one possibility is that interneurones were destroyed due to some kind of selective vulnerability (p. 46), either to the small amounts of kainate that could diffuse from the injection site, or to the excessive excitation from the epileptic discharges from CA3 pyramidal cells before they died.

(iii) Binding studies

Neurochemical analyses can be used to measure the number of sites in a tissue which will bind a transmitter, or related agonists, and the strength with which they will bind. If the receptor numbers or affinity decrease, then this would tend to reduce the effectiveness of transmission. A decrease in receptor numbers also may accompany the loss of synapses. In the case of the GABA system, binding assays often use GABA agonists such as muscimol, or related ligands, such as benzodiazepine. These kinds of study have revealed decreased numbers, or possibly decreased affinity of GABA receptors in several models, such as the Mongolian gerbil in which the substantia nigra and peri-aqueductal grey were affected, and strains of mouse predisposed to audiogenic seizures (p. 64). At best, these changes may well be the basis of the epileptogenesis in these models. However, it should not be forgotten that GABA receptors are under complex control, and these changes may well be a secondary down-regulation in response to an increased level of inhibitory activity.

(iv) Kindling and inhibition

Kindling describes the progressive reduction in seizure threshold associated with the repeated presentation of certain forms of brain stimulation. Once established, these changes in seizure threshold are then usually permanent. We will discuss other aspects of kindling on page 50, but here we will examine the role of changes in inhibition. Repeated stimulation appears to attenuate IPSPs, an effect which may be due to desensitization [132, 133] or to altered ion gradients across neuronal membranes [134]. This 'fading' of inhibition may be important in the development of after-discharges, which appear necessary for effective kindling; it also lends some support to the idea that kindling is due to a progressive weakening of inhibition. However, fading is too short-term a phenomenon to explain the permanent changes of kindling. A more persistent candidate mechanism is the down-regulation of GABA receptors in response to repeated exposure to GABA itself, or to other transmitters, such as noradrenaline.

There is evidence that GABA receptors are down-regulated following kindling with systemic injections of a benzodiazepine 'contragonist', FG 7142, and that this coincides with a persistent reduction in seizure threshold [135, 136]. Kindling with electrical stimulation has been less straightforward. Experiments using a more intensive stimulation protocol than is usual for kindling, over a 24 hour period, do reveal well-defined losses of inhibitory interneurones, and other cells, which correspond to a prolonged reduction in the threshold for epileptic activity [137] (p. 53). However, the evidence is less clear with the more typical kindling protocols, where relatively brief stimulus trains would be given every few hours to days. Binding studies have indicated both increases and decreases in GABA receptors following kindling [138, 139]. The enzyme which synthesizes GABA, glutamic acid decarboxylase (GAD), can be used as a marker for GABAergic neurones. Immunohistochemical studies of GAD in kindling certainly show that GAD is labile. Its density, but not the number of GAD-positive cells or terminals, decreases for one to two days after kindled seizures [140, 141], and subsequently increases, although the physiological evidence from one of these laboratories is of impaired inhibition at this time [142]. That slices from kindled rats release more rather than less GABA, reinforces the idea that any impairments of inhibition in kindling are not presynaptic [143].

Physiological studies of kindling provide evidence both for the enhancement of inhibition [144] and for its depression [142]. Perhaps the most economical speculation on this confusion of data would be that inhibition is indeed impaired, but that the impairment is very localized, and is possibly surrounded by regions where inhibition is strengthened, perhaps helping to contain the seizures. These uncertainties illustrate a general point on the frequently unclear relationship between the observed tissue and the epileptic focus that plagues many types of measurement, particularly in man.

(v)   Loss of inhibitory synapses or neurones
Some of the best evidence for the loss of inhibitory synapses in chronic epilepsy comes from the focus established in animal cortex, usually of the monkey, by intracerebral aluminium hydroxide. In this model, binding studies indicate a decrease in the numbers of GABA receptors. Damage to inhibitory circuits has also been demonstrated by the use of GAD as a marker for inhibitory neurones. It is possible to demonstrate a loss of tissue GAD activity in the alumina focus [145] and, more specifically, to show the loss of GAD-positive terminals, including those of chandelier or axo-axonic cells [146, 147]. Ultrastructural studies of the alumina focus reveal a general loss of synapses, but with the greatest loss in 'inhibitory' synaptic profiles [148] – symmetric or Gray type II synapses. While this evidence is significant, we need to know more about the microcircuitry of this focus before we can safely conclude that the proportionately greater loss of inhibitory vs. excitatory synapses is responsible for the seizures in this model.

Inhibitory synapses appear to be selectively vulnerable in other experimental situations, though in each experimental model the evidence is not entirely complete. Cobalt, like alumina, causes a loss of tissue GAD activity, and also tissue GABA content in rat cortex, though these changes are accompanied by an increase in GABA receptors that might be compensatory [149]. Kainate lesions of the hippocampal CA3 region may damage or destroy inhibitory interneurones in CA1 [113–115] (p. 42). In both these examples, more anatomical studies are needed to show the actual loss of neurones or synapses. On the other hand, a selective loss of symmetric, Gray type II, synapses has been described following hypoxia in monkeys shortly after birth [150], which has led to the suggestion, but unfortunately not the demonstration, that this could cause seizures.

(b)   Inhibition in clinical foci
A question central to this discussion must be whether any of the changes in inhibition or GABAergic synapses can be found in human epileptic tissue. There have been reports of substantial losses of GAD activity and reductions in GABA-related binding sites in epileptic brain tissue, when compared to electrically and/or morphologically normal tissue from the same patient [151, 152], which would be consistent with a selective loss of GABAergic neurones. However, there is some disagreement on these kinds of measurement in man

(see discussion in [5, 153]). Indeed, there are reports of increased GABA levels and GABA binding in epileptic tissue [153]. The clinical situation inevitably is much more complex than the experimental, not only for the variety of cases and the difficulties in the identification of the epileptic tissue, but also in the circumstances under which tissue can be taken ethically. A potentially exciting prospect is the development of non-invasive techniques to monitor functional changes. One example is the development of ligands for the GABA receptor which could be detected by positron emission tomography.

Physiological methods can provide direct evidence on whether inhibitory neurones are still present and effective. This is perhaps best done using intracellular recordings, from brain slices. Human brain slices present significant technical and ethical problems. In spite of the many difficulties in obtaining suitable tissue, several groups have managed to work with brain slices from epileptic patients obtained during surgery. Their results have been very variable, perhaps reflecting the diversity of cases and treatment histories, and of surgical and experimental technique. There has been some dispute about whether the exised 'focus' does [154] or does not [117] generate PDSs. A recent study of human temporal cortex used rather thick (750 μm) slices, in order to preserve more neuronal connections. These slices did not generate all-or-none PDSs, but rather an abnormal, rhythmic, synchronous synaptic activity. This was found in five out of six patients, predominantly in the mesial temporal cortex which is the most likely site for epileptic foci [123] (p. 41 on tetanus toxin foci). The excised tissue probably contained the foci in all these cases, as all showed a significant or total reduction in seizure frequency following surgery. At least some of this synaptic activity was inhibitory, which argues against a major loss of inhibition as the seizure mechanism in these patients.

In summary, evidence for the disruption of inhibition, or at least of GABAergic inhibition, as a cause of chronic or clinical seizures in most cases is weak. Therefore we should consider the possible alternatives.

2.2.3 Mechanisms other than the loss of inhibition

(a) Sprouting of new excitatory connections

Work on the hippocampal slice has pinpointed the excitatory connections between the pyramidal cells of the CA3 region as the basis of the synchronization of epileptic discharges (p. 29). Whilst most of the relevant acute experimental work uses blockade of inhibition to release this mechanism, it is conceivable, indeed likely, that an increase in the numbers of the excitatory interconnections could induce epileptic activity in the presence of normal inhibition. One way that such a rearrangement of excitatory connections could occur is by the 'sprouting' of new synapses in response to a loss of afferent input. We predict that it is not simply a reorganization of afferent inputs on the somato–dendritic surface that is needed to produce an epileptic focus, but rather an increased number of interconnections within a population of neurones.

Sprouting of new recurrent excitatory circuits may be crucial in the development of chronic seizures following lesions of the hippocampal CA3 region made using kainic acid [124] (pp. 42 and 44). This certainly occurs in the dentate area, where the high concentrations of zinc that characterize granule cell axons simplify the demonstration of the new recurrent projection into the inner third of the dentate molecular layer [116]. Although the necessary experiments have not yet been reported, inhibition may also be disrupted in the dentate. This has been demonstrated in the CA1 region of slices from other rats which had received kainate lesions of CA3 [115, 117].

The situation may prove simpler with lesions made by methods which do not cause immediate epileptic fits. Preliminary studies by one of the authors of this chapter (J.J.) suggest that such lesions of the commissural projection to the hippocampal CA3 region lead to the development of chronic epileptic foci after periods of several weeks. The time course of the development of these seizures, and the presence of spontaneous IPSPs in intracellular recordings from slices prepared from these rats, are both consistent with an increase in the numbers of excitatory interconnections, and not a decrease in inhibitory connections, being responsible for epileptogenesis in these rats. Such changes may be particularly significant in post-traumatic epileptic foci, and generally in cases where there has been a loss of the afferent input to particular neuronal populations. These observations further underline the need for quantitative analyses of the microcircuitry of epileptic foci, along the lines of the models of acute foci made by Traub (p. 29), if we are to understand fully the mechanisms of the chronic epilepsies.

(b) Intrinsic neuronal properties

The stability of neuronal systems depends both on their wiring diagrams and on their intrinsic properties. Particularly important amongst these intrinsic properties are the various K^+ currents which have been described in recent years (Table 2.1). We have already referred to mutant insects where the loss of a specific current causes marked behavioural abnormalities. So far there is no evidence of similar genetic abnormalities in mammals. However, K^+ currents may be affected indirectly by changes in neuromodulators (for example in the tottering mouse, p. 62), or alternatively, by exogenous agents such as cholera toxin.

Injecting cholera toxin intracerebrally causes seizures which can recur for many days (for example [126, 127]). This model is reminiscent of the tetanus toxin epilepsy (p. 41), though in our experience the cholera toxin seizures tend not to generalize as often (Williams and Jefferys, unpublished). There is some argument about the primary action of cholera toxin on brain tissue. One line of investigation claims that cholera toxin only needs to bind to GM1-ganglioside in neuronal membranes to cause seizure, by an unspecified mechanism [126].

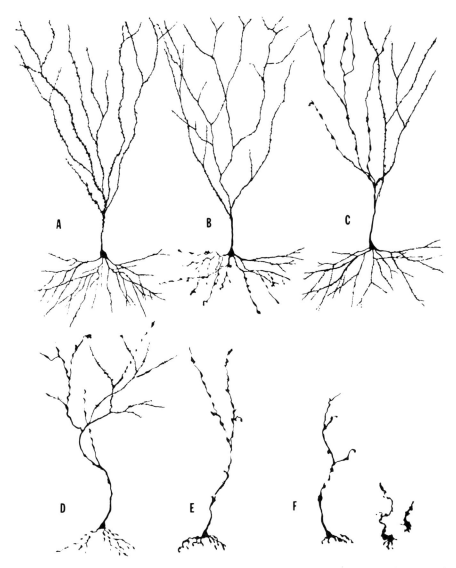

Figure 2.9 Human CA1 pyramidal cells illustrating various stages between the normal neurone (A) and neurones close to death (E,F). The intermediate stages (B–D) may become electrotonically short, resulting in a closer coupling of the slow dendritic Ca^{2+} action potentials with the fast somatic Na^+ action potentials (Figure 2.4), and hence tending to discharge in rapid bursts. Such an increased tendency of neurones to burst may cause, or aggravate, epileptic discharges. Reprinted by permission from Scheibel, Crandall and Scheibel (1974) *Epilepsia*, **15**, 55–80. © Raven Press, New York.

In contrast, another line of work suggests that the cholera toxin acts by causing an accumulation of cyclic adenosine monophosphate (cAMP) [127]; this mechanism has the merits that it mirrors the pathology of cholera in the gut, and that increased cAMP would depress K^+ currents [52]. In either case, the mechanism appears to depend on altering the intrinsic properties of the neurones. We await the results of further experiments on seizures induced by cholera toxin with interest.

Intrinsic burst generators may also become more effective, as suggested by the results of some of the anatomical changes which have been described in chronic models such as the alumina focus, and in the Mongolian gerbil and in man [155, 156]. The hypothesis is that the shortening of dendrites (Fig. 2.9) and the loss of dendritic spines will result in a reduction in the electrotonic length of these neurones, which will result in a closer coupling of soma/axonic Na^+ spike generation with the slow Ca^{2+} spike mechanisms of the dendrites. As a consequence, a single fast somatic spike will be able to trigger a Ca^{2+} spike in the dendrites, which it normally could not because of the attenuation and low-pass filtering on the intervening dendrites. Once the Ca^{2+} spike is triggered, the sustained depolarization will drive the fast Na^+ spike mechanism to generate the rapid burst discharges which are characteristic of this kind of epileptic tissue. This sequence of events specifically explains the occurrence of the 'long-first interval' seen in these bursts [53, 54].

(c) Kindling

Kindling is the phenomenon by which repeated stimulation of parts of the brain results in a progressive and permanent reduction in seizure threshold. A typical kindling stimulus, for example to the amygdala, initially causes little or no response from the animal. As the stimulus is repeated every few hours to days, the response increases progressively, through local myoclonus of the facial muscles and forelimbs, to generalized convulsions. The stimulation can be electrical or chemical (for example muscarinic agonists or benzodiazepine contragonists), focal or systemic. The changes underlying the phenomenon are essentially permanent, but they have not yet been attributed to any discernable histopathology. Kindling can be induced by focal stimulation of many parts of the brain, though the most susceptible appear to be limbic structures, especially the amygdala and piriform cortex.

One possible mechanism is a progressive weakening of inhibitory mechanisms as we have already discussed (p. 45). The evidence for the inhibition hypothesis is strongest for the special case of chemical kindling with benzodiazepine contragonists, and for electrical kindling of the hippocampal CA1 region; contradictory evidence is reported for many other kindling experiments. A large body of work exists which considers other putative mechanisms. This is reviewed in detail elsewhere [157–161]. We confine the discussion here to a brief overview of some of these lines of work. Given the diversity of experimental protocols that can cause kindling, it is entirely possible that more than one mechanism may be at work. In a later section, we consider the wider implications of kindling for the generalization of seizures, and its clinical relevance (p. 56).

Kindling resembles in some respects the physiological phenomenon of long term potentiation (LTP). LTP is the prolonged enhancement of synaptic efficacy which can follow a brief conditioning train of stimuli to presynaptic afferents, particularly in the hippocampus. The physiological basis of LTP has received a great deal of attention in recent years (reviewed in [162]), and while its mechanism has not yet been fully resolved, reduced inhibition does not appear a likely contender. Given the similarities between the stimuli used in these two models, LTP is likely to be a factor in kindling, but recordings from dentate granule cells during perforant path kindling suggest that LTP is not the complete explanation [163]. In particular, kindling continues to develop after LTP has saturated, and may lead to occasional giant population spikes which perhaps reflect fluctuations in neuronal excitability. The search for a mechanism of kindling is complicated by the interactions between increasing numbers of brain structures as the process develops (see p. 57 on generalization and secondary foci). However, insights into the cellular mechanisms probably will come from the discovery of epileptic properties preserved in slices of amygdala/piriform cortex following amygdalar kindling [125] (p. 43).

There exist many neurochemical studies of kindling [159]. The phenomenon is sensitive to a wide variety of neuroactive substances. Such studies can be particularly important in the development of anticonvulsant therapy. However, it is difficult to distinguish any direct effects on the mechanism of kindling from less specific effects on neuronal excitability. An alternative approach is to look for persistent neurochemical changes, which parallel the persistent reductions in seizure threshold characteristic of kindling. Many of the changes which have been described in the literature are transient, and may represent postictal disturbances (for example, see p. 45 for such changes in GAD levels, and p. 55 for possible behavioural significance). Some neurochemical changes induced by kindling are more persistent, lasting at least several weeks; an example is noradrenergic agonist binding in rat neocortex following amygdala kindling [164, 165]. Whilst it is tempting to speculate on a progressive erosion of noradrenergic function in kindling, its physiological significance remains to be established.

(d) Gliosis

A common histological observation in clinical foci is the presence of gliotic scar tissue at the epileptic focus. This pathology is duplicated in chronic experimental models such as the alumina and cobalt foci. The suggestion that gliosis disturbs K^+ regulation, and that this disturbed ionic regulation ultimately results in seizures, has a long history [91, 92, 166–168]. It appears all the more likely in view of recent developments in our understanding of the mechanisms which control $[K^+]_o$ activity within a ceiling of 10 mM, except during spreading depression or anoxia. This regulation depends on K^+ uptake into both neurones and glia, and on the spatial redistribution of K^+ through the syncytium of glia [169, 170]. However, more recent studies of the alumina focus, using ion selective electrodes, have shown that the gliotic tissue has normal baseline levels and buffering of $[K^+]_o$, so that K^+ regulation does not appear to be disrupted in these foci [171]. Whether or not gliosis has other effects on neuronal function remains to be determined, as does the reason for the apparently increased metabolic rate of the gliotic tissue [172].

2.2.4 Structural damage in chronic foci

Pathological changes, such as gliosis or sclerosis, or tumours, are often reported to be associated with clinical epileptic foci; indeed their presence in excised tissue indicates a good prognosis for the surgical treatment of focal seizures [173]. Histological changes can also be found in neurones, including distorted dendrites, the loss of dendritic spines, and the degeneration of synaptic terminals [155, 156] (Fig. 2.9). Often it is difficult to distinguish whether such changes are necessarily involved in causing seizures (p. 50), or whether they are consequences of recurrent epileptic activity over prolonged periods, as will have been experienced by most patients whose excised tissue reaches the pathologist. Certainly there are several chronic experimental foci which are not associated with any discernable histological damage, for instance kindling (p. 50) and tetanus toxin (p. 41). On the other hand, many chronic experimental epilepsies are characterized by gliosis or other histopathology. Examples include the freeze lesion [174], the alumina focus [175], the iron focus [177] and the cobalt focus [178]. Yet others are characterized by the loss of neurones or afferent inputs, such as kainate lesions [124], or commissural lesions (Jefferys, unpublished observations). In these cases it is likely that the histopathological changes precede the onset of the seizures. We have seen that it is unlikely that disturbances of ionic regulation are responsible for seizures, even where there is a clear gliosis. However, it is quite possible that seizures arise from the selective loss of inhibitory neurones under at least some of these conditions (p. 46). Furthermore, it is likely that the rearrangement of excitatory interconnections followed the loss of other excitatory inputs is a critical feature of several of these chronic models (p. 47). Whether or not discernable pathological changes are associated with the development of the epileptic focus, the occurrence of epileptic activity can kill neurones, by mechanisms we discuss next. Depending on the neurones killed, this may cause interictal disturbances of behaviour, or of cognitive or other cerebral functions (p. 55).

(a) What kills epileptic neurones?
It has long been thought that epileptic activity can destroy neurones, and this causes the pathological changes that can be found at sites physically remote

from the primary focus (reviews in [36, 137, 179] and chapters 37–45 in [3]). This loss of neurones is not uniform. A considerable effort has been expended on identifying the reasons why certain types of neurone should be selectively vulnerable. The classic case of this selective loss is the destruction of hippocampal CA1 and CA3 pyramidal cells (and not CA2 pyramidal cells or dentate granule cells) in patients with chronic temporal lobe epilepsy [180]. Similar selective losses of neurones occur following anoxia, hypoglycaemia or ischaemia, which suggested that some metabolic or vascular insufficiency was damaging neurones whilst they were hyperactive. However, the experimental data are, on the whole, against the 'metabolic' hypothesis. Blood flow and glucose consumption both increase during seizures, and the systemic control of various variables such as blood pressure and the partial pressure of O_2 do not prevent the development of histopathological changes [36].

There is now a good deal of evidence to suggest that epileptic damage results from the excessive excitation of the neurones in question during the seizures. This has been called the 'excitotoxic' hypothesis [181, 181a]. Kainic acid is a very effective excitotoxic agent, as we have already seen (for lesions of CA3 pyramidal cells, see p. 42). Kainic acid lesions are not restricted to the vicinity of the injection site; they can also be found in structures 'downstream' of the initial focus, for example in the hippocampus following injection into the amygdala [182]. This distant damage can be prevented by anticonvulsant pretreatment, or by cutting afferent tracts, such as the perforant path or the mossy fibres, to spare hippocampal pyramidal cells [183–185].

The fact that excitation can in itself cause pathological changes was demonstrated directly in experiments where the perforant path of anaesthetized rats was stimulated repetitively for 24 hours. This treatment caused after-discharges of the granule cells, but did not result in generalized motor seizures. It caused a very selective pattern of damage affecting dentate basket and hilar cells, and CA1 and CA3 pyramidal cells, but neither dentate granule cells nor CA2 pyramidal cells [137]. This is the pattern of damage reported in patients with epilepsy. The fact that the granule cells remained excitable over the whole period of these experiments adds further evidence against the metabolic (anoxia/ischaemia) hypothesis of epileptic brain damage. Certainly, the putative transmitters of the pathways involved in the hippocampus, glutamate and aspartate, are neurotoxic in sufficiently large doses [181]. However, it is not entirely clear why the granule cells, and the CA2 pyramidal cells should be spared, given that both receive substantial excitatory amino acid inputs. Several factors have been implicated, as follows.

NMDA receptors form a substantial subset of excitatory amino acid receptors. We have already discussed how they are activated during prolonged depolarizations, such as occur during seizures (p. 31). Activation of these receptors causes an influx of Ca^{2+} ions, both directly and indirectly, by maintaining the depolarization which opens voltage-sensitive Ca^{2+} currents. Abnormally high levels of Ca^{2+} are known to be lethal to many cells, and indeed have been found in degenerating neurones following allylglycine seizures [186]. Therefore the sparing of dentate granule cells may be related to a lack of Ca^{2+} channels, which would also explain the limited epileptic activity that can be obtained from these cells using penicillin [20]. The CA2 pyramidal cells have not been characterized sufficiently to tell whether they might be spared for a similar reason.

The role of Ca^{2+} in neuronal death does not go unchallenged. Experiments on the degeneration of cultured neurones induced by anoxia also show that the release of excitatory amino acids is a necessary step, but they implicate an influx of Cl^- ions rather than Ca^{2+} [187]. It remains to be seen whether Cl^- will prove as important *in vivo* as in experimental epilepsies.

Other mechanisms are involved in different experimental epilepsies. One example is the epileptic syndrome which is induced by intracerebral injections of iron salts, and haemoglobin, which may be particularly relevant to clinical post-traumatic epilepsy [177]. Iron salts are involved in the formation of free radicals, which are extremely toxic [188], and are likely to be responsible for both the damage and the epileptic discharges found in this model [189], and perhaps in anoxic damage too [188].

2.2.5   After-effects of focal seizures

The hypersynchronous, hyperexcitable discharge of the epileptic seizure clearly is the most dramatic aspect of most, if not all, of the epilepsies. However, brain function may be disturbed in more subtle ways for varying periods after seizures (postictal abnormalities), or throughout the period between seizures (interictal abnormalities). The resulting behavioural changes can present significant problems clinically, in particular with temporal lobe epilepsy (see Chapter 18). These include depression, psychosis (mainly with left temporal lobe foci), various changes in personality and impairments of cognitive function. In addition, religiosity, hypergraphia, hyposexuality, excessive concern with philosophical issues, irritability and aggressiveness have been described. Unravelling the mechanisms of these kinds of problems presents immense difficulties. Inevitably the responses of the individual to the psychological stress of having seizures will be a factor, as will the consequences of anticonvulsant medication. Animal models can simplify matters to some extent. We will consider some of these, and their relation to clinical problems, in the next two sections on postictal and interictal changes respectively.

(a)   Transient postictal changes

Patients with epilepsy can exhibit a variety of behavioural changes following their seizures, usually lasting a few minutes, but sometimes longer. A complex partial seizure will often be followed by a period of confusion, automatisms or dysphasia. Such patients may resist restraint, but rarely exhibit unprovoked aggression. A major seizure may be followed by a period of drowsiness. Prolonged seizures or status may lead to Todd's paresis, which can persist for days. Animal experiments have revealed parallels to these postictal abnormalities. There may be, for example, periods of depressed locomotor activity and/or unresponsiveness lasting several minutes to hours. These can last 30 minutes after PTZ seizures, and three hours or more after kindled seizures or electroconvulsive shock [190]. In each of these cases, the behavioural abnormality can be reversed by the administration of naloxone, implicating opiates in the underlying mechanism [190]. It remains to be seen whether any of the clinical postictal changes are mediated by opiates. Generalized seizures induced by intrahippocampal tetanus toxin are also followed by behavioural arrest, lasting about four minutes, and often succeeded by active grooming or exploration [120] (and Jefferys, personal observation).

Behaviours which superficially resemble aggression often occur for several days after experimental seizures originating in limbic structures such as the hippocampus and amygdala, as a result of kindling stimuli or injection of tetanus toxin. As with human epilepsy what appears to be aggression is more an abnormal or hyper-reactive response to unexpected external stimuli. In the animal models, if the stimulus is associated with the experimenter's hand this can appear distinctly aggressive! Rats following intrahippocampal tetanus toxin do not behave aggressively with their peers, rather they become more passive in their interactions with intruder rats [191].

(b) Persistent interictal changes

Impairments of learning and memory are prominent amongst the changes in cognitive function associated with temporal lobe epilepsies. They have the particular merit that they can be measured relatively easily in animals. Clinically, it is difficult to distinguish between the effects of anticonvulsant medication, focal epileptiform activity, losses of neurones associated with the epileptic focus (p. 52) and so on. More subtle mechanisms can be involved, because models, such as intrahippocampal tetanus toxin and kindling, are associated with persistent impairments in learning and memory, but not with any histopathological changes [119, 192–194]. Kindling, by definition, involves a persistent change in neuronal function – the lowering of seizure threshold. This, or indeed the paradoxical increases in inhibitory or GABAergic function (p. 45), may be responsible for the behavioural changes recorded after kindling of the amygdala [194]. Experiments on the tetanus toxin model implicate a reduction in the excitability of hippocampal neurones as a basis for the impairment of learning [119, 192, 195]. This long-term depression may also have had a hand in the remission of seizures because inhibition remains weaker than normal at this stage [196].

These studies have shown that, in the absence of any discernable histopathology, persistent functional changes can follow repeated epileptic seizures. Whether or not these kinds of physiological mechanism are important clinically remains to be seen. The relevant electrophysiological measures are difficult, if not impossible, to make. However, in view of the close relation between neuronal activity and metabolic rate, some indirect support may be derived from observations with positron emission tomography of patients with epilepsy. These reveal that interictal epileptic foci are associated with widespread hypometabolism, which can extend far beyond any areas of pathological involvement, and may include remote regions such as the basal ganglia and the cerebellum [197, 198].

2.2.6   Kindling and secondary epileptogenesis in man

An issue that has been much debated is whether or not seizures beget seizures in man. The possibility has to be considered that seizures could act as a kindling stimulus. That this does not readily occur is suggested by the fact that many seizure disorders spontaneously remit, even after an active epileptic focus has been present for many years – for example, benign centrotemporal epilepsy of childhood (p. 478). Moreover seizures remit in some experimental models of epilepsy, such as those induced by implantation of cobalt or injection of tetanus toxin. There remains the possibility, however, that in other seizure disorders the pattern of occurrence of seizures and of interictal epileptic activity is different, and could produce kindling. There is no direct evidence as to whether or not kindling occurs in man. It does occur in monkeys and baboons, but takes longer to develop than in lower vertebrates, and spontaneous seizures do not occur unless there is an underlying genetic tendency to seizures.

A phenomenon related to kindling is secondary epileptogenesis. This refers to the development of an epileptic focus in a site anatomically connected to the primary focus, which eventually becomes independent of the primary focus, and which can initiate seizures even after the primary focus has been excised [199]. This phenomenon is most commonly recognized contralateral and homotopic to the primary focus. The secondary focus may then be called a 'mirror' focus. The development of this begins with contralateral spikes synchronous with and dependent on spikes in the primary focus. Later the contralateral spikes begin to occur independently of those in the primary focus, and seizures may begin to arise from the secondary focus. At first these will gradually cease after excision of the primary focus, but if a sufficient time is allowed to elapse before such an excision, the secondary focus will persist indefinitely. The development of secondary epileptic foci takes progressively longer as the evolutionary tree is ascended [200]. Independent secondary foci have not been consistently produced in monkeys [201, 202]. In man, the occurrence of bilateral synchronous or independent temporal lobe spikes with unilateral temporal lobe lesions is not uncommon, and the spikes disappear on both sides after unilateral temporal lobectomy [203]. What has not been clear is whether or not the next stage of secondary epileptogenesis, the development of an independent contralateral focus that may initiate a new seizure type, can occur in man. Evidence for this has been sought, and not found [203a]. Recently, however, Morrell [204] has described 16 cases, followed over many years, in which the evidence for the development of secondary foci is quite strong. Each patient had a low grade cerebral tumour associated with the primary focus, and there were no reasons to suspect multiple cerebral lesions. Each developed an independent contralateral EEG focus one to ten years after the onset of the epilepsy, and also developed a new seizure type, which was documented to arise from this secondary focus. Each had surgical excision of the primary focus one to twenty years after the appearance of the secondary focus. This was followed by disappearance of the primary EEG focus and the first seizure type, but the secondary focus and its seizure type persisted either temporarily (11 cases) or permanently (four cases). The former cases all had fewer seizures between the time of onset of the secondary focus and the surgery than the latter cases, who all had many thousands during this time. There is thus some evidence that secondary epileptogenesis may occasionally occur in man, although primates are resistant compared to lower vertebrates. It does not seem to occur in most patients with epilepsy despite frequent seizures for many years. Even if secondary epileptogenesis only occurs rarely in man, it has important implications for the management of epilepsy.

2.2.7 The generalization of seizures

The factors determining why seizures occur when they occur, and determining whether or not partial seizures evolve into generalized tonic-clonic seizures are poorly understood. Synaptic inhibition and possibly depression of neuronal activity (p. 55) usually keep epileptiform discharges spatially restricted. Clinically, the reasons for the occasional failure of these suppressive mechanisms are usually unclear, although in a few patients seizures may be reflexly mediated, or provoked by hormonal or metabolic factors. When a seizure occurs, there is presumably either a reduction in inhibition, or an increased extent of synchronous activity that results in inhibition being overwhelmed.

In human epilepsy and in chronic animal models, the focal interictal spike is the hallmark of the epileptic focus, and it is similar spikes that have been studied in acute models in the hippocampal slice (p. 23). Nevertheless, the relationship between interictal spikes and epileptic seizures is not entirely clear. Clinical seizures usually begin with desynchronization of EEG activity, and not with a spike. The sites of the seizure focus and the spike focus are not always precisely the same. Gotman and Marciani [205] have shown, in one group of patients with epilepsy, that there was no change in the rate of interictal spiking before the onset of a seizure, that the rate of spiking was unrelated to the occurrence of seizures, and that drug levels did not influence the rate of spiking. The rate of spiking was increased, however, for several days following epileptic seizures. They have made the controversial suggestions that spikes and seizures may have different generating mechanisms, and that spiking activity might be a feature of the postictal state.

Seizure activity may spread both locally, and more distantly due to activity in neuronal pathways. Local spread, as in a Jacksonian march, may partly be mediated by terminal depolarization (p. 39). It has been suggested in the past that spreading depression might also have a role, but measurements of changes in extracellular potassium have not supported this (p. 37). The spread of partial seizures has been studied by observation of the effects of physical and chemical lesions on overt seizures [206, 207], recording from multiple implanted electrodes [208–212], and by recording changes in glucose metabolism by autoradiographic techniques [213, 214]. Hayashi [206] demonstrated that severing the pyramidal tracts in dogs did not prevent the motor manifestations of seizures elicited by electrical or chemical stimulation of the cortex. In dogs and monkeys he showed that the descending pathway of seizure activity involved the thalamus and globus pallidus; convulsions were prevented by bilateral globus pallidus lesions or by ipsilateral lesions to both the thalamus and lenticular nucleus (bilateral thalamic lesions were ineffective). He suggested that the pathway descended from the globus pallidus to the homolateral 'substantia nigra and its posterior substantia reticularis', with commissural fibres at both levels. The descending pathways then crossed diffusely in the medulla, since a longitudinal cut in the midline between the pons and caudal medulla prevented clonic convulsions from bilateral cortical application of nicotine. Convulsions elicited by application of nicotine to 'extramotor' cortex were dependent on an intact motor cortex, but convulsions elicited by application to the thalamus, globus pallidus, midbrain or cerebellum were unaffected by removal of the cerebrum. Multiple depth recordings and 2-deoxyglucose studies have confirmed the involvement of the substantia nigra, globus pallidus, thalamic nuclei and other brainstem sites in the spread of seizures from the cerebral cortex or amygdala/hippocampus. Commissural spread between the cerebral hemispheres also occurs. More recent studies of seizures induced by pentylenetetrazol, bicuculline or maximal electroshock have confirmed an important role for the substantia nigra in generalized seizures. Electrolytic and kainic acid lesions of the substantia nigra protect against these seizures [215], and injections of GABA agonists into substantia nigra are also effective, suggesting that this is one site of their anticonvulsant activity [216]. Lesions of midbrain reticular formation may also be effective [217]. It seems likely that pathways from the pars reticulata of the substantia nigra projecting to thalamus, tectum and reticular formation (rather than the nigro–striatal pathway) are involved in these effects. Microinjection of GABA agonists into the substantia nigra not only blocks the motor manifestations of amygdala-kindled seizures, but also attenuates after-discharges in the amygdala itself [218]. Other studies of the generation and spread of amygdala-kindled seizures have suggested particular involvement of the mesencephalic reticular formation [211, 219].

2.3 GENERALIZED EPILEPSIES

The definition and classification of generalized epilepsies is considered in Chapter 3. They are associated with generalized EEG abnormalities, in particular generalized bilaterally synchronous spike and wave activity, although this does not imply that there is generalized involvement of the whole brain in all the seizure types.

Even in the symptomatic cases the mechanisms causing the epilepsy are poorly understood. A variety of seizure types occur, the more common being generalized tonic-clonic seizures, absences, myoclonic jerks and drop attacks. Particular interest has focused on the underlying mechanisms of 3 Hz spike and wave activity. We first consider this in the context of experimental models of absence seizures. We then describe experimental models of photosensitivity and generalized tonic-clonic seizures. Examples are included both of acute and chronic models in normal animals and of genetic models with spontaneous or reflexly induced seizures. We discuss what conclusions can be drawn, and what insights obtained, about the underlying mechanisms of generalized epilepsies in man.

2.3.1 Absences with 3 Hz spike and wave activity

Typical absence seizures associated with generalized 3 Hz spike and wave activity differ profoundly from partial seizures and generalized tonic-clonic seizures in their sensitivity to anticonvulsant drugs. In particular, they respond to ethosuximide and troxidone (trimethadione) but not to phenytoin and carbamazepine, whereas the reverse applies to partial seizures and generalized tonic-clonic seizures. The spikes of the spike and wave activity are associated with EPSPs and action potential generation in cortical neurones, and the waves with IPSPs and neuronal silence [220]. One interpretation of these observations is that absence seizures are a form of 'threshold' seizure, in which excitatory mechanisms are increased or inhibitory mechanisms partially depressed, and in which some inhibitory mechanisms remain intact and limit the intensity of the seizure activity. Threshold seizures in various animal models of epilepsy have a similar pharmacological sensitivity (for example, pentylenetetrazol threshold seizures, p. 65, and minor seizures in Mongolian gerbils, p. 64). Another observation consistent with this interpretation is that absence seizures in man occasionally evolve into generalized tonic-clonic seizures. An alternative hypothesis is that absence seizures are 'inhibitory seizures', and that enhanced inhibition causes synchronization of discharge in cortical neurones, and rhythmic alternation between excitation and inhibition. Possible examples of this mechanism in the rat are provided by the bilaterally synchronous spike and wave activity induced by the GABA agonists muscimol and THIP (4, 5, 6, 7 tetrahydroisoxalo[5,4-C]pyridine

3-0L); the spike and wave bursts are associated with motor arrest and myoclonic twitching of the vibrissae [221].

A question that has been much debated is the location of the site or sites of abnormality that may give rise to 3 Hz spike and wave activity and absences. Penfield and Jasper [222] argued that seizures with loss of consciousness at the onset, and bilaterally synchronous EEG discharges, must have their origin in deep midline structures; they coined the term centrencephalic to describe epilepsies with such seizures. The deep midline structures were presumed to be the ascending reticular activating system and midline thalamic nuclei. Some support for their ideas was provided by the effects of stimulation of the intralaminar thalamic nuclei of the cat at 3 Hz, which produced a generalized cortical 3 Hz spike and wave discharge; the frequency and continuity of the discharge were, however, dependent on continued stimulation [223]. Subsequently Guerrero-Figueroa *et al.* [224] showed that aluminium oxide placed in the intralaminar thalamic nuclei or in the mesencephalic reticular formation (but not elsewhere) of the kitten would give rise to 3 Hz spikes and waves in the thalamus, which later involved the cortex, and were associated with apparent absences. Nevertheless, the centrencephalic concept has since fallen into disfavour. The question has been whether generalized cortical spike and wave activity is driven by abnormal activity in subcortical structures or arises due to an abnormality of the cortex itself. Evidence in favour of the latter is provided by the phenomenon of 'secondary bilateral synchrony'. This refers to the occurrence of bilateral, more or less symmetrical, spike and wave discharges in association with focal (mainly medial frontal) lesions of the cerebral cortex [225]. In addition, Marcus and Watson [226] demonstrated that bilateral symmetrical application of strychnine, PTZ or conjugated oestrogens to the premotor cortex of cats or monkeys would induce bilaterally symmetrical spike and wave discharges associated with behavioural arrest. The discharges persisted and bilateral synchrony was maintained in blocks of cortex isolated from the thalamus, but interconnected by the corpus callosum. Mutani *et al.* [227] obtained similar results in a chronic model with asymmetrical foci. There is thus evidence that 3 Hz cortical spike and wave activity can arise either from abnormal activity in deep midline structures or in the cortex itself. We will now examine in more detail two recently developed animal models of absence seizures associated with spike and wave activity.

(a) Feline generalized penicillin epilepsy [56, 228]

If a cat is given 200 000–400 000 units/kg of penicillin intramuscularly, generalized bilaterally synchronous 3–7 Hz spike and wave discharges will develop 30–60 min later, and will persist for 3–5 hours. The discharges may be associated with arrest of spontaneous activity, blinking, pupillary dilatation and facial myoclonus. They may be precipitated by photic stimulation. They are suppressed by ethosuximide and sodium valproate, but phenytoin is less effective. This model of human petit mal absences has been extensively investigated by Gloor and collaborators [56]. The spike and wave discharges are thought to be an abnormal response of the cortex to normal thalamocortical volleys, which would in the absence of penicillin produce spindle activity. The spike and wave discharges can be provoked by stimulation of midline and intralaminar thalamic nuclei, and abolished by thalamectomy or injection of KC1 into the thalamus. The penicillin appears to act at a cortical level, however, since local application of a very dilute solution of penicillin to the surface of the cortex produces spike and wave discharges, whereas injections of penicillin into the thalamus do not. Spike and wave activity in the cortex always precedes that in the thalamus. The bilateral synchrony is mediated by the corpus callosum. Activity of the brainstem reticular formation modulates the spike and wave discharges; activation by intravertebral pentylenetetrazol suppresses them and inactivation by cooling enhances them. Single unit and intracellular recordings [228, 229] have shown that the spikes are associated with EPSPs and action potentials, and that the waves are associated with IPSPs and neuronal silence. Gloor has proposed that the penicillin causes a mild diffuse increase in the excitability of the cortex. This conclusion is based on the observations that: (1) during the transition from spindle to spike and wave activity, the probability that a cortical neurone generates an action potential during a spindle wave gradually increases, and (2) recurrent inhibition remains intact. Van Gelder *et al.* [230] have shown that the onset of spike and wave activity is preceded by a reduction in the cortical content of glutamate, which presumably leaks into the extracellular space, and might cause a diffuse increase in neuronal excitability. However, penicillin, at larger concentrations than employed in this model, is well known to suppress inhibition. Indeed, occasionally even with the low doses used, recurrent inhibition may be blocked and generalized tonic-clonic seizures ensue. An alternative hypothesis to a diffuse increase in cortical excitability, therefore, is that low doses of penicillin exert a differential effect on inhibitory synapses, suppressing some, but leaving those mediating recurrent inhibition intact. In summary, it is proposed that the generalized spike and wave activity and absences are due to normal thalamic inputs acting upon an abnormally excitable cerebral cortex.

(b) The tottering mouse [231, 232]

Recessive mutations arising from inbred strains of mice have been examined for evidence of epileptic seizure activity, and several mutations have now been identified which have spontaneous generalized or absence seizures [231, 232]. These mutants differ from the parental strains at only single gene loci, the sites of which are multiple and on many different chromosomes. They offer the possibility of precisely identifying genetic factors which lead to the development of epilepsy, and the mechanisms by which they operate. One of the most interesting of these mutants is the 'tottering mouse', which displays from adolescence spontaneous cortical spike and wave discharges, accompanied by behavioural absences, and also simple partial seizures with motor symptoms. The mice are mildly ataxic. In this mutant there is an increase in the terminal axonal arborizations of the noradrenergic neurones arising from the locus coeruleus, and an associated increase in the noradrenaline content of the neocortex, hippocampus, thalamic relay nuclei and cerebellum. Noebels [231] has obtained evidence that this difference is related to the epilepsy. He injected tottering neonatal mice with 6-hydroxydopamine, which destroys the distal terminal projections of the noradrenergic axons; in these animals the development of spike and wave activity and seizures was suppressed, without any apparent ill-effects on behaviour or the EEG. Noradrenaline tends to excite thalamic relay neurones, and inhibit cortical neurones, but the precise mechanism by which the abnormal locus coeruleus innervation causes spike and wave activity has not been established. This model raises the possibility that spike and wave activity and absences may be due to an abnormal innervation of the cortex by a brainstem nucleus.

(c)   Absences and 3 Hz spike and wave activity in the human

The underlying mechanisms of generalized spike and wave activity recorded in human epilepsies remain to be established. There is no doubt that the spike and wave activity is generated in the cortex, and that some powerful inhibitory mechanisms remain intact. It has long been recognized that the spikes are associated with EPSPs and action potential generation, and the waves with IPSPs and silence in cortical neurones, giving rhythmic alternation between excitation and inhibition. In the generalized epilepsies it is not known whether the spike and wave is the response of an abnormal cortex to normal inputs (as in the penicillin model in the cat), the response of a normal cortex to an abnormal input (as in the centrencephalic hypothesis) or a combination of these (as in the tottering mouse, in which there is an abnormal innervation of the cortex by a brainstem nucleus). Generalized spike and wave activity can also arise in response to focal (mainly medial frontal) cortical lesions. Gotman [233] has shown that a small time difference in the spike and wave activity recorded over each hemisphere can usually be detected in such cases of 'secondary bilateral synchrony', but not in patients with generalized epilepsies and 'primary bilateral synchrony'. This observation presumably reflects callosal transfer of the discharge in the secondary cases, and implies additional mechanisms of synchrony in the primary cases. Van Gelder *et al.* [234] have reported that patients with absence attacks and 3 Hz spike and wave have increased plasma levels of glutamate and low levels of taurine. They have suggested that this might be due to excessive neuronal release of these amino acids. The taurine would be lost, leading to a reduced plasma level. The glutamate would be resynthesized, leading to a high plasma level. A corresponding high extracellular glutamate in the brain might cause a diffuse increase in cortical excitability, as suggested for the penicillin model of generalized epilepsy in the cat. This idea is very speculative. In the human generalized epilepsies, it is probable that a variety of different mechanisms can operate to produce spike and wave activity and absences.

2.3.2 Generalized tonic-clonic seizures, myoclonus and photosensitivity

In human generalized epilepsies, the site or sites of abnormality, and the nature of the abnormalities, which give rise to generalized seizure types other than absence are just as uncertain as they are for absence seizures themselves. In animals, including monkeys, generalized convulsive seizures and myoclonus can be evoked by electrical or chemical stimulation of various thalamic, basal ganglia and brainstem sites as well as cerebral cortical ones [206, 235]. Generalized seizures and myoclonus can also be produced by the injection of cobalt powder into the lower brainstem or midline thalamus [236]. The relevance of these acute experiments to chronic epilepsy is uncertain.

We now briefly describe four animal models of chronic generalized epilepsy: photosensitive epilepsy in the baboon, audiogenic seizures in mice, reflex seizures in Mongolian gerbils, and lateral geniculate nucleus kindling in the cat. We also discuss seizures induced by the convulsant drug pentylenetetrazol.

(a) Photosensitive baboons [237–239]
Photosensitive epilepsy in the Senagalese baboon, *Papio papio*, has many similarities with human photosensitive epilepsy. It occurs most frequently in an inbred subpopulation, appears in adolescence and is precipitated by a similar range of flash frequencies. Photic stimulation induces eyelid clonus, which may subsequently involve the face, head and body. Following photic stimulation, clonic jerks may persist or a generalized tonic-clonic seizure may ensue. A major difference from human photosensitive epilepsy lies in the location of the associated polyspike and wave activity; in the baboon it appears in the frontorolandic regions symmetrically, whereas in man it either appears in occipital and posterior temporal regions or is generalized from the onset. The relevant frontorolandic regions of the baboon receive afferents supplying information about vision, eye movement and the periorbital tissues. The visual input alone is insufficient to produce spike and wave activity, as ventilated and paralysed baboons are not photosensitive, and periorbital local anaesthesia is protective. Single cell recordings from paralysed baboons (treated with allylglycine to produce photosensitivity again) have demonstrated that the spikes are associated with burst discharges in frontorolandic units. There is as yet no conclusive evidence as to the mechanisms underlying the photosensitive epilepsy, although it has been speculated that there might be a failure of an intracortical inhibitory system when the excitatory input reaches a critical level [240].

(b) Audiogenic seizures in mice

Audiogenic seizures are generalized convulsions induced by intense sound. Several strains of mice have an inherited susceptibility to these seizures. Although seizures induced by sound are very rare in the human, it has been suggested that audiogenic seizures in mice may represent a model of human generalized photosensitive epilepsy, the different sensory sensitivity being a species difference [232]. A gene has been identified that confers resistance to the spread of audiogenic seizures, but its mode of action is not yet known [241]. Several biochemical differences between susceptible and resistant strains have been reported. One of these is an inverse relationship between the activity in the brainstem of a low affinity calcium adenosine triphosphatase and seizure susceptibility [242].

(c) Seizures in Mongolian gerbils [243]

Some strains of the Mongolian gerbil have reflex seizures in response to handling, a new environment, or puffs of compressed air [243]. Minor myoclonic seizures respond best to diazepam, sodium valproate and ethosuximide, and major generalized tonic-clonic seizures respond best to phenytoin, carbamazepine and phenobarbitone. Recently, Olsen *et al.* [244] have reported that benzodiazepine receptor binding is significantly lower in the midbrain of the seizure-susceptible gerbils than in the midbrain of seizure-resistant strains, whereas there is no difference in binding in other brain areas. This raises the possibility that an alteration in the GABA–A receptor complex might be associated with the occurrence of the epilepsy.

(d) Lateral geniculate nucleus (LGN) kindling in the cat [245]

Shouse and Ryan [245] have demonstrated that generalized tonic-clonic seizures can be kindled from the LGN of the cat after an average of 6.5 subthreshold stimulations. Bilateral eye blinking followed by a generalized tonic-clonic seizure accompanied the first after-discharge, which was associated with generalized 4–5 Hz spike and wave activity. Following LGN kindling, the seizure threshold was reduced by 50% during photic stimulation at 1.5 Hz. These findings contrasted with the results of amygdala kindling, in which focal after-discharges and focal seizures were elicited initially, generalized seizures appearing only after 3–4 weeks, and in which photic stimulation produced no change in seizure theshold. It was suggested that LGN kindling in the cat might be a model of primary generalized seizures. Spontaneous seizures have not been described in this model.

(e) Seizures induced by pentylenetetrazol (PTZ)

The convulsant drug PTZ has been used for many years to induce seizures in a variety of species from mouse to man. Small doses produce 'threshold seizures' consisting of myoclonic jerks with diffuse spike and wave activity, and larger doses will produce severe bilateral myoclonic jerks, generalized tonic-clonic seizures associated with EEG desynchronization, and status epilepticus. The ability of drugs to prevent PTZ threshold seizures shows some correlation with their efficacy at suppressing petit mal seizures in man – ethosuximide, troxidone (trimethadione), sodium valproate, diazepam and phenobarbitone will raise the threshold for these seizures, whereas phenytoin and carbamazepine are ineffective. In contrast, maximal seizures induced by large doses of PTZ are modified by phenytoin and carbamazepine. Rodin [246] demonstrated in cats that the onset of convulsive PTZ seizures was not consistently related temporally to changes in the EEG recorded over the cortex, but was related to high voltage asynchronous spiking in the brainstem, recorded only with a wide bandwidth (30–10 000 Hz). These high frequency discharges in the brainstem usually preceded abnormal activity elsewhere, although sometimes the onset was almost simultaneous in the brainstem, thalamus and cortex. The duration of the high frequency bursts corresponded with the seizure type; bursts of between 50 and 400 ms were associated with myoclonic jerks, those of 500–1500 ms with a fall, and those greater than 1500 ms with a generalized tonic-clonic seizure. This suggests that, in cats, PTZ induced seizures may originate in the brainstem [247]. In the guinea-pig, Mirski and Ferrendelli have also shown that the mamillary bodies are involved in the propagation of generalized seizures induced by PTZ [247a].

(f) Conclusions

There is evidence from these models that primary generalized tonic-clonic seizures and myoclonus (like absences) may arise due to abnormalities in the brainstem, as well as due to abnormalities in the cerebral cortex. Analyses of audiogenic seizures in the mouse, seizures in Mongolian gerbils and seizures induced by cobalt injection into the brainstem suggest that brainstem abnormalities can be involved. Analysis of PTZ-induced seizures suggests a brainstem origin, and implies that, although the drug may act at many sites in the central nervous system, some brainstem structures are particularly sensitive to its action. Nevertheless, the brainstem and thalamus are resistant to kindling [157]. Generalized seizures can be kindled, however, from the LGN of the cat, and they accompany the first after-discharge. In the photosensitive baboon, a cortical origin for the seizures seems most likely, with convergence of visual and somatosensory inputs required for an excitatory threshold to be reached, although subcortical mechanisms may also be important. The first clues as to the underlying neurochemical and cellular abnormalities which give rise to the epilepsy in these animal models are beginning to emerge.

In the human it is probable that different mechanisms operate to produce generalized seizures in different epileptic syndromes. There is evidence in man to suggest that myoclonus may have either a cortical or subcortical origin [248–250]. Drop attacks have been tentatively ascribed to subcortical mechanisms [251]. Investigation of human idiopathic generalized epilepsies has so far not revealed their underlying mechanisms, but a few clues have been found. Analysis of families with several members affected has revealed an association with low levels of plasma haptoglobin [252], and with decreased urinary excretion of taurine [253]. Changes in plasma taurine and glutamate have been reported (p. 62). Neuropathological examination of brains from patients with generalized epilepsy has shown only minor abnormalities [254], the significance of which is uncertain.

Epileptic photosensitivity is associated with a deficiency in cortical dopaminergic neurotransmission [255, 256]. There are three main threads of evidence: first, the effects of apomorphine, a dopamine agonist, which blocks epileptic photosensitivity in man, as in the photosensitive baboon and feline generalized penicillin epilepsy, but is ineffective against spontaneous spike and wave activity. Secondly, high frequency photic stimulation in cats is observed to reduce cortical release of dopamine [257]. Thirdly, the bilateral application of 6-hydroxydopamine to the cortex of cats (which induces cortical catecholamine depletion) is observed to induce epileptic photosensitivity.

Although many single gene mutations in man are associated with epilepsy, and usually with other abnormalities in addition [258], the precise mechanisms underlying the epilepsy in these conditions are almost all poorly understood. Nevertheless, in the future, the further analysis of animal genetic mutants with epilepsy will be of great interest, as they should reveal the mechanisms of action of a variety of single gene mutations. It may subsequently be possible to investigate some of these in the human generalized epilepsies.

2.4   MODELS OF EPILEPSY USED FOR THE ASSESSMENT OF ANTICONVULSANT DRUGS

It will be apparent from the preceding paragraphs that there is a bewildering array of animal models of epilepsy. Drug screening programmes have generally employed just two models of epilepsy, both in the mouse, in the search for new anticonvulsant agents. Maximal electroshock seizures (MES) have been used to search for drugs for partial and generalized tonic-clonic seizures, and PTZ threshold seizures (p. 65) for drugs for petit mal absence [259]. Conventional anticonvulsants are effective in these tests, which are economical, permitting the testing of large numbers of compounds. Nevertheless it can be argued that these tests may only detect drugs that act by mechanisms similar to conventional drugs, and drugs acting by novel mechanisms may remain undetected. It has been suggested, therefore, that a wider range of tests might be employed, particularly utilizing animals with a genetic susceptibility to epilepsy [260].

REFERENCES

1. Jasper, H. H. and van Gelder, N. M. (eds) (1983) *Basic Mechanisms of Neuronal Hyperexcitability*, Alan R. Liss, New York.
2. Schwartzkroin, P. A. and Wheal, H. V. (eds) (1984) *Electrophysiology of Epilepsy*, Academic Press, London.
3. Delgado-Escueta, A. V., Ward, A. A., Woodbury, D. M. and Porter, R. J. (eds) (1986) *Basic Mechanisms of the Epilepsies* (Adv. Neurol. 44), Raven Press, New York.
4. Jefferys, J. G. R. (1984) Review on 'Basic Mechanisms of Neuronal Hyperexcitability' ([1]). *Trends Neurosci.*, **7**, 266.
5. Krnjevic, K. (1983) GABA-mediated inhibitory mechanisms in relation to epileptic discharges, in *Basic Mechanisms of Neuronal Hyperexcitability* (eds H. H. Jasper and N. M. van Gelder), Alan R. Liss, New York, pp. 249–80.
6. Kandel, E. R. and Spencer, W. A. (1961) Excitation and inhibition of single pyramidal cells during hippocampal seizure. *Expl Neurol.*, **4**, 162.
7. Li, C.-L. (1959) Cortical intracellular potentials and their responses to strychnine. *J. Neurophysiol.*, **22**, 436–50.
8. Matsumoto, H. (1964) Intracellular events during the activation of cortical epileptiform discharges. *Electroenceph. Clin. Neurophysiol.*, **17**, 294–307.
9. Matsumoto, H. and Ajmone-Marsan, C. (1964) Cortical cellular phenomena in experimental epilepsy: Interictal manifestations. *Expl Neurol.*, **9**, 286–304.
10. Matsumoto, H. and Ajmone-Marsan, C. (1964) Cortical cellular phenomena in experimental epilepsy: Ictal manifestations. *Expl Neurol.*, **99**, 305–26.
11. Ajmone-Marsen, C. (1969) Acute effects of topical epileptogenic agents, in *Basic Mechanisms of the Epilepsies* (eds H. H. Jasper, A. A. Ward and A. Pope), Little Brown and Co., Boston, pp. 299–319.
12. Prince, D. A. (1969) Microelectrode studies of penicillin foci, in *Basic Mechanisms of the Epilepsies* (eds H. H. Jasper, A. A. Ward and A. Pope), Little, Brown and Co., Boston, pp. 320–8.
13. Dichter, M. and Spencer, W. A. (1968) Hippocampal penicillin 'spike' discharge: Epileptic neuron or epileptic aggregate? *Neurol. (Minneap.)*, **18**, 282.
14. Warburg, O. (1930) Experiments on surviving carcinoma tissue – methods – respiration and glycolysis, in *The Metabolism of Tumours* (ed. O. Warburg; transl. F. Dickens), Churchill, London, pp. 75–93.
14a. Yamamoto, C. and McIlwain, H. H. (1966) Electrical activities in thin sections from the mammalian brain maintained in chemically-defined media *in vitro. J. Neurochem.*, **13**, 1333–43.
15. Li, C.-L. and McIlwain, H. (1957) Maintenance of resting membrane potentials in slices of mammalian cerebral cortex and other tissues *in vitro. J. Physiol.*, **139**, 178–90.
16. Skrede, K. K. and Westgaard, R. H. (1971) The transverse hippocampal slice: a well-defined cortical structure maintained *in vitro. Brain Res.*, **35**, 589–93.
17. Green, J. D. (1964) The hippocampus. *Physiol. Rev.*, **44**, 561–92.
18. Yamamoto, C. (1972) Intracellular study of seizure-like afterdischarges elicited in thin hippocampal sections *in vitro. Expl Neurol.*, **35**, 154–64.
19. Dingledine, R. and Gjerstad, L. (1979) Penicillin blocks hippocampal IPSPs unmasking prolonged EPSPs. *Brain Res.*, **168**, 205–9.

20. Schwartzkroin, P. A. and Prince, D. A. (1978) Cellular and field potential properties of epileptogenic hippocampal slices. *Brain Res.*, **147**, 117–30.

21. Yamamoto, C. and Kawai, N. (1968) Generation of the seizure discharge in thin sections of the guinea pig brain in chloride-free medium *in vitro. Jap. J. Physiol.*, **18**, 620–31.

22. Ransom, B. R. and Goldring, S. (1973) Ionic determinants of membrane potential of cells presumed to be glia in cerebral cortex of cat. *J. Neurophysiol.*, **36**, 855–68.

23. Raabe, W. (1982) Ammonia and postsynaptic inhibition in cat motor cortex, in *Physiology and Pharmacology of Epileptogenic Phenomena* (eds M. R. Klee, H. D. Lux and E. J. Speckman), Raven Press, New York, pp. 73–80.

24. Wood, J. D. (1975) The role of GABA in the mechanisms of seizures. *Prog. Neurobiol.*, **5**, 77–95.

25. Ozawa, S. and Okada, Y. (1976) Decrease of GABA levels and the appearance of a depolarization shift in thin hippocampal slices *in vitro*, in *GABA in Nervous System Function* (eds E. Roberts, T. N. Chase and D. B. Tower), Raven Press, New York, pp. 449–540.

26. Fan, S. G., Wusteman, M. and Iversen, L. L. (1981) 3-Mercaptopropionic acid inhibits GABA release from rat brain slices *in vitro. Brain Res.*, **229**, 379–87.

27. Knowles, W. D., Strowbridge, B. W. and Traub, R. D. (1987) The initiation and spread of epileptiform bursts in the *in vitro* hippocampal slice. Neuroscience (in press).

28. Miles, R. and Wong, R. K. S. (1983) Single neurones can initiate synchronized population discharge in the hippocampus. *Nature*, **306**, 371–3.

29. Mesher, R. A. and Schwartzkroin, P. A. (1980) Can CA3 epileptiform discharge induce bursting in normal CA1 hippocampal neurons? *Brain Res.*, **183**, 472–6.

30. Schwartzkroin, P. A. and Prince, D. A. (1980) Effects of TEA on hippocampal neurones. *Brain Res.*, **185**, 169–81.

31. Schwartzkroin, P. A. and Slawsky, M. (1977) Probable calcium spikes in hippocampal neurons. *Brain Res.*, **133**, 157–61.

32. Wong, R. K. S. and Prince, D. A. (1978) Participation of calcium spikes during intrinsic burst firing in hippocampal neurons. *Brain Res.*, **159**, 385–90.

33. Llinas, R. and Sugimori, M. (1981) Electrophysiological properties of *in vitro* Purkinje cell dendrites in mammalian cerebellar slices. *J. Physiol.*, **305**, 197–213.

34. Wong, R. K. S., Prince, D. A. and Basbaum, A. I. (1978) Intradendritic recordings from hippocampal neurons. *Proc. Natl Acad. Sci.*, **76**, 986–90.

35. Bernardo, L. S., Masukawa, L. M. and Prince, D. A. (1982) Electrophysiology of isolated hippocampal dendrites. *J. Neurosci.*, **2**, 1614–22.

36. Meldrum, B. S. (1981) Metabolic effects of prolonged epileptic seizures and the causation of epileptic brain damage, in *Metabolic Disorders of the Nervous System* (ed. F. C. Rose), Pitman, London, pp. 175– 87.

37. Meldrum, B. S. (1986) Cell damage in epilepsy and the role of calcium in cytotoxicity, in *Basic Mechanisms of the Epilepsies* ([3]) pp. 849–55.

38. Brown, D. A., Docherty, R. J., Gahwiler, B. H. and Halliwell, J. V. (1985) Calcium currents in mammalian central neurones, in *Cardiovascular Effects of Dihydropyridine-Type Calcium Antagonists and Agonists* (Bayer-Symposium IX), Springer-Verlag, Berlin, pp. 74–87.

39. Alger, B. E. and Nicoll, R. A. (1980) Epileptiform burst after hyperpolarization:

calcium-dependent potassium potential in hippocampal CA1 pyramidal cells. *Science*, **210**, 1122–4.

40. Hotson, J. R. and Prince, D. A. (1981) Penicillin- and barium-induced epileptiform bursting in hippocampal neurones: Actions on Ca^{++} and K^{+} potentials. *Ann. Neurol.*, **10**, 11–17.

41. Traub, R. D. (1982) Simulation of intrinsic bursting in CA3 hippocampal neurons. *Neuroscience*, **7**, 1233–42.

42. Carpenter, D. O. (ed.) (1982) *Cellular Pacemakers*, John Wiley and Sons, New York.

43. Schwindt, P. C. and Crill, W. E. (1980) Effects of barium on cat spinal motoneurones studied by voltage clamp. *J. Neurophysiol.*, **44**, 827–46.

44. Schwindt, P. C. and Crill, W. E. (1980) Properties of a persistent inward current in normal and TEA injected motoneurons. *J. Neurophysiol.*, **43**, 1700–24.

45. Voskuyl, R. A. and Albus, H. (1985) Spontaneous epileptiform discharges in hippocampal slices induced by 4-aminopyridine. *Brain Res.*, **342**, 54–66.

46. Galvin, M., Grafe, P. and Ten Bruggencate, G. (1982) Convulsant actions of 4-aminopyridine on the guinea-pig olfactory cortex slice. *Brain Res.*, **241**, 75–86.

47. Eccles, J. C., Libet, B. and Young, R. R. (1958) The behaviour of chromatolysed motoneurones studied by intracellular recording. *J. Physiol.*, **143**, 11–40.

48. Kuno, M. and Llinas, R. (1970) Enhancement of synaptic transmission by dendritic potentials in chromatolysed motoneurones of the cat. *J. Physiol.*, **210**, 807–21.

49. Jan, Y. N., Jan, L. Y. and Dennis, M. J. (1977) Two mutations of synaptic transmission in *Drosophila*. *Proc. R. Soc.Lond. (B)*, **198**, 87–108.

50. Cole, A. E. and Nicoll, R. A. (1984) The pharmacology of cholinergic excitatory responses in hippocampal pyramidal cells. *Brain Res.*, **305**, 283–90.

51. Haas, H. L. and Konnert, A. (1983) Histamine and noradrenaline decrease calcium-activated potassium conductance in hippocampal pyramidal cells. *Nature*, **299**, 432–4.

52. Madison, D. V. and Nicoll, R. A. (1982) Noradrenaline blocks accommodation of pyramidal cell discharge in the hippocampus. *Nature*, **299**, 636–8.

53. Calvin, W. H. (1980) Normal repetitive firing and its pathophysiology, in *Epilepsy: A Window to Brain Mechanisms* (eds J. S. Lockard and A. A. Ward), Raven Press, New York, pp. 97–121.

54. Wyler, A. R. and Ward, A. A. (1986) Neuronal firing patterns from epileptogenic foci of monkey and human, in *Basic Mechanisms of the Epilepsies* ([3]) pp. 967–89.

55. Anderson, P. and Anserson, S. A. (1968) *Physiological Basis of the Alpha Rhythm*, Meredith Corporation, New York.

56. Gloor, P. (1984) Electrophysiology of generalized epilepsy, in *Electrophysiology of Epilepsy* (eds P. A. Schwartzkroin and H. Wheal), Academic Press, London, pp. 107–36.

57. Ayala, G. F., Dichter, M., Gumnit, R. J. *et al.* (1973) Genesis of epileptic interictal spikes. New knowledge of cortical feedback systems suggests a neurophysiological explanation of brief paroxysms. *Brain Res.*, **52**, 1–17.

58. Lebowitz, R. M., Dichter, M. and Spencer, W. A. (1971) Recurrent excitation in the CA3 region of cat hippocampus. *Int. J. Neurosci.*, **2**, 99–108.

59. Dichter, M. and Spencer, W. A. (1969) Penicillin-induced interictal discharges

from the cat hippocampus. II. Mechanisms underlying origin and restriction. *J. Neurophysiol.*, **32**, 663–87.

60. MacVicar, B. A. and Dudek, F. E. (1980) Local synaptic circuits in rat hippocampus: interaction between pyramidal cells. *Brain Res.*, **184**, 220–3.

61. Miles, R. and Wong, R. K. S. (1986) Excitatory synaptic interactions between CA3 neurones in the guinea-pig hippocampus. *J. Physiol.*, **373**, 397–418.

62. Traub, R. D. and Wong, R. K. S. (1982) Cellular mechanism of neuronal synchronization in epilepsy. *Science*, **216**, 745–7.

63. Traub, R. D., Knowles, W. D., Miles, R. and Wong, R. K. S. (1984) Synchronized afterdischarges in the hippocampus: simulation studies of the cellular mechanism. *Neuroscience*, **12**, 1191–200.

64. Finch, D. M., Nowlin, N. L. and Babb, T. L. (1983) Demonstration of axonal projections of neurons in the rat hippocampus and subiculum by intracellular injection of HRP. *Brain Res.*, **271**, 201–16.

65. Miles, R. and Wong, R. K. S. (1986) Multi-synaptic excitatory circuits are released when synaptic inhibition is suppressed in the hippocampus. *J. Physiol.*, (in press).

66. Watkins, J. C. (1984) *Trends Pharmacol. Sci.*, **5**, 373–6.

67. Fagg, G. E. (1985) L-glutamate, excitatory amino acid receptors and brain function. *Trends Neurosci.*, **8**, 207–10.

68. Croucher, M. J., Collins, J. F. and Meldrum, B. S. (1982) Anticonvulsant action of excitatory amino acid antagonists. *Science*, **216**, 899–901.

69. Dingledine, R. (1986) NMDA receptors: what do they do? *Trends Neurosci.*, **9**, 47–9.

70. Herron, C. E., Lester, R. A. J., Coan, E. J. and Collingridge, G. L. (1985) Intracellular demonstration of an *N*-methyl-D-aspartate receptor mediated component of synaptic transmission in the rat hippocampus. *Neurosci. Letters*, **60**, 19–23.

71. Thomson, A. M. (1986) A magnesium-sensitive post-synaptic potential in rat cerebral cortex resembles neuronal responses to *N*-methylaspartate. *J. Physiol.*, **370**, 531–49.

72. Ashwood, T. J. and Wheal, H. V. (1986) D-2-amino 5-phosphonovalerate (D-APV) reduces epileptiform activity in slices of the kainic acid lesioned rat hippocampus. *J. Physiol.*, **373**, 23P.

73. Morris, R. G. M., Anderson, E., Lynch, G. S. and Baudry, M. (1986) Selective impairment of learning and blockade of long-term potentiation by an *N*-methyl-D-aspartate receptor antagonist, AP5. *Nature*, **319**, 774–6.

74. Szente, M. and Pongracz, F. (1979) Aminopyridine-induced seizure activity. *Electroenceph. Clin. Neurophysiol.*, **46**, 605–8.

75. Rutecki, P. A., Lebeda, F. J. and Johnston, D. (1984) Elevated extracellular potassium- and 4-aminopyridine-induced epileptiform activity in CA3 hippocampal neurons. *Soc. Neurosci. Abstr.*, **10**, 1.

76. Dichter, M. and Spencer, W. A. (1969) Penicillin-induced interictal discharges from the cat hippocampus. I. Characteristics and topographic features. *J. Neurophysiol.*, **32**, 649–62.

77. Traub, R. D. (1983) Cellular mechanisms underlying the inhibitory surround of penicillin epileptogenic foci. *Brain Res.*, **261**, 277–84.

78. Jefferys, J. G. R. and Haas, H. L. (1982) Synchronized bursting of CA1

hippocampal pyramidal cells in the absence of synaptic transmission. *Nature*, **300**, 448–50.

79. Taylor, C. P. and Dudek, F. E. (1982) Synchronous neural afterdischarges in rat hippocampal slices without active chemical synapses. *Science*, **218**, 810–12.

80. Yaari, Y., Konnerth, A. and Heinemann, U. (1983) Spontaneous epileptiform activity of CA1 hippocampal neurons in low extracellular calcium solutions. *Expl Brain Res.*, **51**, 153–6.

81. Andersen, P., Gjerstad, L. and Langmoen, I. A. (1978) A cortical epilepsy model *in vitro*, in *Abnormal Neuronal Discharges* (eds N. Chalazonitis and M. Voisson), Raven Press, New York, pp. 29–36.

82. Snow, R. W. and Dudek, F. E. (1984) Synchronous epileptiform bursts without chemical transmission in CA2, CA3 and dentate areas of the hippocampus. *Brain Res.*, **298**, 382–85.

82a. Dudek, F. E., Snow, R. W. and Taylor, C. P. (1986) Role of electrical interactions in synchronization of epileptiform bursts, in *Basic Mechanisms of the Epilepsies* ([3]) pp. 593–617.

83. Dudek, F. E., Andrew, R. D., MacVicar, B. A. *et al.* (1983) Recent evidence for and possible significance of gap junctions and electrotonic synapses in the mammalian brain, in *Basic Mechanisms of Neuronal Hyperexcitability* (eds H. H. Jasper and N. M. van Gelder), Alan R. Liss Inc., New York, pp. 31–73.

84. Korn, H. and Faber, D. S. (1979) Electrical interactions between vertebrate neurons: field effects and electrotonic coupling, in *The Neurosciences: Fourth Study Program* (eds F. O. Schmitt and F. G. Worden), MIT Press, Cambridge, pp. 333–58.

85. Traub, R. D., Dudek, F. E., Taylor, C. P. and Knowles, W. D. (1985) Simulation of hippocampal afterdischarges synchronized by electrical interactions. *Neuroscience*, **14**, 1033–8.

86. Arvanitaki, A. (1942) Effects evoked in an axon by the activity of a contiguous one. *J. Neurophysiol.*, **5**, 89–108.

87. Haas, H. L. and Jefferys, J. G. R. (1984) Low-calcium field burst discharges of CA1 pyramidal neurones in rat hippocampal slices. *J. Physiol.*, **354**, 185–201.

88. Korn, H. and Faber, D. S. (1980) Electric field effect interactions in the vertebrate brain. *Trends Neurosci.*, **3**, 6–9.

89. Jefferys, J. G. R. (1981) Influence of electric fields on the excitability of granule cells in guinea-pig hippocampal slices. *J. Physiol.*, **319**, 143–52.

90. Traub, R. D., Dudek, F. E., Snow, R. W. and Knowles, W. D. (1985) Computer simulations indicate that electrical field effects contribute to the shape of the epileptiform field potential. *Neuroscience*, **15**, 947–58.

91. Tower, D. B. (1969) Neurochemical mechanisms, in *Basic Mechanisms of the Epilepsies* (eds. H. H. Jasper, A. A. Ward and A. Pope), Little, Brown and Co., Boston, pp. 611–48.

92. Fertziger, A. P. and Ranck, J. B. (1970) Potassium accumulation in the interstitial space during epileptiform seizures. *Exp. Neurol.*, **26**, 571–85.

93. Heinemann, U., Lux, H. D. and Gutnick, M. J. (1978) Changes in extracellular free calcium and potassium activity in the somatosensory cortex of cats, in *Abnormal Neuronal Discharges* (eds N. Chalazonitis and M. Voisson), Raven Press, New York, pp. 329–45.

94. Moody, W. J., Futamachi, K. J. and Prince, D. A. (1974) Extracellular potassium activity during epileptogenesis. *Expl Neurol.* **42**, 248–63.
95. Prince, D. A., Lux, H. D. and Neher, E. (1973) Measurement of extracellular potassium activity in cat cortex. *Brain Res.*, **50**, 489–95.
96. Somjen, G. G. and Giacchino, J. L. (1985) Potassium and calcium concentrations in interstitial fluid of hippocampal formation during paroxysmal responses. *J. Neurophysiol.*, **53**, 1098–108.
97. Wadman, W. J. and Heinemann, U. (1985) Laminar profiles of K^+ out and Ca^{2+} out in region CA1 of the hippocampus of kindled rats, in *Ion-Selective Electrodes in Physiology and Medicine* (eds M. Kessler, D. K. Harrison and J. Höper), Springer-Verlag, Berlin, pp. 221–28.
98. Pumain, R., Kurcewicz, I. and Louvel, J. (1983) Fast extracellular calcium transients: involvement in epileptic processes. *Science*, **222**, 177–9.
99. Pumain, R. (1981) Electrophysiological abnormalities in chronic epileptogenic foci: an intracellular study. *Brain Res.*, **219**, 445–50.
100. Connors, B. W. (1984) Initiation of synchronized bursting in neocortex. *Nature*, **310**, 685–7.
101. Ebersole, J. S. and Chatt, A. B. (1986) Spread and arrest of seizures: the importance of layer 4 in laminar interactions during neocortical epileptogenesis, in *Basic Mechanisms of the Epilepsies* ([3]) pp. 515–58.
102. Lockton, J. W. and Holmes, O. (1980) Site of initiation of penicillin-induced epilepsy in the cortex cerebri of the rat. *Brain Res.*, **190**, 301–4.
102a. Gutnick, M. J., Connors, B. W. and Prince, D. A. (1982) Mechanisms of neocortical epileptogenesis *in vitro*. *J. Neurophysiol.*, **48**, 1321–35.
103. Jahnsen, H. and Llinas, R. (1984) Ionic basis for the electroresponsiveness and oscillatory properties of guinea-pig thalamic neurones *in vitro*. *J. Physiol.*, **349**, 227–47.
104. Andersen, P. and Sears, T. A. (1964) The role of inhibition in the phasing of spontaneous thalamocortical discharge. *J. Physiol.*, **173**, 459–80.
105. Noebels, J. L. and Prince, D. A. (1978) Development of focal seizures in cerebral cortex: role of axon terminal bursting. *J. Neurophysiol.*, **41**, 1267–81.
106. Noebels, J. L. and Prince, D. A. (1977) Presynaptic origin of penicillin afterdischarges at mammalian nerve terminals. *Brain Res.*, **138**, 59–74.
107. Lux, H. D., Heinemann, U. and Dietzel, I. (1986) Ionic changes and alterations in the size of the extracellular space during epileptic activity, in *Basic Mechanisms of the Epilepsies* ([3]) pp. 619–39.
108. Kopeloff, L. M., Chusid, J. G. and Kopeloff, N. (1942) Recurrent convulsive seizures in animals produced by immunological and chemical means. *Am. J. Psychiatr.*, **98**, 881–902.
109. Babb, T. L. and Crandall, P. H. (1973) Epileptogenesis of human limbic neurons in psychomotor epileptics. *Electroenceph. Clin. Neurophysiol.*, **40**, 225–43.
110. Calvin, W. H., Ojemann, G. A. and Ward, A. A. (1973) Human cortical neurons in epileptogenic foci: comparison of interictal firing patterns to those of 'epileptic' neurons in animals. *Electroenceph. Clin. Neurophysiol.*, **34**, 337–51.
111. Prince, D. A. and Futamachi, K. J. (1970) Intracellular recordings from chronic epileptogenic foci in the monkey. *Electroenceph. Clin. Neurophysiol.*, **29**, 496–510.
112. Jefferys, J. G. R. (1986) Tetanus toxin chronic epileptic foci in rat hippocampal slices. *J. Physiol.*, **373**, 24P.

113. Ashwood, T. J., Lancaster, B. and Wheal, H. V. (1986) Intracellular electrophysiology of CA1 pyramidal neurones in slices of the kainic acid lesioned hippocampus of the rat. *Expl Brain Res.*, **62**, 189–98.

114. Franck, J. E. and Schwartzkroin, P. A. (1985) Do kainate-lesioned hippocampi become epileptogenic? *Brain Res.*, **329**, 309–13.

115. Wheal, H. V., Ashwood, T. J. and Lancaster, B. (1984) A comparative *in vitro* study of the kainic acid lesioned and bicuculline treated hippocampus: chronic and acute models of focal epilepsy, in *Electrophysiology of Epilepsy* (eds P. A. Schwartzkroin and H. V. Wheal), Academic Press, London, pp. 173–200.

116. Tauck, D. L. and Nadler, J. V. (1985) Evidence of functional mossy fiber sprouting in hippocampal formation of kainic acid treated rats. *J. Neurosci.*, **5**, 1016–22.

117. Schwartzkroin, P. A., Turner, D. A., Knowles, W. D. and Wyler, A. R (1983) Studies of human and monkey 'epileptic' neocortex in the *in vitro* slice preparation. *Ann. Neurol.*, **13**, 249–57.

118. Lighthall, J. W. and Prince, D. A. (1986) quoted in: Prince, D. A. and Connors, B. W. Mechanisms of interictal epileptogenesis, in *Basic Mechanisms of the Epilepsies* ([3]) pp. 275–99.

119. Brace, H. M., Jefferys, J. G. R. and Mellanby, J. (1985) Long-term changes in hippocampal physiology and learning ability of rats after intrahippocampal tetanus toxin. *J. Physiol.*, **368**, 343–57.

120. Mellanby, J., George, G., Robinson, A. and Thompson, P. (1977) Epileptiform syndrome in rats produced by injecting tetanus toxin into the hippocampus. *J. Neurol. Neurosurg. Psychiat.*, **40**, 404–14.

121. Collingridge, G. L. and Herron, C. E. (1985) Effects of tetanus toxin on GABA synapses in the mammalian central nervous system, in *Seventh International Conference on Tetanus* (eds G. Nistico, P. Mastroeni and M. Pitzurra), Gangemi Co., Rome, pp. 127–42.

122. Collingridge, G. L., Thompson, P. A., Davies, J. and Mellanby, J. (1981) *In vitro* effect of tetanus toxin on GABA release from rat hippocampal slices. *J. Neurochem.*, **37**, 1039–41.

123. Schwartzkroin, P. A. and Knowles, W. D. (1984) Intracellular study of human epileptic cortex: *in vitro* maintenance of epileptiform activity? *Science*, **223**, 709–12.

124. Cavalheiro, E. A., Riche, D. A. and Le Gal la Salle, G. (1982) Long-term effects of intrahippocampal kainic acid injection in rats: a method for inducing spontaneous recurrent seizures. *Electroenceph. Clin. Neurophysiol.*, **53**, 581–9.

125. McIntyre, D. C. and Wong, R. K. S. (1985) Modification of local neuronal interactions by amygdala kindling examined *in vitro*. *Expl Neurol.*, **88**, 529–37.

126. Karpiak, S. E., Mahadik, S. P. and Rapport, M. M. (1978) Ganglioside receptors and induction of epileptiform activity: cholera toxin and choleragenoid (B subunits). *Expl Neurol.*, **62**, 256–9.

127. Kuriyama, K. and Kakita, K. (1980) Cholera toxin induced epileptogenic focus: an animal model for studying roles of cyclic AMP in the establishment of epilepsy. *Prog. Clin. Biol. Res.*, **39**, 141–55.

127a. Somogyi, A. D., Smith, M. G., Nunzi, A. *et al.* (1983) Glutamate decarboxylase immuno-reactivity in the hippocampus of the cat: distribution of immunoreactive synaptic terminals with special reference to the axon initial segment of pyrimidal neurons. *J. Neurosci.*, **3**, 1450–68.

128. Gowers, W. R. (1881) *Epilepsy, and Other Chronic Convulsive Disorders: Their Causes, Symptoms and Treatment*, Churchill, London.
129. Duchen, L. W. and Tonge, D. A. (1973) The effects of tetanus toxin on neuromuscular transmission and on the morphology of motor end-plates in slow and fast skeletal muscle of the mouse. *J. Physiol.*, **228**, 157–72.
130. Curtis, D. R. and de Groat, W. C. (1968) Tetanus toxin and spinal inhibition. *Brain Res.*, **10**, 208–12.
131. Bevan, S. and Wendon, L. M. B. (1984) A study of the action of tetanus toxin at rat soleus neuromuscular junctions. *J. Physiol.*, **348**, 1–17.
132. Ben-Ari, Y., Krnjevic, K., Reiffenstein, R. J. and Reinhardt, W. (1981) Inhibitory conductance changes and action of γ-aminobutyrate in rat hippocampus. *Neuroscience*, **6**, 2445–63.
133. Numann, R. E. and Wong, R. K. S. (1984) Voltage-clamp study on GABA response desensitization in single pyramidal cells dissociated from the hippocampus of adult guinea pig. *Neurosci. Letters*, **47**, 289–94.
134. McCarren, M. and Alger, B. E. (1985) Use-dependent depression of IPSPs in rat hippocampal pyramidal cells *in vitro*. *J. Neurophysiol.*, **53**, 557–71.
135. Concas, A., Salis, M., Serra, M. *et al.* (1983) Ethyl-beta-carboline-3-carboxylate decreases (3)H GABA binding in membrane preparations of rat cerebral cortex. *Eur. J. Pharmacol.*, **89**, 179–81.
136. Little, H. J., Nutt, D. J. and Taylor, S. C. (1984) Acute and chronic effects of the benzodiazepine receptor ligand FG 7142: proconvulsant properties and kindling. *Br. J. Pharmacol.*, **83**, 951–8.
137. Sloviter, R. S. (1983) 'Epileptic' brain damages in rats induced by sustained electrical stimulation of the perforant path. I. Acute electrophysiological and light microscopic studies. *Brain Res. Bull.*, **10**, 675–97.
138. Tuff, L. P., Racine, R. J. and Mishra, R. K. (1983) The effects of kindling on GABA-mediated inhibition in the dentate gyrus of the rat. II. Receptor binding. *Brain Res.*, **277**, 91–8.
139. Niznik, H. B., Kish, S. H. and Burnham, W. M. (1983) Decreased benzodiazepine receptor binding in amygdala-kindled rat brains. *Life Sci.*, **33**, 425–30.
140. Babb, T. L., Brown, W. J., Pretorius, J. and Kupfer, W. (1984) Recovery of GABA recurrent inhibition in dentate gyrus after entorhinal kindling in rats. *Soc. Neurosci. Abstr.*, **10**, 345.
141. Kamphuis, W., Wadman, W. J., Buijs, R. M. and Lopes da Silva, F. H. (1985) Loss of gamma-amino butyric acid (GABA) – immunoreactivity in a kindling induced focus of epileptic activity. *Neurosci. Letters*, **Suppl. 22**, S383.
142. Wadman, W. J. and Lopes da Silva, F. H. (1985) Gradual changes in Schaffer-collateral evoked potentials during kindling in the hippocampus in the rat. *Electroenceph. Clin. Neurophysiol.*, **61**, S155.
143. Leibowitz, N. R., Pedley, T. A. and Cutler, R. W. P. (1978) Release of γ-aminobutyric acid from hippocampal slices of the rat following generalized seizures induced by daily electrical stimulation of the entorhinal cortex. *Brain Res.*, **138**, 369–73.
144. Tuff, L. P., Racine, R. J. and Adamec, R. (1983) The effects of kindling on GABA-mediated inhibition in the dentate gyrus of the rat. I. Paired pulse depression. *Brain Res.*, **277**, 79–90.
145. Bakay, R. A. E. and Harris, A. B. (1981) Neurotransmitter, receptor and

biochemical changes in monkey cortical epileptic foci. *Brain Res.*, **206**, 387–404.

146. Ribak, C. E., Harris, A. B., Vaughn, J. E. and Roberts, E. (1979) Inhibitory GABAergic nerve terminals decrease at sites of focal epilepsy. *Science*, **205**, 211–14.

147. Ribak, C. E. (1985) Axon terminals of GABAergic chandelier cells are lost at epileptic foci. *Brain Res.*, **326**, 251–60.

148. Ribak, C. E., Bradburne, R. M. and Harris, A. B. (1982) A preferential loss of GABAergic inhibitory synapses in epileptic foci: A quantitative ultrastructural analysis of monkey neocortex. *J. Neurosci.*, **2**, 1725–35.

149. Ross, S. M. and Craig, C. R. (1981) γ-Aminobutyric acid concentration, L-glutamate-1-decarboxylase activity, and properties of the γ-aminobutyric acid postsynaptic receptor in cobalt epilepsy in the rat. *J. Neurosci.*, **1**, 1388–96.

150. Sloper, J. J., Johnson, P. and Powell, T. P. S. (1980) Selective degeneration of interneurons in the motor cortex of infant monkeys following controlled hypoxia: a possible cause of epilepsy. *Brain Res.*, **198**, 204–9.

151. Lloyd, K. G., Munari, C., Worms, P. *et al.* (1981) The role of GABA mediated neurotransmission in convulsive states, in *GABA and Benzodiazepine Receptors* (eds E. Costa, G. Di Chiara and G. L. Gessa), Raven Press, New York, pp. 199–206.

152. Lloyd, K. G., Bossi, L., Morselli, P. L., Munari, C., Rongier, M. and Loiseau, H. (1986) Alterations in GABA–mediated synaptic transmission in human epilepsy, in *Basic Mechanisms of the Epilepsies* ([3]) pp. 1033–44.

153. Schmidt, D., Cornaggia, C. and Loscher, W. (1984) Comparative studies of the GABA system in neurosurgical brain specimens of epileptic and non-epileptic patients, in *Neurotransmitters, Seizures and Epilepsy II* (eds R. G. Fariello *et al.*), Raven Press, New York, pp. 275–84.

154. Prince, D. A. and Wong, R. K. S. (1981) Human epileptic neurons studied *in vitro*. *Brain Res.*, 210, 323–33.

155. Scheibel, A. B., Paul, L. and Fried, I. (1983) Some structural substrates of the epileptic state, in *Basic Mechanisms of Neuronal Hyperexcitability* (eds H. H. Jasper and N. M. van Gelder), Alan R. Liss, New York, pp. 109–30.

156. Westrum, L. E., White, L. E. and Ward, A. A. (1964) Morphology of the experimental epileptic focus. *J. Neurosurg.*, **21**, 1033–46.

157. Goddard, G. V., McIntyre, D. C. and Leech, C. K. (1969) A permanent change in brain function from daily electrical stimulation. *Expl Neurol.*, **25**, 295–330.

158. Goddard, G. V. (1983) The kindling model of epilepsy. *Trends Neurosci.*, **6**, 275–9.

159. Kalichman, M. W. (1982) Neurochemical correlates of the kindling model of epilepsy. *Neurosci. Biobehav. Rev.*, **6**, 165–81.

160. McNamara, J. O. (1986) Kindling model of epilepsy, in *Basic Mechanisms of the Epilepsies* ([3]) pp. 303–18.

161. Wada, J. A. (ed) (1986) *Kindling 3*, Raven Press, New York.

162. Bliss, T. V. P. (1979) Synaptic plasticity in the hippocampus. *Trends Neurosci.*, **2**, 42–5.

163. Maru, E., Tatsuno, J., Okamoto, J. and Ashida, H. (1982) Development and reduction of synaptic potentiation induced by perforant path kindling. *Expl Neurol.*, **78**, 409–24.

164. McIntyre, D. C. and Roberts, D. C. S. (1983) Long-term reduction in beta-adrenergic receptor binding after amygdala kindling. *Expl Neurol.*, **82**, 17–24.

165. Stanford, S. C. and Jefferys, J. G. R. (1985) Down-regulation of α- and β-

adrenoceptor binding sites in rat cortex caused by amygdalar kindling. *Expl Neurol.*, **90**, 108–17.

166. Lewis, D. V., Matsuga, N., Schuette, W. H. and Van Buren, J. (1977) Potassium clearance and reactive gliosis in the alumina gel lesion. *Epilepsia*, **18**, 499–506.

167. Pedley, T. A., Fisher, R. S., Futamachi, K. J. and Prince, D. A. (1976) Regulation of extracellular potassium concentration in epileptogenesis. *Fed. Proc.*, **35**, 1254–9.

168. Pollen, D. A. and Trachtenberg, M. C. (1970) Neuroglia: gliosis and focal epilepsy. *Science*, **167**, 1252–3.

169. Dietzel, I., Heinemann, U., Hofmeier, G. and Lux, H. D. (1980) Transient changes in the size of the extracellular space in the sensorimotor cortex of cats in relation to stimulus induced changes in potassium concentration. *Expl. Brain Res.*, **40**, 432–9.

170. Gardner-Medwin, A. R. (1983) A study of the mechanism by which potassium moves through brain tissue in the rat. *J. Physiol.*, **335**, 353–74.

171. Heinemann, U. and Dietzel, I. (1984) Extracellular potassium concentration in chronic alumina cream foci of cats. *J. Neurophysiol.*, **52**, 421–34.

172. Duchesne, P. Y., Gheuens, J., Brotchi, J. and Gerebtzoff, M. A. (1979) Normal and reactive astrocytes: a comparative study by immunohistochemistry and by a classical histological technique. *Cell. Mol. Biol.*, **24**, 237–9.

173. Falconer, M. A., Serafetinides, E. A. and Corsellis, J. A. N. (1964) Etiology and pathogenesis of temporal lobe epilepsy. *Arch. Neurol.*, **10**, 233–48.

174. Openchowski, P. (1883) Sur l'action localisée du froid, appliqué à la surface de la région corticale du cerveau. *C. R. Soc. Biol. (Paris)*, **35**, 38–43.

175. Harris, A. B. (1975) Cortical neuroglia in experimental epilepsy. *Expl Neurol.*, **49**, 691–715.

177. Willmore, L. J., Sypert, G. W. and Munson, J. B. (1978) Recurrent seizures induced by cortical iron injection: a model of posttraumatic epilepsy. *Ann. Neurol.*, **4**, 329–36.

178. Fischer, J., Holubar, J. and Malik, V. (1968) Neurohistological study of the development of the cobalt-gelatine foci in rats and its correlation with the onset of epileptic electrical activity. *Acta Neuropath.*, **11**, 45–54.

179. Engel, J. (1983) Epileptic brain damage: how much excitement can a limbic neuron take? *Trends Neurosci.*, **6**, 356–7.

180. Dam, A. M. (1980) Epilepsy and neuron loss in the hippocampus. *Epilepsia*, **21**, 617–29.

181. Olney, J. W. (1978) Neurotoxicity of excitatory amino acids, in *Kainic acid as a Tool in Neurobiology* (eds E. G. McGeer, J. W. Olney and P. L. McGeer), Raven Press, New York, pp. 95–121.

181a. Olney, J. W. (1985) Excitatory transmitters and epilepsy-related brain damage. *Int. Rev. Neurobiol.*, **27**, 337–62.

182. Schwob, J. E., Fuller, T., Price, J. L. and Olney, J. W. (1980) Widespread patterns of neuronal damage following systemic or intracerebral injections of kainic acid: a histological study. *Neuroscience*, **5**, 991–1014.

183. Ben-Ari, Y., Tremblay, E., Ottersen, O. P. and Meldrum, B. S. (1980) The role of epileptic activity in hippocampal and 'remote' cerebral lesions induced by kainic acid. *Brain Res.*, **191**, 79–97.

184. Ben-Ari, Y., Tremblay, E., Ottersen, O. P. and Naquet, R. (1979) Evidence

suggesting secondary epileotogenic lesions after kainic acid: pretreatment with diazepam reduces distant but not local brain damage. *Brain Res.*, **165**, 362–5.

185. Nadler, J. V. and Cuthbertson, G. J. (1980) Kainic acid neurotoxicity towards hippocampus: dependence on specific excitatory pathways. *Brain Res.*, **195**, 47–56.

186. Griffiths, T., Evans, M. C. and Meldrum, B. S. (1982) Intracellular sites of early calcium accumulation in the rat hippocampus during status epilepticus. *Neurosci. Letters*, **30**, 329–34.

187. Rothman, S.-M. (1985) The neurotoxicity of excitatory amino acids is produced by passive chloride influx. *J. Neurosci.*, **5**, 1483–9.

188. Halliwell, B. and Gutteridge, J. M. C. (1985) Oxygen radicals and the nervous system. *Trends Neurosci.*, **8**, 22–6.

189. Willmore, L. J. and Rubin, J. J. (1981) Antiperoxidant pretreatment and iron-induced epileptiform discharges in the rat: EEG and histopathologic studies. *Neurology*, **31**, 63–9.

190. Ehlers, C. L., Koob, G. F. and Bloom, F. E. (1982) Post-ictal locomotor activity in three different rat models of epilepsy. *Brain Res.*, **250**, 178–82.

191. Mellanby, J., Strawbridge, P., Collingridge, G. I. *et al.* (1981) Behavioural correlates of an experimental hippocampal epileptiform syndrome in rats. *J. Neurol. Neurosurg. Psychiat.*, **44**, 1084–93.

192. Jefferys, J. G. R. and Williams, S. F. (1987) Physiological and behavioural consequences of seizures induced in rat by intrahippocampal tetanus toxin. *Brain*, **110**, (in press).

192a. George, G. and Mellanby, J. (1982) Memory deficits in an experimental hippocampal epileptiform syndrome in rats. *Expl Neurol.*, **75**, 678–89.

193. Mellanby, J., Renshaw, M., Cracknell, H. *et al.* (1982) Long-term impairment of learning ability in rats after an experimental hippocampal epileptiform syndrome. *Expl Neurol.*, **75**, 690–9.

194. Boast, C A. and McIntyre, D. C. (1977) Bilateral kindled amygdala foci and inhibitory avoidance behavior in rats: a functional lesion effect. *Physiol. Behav.*, **18**, 25–8.

195. Jefferys, J. G. R. and Williams, S. F. (1985) Long-term depression of CA3 hippocampal pyramidal neurones following intrahippocampal injection of tetanus toxin in rats. *J. Physiol.*, **360**, 33P.

196. Williams, S. F. and Jefferys, J. G. R. (1985) Inhibition and long-term neuronal depression after intra-hippocampal tetanus toxin. *Neurosci. Letters*, **Suppl. 22**, S510.

197. Bernardi, S., Trimble, M. R., Frackowiak, R. S. J. *et al.* (1983) An interictal study of partial epilepsy using positron emission tomography and the oxygen-15 inhalation technique. *J. Neurol. Neurosurg. Psychiatr.*, **46**, 473–7.

198. Engel, J., Brown, W. J., Kuhl, D. E. *et al.* (1982) Pathological findings underlying focal temporal lobe hypometabolism in partial epilepsy. *Ann. Neurol.*, **12**, 518–28.

199. Morell, F. (1960) Secondary epileptogenic lesions. *Epilepsia*, **1**, 538–60.

200. Wilder, B. J., King, R. L. and Schmidt, R. P. (1968) Comparative study of secondary epileptogenesis. *Epilepsia*, **9**, 275–89.

201. Harris, A. B. and Lockard, J. S. (1981) Absence of seizures or minor foci in experimental epilepsy after excision of alumina and astrogliotic scar. *Epilepsia*, **22**, 107–22.

202. Lowrie, M. B. and Ettlinger, G. (1980) The development of independent secondary ('mirror') discharge in the monkey: failure to replicate earlier findings. *Epilepsia*, **21**, 25–30.

203. Goldensohn, E. S. (1984) The relevance of secondary epileptogenesis to the treatment of epilepsy: kindling and the mirror focus. *Epilepsia*, **25** (Suppl. 2), S156–68.

203a. Falconer, M. A. and Kennedy, W. A. (1961) Epilepsy due to small focal temporal lesions with bilateral independent spike-discharging foci. *J. Neurol. Neurosurg. Psychiatry.*, **24**, 205–12.

204. Morrell, F. (1985) Secondary epileptogenesis in man. *Arch. Neurol.*, **42**, 318–35.

205. Gotman, J. and Marciani, M. G. (1985) Electroencephalographic spiking activity, drug levels, and seizure occurrence in epileptic patients. *Ann. Neurol.*, **17**, 597–603.

206. Hayashi, T. (1953) A physiological study of epileptic seizures following cortical stimulation in animals and its application to human clinics. *Jap. J. Physiol.*, **3**, 46–64.

207. Hayashi, T. (1953) The efferent pathway of epileptic seizures for the face following cortical stimulation differs from that for the limbs. *Jap. J. Physiol.*, **3**, 306–20.

208. Faeth, W. H., Walker, A. E. and Andy, O. J. (1956) The propagation of cortical and subcortical epileptic discharge. *Epilepsia*, **3**, 37–48.

209. Wilder, B. J. and Schmidt, R. P. (1965) Propagation of epileptic discharge from chronic neocortical foci in monkey. *Epilepsia*, **6**, 297–309.

210. Walker, A. E. and Udvarhelyi, G. B. (1965) The generalization of a seizure. *J. Nerv. Ment. Dis.*, **140**, 252–71.

211. Wada, J. A. and Sato, M. (1974) Generalized convulsive seizures induced by daily electrical stimulation of the amygdala in cats: Correlative electrographic and behavioural features. *Neurology (Minneap.)*, **24**, 565–74.

212. Gotman, J. (1983) Measurement of small time differences between EEG channels: method and application to epileptic seizure propagation. *Electroenceph. Clin. Neurophysiol.*, **56**, 501–14.

213. Collins, R. C., Kennedy, C., Sokoloff, L. and Plum, F. (1976) Metabolic anatomy of focal motor seizures. *Arch. Neurol.*, **33**, 536–42.

214. Engel, J., Wolfson, L. and Brown, L. (1978) Anatomical correlates of electrical and behavioural events related to amygdaloid kindling. *Ann. Neurol.*, **3**, 538–44.

215. Garant, D. S. and Gale, K. (1983) Lesions of substantia nigra protect against experimentally induced seizures. *Brain Res.*, **273**, 156–61.

216. Iadorola, M. J. and Gale, K. (1982) Substantia nigra: site of anticonvulsant activity mediated by gamma-aminobutyric acid. *Science*, **218**, 1237–40.

217. Browning, R. A., Simonton, R. L. and Turner, F. J. (1981) Antagonism of experimentally induced tonic seizures following a lesion in the midbrain tegmentum. *Epilepsia*, **22**, 595–601.

218. McNamara, J. O., Rigsbee, L. C. and Galloway, M. T. (1983) Evidence that substantia nigra is crucial to the neural network of kindled seizures. *Eur. J. Pharmacol.*, **86**, 485–6.

219. McCaughran, J. A., Corcoran, M. E. and Wada, J. A. (1978) Role of the forebrain commissures in amygdaloid kindling in rats. *Epilepsia*, **19**, 19–33.

220. Pollen, D. A. (1964) Intracellular studies of cortical neurones during thalamic induced wave and spike. *Electroenceph. Clin. Neurophysiol.*, **17**, 398–404.

221. Golden, G. T. and Fariello, R. G. (1984) Epileptogenic action of some direct GABA agonists: Effects of manipulation of the GABA and glutamate systems, in *Neurotransmitters, Seizures and Epilepsy II* (eds R. G. Fariello *et al.*), Raven Press, New York.

222. Penfield, W. and Jasper, H. (1954) *Epilepsy and Functional Anatomy of the Human Brain.* Little, Brown and Co., Boston.

223. Jasper, H. and Drooglever-Fortuyn, J. (1947) Experimental studies on the functional anatomy of petit mal. *Res. Publ. Assoc. Nerv. Ment. Dis.*, **26**, 272–98.

224. Guerrero-Figueroa, R., Barros, A., de Balbian Verster, F. and Heath, R. G. (1963) Experimental 'petit mal' in kittens. *Arch. Neurol.*, **9**, 297–306.

225. Tukel, K. and Jasper, H. (1952) The electroencephalogram in parasagittal lesions. *Electroenceph. Clin. Neurophysiol.*, **4**, 481–94.

226. Marcus, E. M. and Watson, C. W. (1968) Symmetrical epileptogenic foci in monkey cerebral cortex. *Arch. Neurol. (Chic.)*, **19**, 99–116.

227. Mutani, R., Bergamini, L., Fariello, R. and Quattrocole, G. (1973) Bilateral synchrony of epileptic discharge associated with chronic assymmetrical cortical foci. *Electroenceph. Clin. Neurophysiol.*, **34**, 53–9.

228. Prince, D. A. and Farrell, D. (1969) 'Centrencephalic' spike and wave discharges following parenteral penicillin injection in the cat. *Neurology (Minneap.)*, **19**, 309–10.

229. Fisher, R. S. and Prince, D. A. (1977) Spike-wave rhythms in cat cortex induced by parenteral penicillin. II. Cellular features. *Electroenceph. Clin. Neurophysiol.*, **42**, 625–39.

230. Van Gelder, N. M., Siatitsas, I., Menini, C. and Gloor, P. (1983) Feline generalized penicillin epilepsy: changes of glutamic acid and taurine parallel the progressive increase in excitability of the cortex. *Epilepsia*, **24**, 200–13.

231. Noebels, J. L. (1984) Single gene control of excitability in central neurones, in *Electrophysiology of Epilepsy* (eds P. A. Schwartzkroin and H. Wheal), Academic Press, London, pp. 201–18.

232. Seyfried, T. N. and Glaser, G. H. (1985) A review of mouse mutants as genetic models of epilepsy. *Epilepsia*, **26**, 143–50.

233. Gotman, J. (1981) Interhemispheric relations during bilateral spike-and-wave activity. *Epilepsia*, **22**, 453–66.

234. Van Gelder, N. M., Janjua, N. A., Metrakos, K. *et al.* (1980) Plasma amino acids in 3/sec spike-wave epilepsy. *Neurochem. Res.*, **5**, 659–71.

235. Kreindler, A., Zuckermann, E., Steriade, M. and Chimian, D. (1958) Electro-clinical features of the convulsive fit induced experimentally through stimulation of the brainstem. *J. Neurophysiol.*, **21**, 430–6.

236. Cesa-Bianchi, M. G., Mancia, M. and Mutani, R. (1967) Experimental epilepsy induced by cobalt powder in lower brainstem and thalamic structures. *Electro-enceph. Clin. Neurophysiol.*, **22**, 525–36.

237. Naquet, R. and Meldrum, B. S. (1972) Photogenic seizures in baboon, in *Experimental Models of Epilepsy* (eds D. P. Purpura *et al.*), Raven Press, New York, pp. 373–406.

238. Menini, Ch., Silva-Comte, C., Stutzmann, J. M. and Dimov, S. (1981) Cortical unit activity during intermittent photic stimulation in *Papio papio*. Relationship

with paroxysmal fronto-rolandic activity. *Electroenceph. Clin. Neurophysiol.*, **52**, 42–9.

239. Silva-Comte, C., Velluti, J. and Menini, Ch. (1982) Characteristics and origin of frontal paroxysmal responses induced by light stimulation in the *Papio papio* under allylglycine. *Electroenceph. Clin. Neurophysiol.*, **53**, 479–90.

240. Meldrum, B. S. and Wilkins, A. J. (1984) Photosensitive epilepsy in man and the baboon: Integration of pharmacological and psychophysical evidence, in *Electrophysiology of Epilepsy* (eds P. A. Schwartzkroin and H. Wheal), Academic Press, London, pp. 51–77.

241. Seyfried, T. N. and Glaser, G. H. (1981) Genetic linkage between the Ah locus and a major gene that inhibits susceptibility to audiogenic seizures in mice. *Genetics*, **99**, 117–26.

242. Palayoor, S. T. and Seyfried, T. N. (1984) Genetic association between calcium adenosine triphosphatase activity and audiogenic seizures in mice. *J. Neurochem.*, **42**, 1771–4.

243. Loskota, W. J., Lomax, P. and Rich, S. T. (1974) The gerbil as a model for the study of the epilepsies. *Epilepsia*, **15**, 109–19.

244. Olsen, R. W., Wamsley, J. K., Lee, R. and Lomax, P. (1984) Alterations in the benzodiazepine/GABA receptor-chloride ion channel complex in the seizure-sensitive Mongolian gerbil, in *Neurotransmitters, Seizures and Epilepsy II* (eds R. G. Fariello *et al.*), Raven Press, New York, pp. 210–13.

245. Shouse, M. N. and Ryan, W. (1984) Thalamic kindling: Electrical stimulation of the lateral geniculate nucleus produces photosensitive grand mal seizures. *Expl Neurol.*, **86**, 18–32.

246. Rodin, E., Onuma, T., Wasson, J. *et al.* (1971) Neurophysiological mechanisms involved in grand mal seizures induced by metrazol and megimide. *Electroenceph. Clin. Neurophysiol.*, **30**, 62–72.

247. Rodin, E., Kitano, H., Wasson, S. and Rodin, M. (1975) The convulsant effects of bicuculline compared with metrazol. *Electroenceph. Clin. Neurophysiol.*, **38**, 106.

247a. Mirski, M. A. and Ferrendelli, J. A. (1984) Interruption of the mamillo-thalamic tract prevents seizures in guinea-pigs. *Science*, **226**, 72–4.

248. Hallett, M., Chadwick, D., Adams, J. and Marsden, C. D. (1977) Reticular reflex myoclonus: a physiological type of human post hypoxic myoclonus. *J. Neurol. Neurosurg. Psychiat.*, **40**, 253–64.

249. Hallett, M., Chadwick, D. and Marsden, C. D. (1979) Cortical reflex myoclonus. *Neurology (Minneap.)*, **29**, 1107–25.

250. Wilkins, D. E., Hallett, M. and Erba, G. (1985) Primary generalized epileptic myoclonus: a frequent manifestation of minipolymyoclonus of central origin. *J. Neurol. Neurosurg. Psychiatr.*, **48**, 506–16.

251. Egli, M., Mothersill, I., O'Kane, M. and O'Kane, F. (1985) The axial spasm – The predominant type of drop seizure in patients with secondary generalized epilepsy. *Epilepsia*, **26**, 401–15.

252. Panter, S. S., Sadrzadeh, S. M. H., Hallaway, P. E. *et al.* (1985) Hypohaptoglobinemia associated with familial epilepsy. *J. Expl Med.*, **161**, 748–54.

253. Goodman, H. O. and Connolly, B. M. (1982) Taurine transport alleles: dissecting a polygenic complex, in *Genetic Basis of the Epilepsies* (eds V. E. Anderson *et al.*), Raven Press, New York, pp. 171–80.

254. Meencke, H. J. (1985) Neuron density in the molecular layer of the frontal cortex in primary generalized epilepsy. *Epilepsia*, **26**, 450–4.

255. Quesney, L. F. (1981) Dopamine and generalized photosensitive epilepsy, in *Neurotransmitters, Seizures and Epilepsy* (eds P. L. Morselli *et al.*), Raven Press, New York, pp. 263–74.

256. Quesney, L. F. and Reader, T. A. (1984) Role of cortical catecholamine depletion in the genesis of epileptic photosensitivity (eds R. G. Fariello *et al.*), Raven Press, New York, pp. 11–21.

257. Reader, T. A., de Champlain, J. and Jasper, H. (1976). Catecholamines released from cerebral cortex in the cat; decrease during sensory stimulation. *Brain Res.*, **111**, 95–108.

258. Newmark, M. E. and Penry, J. K. (1980) *Genetics of Epilepsy: A Review*, Raven Press, New York.

259. Krall, R. L., Penry, J. K., White, B. G. *et al.* (1978) Antiepileptic drug development: II. Anticonvulsant drug screening. *Epilepsia*, **19**, 409–28.

260. Loscher, W. and Meldrum, B. S. (1984) Evaluation of anticonvulsant drugs in genetic animal models of epilepsy. *Fed. Proc.*, **43**, 276–82.

CHAPTER THREE

The Different Types of Epileptic Seizures, and the International Classification of Epileptic Seizures and of the Epilepsies

Fritz E. Dreifuss

The brain has a very limited repertoire of response to inimical influences. One of these responses is a breakdown of the normal ionic membrane equilibrium leading to an abnormal discharge of neurones which, if it propagates in such a manner as to mobilize a sufficient number of cells, will lead to the clinical manifestation of a seizure. It is evident that epilepsy is not a disease but a phenotypic expression whose nuances are dictated by the manner of its precipitation, by its route and rapidity of propagation through the nervous system, as well as by the balance between excitatory and inhibitory phenomena. For example, the man who has consumed a litre of whisky every day for 40 years with resultant brain atrophy, the young woman whose cortex harbours a slowly growing tumour, the child who for no apparent reason blinks his eyes, smacks his lips and then resumes normal activity, and the child who falls to the ground, convulses, bites his tongue and becomes incontinent because his body is unable to metabolize certain amino acids, clearly, do not suffer from the same disease. A realization of this and resulting attempts at classification have occupied physicians since the days of Galen. The availability of intensive EEG and video monitoring, the development of newer antiepileptic drugs with great specificity for certain seizure types, and the immediate application of improved diagnostic technology to more specific pharmacological treatment, have all dictated a pragmatic rather than a purely academic approach to the problem of defining epileptic seizures as well as the different syndromes of epilepsy. Neurologists have increasingly realized that the administration of medication represents a compromise between control of seizures and the side-effects of medication. This realization has led to the re-evaluation of those seizures which do not constitute true epilepsy and which require methods for control other than anticonvulsant drugs. There has also been a re-evaluation of those epilepsies which are benign, have a self-limited course, and in which the balance of risks and benefits might tilt towards withholding treatment rather than the willy-nilly administration of medication. Furthermore, there has been a need to define those epilepsies which have a tendency to be progressive and in which early and vigorous treatment might curtail the development of secondary epileptogenesis, including the development of mirror foci and kindling [1, 2] (see also p. 50), with the prospect of seizures intractable to treatment. The recognition of different seizure types and classification, then, has pragmatic goals, namely the most appropriate utilization of treatment, the judicious withholding of treatment and the assessment of prognosis, on which may be based the decision as to whether and when to begin the withdrawal of medication.

3.1   HISTORICAL REVIEW

By 175 AD Galen had recognized the difference between seizures originating in the brain (idiopathic), seizures originating 'in the cardia' and seizures the origin of which were in diseases elsewhere in the body (sympathetic) [3]. He also coined the term aura, referring to a sensation like a 'rising breeze'. The distinction between 'grand accès' and 'petit accès' dates from Tissot in 1770 [4]. This author also recognized that seizures were triggered by precipitating factors (causes procatartiques) supervening upon predisposing factors (causes proégumènes). Calmeil in his well known thesis of 1824 [5] divided epilepsies into grand mal, a petit mal syndrome known as 'des vertiges' and absences (which we now call petit mal). The word absence was coined to describe the peculiar blank stare which gives the expression a sense of 'absence d'esprit'. Esquirol in 1838 recognized that seizures might be 'essential' or 'idiopathic', 'sympathetic' or 'symptomatic' thus reiterating what Galen had suggested 1500 years earlier. The first distinction between generalized seizures and partial seizures was made by Delasiauve [6] who in 1854 wrote about 'accès intermediaires' referring to partial seizures and 'accès completes' referring to generalized seizures. Hughlings Jackson [7] in 1863 coined the words 'epileptiform' or 'epileptoid' for the former and 'epilepsy proper' for the latter. It was also Hughlings Jackson who realized that there might have to be, for a time, two classifications – one based on anatomy and pathology, which he referred to as akin to a botanist's classification of plants, and one based pragmatically on phenomenological observation, which he likened to a gardener's classification. With the introduction of anatomical concepts into the analysis of partial and generalized seizures, for which the Montreal School was largely responsible, an approximation of these two types of classification has now become possible.

This chapter will describe seizures and epilepsies according to the International classification of Epileptic Seizures of 1981 [8] and the Proposed Classification of Epileptic Syndromes, 1985 [9].

3.2   DIFFERENTIAL DIAGNOSIS OF EPILEPSY

Episodes of loss of consciousness may occur for reasons other than epilepsy. Syncope, whether cardiac, vasovagal or reflex, may present with loss of consciousness, and such episodes, attended with pallor, with sensations of fainting or with evidence of severe increase in vagal tone (pallor, sweating, bradycardia) should be fully evaluated (pp. 157–61). Any event in which cerebral vascular perfusion is impaired may be associated with convulsive seizures. Some of these episodes, particularly if based on ventricular tachy-arrhythmias, may have a fatal outcome, as, for example, the syndrome associated with prolonged Q-T interval [10].

Severe vertigo needs to be distinguished from epilepsy [11] as do the various periodic syndromes of childhood, including recurrent abdominal pain with or without headaches, more often due to childhood migraine than epilepsy [12, 13]. Hyperventilation is commonly seen in adolescent girls (p. 161), and breathholding in infants (p. 163 and [14]). Various episodic attacks occurring during sleep include night terrors, somnambulism and other parasomnic experiences, and these should be carefully evaluated in the differential diagnostic consideration of epilepsy (p. 163).

Simulated or pseudoseizures are relatively common, especially among those who have true epilepsy (p. 537–40). Their 'seizures' may become intractable, not because of resistance of the epilepsy to treatment, but because of the superimposition of pseudoseizures [15, 16]. These points suggest the possibility of pseudoseizures: (1) the absence of ictal EEG abnormality; (2) the absence of incontinence with seizures; (3) the absence of a postictal confusional state but rather a state of combativeness; (4) resistance to medication; and (5) exacerbation by stress. A particularly distressing syndrome is the von Munchausen syndrome by proxy [17]. Children are brought for treatment with a convincing history of seizures which in fact they have never had.

Should the clinical history not clearly identify the problem as one of epileptic seizures, then intensive monitoring with video visualization of the episodes may accurately identify the type of episode presented. Closed circuit television with simultaneous EEG (CCTV-EEG) can be easily accomplished at moderate cost with equipment which is increasingly simple to operate; with special-effects generators allowing the video screen to be split, one or two cameras can be focused on the patient including close-up with zoom attachment. The EEG can be a conventional 'hard-wired' record or recorded by FM radio telemetry and displayed electronically through a reformatter. Video monitors can be located at the nurses' station on the ward. Refinements including patient activated signalling equipment to identify the subjectively experienced beginning of seizures can be added. Such monitoring is relatively economical in that it is not particularly labour intensive though the capital outlay for the equipment may involve $10–40 000 depending on the sophistication, the sensitivity of the cameras and the number of telemetry channels. In instances of difficulty in documenting the nature of seizures, which is the case with increasing frequency in specialized diagnostic units, accuracy of diagnosis is so crucial to the early institution of the appropriate treatment plan that the cost effectiveness of such an installation is readily demonstrable.

3.3 THE CLASSIFICATION OF EPILEPTIC SEIZURES

The main feature of the present Classification [8] is a distinction between those seizures that are clinically and electrographically generalized from the beginning, and those that are partial or focal at onset, and which may become generalized secondarily. This distinction, which is frequently difficult to make on clinical grounds alone, can be validated by simultaneous video display of a seizure and the EEG. An important distinction from previous classifications is the separation of partial seizures into simple partial seizures, in which consciousness is retained, and complex partial seizures, in which consciousness is impaired. In simple partial seizures the seizure presumably arises from, and is confined to, neocortical structures. In complex partial seizures the spread of the seizure involves allocortical structures and, traversing the limbic system, achieves bilaterality. Consciousness in this context implies awareness and/or responsiveness of the patient to externally applied stimuli. A responsive person has the ability to carry out simple commands or willed movements. Awareness refers to the person's contact with events during the period in question, and their subsequent recall.

Table 3.1 sets out the classification of seizures and epilepsies according to the International Classification of Epileptic Seizures of 1981 [8].

3.3.1 Simple partial seizures

(a) With motor symptoms
The portion of the body involved will depend on the anatomical site of the focal seizure activity. As shown by Penfield and Jasper [18] in the human brain, the hand and the region of the mouth have the largest cortical representation, which reflects the specialization of hand-related activities and communication by language in man. Hence the majority of localization related seizures (as defined on p. 100) will begin in the face or upper extremity. Such seizures may remain strictly localized or they may spread and even become generalized. Spread to contiguous brain areas will result in a Jacksonian march. Other motor seizures may result in adversion of the head, and there may be associated tonic deviation of the eyes. In seizures arising from the supplementary motor area, the hand may elevate as the head and eyes turn, so that the subject appears to gaze at his elevated hand. In childhood, very localized twitching in face and hand may characterize the so-called Rolandic epilepsy syndrome [19–21] (p. 478). Other childhood discrete motor seizures are seen in children with hemiplegia in the so-called HHE syndrome (hemiplegia and hemiconvulsions) [22]. Focal seizures affecting the dominant hemisphere frequently result in arrest of speech. Following a partial seizure, there may be a transient paralysis of the involved part of the body, lasting for minutes to hours; this is known as a Todd's paralysis. This postictal paralysis may result from neuronal exhaustion, or from an excess of inhibitory activity engendered

Table 3.1 International classification of epileptic seizures of 1981 [8]

---

1. Partial (focal, local) seizures

Partial seizures are those in which, in general, the first clinical electroencephalographic changes indicate initial activation of a system of neurones limited to part of one cerebral hemisphere. A partial seizure is classified primarily on the basis of whether or not consciousness is impaired during the attack. When consciousness is not impaired, the seizure is classified as a simple partial seizure. When consciousness is impaired, the seizure is classified as a complex partial seizure. Impairment of consciousness may be the first clinical sign, or simple partial seizures may evolve into complex partial seizures. In patients with impaired consciousness, aberrations of behaviour (automatisms) may occur. A partial seizure may not terminate, but instead progress to a generalized motor seizure. Impaired consciousness is defined as the inability to respond normally to exogenous stimuli by virtue of altered awareness and/or responsiveness. (*vide infra:* Definition of Terms)

There is considerable evidence that simple partial seizures usually have unilateral hemispheric involvement and only rarely have bilateral hemispheric involvement; complex partial seizures, however, frequently have bilateral hemispheric involvement.

Partial seizures can be classified into one of the following three fundamental groups:
A. Simple partial seizures
B. Complex partial seizures
   1. With impairment of consciousness at onset
   2. Simple partial onset followed by impairment of consciousness
C. Partial seizures evolving to generalized tonic-clonic convulsions (GTC)
   1. Simple evolving to GTC
   2. Complex evolving to GTC (including those with simple partial onset)

Clinical seizure type	EEG seizure type	EEG interictal expression
A. *Simple Partial Seizures* (consciousness not impaired)	local contralateral discharge starting over the corresponding area of cortical representation (not always recorded on the scalp)	local contralateral discharge

   1. With motor signs
      (a) Focal motor without march
      (b) Focal motor with march (Jacksonian)
      (c) Versive
      (d) Postural
      (e) Phonatory (vocalization or arrest of speech)
   2. With somatosensory or special-sensory symptoms (simple hallucinations, e.g., tingling, light flashes, buzzing)
      (a) Somatosensory
      (b) Visual
      (c) Auditory

Table 3.1–cont.

Clinical seizure type	EEG seizure type	EEG interictal expression

   (d) Olfactory
   (e) Gustatory
   (f) Vertiginous
 3. With autonomic symptoms or signs (including epigastric sensation, pallor,
    sweating, flushing, piloerection and pupillary dilatation)
 4. With psychic symptoms (disturbance of higher cerebral function). These
    rarely occur without impairment of consciousness and are much more
    commonly seen as complex partial seizures.
    (a) Dysphasic
    (b) Dysmnesic (e.g. déjà-vu)
    (c) Cognitive (e.g. dreamy states, distortions of time sense)
    (d) Affective (fear, anger, etc.)
    (e) Illusions (e.g. macropsia)
    (f) Structured hallucinations (e.g. music, scenes)

B. *Complex Partial Seizures*
(with impairment of   unilateral or, frequently,   unilateral or bilateral
consciousness; may   bilateral discharge, diffuse   generally asynchronous
sometimes begin with   or focal in temporal or   focus; usually in the
simple symptomatology)   fronto-temporal regions   temporal regions
    1. Simple partial onset followed by impairment of consciousness
          (a) With simple partial features (A1–A4) followed by impaired consciousness
          (b) With automatisms
    2. With impairment of consciousness at onset
          (a) With impairment of consciousness only
          (b) With automatisms

C. *Partial Seizures Evolving to Generalized Tonic-Clonic Seizures (GTC)*
(GTC with partial or   above discharges become
focal onset)   secondarily and rapidly
                               generalized
    1. Simple partial seizures (A) evolving to GTC
    2. Complex partial (B) evolving to GTC
    3. Simple partial seizures evolving to complex partial seizures evolving to GTC

2. Generalized seizures (convulsive or non-convulsive)
Generalized seizures are those in which the first clinical changes indicate initial
involvement of both hemispheres. Consciousness may be impaired and this impairment may be the initial manifestation. Motor manifestations are bilateral. The ictal
electroencephalographic patterns initially are bilateral and presumably reflect
neuronal discharge which is widespread in both hemispheres.
A.1. *Absence Seizures*
                               usually regular and   background activity
                               symmetrical 3 Hz but   usually normal although

Table 3.1–cont.

Clinical seizure type	EEG seizure type	EEG interictal expression
	may be 2–4 Hz spike-and-slow wave complexes and may have multiple spike-and-slow wave complexes. Abnormalities are bilateral.	paroxysmal activity (such as spikes or spike-and-slow wave complexes) may occur. This activity is usually regular and symmetrical.

    (a) impairment of consciousness only
    (b) with automatisms
    (c) with mild clonic components
    (d) with atonic components
    (e) with tonic components
    (f) with autonomic components
    (b through f may be used alone or in combination)
  2. *Atypical Absence*

| | EEG more heterogeneous, may include irregular spike-and-slow wave complexes, fast activity or other paroxysmal activity. Abnormalities are bilateral but often irregular and asymmetrical. | background usually abnormal; paroxysmal activity (such as spikes or spike-and-slow wave complexes) frequently irregular and asymmetrical. |

    May have:
    (a) changes in tone which are more pronounced
    (b) onset and/or cessation which is not abrupt

B. *Myoclonic Seizures*

| Myoclonic jerks (single or multiple) | polyspike and wave, or sometimes spike and wave or sharp and slow waves | same as ictal |

C. *Clonic Seizures*

| | fast activity (10 c/s or more) and slow waves; occasional spike and wave patterns | spike and wave or polyspike and wave discharges |

D. *Tonic Seizures*

| | low voltage fast activity or a fast rhythm 9–10 c/s or more decreasing in frequency and increasing in amplitude | more or less rhythmic discharges of sharp and slow waves, sometimes asymmetrical |

Table 3.1–cont.

Clinical seizure type	EEG seizure type	EEG interictal expression
E. *Tonic-Clonic Seizures*	rhythm at 10 or more c/s decreasing in frequency and increasing in amplitude during tonic phase, interrupted by slow waves during clonic phase	polyspike and waves or spike and wave, or, sometimes, sharp and slow wave discharges
F. *Atonic Seizures*	polyspikes and wave or flattening or low-voltage fast activity	polyspikes and wave

3. Unclassified epileptic seizures

Includes all seizures which cannot be classified because of inadequate or incomplete data and some which defy classification in hitherto described categories. This includes some neonatal seizures, e.g. rhythmic eye movements, chewing and swimming movements.

4. Addendum

(1) Repeated epileptic seizures occur under a variety of circumstances:
  (i) as fortuitous attacks, coming unexpectedly and without any apparent provocation:
  (ii) as cyclic attacks, at more or less regular intervals (e.g. in relation to the menstrual cycle, or the sleep-waking cycle):
  (iii) as attacks provoked by: (a) non-sensory factors (fatigue, alcohol, emotion, etc.), or (b) sensory factors, and sometimes referred to as 'reflex seizures'.
(2) Prolonged or repetitive seizures (status epilepticus). The term 'status epilepticus' is used whenever a seizure persists for a sufficient length of time or is repeated frequently enough that recovery between attacks does not occur. Status epilepticus may be divided into partial (e.g. Jacksonian), or generalized (e.g. absence status or tonic-clonic status). When very localized motor status occurs, it is referred to as epilepsia partialis continua.

by the seizure [23]. A spreading motor seizure can sometimes be inhibited or aborted by forced thinking, or by application of pressure on the involved limb. The nature of this inhibitory activity is not understood.

(b) With sensory or somatosensory phenomena

Somatosensory symptoms arise from seizures affecting the postcentral cortex.

Seizures usually consist of paresthetic or pins-and-needles sensations in the affected part, or a sense of distortion, such as metamorphopsia, foreshortenings and elongations. These are more frequently seen in non-dominant hemisphere discharges. Negative phenomena include a feeling as if the body part were absent. Somatosensory seizures may march in the manner described for motor seizures, and they also may become generalized. Sensory seizures may also be followed by a Todd's paralysis. Seizures arising from the suprasylvian parietal region may be associated with severe focal pain [24]. Visual seizures vary in their elaboration depending on the area involved; in parieto-occipital seizures, there are relatively crude perceptions of flashing, whereas if a seizure begins in the temporoparietal association cortex, elaborate visual hallucinatory phenomena, including shapes, scenes or remembered faces may be perceived. Auditory seizures, again, may range from experiences of crude rushing sound to formed musical or prosodic sounds.

(c) Autonomic seizures
These usually arise from the temporal regions or insula, and may accompany other seizure types. Nausea, pallor, flushing, borborygmi, vomiting, dilatation of the pupils and changes in heart rate may occur. Goose-flesh is prominent in the so-called pilomotor seizures [25].

3.3.2 Complex partial seizures

(a) Impairment of consciousness only
These may resemble absence seizures, but they are more prolonged, and are often followed by a period of postictal confusion [26]. Intensive monitoring may be necessary for definitive distinction between these seizure types [27].

(b) Visceral manifestations
Olfactory or gustatory hallucinatory experiences may occur in association with a dreamy state which characterizes some forms of complex partial seizures [7]. Patients complain of a vague, unpleasant odour or taste, such as of garlic, burnt rubber or something metallic. Lip smacking may be the consequence of such an experience [28], but may also occur without reported hallucinations. Visceral sensations may occur with or without affective concomitants such as fear or anxiety [29]. These sensations include hollow feelings in the pit of the stomach, sensations of rising and choking. Salivation may accompany such visceral phenomena. So-called cursive seizures, or running fits, may occur without any warning and the patient may find himself far from where he was; this phenomenon may be preceded by a feeling of fear.

(c) With dysmnesic disturbances
Distortions of memory may accompany complex partial seizures. Again, they may be part of a dreamy state of altered consciousness, which is what sets

complex partial seizures apart from similar experiences seen in some simple partial seizures with psychic disturbances. Déjà vu, déjà entendu, jamais vu and depersonalization experiences may occur. Occasionally, a prolonged dreamy state, a flash-back to a long-forgotten scene or tune may characterize the attack which, to an observer, might just consist of lip smacking, fumbling with clothes, humming or aimless walking. Postictal confusion is the rule.

(d)   With affective symptoms

Fear, displeasure, vague pleasurable sensations, depression or anger may characterize such attacks. Unlike psychiatric states, these last for a few minutes and are of sudden onset and paroxysmal occurrence. Of these, fear is the most frequent symptom.

3.3.3   Automatisms

In the *Dictionary of Epilepsy* [30], automatisms are described as 'more or less coordinated adapted (eupractic or dyspractic) involuntary motor activity occurring during the state of clouding of consciousness either in the course of, or after an epileptic seizure, and usually followed by amnesia for the event. The automatism may be simply a continuation of an activity that was going on when the seizure occurred, or, conversely, a new activity developed in association with the ictal impairment of consciousness. Usually, the activity is commonplace in nature, often provoked by the subject's environment, or by his sensations during the seizure; exceptionally, fragmentary, primitive, infantile, or antisocial behaviour is seen. From a symptomatological point of view the following are distinguished: (1) eating automatisms (chewing, swallowing); (2) automatisms of mimicry, expressing the subject's emotional state (usually of fear) during the seizure; (3) gestural automatisms, crude or elaborate, directed towards either the subject or his environment; (4) ambulatory automatisms; (5) verbal automatisms.'

Automatism may be ictal or postictal. Ictal epileptic automatisms usually represent the release of automatic behaviour under the influence of the clouding of consciousness that accompanies a generalized or partial epileptic seizure (confusional automatisms). They may occur in complex partial seizures as well as in absence seizures. Postictal epileptic automatisms may follow any severe epileptic seizure, especially a tonic-clonic one, and are usually associated with confusion [31].

Some workers regard masticatory or oropharyngeal automatisms as arising from the amygdala or insula and opercular regions, but these movements are occasionally seen in the generalized epilepsies, particularly absence seizures, and are not of localizing help. The same is true of mimicry and gestural automatisms. In the latter, fumbling of the clothes, scratching and other complex motor activity may occur both in complex partial and absence seizures. Ictal speech automatisms are occasionally seen. Ambulatory seizures again may occur either as prolonged automatisms of absence, particularly a continuing prolonged absence, or of complex partial seizures. In the latter, a patient may occasionally continue to drive a car, though they may contravene traffic light regulations. Clinical features of automatisms are discussed further on pp. 519–20.

Automatisms are a common feature of different types of epilepsy. While they do not lend themselves to simple anatomic interpretation, they appear to have in common a discharge involving various areas of the limbic system. Both crude and elaborate automatisms do occur in patients with absence as well as complex partial seizures. Of greater significance is a precise descriptive history of the seizures, the age of the patient, the presence or absence of an aura and of postictal behaviour, including the presence or absence of confusion. The EEG is of cardinal importance in localizing the origin of the automatism.

3.3.4 Partial seizures secondarily generalized

These seizures spread from an originally focal origin. Such spread may take different routes dependent on such factors as age, previous seizure occurrence with the development of facilitated (kindled) pathways, the presence and degree of inhibition, the area of brain originating the seizure and the underlying epileptic predisposition. Spread to generalization may be by callosal connections [32] or by involvement of subcortical reticular pathways [33]. Some areas of cortex, particularly parasagittal and orbitofrontal regions, appear to be more liable to foster secondary generalization [34]. Seizures arising there may generalize with such rapidity that clinically they appear to be primarily generalized from the beginning [35] (Fig. 3.1). It is likely that many generalized epilepsies result from a combination of increased cortical irritability and a discharge involving a central pace-setting mechanism, as postulated in the concept of corticoreticular epilepsy [33].

When a localization-related seizure becomes generalized, the portion of the attack for which awareness is retained and for which the patient is not amnesic, is referred to as the aura.

3.3.5 Generalized seizures

Generalized seizures are those in which the first clinical changes indicate initial involvement of both hemispheres. Consciousness may be impaired and this impairment may be the initial manifestation. Motor manifestations are bilateral. The ictal EEG patterns initially are bilateral, and presumably reflect neuronal discharge which is widespread in both hemispheres. Primary generalized seizures frequently have their onset in childhood or adolescence, and there is frequently an element of heritability (p. 142). While most primary generalized epilepsies arise in the absence of focal cerebral disease, secondary generalization from a lesion, particularly if located near midline structures, for

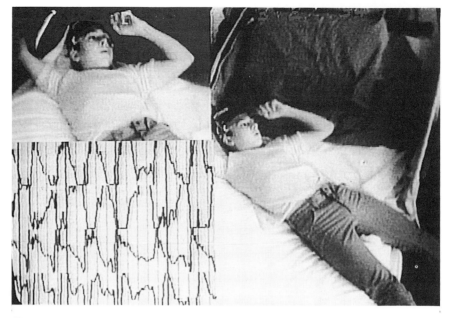

Figure 3.1 Partial seizure (supplementary motor seizure) with rapid secondary generalization.

example in the parasagittal region, may be sufficiently rapid to present clinically and electroencephalographically as a primary generalized seizure.

3.3.6   Absence seizures [36, 37]

The paradigm of generalized seizures is the absence attack [27, 36, 37]. The hallmark of the absence attack is a sudden onset, interruption of ongoing activities, a blank stare, and possibly a brief upward rotation of the eyes. If the patient is speaking, speech is interrupted; if walking, he stands transfixed; if eating, the food will stop on his way to the mouth. Usually the patient will be unresponsive when spoken to. The attack lasts from a few seconds to half a minute and evaporates as rapidly as it commenced [27].

(1) *Absence with impairment of consciousness only.* The above description fits the description of absence simple, in which no other activities take place during the attack.
(2) *Absence with mild clonic components.* Here the onset of the attack is indistinguishable from the above, but clonic movements may occur in the eyelids, at the corner of the mouth or in other muscle groups; these may vary in severity from almost imperceptible movements to generalized myoclonic jerks. Objects held in the hand may be dropped.
(3) *Absence with atonic components.* Here there may be a diminution in tone of

muscles subserving posture as well as in the limbs, leading to drooping of the head, occasionally slumping of the trunk, dropping of the arms and relaxation of the grip. Rarely, tone is so diminished that the patient falls.

(4) *Absence with tonic components.* During such an attack, tonic muscular contraction may occur, affecting extensor muscles or flexor muscles symmetrically or asymmetrically. If the patient is standing, the head may be drawn backwards and the trunk may arch, leading to a backwards fall. The head may be tonically drawn to one or other side.

(5) *Absence with automatisms.* (See also prior discussion on automatisms on pp. 92–93.) Purposeful or quasi-purposeful movements occurring in the absence of awareness during an absence attack are frequent; these may range from licking of the lips, swallowing, to fumbling with the clothes, or aimless walking. If spoken to, the patient may grunt òr turn to the spoken voice, when touched or tickled, may rub that site. Automatisms may be elaborate, and often consist of combinations of such movements, or they may be so simple as to be missed on casual observation.

Mixed forms of absence frequently occur.

The EEG during an absence seizure consists of a 3 Hz spike and wave episode (p. 175, 185) more or less contemporaneous with the clinical attack. However, if carefully tested it can be shown that the response time may lengthen even before the electrographic pattern is noted [38], and responsiveness may be regained while the electrographic attack is still in progress [39].

3.3.7 Myoclonic seizures

Myoclonic jerks (single or multiple) are sudden, brief contractions which may be generalized, or confined to the face, or to one or more extremities, or to individual muscles or groups of muscles. They may occur predominantly around the time of going to sleep or awakening from sleep. Myoclonus is frequently associated with giant evoked potentials in response to a somatosensory stimulus. In association with the cortical giant evoked potentials there is frequently enhancement of the response at the thalamic level. Some types of myoclonus may be produced at the spinal level and then the myoclonus is, of course, not an epileptic phenomenon. In the majority of cases, however, the impulses responsible for myoclonus travel to the cerebral hemispheres and then caudally to the spinal level, with the appropriate latencies. These latencies are characteristic of the modality involved whether this is photic, auditory or somatosensory. Sometimes stimulus-sensitive myoclonus is asymmetrical as is seen in some cases of hemiplegia where the reflex myoclonic jerk occurs in response to tapping the affected limb.

Many instances of myoclonus are not associated with alteration in the conscious state although these may be associated with generalized epileptic discharge. This is particularly the case in so-called myoclonic absence which is a childhood epileptic syndrome with generalized spike-wave discharge and a rather prominent jerking and tonic flexion of the trunk. Preservation of awareness during generalized spike-wave discharge is also frequently seen in older persons with absence but in all these instances there is impaired responsiveness. If the characteristic of consciousness is operationally defined as impairment of awareness and/or responsiveness, then, thus defined, consciousness is impaired though awareness may be relatively preserved.

The ictal EEG shows symmetrical spike and wave or multiple spike and wave episodes in association with the jerks. Myoclonic seizures may occur as part of the syndrome of primary generalized epilepsy as is seen in the myoclonus of infancy, myoclonic absence or juvenile myoclonic epilepsy (as described under epileptic syndromes, p. 101). On the other hand, myoclonus may be part of a more widespread encephalopathy as occurs in lipid storage diseases, in subacute sclerosing panencephalitis, Creutzfeldt-Jakob disease or progressive poliodystrophy. The syndrome may be part of a metabolic encephalopathy, a postanoxic encephalopathy or part of a progressive myoclonic epilepsy with or without Lafora bodies [39a].

3.3.8   Clonic seizures, tonic seizures and tonic-clonic seizures

Clonic seizures are characterized by the sudden onset of rhythmic clonic movements in which there is very often a tonic extension or flexion component. Consciousness may be preserved. The EEG shows either generalized spike-wave activity or fast activity (10 Hz or more) and slow waves. In tonic seizures, there is usually sudden loss of consciousness and contraction of muscles leading either to slow forward flexion or hyperextension, usually predominantly axial. The EEG shows low voltage fast activity which, during the seizure, decreases in frequency and increases in amplitude (Fig. 3.2).

Tonic-clonic seizures frequently begin with a clonic component followed by a tonic component but may also begin with a tonic component. Loss of consciousness is abrupt, there is a severe tonic extensor spasm which may be associated with a loud cry, the patient is then rigid and opisthotonic, respiration is inhibited and cyanosis may occur. A tonic stage then gives way to clonic convulsive movements which last for a variable period of time. Small gusts of grunting respiration may occur between the convulsive movements, though the patient may remain cyanotic, saliva issuing from the mouth.

If the tongue has been bitten, the saliva may be tinged with blood. At the end of this stage, deep respiration occurs, the muscles relax, though the patient remains unconscious for variable periods; he then awakes feeling stiff and sore all over. Sometimes, the attack is preceded by an aura, usually a vague foreboding or epigastric sensation, occasionally a series of myoclonic jerks, or an exacerbation of absence attacks [40, 41].

Secondary generalized seizures beginning as partial seizures and rapidly projecting to become generalized may be difficult to distinguish from primary

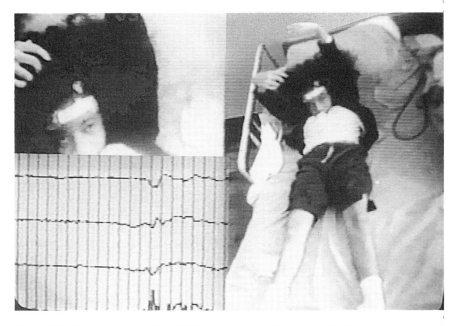

Figure 3.2 Tonic seizure. The EEG is attenuated in amplitude (electrodecremental attack).

generalized tonic-clonic seizures if the aura is short, or if amnesia for the aura takes place as a result of the seizure. In most partial seizures that become secondarily generalized, the aura provides the focal signature, be it motor, somatosensory, autonomic or psychic.

In primary generalized tonic-clonic seizures, the EEG shows rhythms at ten or more cycles per second (Hz) decreasing in frequency and increasing in amplitude during the tonic phase, and interrupted by slow waves during the tonic-clonic phase.

In juvenile myoclonic epilepsy, which is an epileptic syndrome rather than a seizure type, myoclonic seizures and generalized tonic-clonic seizures occur in the same individual. A flurry of myoclonic seizures frequently ushers in a generalized tonic-clonic attack, after which the seizures tend to go into abeyance until the next flurry [40, 42].

Many patients with myoclonic seizures, with tonic-clonic seizures or with juvenile myoclonic epilepsy show photosensitivity (p.129). Photically induced generalized tonic-clonic seizures are particularly commonly seen during adolescence, and are more frequently encountered in females. Flash frequencies which are harmonics of eight most often provoke attacks [43, 44].

Atonic seizures are associated with the sudden onset of diminished muscular tone; this results in the patient dropping objects from the hand and occasionally falling. Consciousness may be lost only briefly. Some patients may be unaware of lost consciousness, but are usually not aware of hitting the ground. The EEG is characterized by polyspike and wave activity or flattening of the EEG with low voltage fast activity.

It is very important in accurately classifying a seizure to recognize those attacks which are superficially indistinguishable but which with intensive monitoring may be identified. This has important implications for the appropriate therapy. The development of more specific anticonvulsant drugs for individual seizure types requires accurate identification. The recognition of the deleterious effects of some anticonvulsant medications has emphasized the importance of their judicious use and most appropriate application. One important example of the need to distinguish seizures which may resemble each other is the differentiation between absence seizures and complex partial seizures with impairment of consciousness only. Similarly, absence seizures with automatisms and complex partial seizures with automatisms may be difficult to distinguish without resorting to intensive video monitoring with simultaneous EEG display. Despite their resemblance the treatment for these two varieties of seizures is so different and the results of giving the wrong treatment so inimical to the patient's welfare that early accurate identification of the seizure type is of critical, and of very much more than academic importance [45, 46].

3.4 CLASSIFICATION OF EPILEPTIC SYNDROMES AND THE EPILEPSIES

A classification of epileptic syndromes so that the terminology can be used daily in communication between colleagues, and as diagnostic entries in hospital records and in clinical trials and other investigations, is a further elaboration. An epileptic syndrome may be defined as a disorder characterized by a cluster of signs and symptoms customarily occurring together [9]. Such signs and symptoms may be clinical – such as the history, seizure type, the modes of seizure recurrence and neurological findings on examination – or they may be those detected by ancillary studies such as electroencephalography, computed tomography or nuclear magnetic resonance imaging. The first major dichotomy used to shape syndromes is the separation of the epilepsies

Table 3.2 International classification of epilepsies and epileptic syndromes [9]

---

1. *Localization-related (focal, local, partial) epilepsies and syndromes*
1.1 Idiopathic (with age-related onset)
At present, two syndromes are established but more may be identified in the future.
– benign childhood epilepsy with centro-temporal spike
– childhood epilepsy with occipital paroxysms

*Table 3.2–*cont.

1.2 Symptomatic
This comprises syndromes of great individual variability which will mainly be based on anatomical localization, clinical features, seizure types and aetiological factors (if known).

2. *Generalized epilepsies and syndromes*
2.1 Idiopathic (with age related onset – listed in order of age)
    – benign neonatal familial convulsions
    – benign neonatal convulsions
    – benign myoclonic epilepsy in infancy
    – childhood absence epilepsy (pyknolepsy)
    – juvenile absence epilepsy
    – juvenile myoclonic epilepsy (impulsive petit mal)
    – epilepsy with grand mal seizures (GTCS) on awakening
    Other generalized idiopathic epilepsies, if they do not belong to one of the above syndromes, can still be classified as generalized idiopathic epilepsies.
2.2 Idiopathic and/or symptomatic (in order of age)
    – West syndrome (infantile spasms, Blitz-Nick-Salaam Krämpfe)
    – Lennox-Gastaut syndrome
    – Epilepsy with myoclonic-astatic seizures
    – Epilepsy with myoclonic absences
2.3 Symptomatic
2.3.1 Non-specific aetiology
    – Early myoclonic encephalopathy
2.3.2 Specific syndromes
    – Epileptic seizures may complicate many disease states
    Under this heading are included those diseases in which seizures are a presenting or predominant feature.

3. *Epilepsies and syndromes undetermined whether focal or generalized*
3.1 With both generalized and focal seizures
    – Neonatal seizures
    – Severe myoclonic epilepsy in infancy
    – Acquired epileptic aphasia (Landau-Kleffner syndrome)
3.2 Without unequivocal generalized or focal features
    All cases with generalized tonic-clonic seizures where clinical and EEG findings do not permit classification as clearly generalized or localization-related such as in many cases of sleep grand mal.

4. *Special syndromes*
4.1 Situation-related seizures (Gelegenhesitsanfälle)
    – Febrile convulsions
    – Seizures related to other identifiable situations such as stress, hormonal, drugs, alcohol, sleep deprivation, etc.
4.2 Isolated apparently unprovoked epileptic events
4.3 Epilepsies characterized by specific modes of seizure precipitation
4.4 Chronic progressive epilepsia partialis continua of childhood

with generalized seizures from those with partial or focal seizures. The second dichotomy is that which separates epilepsies of known aetiology (symptomatic) from those that are idiopathic (or primary). The Proposal for a Classification of Epileptic Syndromes (1985) [9] recognized that the words focal or partial did not adequately describe the potentially localizational element of epileptic seizures. The term 'localization-related' has been proposed, which will be used in this discussion. This Classification also includes a category of special syndromes such as those occurring only in specific situations, those that result from specific triggering devices and those that have peculiar periodicity which determine the nature of the syndrome.

3.4.1 Localization-related epilepsies

This syndromic classification recognizes that localization-related seizures may be *idiopathic or primary* as exemplified in *benign childhood epilepsy with centrotemporal spikes*, or *childhood epilepsy with occipital paroxysms*. *Benign childhood epilepsy with centrotemporal spikes* (p. 478) is a syndrome of brief simple partial hemifacial motor seizures, frequently with associated somatosensory symptoms. The syndrome has a tendency to evolve into generalized tonic-clonic seizures; seizures are often related to sleep. The seizures occur between the ages of 3 and 13, with a tendency to spontaneous resolution by adolescence. There is frequently a genetic predisposition. The EEG has blunt, high voltage centrotemporal spikes, often followed by slow waves, and activated by sleep. *Epilepsy with occipital paroxysms* is a similar childhood syndrome beginning with visual symptoms followed by hemiclonic seizures or automatisms, and is frequently associated with migrainous headaches. The EEG shows paroxysms of high amplitude spikes or sharp waves occurring rhythmically in the occipital and posterior temporal areas.

Most localization-related epilepsies are, however, *symptomatic*. The epileptic lesion can be traced to one part of one cerebral hemisphere. Symptomatic epilepsies are considered to be the consequence of known or suspected disorders of the central nervous system. The individual seizure type will be largely determined by anatomical localization of the seizure discharge and the rapidity and direction of its spread.

3.4.2 Generalized epilepsies

Generalized epilepsies may again be either idiopathic or symptomatic. They are often defined in relation to the person's age.

(a) Generalized idiopathic epilepsies
These include a number of different seizures. *Benign neonatal convulsions* are frequently repeated clonic or apnoeic seizures occurring during the first few days of life. The syndrome may be familial or sporadic [47–49].

Benign myoclonic epilepsy in infancy [50] is characterized by brief bursts of generalized myoclonus occurring during the first or second year of life in otherwise normal children. The EEG shows generalized spike-wave occurring in brief bursts during the early stages of sleep. These seizures carry a good prognosis for control with appropriate medications.

Childhood absence epilepsy or *pyknoleptic petit mal* [36, 37] occurs in children of school age. There is a strong genetic predisposition. There are frequent absence seizures and the EEG reveals bilateral, synchronous, symmetrical spike-wave activity at 3 Hz with a normal interictal background.

The absence seizure types were previously described in detail (p. 94). In the pyknoleptic petit mal syndrome, there appears to be an autosomal dominant type of inheritance with age-related penetrance. Both seizures and EEG trait tend to disappear after adolescence (pp. 138, 142). In this syndrome, neurological development is normal prior to the development of seizures. Other seizure types rarely occur except occasionally generalized tonic-clonic seizures. The child's school performance is normal as is the intellect.

Juvenile myoclonic epilepsy [40, 51] appears around puberty. Seizures are ushered in by bilateral, single or repetitive irregular myoclonic jerks predominantly in the arms, and are interspersed with the development of generalized tonic-clonic seizures. These seizures frequently occur shortly after awakening and are frequently precipitated by sleep deprivation. The interictal and the ictal EEGs have rapid generalized irregular polyspike and wave discharges. There is frequently photosensitivity.

Juvenile myoclonic epilepsy is one of the commonest varieties of primary generalized epilepsy. When an adolescent presents with a generalized tonic-clonic convulsion, inquiry should be made concerning the possibility of antecedent myoclonic jerks which may have preceded the onset of convulsions by as long as several years. Absence attacks may also occur in this syndrome. EEG abnormalities persist well into adult life and withdrawal from medication is frequently followed by recurrence of seizures. This condition shows a strong heritable pattern.

Some patients have *epilepsy with generalized tonic-clonic seizures on awakening*; this is very similar to juvenile myoclonic epilepsy [40, 52, 53].

(b) Generalized, idiopathic and/or symptomatic seizures

West syndrome or infantile spasms (pp. 473–75) consists of the triad of infantile spasms, arrest of psychomotor development and the EEG finding of hypsarrhythmia [54–60]. The spasms may be flexor, extensor or nodding in type; most subjects have mixed types. The age of onset peaks between four and seven months.

In the idiopathic form of West syndrome, neurological development is usually normal prior to the onset of seizures, after which development appears to slow. Indeed, there may be regression of attained capabilities. The spasms usually occur in clusters of perhaps 30 or 40 spasms per cluster. Each spasm

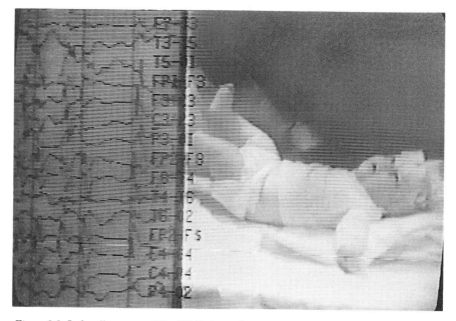

Figure 3.3 Infantile spasm. The EEG shows hypsarrhythmia, decremental activity at onset of seizure followed by a spike-wave complex.

lasts for one or two seconds although in some there may be a more prolonged tonic component. German neurologists have called this syndrome 'Blitz-Nick-Salaam-Krämpfe'. The early sudden flexion is the 'Blitz' and the more prolonged tonic component the 'Salaam' portion of the attack (Fig. 3.3).

In the symptomatic form, neurological development may be abnormal from birth. There is frequently an identified cause such as a metabolic disorder, an intrauterine infection, a severe perinatal anoxic episode or tuberous sclerosis. While either variety may respond favourably to the administration of ACTH, in the symptomatic variety, recurrence of seizures is usual after a course of therapy, intellectual development remains severely impaired, and other seizure syndromes such as the Lennox-Gastaut syndrome may emerge. The prognosis for intellectual development is better in the truly idiopathic form (pp. 344–48).

The Lennox-Gastaut syndrome may also occur in idiopathic or symptomatic forms, with the former again carrying a somewhat better prognosis. This syndrome manifests itself in children between the ages of one and eight years. The common seizure types include tonic, atonic or absence seizures. Other types such as myoclonic, generalized tonic-clonic and partial seizures also occur [61–63]. Status epilepticus in the form of stuporous states with myoclonus, tonic and atonic seizures may occur. The EEG is characterized by an abnormal background, with slow spike-waves of less than 3 Hz occurrence.

The Lennox-Gastaut syndrome is frequently preceded by infantile spasms. Only in its idiopathic form does it fall into the category of the primary epilepsies. It is more commonly the result of a severe progressive encephalopathy, symptomatic of perinatal hypoxia, intracranial haemorrhage, infections or metabolic disorder. Patients with this condition are usually severely mentally retarded as a consequence of the severity of the underlying cause.

Epilepsy with myoclonic/astatic seizures is very similar except that the background rhythms in the EEG are usually normal. The child's development is usually more normal. Myoclonic and astatic seizures are common [64].

Epilepsy with myoclonic absences is characterized by bilateral, rhythmic clonic jerks. These are accompanied by bilateral synchronous symmetrical 3 Hz discharges on the EEG. There is less impairment of consciousness than during typical absence seizures. On the other hand, the prognosis is less favourable for control of seizures and for cognitive development.

(c) Generalized symptomatic epilepsies

Generalized symptomatic epilepsies may also be age related and have considerably graver prognosis than the idiopathic variety.

Early myoclonic encephalopathy is a syndrome with onset before three months of age, usually fragmentary myoclonus, and tonic spasms. The EEG shows suppression burst activity. Psychomotor development is severely delayed. The condition is frequently fatal in the first year of life [65, 66]. Many of these cases arise on the basis of intrauterine infection, neonatal asphyxia or metabolic disorders, including such conditions as non-ketotic hyperglycinaemia [67]. As already mentioned, the West syndrome and the Lennox-Gastaut syndrome are frequently seen in symptomatic forms and here the prognosis is bad as regards intellectual development and the ability to achieve long standing seizure control, even with the early administration of the drugs of choice.

A syndrome superficially clinically and electrographically indistinguishable from pyknoleptic *petit mal* may be seen in symptomatic form. Unlike pyknoleptic petit mal epilepsy, the child's early development may be abnormal, there may be an earlier onset of absence seizures, there may be abnormal neurological findings on examination, and the child's intelligence will be less than in the pyknoleptic form. The EEG may show interictal slow wave abnormalities. The seizures may be admixed with other seizure types such as generalized tonic-clonic seizures or partial seizures.

The principal distinctions between idiopathic and symptomatic epilepsies are that the former commence more often on a background of normal development and are not associated with abnormal neurological signs or abnormal interictal EEG disturbances. Intellect is normal, and there may be a family history of a similar disorder. Spontaneous resolution, good response to treatment and continuing remission on ultimate drug withdrawal are features of the idiopathic group. The converse is true of the symptomatic epilepsies which are less likely to occur on a normal developmental background, and are often associated with abnormal neurological findings and abnormal interictal EEG disturbances; there is frequently a lack of a family history of similar disorder. If untreated, they tend to become intractable. The prognosis for cessation of treatment is poor. There is often impaired development or deterioration of intellect.

The distinction between individual epileptic syndromes is of critical importance. The designation of a syndrome as being symptomatic sets off a train of investigations searching for the underlying process or lesion. The designation carries with it the prognostic significance of the underlying condition. The idiopathic label frequently implies an inherited disorder, a predictable course, a relatively predictable treatment response, and a particular treatment with specific medications usually given for finite periods of time.

3.4.3   Partial or generalized epilepsies

It is not certain whether some specific seizure syndromes are focal or generalized.

Neonatal seizures [68, 69] differ from seizures of older children in that they are more likely to be subtle, with frequently overlooked clinical manifestations (pp. 471–72).

The types of seizures seen in the neonate largely defy classification in the terminology of the Internal Classification of Epileptic Seizures because of the relative lack of recorded clinical material.

In general, neonatal seizures are classified as:

(1) *Subtle seizures*. Here there may be tonic eye deviation sometimes accompanied by rhythmic nystagmoid jerking, fluttering of the lids or repetitive blinking. Sucking, buccolingual movements may occur, usually in a rhythmic manner and more vigorous than spontaneous sucking. Swimming arm movements, or pedalling leg movements may indicate seizures. Apnoea is sometimes a subtle seizure manifestation. EEG changes accompany the above seizures and may be confirmatory of a seizure disorder.

(2) *Tonic seizures*. Here there is tonic extension of the limbs and sometimes opisthotonic posturing. Occasionally, the upper limbs will be flexed. Signs of subtle seizures may accompany the tonic attacks. This symptom is often an indication of intraventricular haemorrhage, and occurs predominantly in premature infants.

(3) *Multifocal clonic jerking*. This type of seizure, most often seen in full-term infants is the most frequent seizure type in the neonate.

(4) *Focal clonic jerking*. This often denotes a localized lesion, but may also occur in metabolic encephalopathies.

(5) *Myoclonic seizures*. These seizures are associated with an EEG showing

burst-suppression. They are indicative of a severe infantile encephalopathy due, for example, to perinatal asphyxia, metabolic disorders such as non-ketotic hyperglycinaemia, or intrauterine infections, for example Cytomegalovirus.

It is undetermined whether *epilepsy with continuous spike waves during slow wave sleep* [70] is of focal or predominantly generalized origin. The characteristic feature is the occupation of stage 3 and 4 sleep by irregular spike and wave epileptic pattern which is seen night after night for months or years. The clinical manifestation is of nocturnal generalized tonic-clonic seizures, and occasionally atypical absence when awake.

Acquired epileptic aphasia (Landau-Kleffner syndrome) is a childhood disorder in which acquired aphasia, multifocal epileptic spikes, and seizures occur with behavioural and psychomotor disturbances. The seizures usually remit spontaneously but the speech disturbance may remain for a long period [71, 72].

3.4.4 Special epileptic syndromes

Special epileptic syndromes include the epilepsies whose occurrence depends upon the presence of certain specific situational factors. This is the case in *febrile seizures* which occur only in the presence of fever. These are age related, almost always characterized by brief and uncomplicated generalized seizures [73–77] (and see Chapter 15). There is a tendency for these to recur. The risk of subsequent epilepsy depends upon the factors reviewed on pp. 350–51 and 458–59, but in the majority this is a relatively benign disorder of early childhood. Other special syndromes include the epilepsies triggered by specific precipitants. These include *photic sensitive epilepsies* where the intensity of the stimulus, the frequency of the stimulus and occasionally the elaboration of the stimulus are characteristic (pp. 129–30) [41, 78, 79]. In the case of epilepsies triggered by auditory stimuli, the nature of the adequate stimulus may include music, the sound of certain voices or certain specific noises such as the ringing of bells [80].

3.5 SPECIFIC DISEASES [82–88]

Other than epileptic syndromes, there are certain diseases in which epilepsy may be a complicating factor and in which seizures are a presenting or predominant feature [39a, 82–88]. Such diseases include certain malformations such as phacomatoses, lissencephaly and Aicardi's syndrome as examples. Some diseases which are based on inborn errors of metabolism may have epilepsy as a predominant feature; these include the amino acidopathies, the lipoidoses, the progressive myoclonic epilepsies [39a] (Lafora disease, non-Lafora progressive myoclonic epilepsy and dyssynergia cerebellaris

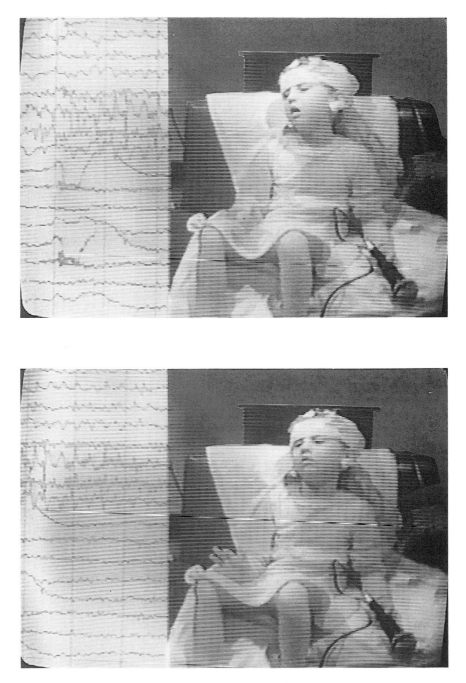

Figure 3.4 Epilepsia partialis continua sequence showing left cerebral EEG spiking, contralateral face and hand clonic movement in (A) and (B).

myoclonica) and the Kojewnikow syndrome of epilepsia partialis continua on the basis of chronic encephalitis. Two types of Kojewnikow syndrome are recognized [88–91]. The first type represents a particular form of rolandic partial epilepsy in both adults and children, and is related to a lesion of the motor cortex. Well localized partial motor seizures occur, and the EEG has normal background activity and focal paroxysmal abnormalities. One type may occur at any age in childhood or adult life and there is no progression. The second type occurs in childhood, and is thought to be on the basis of chronic encephalitis. The onset is between the age of two and ten years, with seizures that are partial motor seizures which tend to progress, leading to a progressive motor deficit and ultimately mental deterioration. The EEG discharges are not usually confined to the rolandic area (Fig. 3.4).

3.5.1 Status epilepticus (see Chapter 14)

Status epilepticus may be defined as a seizure that persists for a sufficient length of time or is repeated frequently enough that recovery between attacks does not occur. It may be divided into two principal seizure types: partial (for example, Jacksonian) or generalized (for example, absence status or tonic-clonic status). A series of attacks in which consciousness is regained between the episodes is called serial seizures. These may evolve into status epilepticus and from the practical point of view they should be treated with the same concern as status epilepticus [92]. One usually regards status as occurring when seizures continue for 30 min [93], though some would call the condition status when two or more seizures occur without the regaining of consciousness.

Status epilepticus may be divided into the following seizure types.

(1) Generalized status epilepticus including:
    (a) convulsive seizures such as tonic-clonic, tonic, clonic and myoclonic;
    (b) nonconvulsive generalized status epilepticus including absence status and so-called spike wave stupor.
(2) Partial status epilepticus:
    (a) simple partial status including somatosensory status epilepticus,
        (i) epilepsia partialis continua,
        (ii) a condition characterized by paroxysmal lateralized epileptic discharges (PLEDS),
        (iii) dysphasic status epilepticus may also occur [94];
    (b) complex partial status epilepticus or 'psychomotor status' is characterized by a nonconvulsive confusional state with automatisms which may be the result of frequently repeated seizures or of continuous complex partial seizure activity.

The cause of status epilepticus has differed in various studies and has depended on the age group under review. In the adult, tumour, trauma, vascular disease and infection are the commonest causes. In children status is frequently seen with chronic static encephalopathy, progressive encephalopathy, the sudden withdrawal of anticonvulsant medication and acute brain injury such as meningitis, encephalitis or dehydration. The majority of lesions to which status epilepticus may be attributed lie in the frontal lobes [95].

3.6 CONCLUSION

In a general neurological practice, complex partial seizures are those most frequently encountered, particularly among adults; in a comprehensive epilepsy programme one is more likely to see the various difficult varieties of generalized seizures both of the primary, or idiopathic, and secondary, or symptomatic variety, including atypical absence, the Lennox-Gastaut syndrome and various combinations of seizures in which pseudoseizures may play a part. In our experience pseudoseizures are seen in approximately 20% of difficult-to-control epilepsies and, as previously mentioned, for the most part complicate true seizure disorders and only relatively rarely exist in isolation.

Accurate diagnosis of seizure type and syndromic classification are essential for the utilization of the most appropriate therapy in the prevention of intractability of epileptic seizures. This is the main thrust of this chapter. One of the principal means of achieving accuracy in diagnosis is visualization of seizures, using closed circuit TV recording of seizures (CCTV) with simultaneous display of the EEG as an essential aid to diagnosis (p. 85). Incorrect identification of seizure types is one of the principal reasons for the development of intractability, leading as it does to inappropriate management for prolonged periods of time. Failure to distinguish epileptic seizures from nonepileptic seizures or pseudoseizures is a common cause for lack of seizure control, and this in turn may lead to inappropriate- or over-medication. Failure to recognize underlying disease processes such as porphyria, hyperglycaemia and other potentially remediable causes may lead to apparent intractability, and failure to recognize precipitating factors may result in difficulty in obtaining seizure control. In difficult circumstances, it is essential that seizures be viewed. This may require CCTV-monitoring for a prolonged period, with attacks precipitated by withdrawal of anticonvulsant drugs and deprivation of sleep.

REFERENCES

1. Morrell, F. (1959/1960) Secondary epileptogenic lesions. *Epilepsia*, **1**, 538–60.
2. Goddard, G. V., McIntyre, D. C. and Leech, C. K. (1969) A permanent change in brain function resulting from daily electrical stimulation. *Expl. Neurol.*, **25**, 295–330.
3. Galen, cited by Temkin, O. (1971) *The Falling Sickness: A History of Epilepsy from the Greeks to the Beginnings of Modern Neurology*, 2nd edn, Johns Hopkins Press, Baltimore.

4. Tissot, S. A. (1770) *Traité de l'épilepsie, faisant le Tome Troisième du traité des nerfs et de leurs maladies*, Paris.

5. Calmeil, L. F. (1824) *De l'epilepsie, étudiée sous le rapport de son siège et de son influence sur la production de l'aliénation méntale*, thesis, Paris.

6. Delasiauve, F. J. F. (1854) *Traité de l'Epilepsie*, Paris.

7. Jackson, J. H. (1931) On epilepsy and epileptiform convulsions, in *Selected Writings of J. Hughlings Jackson*, Vol. 1 (ed. J. Taylor), Hodder & Staughton, London.

8. Commission on Classification and Terminology, International League Against Epilepsy (1981) Proposed revisions of clinical and electroencephalographic classification of epileptic seizures. *Epilepsia*, **22**, 480–501.

9. Commission on Classification and Terminology, International League Against Epilepsy (1985) Proposal for classification of epilepsies and epileptic syndromes. *Epilepsia*, **26**, 268–78.

10. Ward, O. C. (1964) A new familial cardiac syndrome in children. *J. Ir. Med. Assoc.*, **54**, 103–6.

11. Eviatar, L. and Eviatar, A. (1977) Vertigo in childhood: Differential diagnosis and management. *Pediatrics*, **59**, 833–8.

12. Brown, J. K. (1977) Migraine and migraine equivalents in childhood. *Devl. Med. Child. Neurol.*, **19**, 683–92.

13. O'Donohoe, N. V. (1971) Abdominal epilepsy. *Devl. Med. Child. Neurol.*, **13**, 798–800.

14. Lombroso, C. T. and Lerman, P. (1967) Breath holding spells (cyanotic and pallid infantile syncope). *Pediatrics*, **39**, 563–81.

15. Finlayson, P. E. and Lucas, A. R. (1979) Pseudoepileptic seizures in children and adolescents. *Mayo Clin. Proc.*, **54**, 83–7.

16. Holmes, G., Sackellares, J. C., McKiernan, J. *et al.* (1980) Evaluation of pseudoseizures using EEG telemetry and videotape monitoring. *J. Pediatr.*, **97**, 554–8.

17. Meadow, R. (1984) Fictitious epilepsy. *Lancet*, **ii**, 25–8.

18. Penfield, W. and Jasper, H. (1954) *Epilepsy and the Functional Anatomy of the Human Brain*, Little Brown & Co., Boston.

19. Beaussart, M. (1972) Benign epilepsy of children with rolandic (centrotemporal) paroxysmal foci: A clinical entity. Study of 221 cases. *Epilepsia*, **13**, 793–6.

20. Beaussart, M. and Faou, R. (1978) Evolution of epilepsy with rolandic paroxysmal foci: A study of 324 cases. *Epilepsia*, **19**, 337–42.

21. Blom, S., Heijbel, J. and Bergfass, I. G. (1972) Benign epilepsy of children with centrotemporal electrographic foci. *Epilepsia*, **13**, 609–19.

22. Gastaut, H., Poirier, F., Salamon, G. *et al.* (1959/1960) H.H.E. syndrome. *Epilepsia*, **1**, 418–47.

23. Efron, R. (1961) Post-epileptic paralysis: Theoretical critique and report of a case. *Brain*, **84**, 381–94.

24. Young, G. B. and Blume, W. T. (1983) Painful epileptic seizures. *Brain*, **106**, 537–54.

25. Green, J. (1984) Pilomotor seizures. *Neurology*, **34**, 837–9.

26. Caffi, J. (1973) Zur Frage klinischer Anfallsformen der psychomotorischer Epilepsie. *Schweiz Med. Wochenschr.*, **103**, 469–75.

27. Penry, J. K., Porter, R. J. and Dreifuss, F. E. (1975) Simultaneous recording of

absence seizures in video tape and electroencephalography. A study of 374 seizures in 48 patients. *Brain*, **98**, 427–40.

28. Penry, J. K. and Dreifuss, F. E. (1969) Automatisms associated with the absence of petit mal epilepsy. *Arch. Neurol.*, **21**, 142.
29. Daly, D. D. (1975) Ictal clinical manifestations, in *Advances in Neurology*, Vol. 2 (eds J. K. Penry and D. D. Daly), Raven Press, New York, pp. 57–83.
30. Gastaut, H. (1973) *Dictionary of Epilepsy, Part 1: Definitions*, World Health Organization, Geneva.
31. Dreifuss, F. E. (1975) The differential diagnosis of partial seizure with complex symptomatology, in *Advances in Neurology*, Vol. 2 (eds J. K. Penry and D. D. Daly), Raven Press, New York, pp. 187–99.
32. Marcus, E. M. and Watson, C. W. (1966) Bilateral synchronous spike-wave electrographic patterns in the cat. *Arch. Neurol.*, **14**, 601–10.
33. Gloor, P. (1968) Generalized cortico-reticular epilepsies. Some considerations on the pathophysiology of generalized bilaterally synchronous spike and wave discharge. *Epilepsia*, **9**, 245–63.
34. Tückel, K. and Jasper, H. H. (1952) The electroencephalogram in parasagittal lesions. *Electroenceph. Clin. Neurophysiol.*, **4**, 481–94.
35. Stewart, F. F. and Dreifuss, F. E. (1964) 'Centrencephalic' seizure discharges in focal hemispheric lesions. *Arch. Neurol.*, **17**, 60–8.
36. Drury, I. and Dreifuss, F. E. (1985) Pyknoleptic petit mal. *Acta Neurol. Scand.*, (in press).
37. Loiseau, P. (1985) Childhood absence epilepsy. In *Epileptic syndromes in Infancy, Childhood and Adolescence* (eds J. Roger *et al.*), John Libbey Eurotext, London and Paris, pp. 106–20.
38. Browne, T. R., Penry, J. K., Porter, R. J. *et al.* (1974) Responsiveness before, during and after spike-wave paroxysms. *Neurology*, **24**, 659–65.
39. Goode, D. J., Penry, J. K. and Dreifuss, F. E. (1970) Effects of paroxysmal spike-wave on continuous visual-motor performance. *Epilepsia*, **11**, 241–54.
39a. Berkovic, S. F., Andermann, F., Carpenter, S. and Wolfe, L. S. (1986) Progressive myoclonus epilepsies: specific causes and diagnosis. *New Engl. J. Med.*, **315**, 296–305.
40. Janz, D. (1969) *Die Epilepsien. Spezielle Pathologie und Therapie*. Georg Thieme, Stuttgart.
41. Dreifuss, F. E. (1983) Generalized tonic-clonic seizures, in *Antiepileptic Drug Therapy in Pediatrics* (eds P. L. Morselli, C. E. Pippenger and J. K. Penry), Raven Press, New York, pp. 145–51.
42. Wolf, P. (1985) Juvenile myoclonic epilepsy, in *Epileptic Syndromes in Infancy, Childhood and Adolescence* (eds J. Roger *et al.*), John Libbey Eurotext, Paris and London.
43. Jeavons, P. M. and Harding, G. F. A. (1975) Photosensitive epilepsy, in *Clinics in Developmental Medicine*, No. 56, Heinemann, London.
44. Newmark, M. E. and Penry, J. K. (1979) *Photosensitivity and Epilepsy: A Review*, Raven Press, New York.
45. Dreifuss, F. E. (1980) The development of a comprehensive epilepsy program, in *Epilepsy Updated: Causes and Treatment* (ed. P. Robb), Year Book Medical Publishers, Chicago, pp. 303–12.
46. Dreifuss, F. E. (1987) The role of intensive monitoring in classification of

epilepsies, in *Intensive Monitoring* (ed. R. Gumnit), Raven Press, New York, (in press).

47. Bjerre, I. and Corelius, E. (1968) Benign familial neonatal convulsions. *Acta Paediatr. Scand.*, **57**, 557–61.

48. Tibbles, J. A. R. (1980) Dominant benign neonatal seizures. *Devl. Med. Child. Neurol.*, **22**, 664–7.

49. Plouin, P. (1985) Benign neonatal convulsions, in *Epileptic Syndromes in Infancy, Childhood and Adolescence* (eds J. Roger *et al.*), John Libbey Eurotext, London and Paris, pp. 2–11.

50. Dravet, C., Bureau, M. and Roger, J. (1985) Benign myoclonic epilepsy in infants, in *Epileptic Syndromes in Infancy, Childhood and Adolescence* (eds J. Roger *et al.*), John Libbey Eurotext, London and Paris, pp. 51–7.

51. Asconape, J. and Penry, J. K. (1984) Some clinical and EEG aspects of benign juvenile myoclonic epilepsy. *Epilepsia*, **25**, 108–14.

52. Janz, D. and Neimanis, G. (1961) Clinico-anatomical study of a case of idiopathic epilepsy with impulsive petit mal and grand mal on awakening. *Epilepsia*, **2**, 251–69.

53. Touchon, J. (1982) Effect of awakening on epileptic activity in primary generalized myoclonic epilepsy, in *Sleep and Epilepsy* (eds M. B. Sterman, M. N. Shouse and P. Passouant), Academic Press, New York, pp. 239–48.

54. West, W. J. (1841) On a peculiar form of infantile convulsions. *Lancet*, **i**, 724–5.

55. Gastaut, H., Roger, J., Soulayrol, R. and Pinsard, N. (1964) *Encephalopathie myoclonique infantile avec hypsarythmie (syndrome de West)*. Masson, Paris.

56. Jeavons, P. M. and Bower, B. D. (1964) *Infantile Spasms. A Review of the Literature and a Study of 112 cases*. Heinemann, London.

57. Jeavons, P. M., Bower, B. D. and Dimitrakoudi, M. (1973) Long term prognosis of 150 cases of 'West Syndome'. *Epilepsia*, **14**, 153–64.

58. Kellaway, P., Hrachovy, R. A., Frost, J. D. and Zion, T. (1979) Precise characterization and quantification of infantile spasms. *Ann. Neurol.*, **6**, 214–18.

59. Lacy, J. R. and Penry, J. K. (1976) *Infantile Spasms*, Raven Press, New York.

60. Lombroso, C. T. (1983) A prospective study of infantile spasms: clinical and therapeutic correlations. *Epilepsia*, **24**, 135–58.

61. Lennox, W. G. and Davis, J. P. (1950) Clinical correlates of the fast and slow spike wave electroencephalogram. *Pediatrics*, **5**, 626–44.

62. Gastaut, H., Roger, J., Soulayrol, R. *et al.* (1966) Childhood epileptic encephalopathy with diffuse slow spike-waves (otherwise known as 'petit mal variant') or Lennox syndrome. *Epilepsia*, **7**, 139–79.

63. Chevrie, J. J. and Aicardi, J. (1972) Childhood epileptic encephalopathy with slow spike wave. A statistical study of 80 cases. *Epilepsia*, **13**, 259–71.

64. Doose, H., Gerken, H., Leonhart, R. *et al.* (1970) Centrencephalic myoclonic astatic petit mal. *Neuropädiatrie*, **2**, 59–78.

65. Aicardi, J. and Goutieres, F. (1978) Encephalopathie myoclonique neonatale. *Rev. EEG Neurophysiol.*, **8**, 99–101.

66. Ohtahara, S., Ishida, T., Oka, E. *et al.* (1976) On the age-dependent epileptic syndromes: the early infantile encephalopathy with suppression-burst. *Brain Dev.*, **8**, 270–88.

67. Dalla Bernardina, B., Aicardi, J., Goutieres, F. and Plouin, P. (1979) Glycine encephalopathy. *Neuropadiatrie*, **10**, 209–25.

68. Freeman, J. M. (1983) Neonatal seizures, in *Pediatric Epileptology*, (ed. F. E. Dreifuss), John Wright PSG, Boston, pp. 159–72.
69. Volpe, J. J. (1981) *Neurology of the Newborn*, W. B. Saunders Co., Philadelphia.
70. Tassinari, C. A., Bureau, M., Dravet, C. *et al.* (1982) Electrical status epilepticus during sleep in children (ESES), in *Sleep and Epilepsy*, (eds M. B. Sterman, M. N. Shouse and P. Passouant), Academic Press, London and New York, pp. 465–79.
71. Landau, W. M. and Kleffner, F. R. (1957) Syndrome of acquired aphasia with convulsive disorder in children. *Neurology*, **7**, 523–30.
72. Gascon, G., Victor, D., Lombroso, C. T. and Goodglass, H. (1973) Language disorder, convulsive disorder and electroencephalographic abnormalities. Acquired syndrome in children, *Arch. Neurol.*, **28**, 156–62.
73. Lennox-Buchthal, M. A. (1973) Febrile convulsions: A reappraisal. *Electroenceph. Clin. Neurophysiol.*, **32** (Suppl.), 1–138.
74. Frantzen, E., Lennox-Buchthal, M. and Nygaard, A. (1968) Longitudinal EEG and clinical study of children with febrile convulsions. *Electroenceph. Clin. Neurophysiol.*, **24**, 197–212.
75. Nelson, K. B. and Ellenberg, J. H. (1976) Predictors of epilepsy in children who have experienced febrile seizures. *N. Engl. J. Med.*, **295**, 1029–33.
76. Nelson, K. B. and Ellenberg, J. H. (1978) Prognosis in children with febrile seizures. *Pediatrics*, **61**, 720–7.
77. Nelson, K. B. and Ellenberg, J. H. (1981) The role of recurrences in determining outcome in children with febrile seizures, in *Febrile Seizures*, (eds K. B. Nelson and J. H. Ellenberg), Raven Press, New York, pp. 19–25.
78. Newmark, M. E. and Penry, J. K. (1979) *Photosensitivity and Epilepsy: A Review*, Raven Press, New York.
79. Ames, F. R. (1971) Self-induction in photosensitive epilepsy. *Brain*, **94**, 781–98.
80. Newmark, M. E. (1983) Sensory-evoked seizures, in *Pediatric Epileptology*, (ed. F. E. Dreifuss), John Wright/PSG, Boston, pp. 199–219.
81. O'Brien, J. S. (1969) Five gangliosidoses. *Lancet*, **ii**, 805.
82. Okada, S. and O'Brien, J. S. (1968) Generalized gangliosidosis β-galactosidase deficiency. *Science*, **160**, 1002.
83. Pilz, H., Sandhoff, K. and Jatzkewitz, G. (1966) A disorder of ganglioside metabolism with storage or ceramide lactoside, monosialoceramide lactoside and tsd ganglioside in brain. *J. Neurochem.*, **13**, 1273–82.
84. Suzuki, Y. and Suzuki, K. (1970) Partial deficiency of hexosaminidase A in juvenile GM_2 gangliosidosis. *Neurology*, **20**, 848–51.
85. Van Heycopten Ham, M. W. and De Jager, H. (1963) Progressive myoclonic epilepsy with Lafora bodies. Clinical and pathological features. *Epilepsia*, **4**, 95–119.
86. Janeway, R., Ravens, J. R. and Pearce, L. A. (1967) Progressive myoclonic epilepsy with Lafora bodies: Clinical, genetic, histopathological and biochemical study. *Arch. Neurol.*, **16**, 565–82.
87. Horenko, A. and Toivakka, E. (1961) Myoclonic epilepsy in Finland. *Acta Neurol. Scand.*, **27**, 282–96.
88. Kojewnikow, L. (1895) Eine besondere Form von corticaler Epilepsie. *Neurologisch. Centralblatt.*, **14**, 47–8.
89. Bancaud, J., Bonis, A., Trottier, S. *et al.* (1982) L'epilepsie partielle continue: syndrome et maladie. *Rev. Neurol.*, **138**, 802–14.

90. Thomas, J., Reggan, J. and Klass, D. (1977) Epilepsia partialis continua. A review of 32 cases. *Arch. Neurol.*, **34**, 266–75.

91. Juul-Jensen, P. and Denny-Brown, D. (1966) Epilepsia partialis continua. *Arch. Neurol.*, **15**, 563–78.

92. Heintel, H. (1972) *Der Status Epilepticus. Seine Atiologie, Klinik und Letalitat.* Fischer, Stuttgart.

93. Rothner, A. D. and Erenberg, J. (1980) Status epilepticus. *Pediatr. Clin. N. Am.*, **27**, 593–602.

94. Sato, S. and Dreifuss, F. E. (1973) Electroencephalographic findings in a patient with developmental expressive aphasia. *Neurology*, **23**, 181–5.

95. Janz, D. (1964) Status epilepticus and frontal lobe lesions. *J. Neurol. Sci.*, **1**, 446–57.

CHAPTER FOUR

The Causes and Precipitation of Seizures

The causes of epilepsy in infancy and early childhood are considered in Chapter 16. The special contribution of genetic factors is considered in Chapter 5. This section is devoted to a consideration of the aetiologies of epilepsy in later childhood and adult life. By 'cause' is meant more or less steady-state background factors such as the scarring of a brain following meningitis; by 'precipitation' is meant short term stimuli such as exposure to television sets in susceptible people. Table 4.1 lists some of the 'steady state' factors that might reasonably be supposed to cause epilepsy, and Table 4.3 on p. 124 some common precipitants of seizures.

4.1 CAUSES OF EPILEPSY

Anthony Hopkins

4.1.1 Genetic factors

These are reviewed in Chapter 5. Many of the recessively inherited disorders of lipid and amino acid metabolism may be associated with seizures [1]. Other recessively inherited disorders associated with epilepsy include tuberous sclerosis and neurofibromatosis. The studies of Metrakos and Metrakos [2, 3] suggest that primary generalized epilepsy is inherited as an autosomal dominant.

A 'convulsive threshold' may be inherited, perhaps polygenically. The best evidence for this would be an increased risk of seizures amongst members of a population with a family history of epilepsy following some additional neurological insult, such as cranial injury, compared to the risk of those similarly injured without a family history. No such controlled study has been carried out on patients with cranial injury. Jennett [4] reports an increased incidence of a positive family history among his injured patients who develop epilepsy, though this did not reach significance for either early (within one week) or late post-traumatic epilepsy. In these and similar studies in which the family history is recorded as a side-line to the main thrust of the study, the extent of enquiry about a family history to relatives of lesser degree is never defined. In Chapter 5, Bundey reviews on p. 141 a study that shows that

Table 4.1 The 'causes' of epilepsy

Genetic propensity
  Recessively inherited disorders of lipid and amino acid metabolism
  Recessively inherited 'developmental' disorders – tuberous sclerosis;
    neurofibromatosis
  Dominantly inherited disorders – primary generalized epilepsy
  Polygenic inherited propensity (probable)
Congenital abnormalities
  Microgyria
  Focal cortical dysplasia
  Megaloencephaly
Ante- and perinatal injury
  Anoxia
  Intracerebral haemorrhage
  Infarction; porencephalic cyst
Effects consequent to prolonged febrile convulsions
Trauma
  Accidental
  Following elective neurosurgery
Infections
  Bacterial meningitis
  Cerebral abscess
  Viral encephalitis
  Parasitic infections
Immunization
  Pertussis vaccine
Vascular causes
  Infarction
  Hypertensive encephalopathy
  Cerebral venous thrombosis
  Arteriovenous malformations
  Postanoxic encephalopathy
Toxic causes
  Alcohol ingestion and withdrawal; chronic alcoholic encephalopathy
  Heavy metals, particularly lead
Metabolic causes
  Hypoglycaemia   Hyperglycaemia
  Hypoxia   Hyperbaric oxygenation
  Hypocalcaemia   Hypercalcaemia
  Hyponatraemia   Hypernatraemia
                             Uraemia
  Deficiency of pyridoxine
Degenerative causes
  Alzheimer's disease

patients who convulse after stroke are more likely to have a family history of seizures than those who do not.

4.1.2 Congenital abnormalities

Epilepsy may be associated with the congenital dysplasias, microgyria, macrogyria, etc., but it is sometimes difficult to distinguish congenital abnormalities in association with hydrocephalus from cerebral damage sustained in the antenatal and perinatal period. The Sturge-Weber syndrome with both facial and cortical angiomata, and the Aicardi syndrome of agenesis of the corpus callosum, in association with cortical and retinal dysplasia, are other examples of epilepsy in association with congenital abnormalities.

4.1.3 Antenatal and perinatal injury

Cerebral palsy is commonly associated with epilepsy. In a community survey Kudrjavcev and colleagues [5] found that epilepsy was present in 52% of patients with severe or very severe palsy, but only 23% of those with mild or moderate palsy. The occurrence of epilepsy correlated not only with the degree of motor disability but also with the level of cognitive handicap.

Epilepsy in association with birth injury may arise on a basis of intracerebral or intraventricular haemorrhage, or infarction. The evidence in later life of infarction in the neonatal period is often a porencephalic cyst.

4.1.4 The effects subsequent to prolonged febrile convulsions

The epidemiological evidence of Ounsted and his colleagues [6] (reviewed on pp. 448–49), and the experimental evidence of Meldrum and colleagues [7, 8] on seizures induced in young baboons, leaves no doubt that prolonged seizures can induce neuronal damage that is prominent in the mesial temporal lobe, with loss of cells and glial sclerosis that is particularly prominent in the H1 sector of the hippocampus (p. 313). Such a sclerotic scar then forms a focus for the subsequent development of complex partial and secondarily generalized seizures.

4.1.5 Trauma and the effects of craniotomy

These aspects are fully reviewed in Chapter 13. Here, as brief examples, it may be noted that late post-traumatic epilepsy is particularly likely to develop after head injury if the injury is associated with a depressed fracture, with a dural tear, with focal neurological signs, with a long post-traumatic amnesia, and, particularly, if seizures occur in the first week after injury. Such early epilepsy in response to trauma may be an important marker of an innate propensity to seizures. If all such factors are associated with a head injury, then the patient has a greater than 60% probability of developing epilepsy. If none of these factors are present, then the incidence of late post-traumatic epilepsy is probably barely higher than that of the population as a whole.

As an example of the risks of epilepsy after neurosurgical intervention, also reviewed in Chapter 13, epilepsy is particularly likely after aneurysmal surgery if the aneurysm lies on the middle cerebral system, if the patient were obtunded or stuperose before surgery, and if the procedure were complicated by spasm, a haematoma, or the need, postoperatively, for a shunt.

4.1.6   Infections

Bacterial meningitis is often followed by the development of epilepsy. The usual organisms in western countries are *Haemophilus influenzae, Pneumococcus, Meningococcus*, and, in developing countries, *Mycobacterium tuberculosis*. Energetic early treatment minimizes the risk of later epilepsy. A cerebral abscess, particularly if in the frontal region, is particularly likely to be followed by epilepsy [9]. Granulomas, often tuberculous, are frequent causes of epilepsy in developing countries [9a].

Seizures may be a presenting feature of viral infections such as *Herpes simplex* encephalitis. It is conceivable that less severe infections may not be recognized as an encephalitic illness as such, but provide a focus from which epilepsy may subsequently develop. Gannicliffe and colleagues [10] have detected by molecular hybridization *Herpes simplex* type 1 DNA sequences in operative specimens of temporal lobe from epileptic patients. Whether this is evidence that *H. simplex* 'causes' some cases of temporal lobe epilepsy remains uncertain, as the presence of the DNA sequences could be merely evidence of past asymptomatic exposure to the virus, of no aetiological significance. Although it is recognized that there are less fulminant forms of *H. simplex* encephalitis, the spectrum of clinical disease does not seem to extend to 'mild' forms, and hence, by implication, not to 'asymptomatic' forms.

There is no doubt, however, that persistent viral replication occurs in subacute sclerosing panencephalitis, and myoclonic jerks and tonic-clonic seizures are cardinal features of this illness.

Seizures are also a feature of infection with *Toxoplasma gondii*, and, in particular, in cysticercosis. Patients with cysticercosis who present with seizures often have a relatively benign disorder, with parenchymal cysts or calcification [11].

4.1.7   Immunization

In the last decade, there has been some anxiety about pertussis vaccine, encephalopathy, and seizures. The question has been carefully analysed by Cherry and Shields [12]. They quote three studies. In one, Melchior analysed the incidence of infantile spasms in Denmark in two different time periods –

when pertussis vaccine was administered to children at the ages of five, six and 15 months, and at five weeks, nine weeks and ten months. If pertussis vaccine were a significant cause of infantile spasms, then it would be expected that the incidence prior to age five months would be greater in the second epoch, whereas in the event the incidence in the two epochs proved identical. In another, British, study quoted by Cherry and Shields, the incidence of neurological disturbances in over 133 000 children who received diphtheria and tetanus vaccine alone (DT) was compared to that in a similar number of children who received diphtheria, tetanus and pertussis vaccine together (DTP). A greater frequency of neurological events was recorded after DTP than DT but, when individual cases were analysed, it was clear that in most instances there was another cause for the problem noted, and that the difference was probably due to a reporting bias caused by adverse publicity to pertussis vaccine.

One study, however, the National Childhood Encephalopathy study, quoted by Cherry and Shields, showed that DTP immunization occurred significantly more frequently within 72 hours and within seven days before neurological illness than such illness occurred in the control subjects following within 72 hours and within seven days of the index date. After making various assumptions, the risk of neurological illness for previously normal children was 1 per 310 000 pertussis immunizations – but the 95% confidence limits were 1:54 000–1:53 000 000.

4.1.8 Vascular causes

Seizures may follow atheroembolic brain infarction, but do not commonly do so. Seizures occur in the acute period after stroke in some patients [13]. Seizures may be partial or generalized (presumably secondarily), but if partial are often motor in type. Hauser and colleagues have shown in a prospective study of 206 stroke patients that 15% developed seizures in the first week after stroke, and the cumulative risk for survivors, by life table analysis to six years, was 19% for subsequent seizures [14]. In studies that have compared embolic with other strokes, seizures are more likely to follow embolic events, including emboli from the mitral valve or left atrium.

One useful clinical point raised in Lesser's review [13] is that stroke may result in paroxysmal lateralizing epileptiform discharges (PLEDs) on the EEG, and, if seizures accompany these, they may prove extremely difficult to control, even with high doses of anticonvulsants. Fortunately however, seizures associated with PLEDs tend to remit over several days, and, if seizures are partial, or partialis continua, it may be better to wait for remission rather than depress consciousness by the use of large doses of anticonvulsants.

Although *overt* cerebrovascular incidents are associated with epilepsy as described above, a more common clinical situation is the attribution of seizures of late onset to ischaemic lesions seen on the cranial CT scan. This has been placed on a more quantitative basis by Shorvon and colleagues [15]. These authors compared the CT scans of 74 patients with epilepsy over the age of 40 with an age and sex matched group of controls. Patients with tumours were excluded. Thirteen of the patients and only two of the controls showed ischaemic lesions on the scan ($p < 0.0005$). All patients with ischaemic lesions were over the age of 55; they had more evidence of vascular disease than the controls. Although the ischaemic lesions imaged were often lacunar infarctions in the deep white matter, the authors conclude that these lacunes are indicative of more widespread cerebrovascular disease rather than being themselves directly responsible for the seizures. In this study of selected patients, neither clinical nor EEG features proved useful in predicting the presence of ischaemic lesions in the CT scan. The prevalence of prior epilepsy in patients with first strokes has been shown to be considerably higher than that for age-matched controls – again evidence that vascular disease in older subjects may cause seizures [15a].

Small venous infarctions in the cortex are particularly epileptogenic [16]. Such infarctions on a small scale are probably responsible for the epilepsy which is often the presenting feature of arteriovenous malformations. A recent careful study of 343 consecutive patients with cerebral angiomas seen in one large British neurological and neurosurgical unit has given much information about the natural history of angiomas, and the risk of epilepsy [17]. Sixty-one (19%) had seizures as a major symptom leading to diagnosis; 20 of these had physical signs. In 247, the diagnosis was reached after haemorrhage. Those angiomas that were diagnosed as a result of epilepsy tended to be larger and more superficial than those diagnosed as a result of haemorrhage. Of those who had not had seizures at the time of diagnosis the risk of subsequent seizures was only approximately 1% per year, declining with age. Surgical treatment of angiomas, rather than reducing the risk of epilepsy, was shown in this study to treble it [17].

Seizures may also occur consequent to subarachnoid haemorrhage (Chapter 13), particularly if aneurysm lies on the middle cerebral artery [17a]. The vascular encephalopathy of accelerated hypertension is particularly likely to cause seizures. The encephalopathy of eclampsia has some similar features. The encephalopathy resulting from an only partially successful resuscitation following cardiopulmonary arrest may result in myoclonus and seizures. Although there are many reports of neurological complications following coronary bypass surgery, and other cardiac surgery, epilepsy does not seem a common consequence [13].

4.1.9 Cerebral tumours

Traditional teaching held that epilepsy of 'late' onset was usually due to a tumour, and many patients were evaluated by contrast radiology with this in mind in the 1950s and 1960s. However a number of careful studies, and the advent of CT scanning, have shown that this is clearly incorrect. The proportion varies in different studies (for references see [18]). One recent study may be taken as an example [18]. Of 221 patients with onset of seizures at age 25 or over, 36 (16%) proved to have tumours. Another aspect is the incidence of tumours found during very careful evaluation of subjects with intractable partial seizures preparatory to surgery. In one study [19], 15% of patients had intracranial mass lesions found during preoperative evaluation, and which had escaped discovery during more conventional routine screening. In another, Rich and colleagues [20] underline the probability that well differentiated gliomas account for calcified or hypodense lesions on the scan that had been assumed to be heterotopic lesions or old infarcts.

Epilepsy may arise as a presenting symptom or during the course of development of primary tumours, both benign and malignant, and metastases. Thomas and Graham [21] found that epilepsy was the initial symptom in 39% of the National Hospital series of gliomas, and had occurred in 54% by the time of neurological assessment and diagnosis. These authors highlight those features that should, in their opinion, alert a neurologist to the possibility of an underlying tumour being responsible for epilepsy. Headaches, and the new development of focal neurological signs, or a postictal paresis, are obvious warning signals. Other signals include a change in the character of the epilepsy, undue resistance to drug therapy, and the occurrence of status epilepticus.

Tumours in different areas of the brain declare themselves by the onset of epilepsy with different characteristics. Tumours in the central sensorimotor strip are particularly likely to present with focal motor or aphasic partial seizures. Tumours in the frontal lobe are likely to present with tonic-clonic seizures. A patient whose epilepsy begins with tonic-clonic status epilepticus is particularly likely to have frontal tumour. Tumours in the occipital lobe seldom cause seizures.

Oligodendrogliomas are particularly likely to cause seizures. However, astrocytomas, glioblastomas, meningiomas and metastases may also produce epilepsy. Rarely a large pituitary adenoma can cause epilepsy by lateral extension into a temporal lobe.

4.1.10 Toxic causes

Seizures may result from chronic intoxication with lead and other heavy metals; children seem particularly liable. Acute alcohol ingestion may precipitate seizures, and recurrent seizures may occur as the result of chronic alcohol abuse. The effects of alcohol and drugs are further considered on p. 127.

4.1.11 Metabolic causes

Seizures may occur in chronic renal failure, although the exact metabolic cause is uncertain. They may also result in association with hypoxia (and hyperbaric oxygenation), from overhydration, from hypoglycaemia, from non-ketotic hyperglycaemia [22], from hyponatraemia, hypernatraemia, hypocalcaemia, hypercalcaemia, and pyridoxine deficiency. The complex field of seizures induced by such metabolic derangements in children is covered in Chapter 16.

4.1.12 Alzheimer's disease and other dementias

Seizures do not figure at all in the longitudinal study over five years of 199 demented patients by Barclay and his colleagues [23]. A different perspective, however, has recently been reported by Hauser [23a], who reported a ten fold risk of seizures in patients with Alzheimer's disease. The difference between the two studies presumably reflects two different approaches – longitudinal [23], and cross-sectional [23a].

In Jakob-Creutzfeldt disease, in which myoclonus is common, seizures are not a common feature.

Although the preceding pages have described various neurological disorders in which epilepsy is a not infrequent symptom, the question arises as to how often, in a population of people with epilepsy in the community, can a cause of epilepsy be assigned with any degree of confidence? This point is best considered using the example of cranial injury. No-one doubts that epilepsy is much commoner than in the general population after penetrating missile injuries to the cranium, or after a depressed fracture with a dural tear (see Chapter 13). At the other extreme, if a child has a trivial head injury at school, and then has his first seizure two weeks later, many parents will link the two events, and remain firmly convinced that the injury 'caused' the epilepsy, though most neurologists would suspect that the two events were only coincidentally linked. It follows that somewhere along the continuum of mild to moderate to severe cranial injuries there must be a zone in which there is reasonable doubt, even amongst neurologists, as to whether or not the epilepsy was 'caused' by the head injury.

Hauser and Kurland [24] assigned causes to the epilepsy of 516 unselected patients from the community of Olmstead County, whose medical care is undertaken by the excellent facilities of the Mayo Clinic. In spite of a review of all available medical records, and a mean follow-up time exceeding ten years, a cause of epilepsy could only be defined in 23.3% of the 516 cases. A summary of their findings is presented in Table 4.2, which also shows the similar findings in other community surveys. The small proportion of epilepsies in the community caused by tumours (4.1% and 3.2%) contrasts with the different perspective held by neurosurgeons. As already noted on p. 121, 54% of all

Table 4.2 Identified causes of epilepsy in six studies (%)

	Study (Reference)				
	[24]	[25]	[18]	[18a]	[18b]
	Adults			Children	Elderly
Birth trauma, anoxia	2.5	6.3	with miscellaneous	7.8	—
Cranial injury, postoperative	3.6	7.0	4.1	3.3	3.9
Vascular	5.2	3.2	14.0	—	32.4
Tumours	4.1	3.2	16.3	—	13.9
Infections	2.9	3.2	with miscellaneous	6.3	—
Congenital	2.3	1.1	with miscellaneous	4.7	—
Alcohol	excluded	0	23.1	—	9.9
Miscellaneous	excluded	0	4.5	—	15.2
Unknown	79.4	76.0	38.0	76.7	24.5

(24) – 516 cases of epilepsy, community study, all ages, some EEG, no CT.
(25) – 94 cases, community study, age 16 or over, some EEG, no CT.
(18) – 221 cases, age 25 or over, all EEG and CT.
(18a) – longitudinal study of a national population sample, including all 15496 children born in one week in March, 1958, in the UK; 64 cases of epilepsy by age 11.
(18b) – 151 cases of epilepsy over the age of 60, some EEG, some CT. In this study 'alcohol' also includes 5 cases of epilepsy induced by drugs.

patients with tumours have epilepsy at the time of initial assessment and diagnosis. Since the publication of these community surveys, the advent of CT and magnetic resonance imaging has led to the more extensive investigation of patients presenting with epilepsy. Although abnormalities such as focal atrophy are often seen in the scans of patients with epilepsy, the cause still often remains obscure. Even in patients over 25 investigated fully by CT scanning and EEG by Dam and colleagues [18] the cause was unknown in 38% (Table 4.2).

Table 4.2 also shows the identified causes of epilepsy in a very careful longitudinal study of a national sample of children in the U.K. [18a], and a recent survey [18b] of causes of epilepsy in older people (age over 60) which shows the greater proportion of cases attributable to stroke and tumour. It must however be remembered that these are surveys in developed communities. In the developing countries, a far higher number of patients with epilepsy will have seizures due to infections and parasitic causes – particularly tuberculomas and cysticercosis.

If it is not possible to find a cause for seizures, it does not follow that the epilepsy is 'idiopathic'. This term is best reserved for primary generalized epilepsy. Patients who have partial seizures, clearly arising from some structural focus which is not successfully imaged or 'diagnosed', are sometimes described as having 'cryptogenic' epilepsy.

4.2 PRECIPITATION OF SEIZURES

Anthony Hopkins and Andrea Garman

The foregoing paragraphs have shown that the assignation of a definite 'cause' for epilepsy is impossible for about 40–70% of all subjects. Patients often have firm beliefs about the immediate precipitant of their seizures. However, neurologists should not be trapped by patients' understandable desires to make sense of their world, by establishing cause and effect, into firmly allocating precipitating causes for epilepsy. The very fact of the genetic predispositions reviewed in Chapter 5 indicates that there is a whole range of propensities to epilepsy, and on this foundation the effects of one, or probably more often several, factors summate to precipitate a seizure. A hypothetical example illustrates this point. Take a man with a moderate genetic predisposition to seizures. Add the effects of a moderate cranial injury some two years before. Add also the effects of 'stress' at the office during the preceding month. Add also the effects of amitriptyline prescribed to help the depression associated with this stress. If this man then has a seizure after consuming a moderate amount of alcohol the night before, what caused it – the genetic

Table 4.3 Suggested precipitants of seizures

Sleep
Waking
Deprivation of sleep

Menstrual cycle

Toxic and metabolic causes
   Acute alcohol intoxication
   Withdrawal from alcohol
   Drugs
   Hypoglycaemia
   Hypoxia

Reflex causes
   glare, flashing lights, television
   reading
   sounds
   thinking
   startle
   movement

Stressful life events

propensity, the cranial injury, the stress, the alcohol and associated metabolic changes, the disturbance of sleep associated with the depression, or the amitriptyline? Depending upon the perspective of the world of both patient and neurologist, agreement may be reached to blame just one of all these factors, quite illogically. The above example also shows the difficulty in distinguishing between 'cause' and 'precipitant', although the distinction suggested on p. 115 is useful. The whole question of precipitation of seizures is next considered. Some of the commoner suggested precipitants are listed in Table 4.3.

4.2.1 Sleep, waking and deprivation of sleep

Classic observations on the relation between the sleep cycle and seizures were made by Langdon-Down and Brain in 1929 [27]. They studied the time of day at which no fewer than 2524 seizures occurred in 66 subjects with severe epilepsy. When data for all subjects were pooled, several peak times of occurrence were noted. Of those who tended to have nocturnal seizures, peak times of occurrence occurred about two hours after going to bed, and between 5 and 6 am. The group who tended to have daytime seizures had a high propensity to seizures in the first hour after waking.

The whole relationship between epilepsy, drowsiness, sleep, arousal and deprivation of sleep has been reviewed in a monograph of nearly 400 pages in 1984 [28] and only a few aspects will be considered here. The usefulness of drowsiness in eliciting epileptiform activity on the EEG is considered in Chapter 7.

(a) The effect of sleep on different types of seizure

Most generalized epilepsies are enhanced by non-rapid eye movement or slow wave (NREM) sleep. Generalized seizures occur predominantly during the first or last hour of sleep, most often during stage 2 NREM sleep, during a transitional stage, or upon waking spontaneously. Tonic-clonic seizures do not occur during rapid eye movement (REM) sleep, nor does REM sleep immediately follow a tonic-clonic seizure.

Typical absences are difficult to identify clinically during sleep, although they may be accompanied by some myoclonic jerks. However, the EEG shows that 3 Hz paroxysms occur during REM sleep. If discharges do occur during NREM sleep, they are degraded into polyspike and wave discharges [28]. Drowsiness and induction of NREM sleep is the most useful activator of epileptiform activity in the case of complex partial seizures [29]. Clinically, complex partial seizures during sleep are deprived of one of their principal nosological characteristics – the altered conscious experience. However it has been shown that epileptic auras in REM sleep may be incorporated into dreams (for references, see [29]). Wieser [30] has shown with depth recording that seizure discharges may precede awakening. Some groups of workers (see

[29]) have found that hippocampal, amygdaloid, frontal and supplementary motor epileptic foci may be selectively activated during REM sleep. In the evaluation of patients for temporal lobe surgery, it has been proposed that the principal focus can be identified as being that which is most autonomous across all sleeping/waking states. Generalization of seizures from a partial focus is however most likely to occur in NREM sleep.

The rolandic spikes associated with the benign partial epilepsies of childhood increase in frequency in NREM sleep, and decrease again in REM sleep, though they remain more frequent than when the child is awake [31]. Some 50–60% of children with this form of epilepsy have seizures only during sleep.

A common practical clinical problem is the prediction of the likelihood of seizures recurring in the day time in a patient who has until then only had seizures whilst asleep. Gibberd and Bateson [32] followed up 38 patients who had had only attacks whilst asleep for the first six months of their epilepsy. The tables in this paper are not easy to understand, but it is clear that a significant proportion went on to develop seizures whilst awake.

(b)   The effect of arousal

Seizures on awakening were delineated by Janz in 1953, and have been reviewed by Niedermeyer [33]. The patients are usually adolescents or young adults. One or more brief myoclonic jerks occur on arousal. These may or may not then be followed by a tonic-clonic seizure. Those affected have 3–4 Hz generalized synchronous spike waves in the waking record. During stage 2 NREM sleep, such spikes and polyspikes are superimposed upon K-complexes, which in the normal subject are in themselves related to arousal. Patients may have associated typical absences and/or tonic-clonic seizures, or be photosensitive. All these phonemena show that epilepsy on waking is related to primary generalized epilepsy.

(c)   The effect of deprivation of sleep

Sleep deprivation undoubtedly precipitates seizures. Although known for many years, this was illustrated in a controlled way amongst US veterans returning from Vietnam [34]. The authors compared different batches of veterans exposed to different patterns of 'processing' by the Army administration, and subject therefore to different degrees of deprivation of sleep. In the most deprived group, the incidence of seizures in this healthy male population was 4330 per 100 000 per year, several hundred times than that expected in the general population [34]. The authors acknowledge that excitement and alcohol may have played some part, and indeed these are factors commonly accompanying deprivation of sleep.

Young people seem particularly prone to have their seizures exacerbated by deprivation of sleep, and light sensitive and other reflex epilepsies are particularly affected, as are those with typical absences, and generalized seizures on awakening [29].

4.2.2 The menstrual cycle

The effect of different phases of the menstrual cycle upon epilepsy is reviewed in Chapter 12, pp. 373–77.

4.2.3 Toxic and metabolic precipitants

(a) Alcohol

Seizures in association with alcohol may occur as a result of acute intoxication or during a period of withdrawal of alcohol. Withdrawal seizures may occur as an isolated phenomenon, or as part of an acute alcoholic hallucinosis (delirium tremens). Finally, seizure may arise after some years of alcohol abuse as a feature of alcohol-induced brain damage.

Much has been written on withdrawal seizures, first described as early as 1848 by Huss. Victor and Brausch studied a group of 241 alcoholic patients presenting with convulsive seizures [35]. They found that 90% of the patients had tonic-clonic seizures beginning in adult life. Seizures occurred singly or in short bursts on withdrawal of alcohol after a period of chronic intoxication. The EEG was usually normal except transiently between the 15th and 19th hours after withdrawal. This coincided with the time of peak incidence of seizures. Deisenhammer and coworkers in 1984 [36] distinguished two groups clinically and by EEG. In one group, seizures occurred only during a time during which alcohol was being withdrawn, or partially withdrawn. Seizures then were attributed solely to alcohol withdrawal. In the other group seizures occurred spontaneously as well as during alcohol withdrawal. Other epileptogenic factors, such as brain damage after trauma, and a family history of seizures probably play some part in the genesis of seizures. Paroxysms or focal abnormalities are rarely seen in the first group; in the second group, EEG abnormalities are seen approximately as frequently as in other epileptic conditions.

These observations on humans are compatible with animal experiments. Chronic administration of alcohol leads to suppression, and withdrawal to an increase of neuronal excitability lasting from hours to days [37, 38]. Other factors which may play a part in seizures associated with alcohol abuse include magnesium deficiency [39], pyridoxine deficiency [40] and hypoglycaemia. Of seizures associated with drinking, overhydration by drinking large volumes of, for example, beer also certainly play a part [41].

The published work principally concerns abuse of alcohol, and its effects upon seizures [42]. There is little work on the effect of the social consumption of alcohol on seizures, with the exception of the work of Höppener and colleagues [43] who demonstrated that social alcohol intake does not affect the frequency of either partial or tonic-clonic seizures. Furthermore, serum levels of anticonvulsant medication were not significantly influenced, nor were any changes seen in the EEG following alcohol in quantities often consumed in social circumstances.

(b) Drugs

Many different drugs have been suspected of precipitating seizures. The evidence that the association is other than coincidental rests upon the frequency of reported occurrence. The underlying illness for which the drug is being given, or non-specific events such as fever, may often be more relevant factors. Nevertheless, some drugs figure so prominently in reported series [44, 45] that a causal relation is likely.

Antidepressant drugs precipitate seizures, and, by reason of their frequent prescription are the drugs most likely to be thought to be responsible for precipitating seizures in everyday practice. Tricyclic drugs such as imipramine and amitriptyline seem more likely to precipitate seizures than viloxazine. Myoclonic jerks and tonic-clonic seizures are frequent manifestations of overdose with these drugs in attempted suicide, but some patients appear to have seizures precipitated by low dosages, such as 25–50 mg of amitriptyline at night. Antipsychotic drugs such as chlorpromazine or haloperidol may also precipitate seizures. Patients under psychiatric care, but with organic brain disease, are particularly likely to have seizures precipitated by chlorpromazine [46].

In the report of Messing and colleagues [45], isoniazid accounted for about 20% of all seizure episodes attributed to drugs. Isoniazid depletes the body of pyridoxine, a necessary constituent of the coenzyme required for synthesis of gamma-amino butyric acid, by increasing renal clearance as xanthenuric acid. Pyridoxine supplements should be given to all those on isoniazid therapy. This would probably prevent all seizures due to isoniazid.

Penicillin directly applied to the cortex is a popular method of inducing focal seizures in experimental animals (Chapter 2). Very high blood levels of benzyl penicillin, caused by impaired renal clearance and massive dosage, may precipitate convulsions [44]. Unfortunately all too often seizures, or death, may be precipitated by the unwise excessive intrathecal injection of penicillin. No more than 10 000 units should be given as a single dose.

Lignocaine and lidocaine given intravenously as antiarrhythmic agents have been reported to induce seizures, and these agents, and bupivacaine, have also precipitated seizures when given in excess as local anaesthetic agents. Bronchodilators such as theophylline, aminophylline and terbutaline have all been reported to cause seizures (see [45] for references).

Another group of epileptogenic agents that is particularly close to the heart of neurologists is iodine-containing radiographic contrast medium. The original use of meglumine iothalamate (Conray) for lumbar radioculography was associated with a risk of convulsions as high as 11% and meglumine iocarmate (Dimer-X) was little safer. Metrizamide (Amipaque) appears to be virtually free from risk of precipitating seizures if confined to the lumbar subarachnoid space, but may precipitate seizures in 0.4% of cases if taken up into the cervical region [47]. Patients who undergo metrizamide radiculography or myelography should be nursed with the head and neck raised for eight hours after the examination, in order to prevent the seepage of contrast medium into the head.

(c) Hypoglycaemia

The precipitation of seizures by hypoglycaemia is discussed on p. 163.

4.2.4 Reflex precipitants of seizures

(a) Visually induced seizures [48]

About 3% of patients with epilepsy have seizures induced by viewing intermittent light, steady bright light, patterns or television. Most of the subjects are young, the modal age of first referral being 12 years. The male:female ratio is 2:3. Visually induced seizures are a variant of primary generalized epilepsy. Seizure types include absences, myoclonic jerks and tonic-clonic seizures, so there may well be a family history of epilepsy.

If the subject is asked to view a gas discharge lamp during photic stimulation at slow frequencies, a visual evoked potential will be seen in the occipital EEG. Flashes of light evoke potentials which follow the frequency of the flash, up to 10–20 Hz. In about 5% of those with seizure disorders, and a proportion of the relatives of those with seizure disorders, this 'following response' is replaced by or followed by a photoconvulsive response, consisting of regular or irregular single or multiple spikes interspersed with slow waves. The amplitude of these discharges, which are not time-locked to the flash frequency, is maximal in the frontal and central regions. The discharges outlast the photic stimulation, may be associated with myoclonic jerks, or may spread and result in a generalized tonic-clonic seizure. If so defined, the EEG findings are strongly associated with epilepsy. Large amplitude following responses, occipital spikes or slow waves are seen in some normal subjects. Confusion may also be caused by the electrical recording of rhythmic contractions of scalp muscles in time with the flash – a so-called photomyoclonic response.

Photosensitivity is increased following deprivation of sleep. The response is attenuated if the flash is directed away from the fovea, and very considerably attenuated if one eye is covered. Occasional patients are more sensitive if the stimulus is diffused through closed eyelids but most patients are most sensitive with the eyes open. The most effective flash frequency varies between patients, but is usually 15–20 Hz.

In some photosensitive patients, paroxysmal EEG discharges will be induced by viewing static, continuously illuminated patterns. The patterns are even more evocative if oscillated in a direction orthogonal to its lines. Although these observations are principally of laboratory interest, discharges may be induced by striped patterns found in everyday life – such as escalator treads and fence palings. There may be some relation between these responses and the sense of discomfort experienced when viewing certain modern paintings, such as some of those of Brigid Riley.

Some photosensitive patients induce seizures in themselves, usually by waving the outstretched fingers in front of their eyes. Others may slowly close their eyelids, a stimulus which in them seems sufficient. Although some patients confess that they gain pleasure from the effects of the seizure discharge, this does not always seem to be the case.

Seizures in photosensitive subjects are commonly induced by television. Studies reviewed by Wilkins and colleagues [48] suggest that the evocative stimulus is the pattern of interlacing lines formed by the flying spot from the electron gun. The interlace is at half mains frequency (25 or 30 Hz). With large screens, or small screens viewed closely, the interlace has spatial characteristics that evoke seizure discharges. Preventive measures include viewing the screen from a greater distance, changing the set to one with a smaller tube or occluding one eye while viewing. This last suggestion is not really practical, but should certainly be considered if the set is approached closely for adjustment – though this can now largely be avoided by the use of infrared beams for controlling functions.

Although changes in light, or alternating light and dark stripe (pattern) are the most effective stimulus, some subjects have seizure discharges if they are exposed to sustained bright light after darkness, or vice versa – for example, on entering or leaving the cinema [49]. Morimoto and colleagues [50] have described such a patient though in this case the subject's propensity to reflex seizures extended to seizures induced by movement (p. 131) and by immersion in hot water.

Experimental studies reviewed by Anlezark [51] show that the photo-convulsive response can be abolished by the dopamine agonist, apomorphine, though the normal evoked potentials are unaffected. If clinical treatment is required, photosensitive epilepsy responds best to treatment with sodium valproate.

(b) Reading epilepsy

Primary reading epilepsy has recently been reviewed at length [52]. First described by Bickford in 1956, the seizures, triggered by reading, begin with myoclonic jerks in the region of the mouth and throat; sometimes these jerks are followed by a generalized convulsion if the subject persists in reading. In a few cases, seizures have been induced by asking the patients to perform articulatory or chewing movements, suggesting that afferent feedback from buccal and lingual muscles is important. In the majority of cases, however, it is the cortical elaboration of internal or external language that is important in precipitating seizures. The evidence for this is that in some patients an interesting conversation or heated argument, or writing, may also precipitate attacks [52].

During reading, the EEG usually shows focal epileptiform activity in the left frontotemporal region, or synchronous activity over both hemispheres.

Reading epilepsy usually begins in the second decade of life and may settle subsequently as the patient learns personal tricks to avoid the onset of facial jerks. Seizures may be controlled by clonazepam or sodium valproate [52].

(c) Reflex auditory epilepsy
The suggestion that it is 'cortical elaboration' of internal or external language that is the key to reading epilepsy is supported by parallel obervations in auditory epilepsy. Seizures have been reported to be caused by hearing bells and by music. In other instances, a stereotyped sound such as a frog croaking may precipitate a seizure after many repetitions (see [49] for references). Seizures produced by loud sounds occur in particular strains of mice and provide a model on which potential anticonvulsants can be tried.

(d) Reflex 'thinking' epilepsy
Seizures have been reported to be induced by playing chess or cards [49] and by mental arithmetic [53]. As in reading epilepsy, the specificity of the task is related to the probability of seizure discharge.

(e) Startle epilepsy
A sudden unexpected loud noise, or an unexpected hand on the shoulder when one thinks one is alone, produces a characteristic involuntary muscle response with eyelid closure and knee flexion. Some patients have an exaggerated response resulting in falls [54]. Other features of this syndrome include generalized muscle rigidity and prominent nocturnal myoclonus. This syndrome of hyperexplexia seems to differ from a true startle response, and is probably one of the stimulus-sensitive myoclonic disorders [54a]. In startle epilepsy [55], a sudden noise or other unexpected stimulus results in a sudden brief flattening of background activity of the EEG, followed by a seizure discharge. Reported patients may have either diffuse or hemispheric brain disease. If the latter, some at least of the seizures may be confined to the contralateral limbs. In startle epilepsy a non-habituating startle response seems to be followed by cortical embellishment [54a].

(f) Seizures induced by movements and other actions
Some subjects have seizures induced by movement and these movements may be stereotyped. Seizures have, for example, been reported on eating [56]. In this instance, for example, it has to be explored whether the seizures are due to mastication, swallowing, the resulting gastric distension, or the many bodily manoeuvres associated with eating. Such difficulties of analysis are common to many types of reflex epilepsy.

4.2.5 Emotional stress

A first seizure is such an alarming event that the patient will search for an explanation or 'cause' in order to make sense of his world. In the case of recurrent attacks, he will analyse day-to-day activities in an attempt to detect factors which precipitate seizures. Often seizures will be linked to a stressful event or period in the patient's life. Patients commonly cite overwork, a family row, a divorce or other personal factors. There has been little research to justify the presumption that such events precipitate seizures. The dearth of adequate research of the result of two factors: first, stress is difficult to quantify, varies from patient to patient, and in the same patient at different times; secondly, the widespread introduction of anticonvulsants in the late 1930s diverted attention from stress factors and de-emphasized their importance.

The literature does contain a few reports on stress as an aetiological factor for both single and recurrent seizures, and several workers have also looked at modification of stress factors as a possible method of control of epilepsy in patients with refractory seizures. Livingston [57] described six patients who only ever had seizures under emotionally stressful conditions. Interestingly, these 6 patients all had normal EEGs. Friis and Lund [58] found emotional stress to be the third most common relevant factor in a group of patients who only ever had what they termed 'provoked seizures'. Two-thirds of a group of 200 patients studied by Mattson and colleagues [59] reported that emotional stress precipitated their attacks. Feldman and Paul [60] identified specific emotional triggers in five patients with epilepsy. They played to the patients various recorded tapes of stressful events – for example, a domestic row. Some of the patients were seen to have seizures in response to certain tapes. When this occurred the seizure was recorded on video by the research workers. The video was then played back to the patient who then identified exactly what it was on the tape to which he was reacting. Feldman and Paul felt that once the association had been acknowledged, periodic reinforcement would lead to 'anticipatory inhibition' of seizures. They did find that after these video tape replay sessions there was some decrease in seizure frequency.

Aird [61] studied a group of 500 patients with drug-resistant epilepsy, and found that intense emotional reactions were the most common precipitating factors reported. He pointed out that such an evaluation is complicated by other seizure-inducing factors, such as sleep deprivation (p. 126), excessive use of stimulant drugs and alcohol (p. 127) which are often associated with stress.

Most of the work discussed above has been based on clinical observations and is largely anecdotal. Temkin and Davis [62] have, however, attempted to quantify stress as a risk factor for seizures. They studied 12 patients with severe epilepsy. The patients monitored the occurrence of seizures and stress levels over three months. High stress levels and stressful events were associated with more frequent seizures for most participants.

One proposed mechanism for the association between stress and seizures is hyperventilation. Mattson and colleagues [63] reported three patients who, when anxious, tended to hyperventilate unconsciously. At these times, EEG and clinical seizure activity increased, correlating with a reduction in alveolar

$p\text{CO}_2$. The hypothesis that anxiety leads to hyperventilation and, by lowering $p\text{CO}_2$, triggers the seizure activity was supported by their observation that administration of 5% carbon dioxide could prevent or terminate the seizure activity, even though anxiety and overbreathing continued. This is one of several mechanisms that might explain the precipitation of seizures by stress. Another might be alteration in neurotransmitter levels. However, since the 1940s, and particularly in the 1970s, attention has been drawn to the fact that episodic stresses can be linked with an increase in illness risk through less direct pathways.

In 1946, Hans Selye [64] proposed a mechanism for the link between episodic stresses and increases in the risk of illness. He claimed that when men or women identify change as threatening, they attempt to adapt to the adverse event. When the adaptation is difficult or unsuccessful, there is prolonged arousal, with chronic changes in autonomic function, hormonal levels and immune competence which leads to premature onset of illness. Rahe and colleagues [65] formulated in 1974 a model relating stress and illness. They assume that a subject's recent exposure to life stress is composed of events of varying significance. A subject's past experience may alter perceptions of the significance of these recent events. Ego defence mechanisms such as denial may diffract away the impact of certain events. Events not diffracted away may stimulate psychophysiological processes, that eventually lead to organ system dysfunction and bodily disease. There has since been much research on the relationship between stressful life events and physical and psychiatric illness, but as yet very little on psychosocial stress and the onset of epilepsy, or increases in seizure frequency in established epilepsy [62].

REFERENCES

1. Adams, R. D. and Lyon, G. (1982) *Neurology of Hereditary Metabolic Diseases of Children*. McGraw-Hill, St Louis.
2. Metrakos, J. D. and Metrakos, K. (1960) Genetics of convulsive disorders I. Introduction, problems, methods and baselines. *Neurology (Minneap.)*, **10**, 228–40.
3. Metrakos, K. and Metrakos, J. D. (1961) Genetics of convulsive disorders II. Genetic and electroencephalographic studies in centrencephalic epilepsy. *Neurology (Minneap.)*, **11**, 474–83.
4. Jennett, W. B. (1975) *Epilepsy after Non-Missile Head Injuries*, Heinemann, London.
5. Kudrjavcev, T., Schoenberg, B. S., Kurland, K. T. and Groover, R. V. (1985) Cerebral palsy: survival rates, associated handicap and distribution by clinical sub-type (Rochester, Mn, 1950–76). *Neurology*, **35**, 900–3.
6. Ounsted, C. (1967) Temporal lobe epilepsy: the problem of aetiology and prophylaxis. *J. R. Coll. Phys. Lond.*, **1**, 273–84.
7. Meldrum, B. S. and Brierley, J. B. (1973) Prolonged epileptic seizures in primates. Ischaemic cell change and its relations to ictal physiological events. *Arch. Neurol.*, **28**, 10–17.
8. Meldrum, B. S., Horton, R. W. and Brierley, J. B. (1974) Epileptic brain damage

in adolescent baboons following seizures induced by allylglycine. *Brain*, **97**, 407–18.

9. Legg, N. J., Gupta, P. C. and Scott, D. F. (1973) Epilepsy following brain abscess. A clinical and EEG study of 70 patients. *Brain*, **96**, 259–68.

9a. Yaqub, B. A., Panayiotopoulos, C. P., al Nozha, M. *et al.* (1987) Causes of late onset epilepsy in Saudi Arabia: the role of cerebral granuloma. *J. Neurol. Neurosurg. Psychiatr.*, **50**, 90–92.

10. Gannicliffe, A., Saldanha, J. A., Itzhaki, R. F. and Sutton, R. N. P. (1985) *Herpes simplex* viral DNA in temporal lobe epilepsy. *Lancet*, **i**, 214–15.

11. Estanol, B., Corona, T. and Abad, P. (1986) A prognostic classification of cerebral cysticercosis: therapeutic implications. *J. Neurol. Neurosurg. Psychiatr.*, **49**, 1131–34.

12. Cherry, J. D. and Shields, W. D. (1984) Recurrent seizures after diphtheria, tetanus and pertussis immunization. Cause and effect *v.* temporal association. *Am. J. Dis. Child.*, **138**, 904–7.

13. Lesser, R. P., Lüders, H., Dinner, D. S. and Morris, H. H. (1985) Epileptic seizures due to thrombotic and embolic cerebrovascular disease in older patients. *Epilepsia*, **26**, 622–30.

14. Hauser, W. A., Ramirez-Lassepas, M. and Rosenstein, R. (1984) Risk for seizures and epilepsy following cerebrovascular insults. *Epilepsia*, **25**, 666.

15. Shorvon, S. D., Gilliatt, R. W., Cox, T. C. S. and Yu, Y. L. (1984) Evidence of vascular disease from CT scanning in late onset epilepsy. *J. Neurol. Neurosurg. Psychiat.*, **47**, 225–30.

15a. Shinton, R. A., Gill, J. S., Zezulka, A. V. and Beavers, D. G. (1987) The treatment of epilepsy preceding stroke. *Lancet*, **i**, 11–12.

16. Kalbag, R. M. and Woolf, A. L. (1967) *Cerebral Venous Thrombosis: With Special Reference to Primary Aseptic Thrombosis*, Oxford University Press, London and New York.

17. Crawford, P. M., West, C. R., Shaw, M. D. M. and Chadwick, D. W. (1986) Cerebral arteriovenous malformations and epilepsy: factors in the development of epilepsy. *Epilepsia*, **27**, 270–5.

17a. Keranen, T., Tapaninaho, A., Hernesniemi, J. and Vapalahti, M. (1985) Late epilepsy after aneurysm operations. *Neurosurgery*, **17**, 897–900.

18. Dam, A., Fuglsang-Frederiksen, A., Svarre-Olsen, U. and Dam, M. (1985) Late onset epilepsy: etiologies, types of seizure and value of clinical investigation, EEG and computerised tomography scan. *Epilepsia*, **26,** 277–31.

18a. Kurtz, Z., Tookey, P. and Ross, E. M. (1986) The epidemiology of epilepsy in childhood, in Epilepsy in young people (eds E. Ross *et al.*) John Wiley, Chichester, pp. 13–21.

18b. Lühdorf, K., Jensen, L. K. and Plesner, A. M. (1986) Etiology of seizures in the elderly. *Epilepsia*, **27**, 458–63.

19. Spencer, D. D., Spencer, S. S., Mattson, R. H. and Williamson, P. D. (1984) Intracerebral masses in patients with intractable partial epilepsy. *Neurology*, **34**, 432–6.

20. Rich, K. M., Goldring, S. and Gado, M. (1985) Computed tomography in chronic seizure disorder caused by glioma. *Arch. Neurol.*, **42**, 26–7.

21. Thomas, D. G. T. and Graham, D. I. (1980) *Brain Tumours: Scientific Basis, Clinical Investigation and Current Therapy*, Butterworths, London.

22. Grant, C. and Warlow, C. (1985) Focal epilepsy in diabetic non-ketotic hypergly-caemia. *Br. Med. J.*, **290**, 1204–6.

23. Barclay, L. L., Zemcov, A., Blass, J. P. and Sansone, J. (1985) Survival in Alzheimer's disease and multi-infarct dementia. *Neurology*, **35**, 834–40.

23a. Hauser, W. A., Morris, M. L., Heston, L. L. and Anderson, V. E. (1986) Seizures and myoclonus in patients with Alzheimer's disease. *Neurology*, **36**, 1226–29.

24. Hauser, W. A. and Kurland, L. T. (1975) The epidemiology of epilepsy in Rochester, Minnesota, 1935 through 1967. *Epilepsia*, **16**, 1–66.

25. Hopkins, A. and Scambler, G. (1977) How doctors deal with epilepsy. *Lancet*, **i**, 183-6.

26. Rutter, M., Graham, P. and Yule, W. (1970) *A Neuropsychiatric Study of Childhood*. Spastics Medical Publications, London, and J. B. Lippincott, Philadelphia.

27. Langdon-Down, M. and Brain, W. R. (1929) Time of day in relation to convulsions in epilepsy. *Lancet*, **2**, 1029–32.

28. Broughton, R. J. (1984) Epilepsy and sleep: a synopsis and prospectus, in *Epilepsy, Sleep and Sleep Deprivation* (eds R. Degen and E. Niedermeyer), Elsevier, Amsterdam, pp. 317–56.

29. Degen, R. and Niedermeyer, E. (eds) (1984) *Epilepsy, Sleep and Sleep Deprivation*, Elsevier, Amsterdam.

30. Wieser, H. G. (1984) Temporal lobe epilepsy, sleep and arousal: Stereo-EEG findings, in *Epilepsy, Sleep and Sleep Deprivation* (eds R. Degen and E. Niedermeyer), Elsevier, Amsterdam, pp. 137–68.

31. Bernadina, B. D., Colamaria, V., Caponilla, G. and Bondavalli, S. (1984) Sleep and benign partial epilepsies of childhood, in *Epilepsy, Sleep and Sleep Deprivation* (eds R. Degen and E. Niedermeyer), Elsevier, Amsterdam, pp. 119–36.

32. Gibberd, F. B. and Bateson, M. C. (1974) Sleep epilepsy: its pattern and prognosis. *Br. Med. J.*, **1**, 403–5.

33. Niedermeycr, E. (1984) Awakening epilepsy ('Aufwach-Epilepsie') revisited 30 years later, in *Epilepsy, Sleep and Sleep Deprivation* (eds R. Degen and E. Niedermeyer), Elsevier, Amsterdam, pp. 85–96.

34. Gunderson, C. H., Dunne, P. B. and Feyer, T. L. (1973) Sleep deprivation seizures. *Neurology*, **23**, 678–86.

35. Victor, M. and Brausch, C. (1967) The role of abstinence in the genesis of alcoholic epilepsy. *Epilepsia*, **8**, 1–20.

36. Deisenhammer, E., Klinger, D. and Trägner, H. (1984) Epileptic seizures in alcoholism and diagnostic value of EEG after sleep deprivation. *Epilepsia*, **25**, 526–30.

37. McQuarrie, D. G. and Fingl, E. (1958) Effects of single doses and chronic administration of ethanol on experimental seizures in mice. *J. Pharmacol. Exp. Therapeut.*, **124**, 264–71.

38. Gibbins, R. J., Kalant, H., LeBlanc, A. E. and Clark, W. (1971) Sound induced seizures during ethanol withdrawal in mice. *Psychopharmacologia*, **22**, 24–49.

39. Klingman, W. O., Suter, C., Green, R. and Robinson, I. (1955) Role of alcoholism and magnesium deficiency in convulsions. *Trans. Am. Neurol. Assoc.*, **80**, 162–5.

40. Lerner, A. M., De Carli, L. M. and Davidson, C. S. (1958) Association of pyridoxine deficiency and convulsions in alcoholics. *Proc. Soc. Exp. Biol.*, **98**, 841–3.

41. Garland, H. G., Dick, A. P. and Whitty, C. W. M. (1943) Water-pitressin test in the diagnosis of epilepsy. *Lancet*, **ii**, 566–9.

42. Chan, A. W. K. (1985) Alcoholism and epilepsy. *Epilepsia*, **26**, 323–33.
43. Höppener, R. J., Kuyer, A., Van der Lugt, P. J. M. (1983) Epilepsy and alcohol: the influence of social alcohol intake on seizures and treatment in epilepsy. *Epilepsia*, **24**, 459–71.
44. Boston Collaborative Drug Surveillance Program (1972) *Lancet*, **ii**, 677–9.
45. Messing, R. O., Closson, R. G. and Simon, R. P. (1984) Drug induced seizures: A 10 year experience. *Neurology (Clevel.)*, **34**, 1582–6.
46. Logothetis, J. (1967) Spontaneous epileptic seizures and electroencephalographic change in the course of phenothiazine therapy. *Neurology (Minneap.)*, **17**, 869–77.
47. Convulsions associated with drug therapy (1981) *Adverse Drug React. Bull.* **87**, 316–19.
48. Wilkins, A. J., Binnie, C. D. and Darby, C. E. (1980) Visually induced seizures. *Prog. Neurobiol.*, **15**, 85–117.
49. Symonds, C. (1959) Excitation and inhibition in epilepsy. *Brain*, **82**, 10–146.
50. Morimoto, T., Hayakawa, T., Sugie, H. *et al.* (1985) Epileptic seizures precipitated by constant light, movement in daily life and hot water immersion. *Epilepsia*, **26**, 237–42.
51. Anlezark, G. M. (1984) Dopamine and serotonin in reflex epilepsy, in *Research Progress in Epilepsy* (ed. F. C. Rose), Pitman, London, pp. 126–34.
52. Saenz-Lope, E., Herranz-Tanarro, F. J. and Masdeu, J. C. (1985) Primary reading epilepsy. *Epilepsia*, **26**, 649–56.
53. Wilkins, A. J., Zifkin, B., Andermann, F. and McGovern, E. (1982) Seizures induced by thinking. *Ann. Neurol.*, **11**, 608–12.
54. Kurczynski, T. W. (1983) Hyperekplexia. *Arch. Neurol.*, **40**, 246–8.
54a. Wilkins, D. E., Hallet, M. and Wess, M. M. (1986) Audiogenic startle reflex of man and its relationship to startle syndromes: a review. *Brain*, **109**, 561–73.
55. Saenz-Lope, E., Herranz, F. J. and Masdeu, J. C. (1984) Startle epilepsy: a clinical study. *Ann. Neurol.*, **16**, 78–81.
56. Fiol, M. E., Leppik, I. E., Pretzel, K. L. (1986) Eating epilepsy: electroencephalographic and clinical study. *Epilepsia*, **27**, 441–5.
57. Livingston, M. D. (1956) Etiological factors in adult convulsions. *N. Engl. J. Med.*, **254**, 1211–16.
58. Friis, M. L. and Lund, M. (1974) Stress convulsions. *Arch. Neurol.*, **31**, 155–9.
59. Mattson, R., Lerner, E. and Dix, G. (1974) Precipitating and inhibiting factors in epilepsy: a statistical study. *Epilepsia*, **15**, 271–2.
60. Feldman, R. G. and Paul, N. L. (1976) Identity of emotional triggers in epilepsy. *J. Nerv. Ment. Dis.*, **162**, 345–53.
61. Aird, R. B. (1983) The importance of seizure-inducing factors in the control of refractory forms of epilepsy. *Epilepsia*, **24**, 567–83.
62. Temkin, N. R. and Davis, G. R. (1984) Stress as a risk factor for seizures among adults with epilepsy. *Epilepsia*, **24**, 450–6.
63. Mattson, R. H., Heninger, G. R., Gallagher, B. B. and Glaser, G. H. (1970) Psychophysiologic precipitates of seizures in epileptics. *Neurology*, **20**, 407.
64. Selye, H. (1946) The general adaptation syndrome and the diseases of adaptation. *J. Clin. Endocrinol.*, **6**, 117–230.
65. Rahe, R. H., Floistad, I., Bergan, T. *et al.* (1974) A model for life changes and illness research. *Arch. Gen. Psychiat.*, **31**, 172–7.

CHAPTER FIVE

The Genetic Basis of the Epilepsies

Sarah Bundey

5.1 INTRODUCTION

5.1.1 Inheritance of normal EEG patterns

Since EEG abnormalities are important in assessing the type, cause and prognosis of epilepsy, it is useful first to consider the normal EEG, its inheritance and the frequency of variations in the population.

Notable family studies on EEG patterns have been carried out by Vogel [1], summarized by Vogel and Motulsky [2]. Firstly, Vogel studied EEG patterns in 98 dizygous and 110 monozygous twin pairs. Such a study inevitably controls for age, which is a major cause of variability of EEG patterns, presumably due to degree of brain maturation. Vogel [1] found that there were 'no constant differences between monozygous twins in measurable (electro-encephalographic) traits'. In other words, the variability of the EEG in normal cicumstances is exclusively determined by heredity. A study from Denmark [3] showed that a small group of monozygous twins who had been separated from their co-twin shortly after birth, had very similar EEG recordings in adult life.

Table 5.1 summarizes some of the findings in Vogel's family studies.

Table 5.1 Family studies of normal EEG patterns [1]

EEG pattern in index case	Frequency in first degree relatives %		Frequency in healthy adult males
	At all ages	At age of greatest manifestation*	
Low voltage EEG	37	48 (over 19)	4.2
Occipital beta waves (frequenccy 16–19 Hz)	—	50 (over 19)	0.6
4–5 Hz rhythm in occipital region	10	—	0.12
Monotonous high alpha waves	—	57 (parents)	3.8
Variants of beta waves	Variable, according to precise pattern in proband; all influenced by age and sex		

*This age is given in brackets.

Approximately one-half of first degree relatives, if tested at the appropriate age, showed similar alpha wave rhythms as those in the index patient, suggesting autosomal dominant inheritance. There were two additional observations of interest. Firstly, for the relatively common alpha rhythm variant with low voltage, there was a frequency of 75% in children if both parents were affected, consistent with autosomal dominant inheritance, with half the children being heterozygous and a quarter of them being homozygous. Secondly, for the pattern of monotonous and regular alpha waves there was a frequency of affected parents that was greater than expected, suggesting that there might be assortative mating for this feature.

The family patterns and the relationships with age and sex seen with the beta wave variants suggested to Vogel that some of these traits were likely to have a multifactorial aetiology rather than a simple autosomal dominant one.

5.1.2   Inheritance of abnormal EEG patterns

There are certain distinctive EEG patterns that are found in patients with idiopathic epilepsy (although not at all ages) but which may also occur in non-epileptic individuals. Like the normal patterns described above, these abnormal ones also appear to be inherited. Generally they breed true within families, although by chance a relative may also have another EEG pattern because of the frequency of these in the normal population (Table 5.2).

Observations from family studies on five different types of EEG abnormalities are presented in Table 5.2, and the 40–50% occurrence in the first degree relatives of four of them suggest that these patterns too are inherited as

Table 5.2   Family studies of abnormal EEG patterns

EEG pattern in epileptic index patient	Frequency (%) of similar EEG pattern in:		
	Siblings of all ages	Siblings of a certain age range (given in brackets)	Controls
'Centrencephalic' trait: 3 Hz spike and wave [4]	37	>40 (5–16 years)	6
Centrotemporal focus [5, 6]	36	56 (6–10 years)	2
Spike-waves with theta background activity: 4–7 Hz rhythms [7]	46	56 (2–6 years)	10 (2–6 years)
Photoconvulsive reaction [8, 9]	23	41 (5–16 years)	7.6
Occipital delta 2–4 Hz rhythms [10]	10	21 (5–6 years)	6.8 (3–4 years)

distinct, age-dependent, autosomal dominant traits. However the development of the photoconvulsive reaction appears to depend on additional factors such as the presence or absence of occipital delta rhythms [8]. These delta rhythms probably also reflect a genetically determined function of the brain, and may protect against the development of some abnormal EEG patterns [10].

5.1.3 Inheritance of convulsions

Those first degree relatives who have not inherited the same abnormal EEG pattern that is present in the index patient do not appear to be at increased risk for epilepsy [4]. However, reference to Tables 5.2 and 5.4 shows that only about one-quarter of relatives with abnormal EEG patterns actually develop epilepsy. Therefore, for those relatives who have inherited the EEG abnormality, other factors must be important in determining whether or not that particular individual convulses. These are likely to be a mixture of both genetic and environmental factors.

The twin studies of Lennox [11] and Gedda and Tatarelli [12] demonstrated that genetic factors must be of great importance. These workers observed high concordance rates of monozygous (MZ) twins compared to dizygous (DZ) twins for convulsions, for the same clinical type of convulsion and for the same type of EEG abnormality; the figures are summarized in Table 5.3. It is unusual to find such high concordance rates in monozygotic twins for a trait that has a multifactorial aetiology [13] suggesting that the genetic component must be very high.

Table 5.3   Epilepsy in twins [11, 12]

	Concordance (%) in	
	MZ twins n = 64	DZ twins n = 66
Any type of epilepsy	87	12
Same type of epilepsy	82	
Same type of EEG pattern	61	

Doose *et al.* [14] have analysed families of index patients who had suffered from absence epilepsy associated with spike-wave patterns on their EEGs. They concluded that the different EEG patterns of photically evoked spike waves, theta rhythms, and spike-waves at rest and during hyperventilation, all influenced the course, onset and development of epilepsy in their subjects. Since these EEG patterns are more frequently found in the siblings of epileptic index patients who also possess them, rather than in the siblings of other epileptic index patients, they are presumably genetically caused. These associated EEG features provide some examples of how other genetic factors influence the development of convulsions. The maturation of EEG patterns has been shown to depend upon age. Another constitutional factor affecting the development of epilepsy is sex. Some types of epilepsy, such as childhood absence epilepsy, and benign childhood epilepsy with centrotemporal spikes, are more common in females, and the relatives of female probands are at greater risk for epilepsy [14, 15]. In contrast, myoclonic astatic epilepsy of childhood is commoner in males [16].

It is possible that for some types of epilepsy, perinatal hypoxia is one environmental factor which may encourage the development of overt epilepsy in an individual who is genetically predisposed [17, 18].

The environmental trigger of a high fever does not produce convulsions in all children with an inherited predisposition to generalized epilepsy. The tendency to convulse after a fever is a specific genetic trait, and is described in the next section.

5.2 EPILEPSY PRODUCED BY ENVIRONMENTAL EVENTS

5.2.1 Convulsions produced by fever

Febrile convulsions are largely a benign condition, in which brief convulsions occur with upper respiratory tract infection complicated by a temperature greater than 39°C (Chapter 15). The disorder occurs in 3–7% of children aged between six months and five years. About 40% of these children can be shown to have EEG abnormalities that are characteristic of idiopathic epilepsy [19]. About 4% of index patients develop chronic epilepsy, due either to damage of the temporal lobe during a prolonged fit, or due to a genetic predisposition to generalized epilepsy. In the case of the latter, the febrile convulsion appears to be merely a manifestation of the genetic predisposition. The small risk of 4% for chronic epilepsy makes it clear that the occurrence of febrile convulsions has not worsened the prognosis for an individual who has an inherited epileptic trait.

There appears to be a specific genetic predisposition to convulse with fever, because the risk of epilepsy in relatives of index patients with febrile convulsions relates mainly to febrile convulsions only, and there is only a small risk for other forms of epilepsy. Van den Berg [20] demonstrated in a large prospective study that the risk of febrile convulsions occurring in the siblings of index patients was 37/432 (8.5%). Higher recurrence risks had been given by two series from Japan, where the incidence of febrile convulsions in the population appears to be higher than in America and Europe. In Japan, the incidence of febrile convulsions in siblings of index patients was between 16% and 19% if neither parent was affected, between 23% and 36% if one parent was affected, and was between 52% and 66% if both parents were affected [19, 21]. The incidence in siblings was greater if the index case was a male, or if the index case had more than four febrile convulsions. These observations led Tsuboi [19] and Fukuyama *et al.* [21] to postulate that the predisposition to febrile convulsions is polygenic in nature.

There is a small but definite increased risk of siblings of index patients with febrile convulsions developing unprovoked epilepsy. In a useful study from Rochester [22] this risk was three times the population risk. This risk presumably reflects the fact that many children with febrile convulsions have a predisposition to generalized epilepsy, a predisposition which is shared by half their first degree relatives.

5.2.2 Convulsions produced by trauma

The prognosis for epilepsy following head injury, perinatal problems or other cerebral insult depends in part upon whether the individual concerned has or has not a genetic predisposition to epilepsy. This was clearly shown by Rimoin and Metrakos [23] who studied two groups of hemiplegic patients, the first of which suffered from convulsions and the second did not. Both groups were similar with regard to the cause and severity of their hemiplegia. The frequency of convulsions or an epileptiform EEG was significantly higher in the relatives of the first group of hemiplegics than for the relatives of the second group. The authors concluded that a genetic predisposition to epilepsy played a significant role in determining whether or not a particular cerebral insult was sufficient to cause convulsions. Moreover, they found that the relatives of hemiplegics who did not convulse themselves had a lower incidence of epilepsy than the relatives of controls, suggesting that the non-convulsing hemiplegics had less innate tendency to convulse than the population at large.

5.2.3 Convulsions produced by flickering light or by reading

The occurrence of photosensitive epilepsy in the first degree relatives of index cases who have clinical epilepsy produced by flickering light is about 2–3% [24]. However, the occurrence of a photosensitive EEG in the relatives of index cases is higher than this, rising to 35–50% in teenage brothers and sisters [8, 9]. A different trait results in a tendency to convulse on reading, in which the convulsion may be averted if the individual ceases to read. This condition also appears to be autosomal dominant, with variable penetrance [25].

5.3 EPILEPTIC SYNDROMES

The following classification of specific epileptic syndromes is taken from Dreifuss *et al.* [26]. Their clinical and EEG features are described in Chapter 3, and, in more detail, in a monograph [27]. Here, I shall describe mainly the genetic aspects.

5.3.1   Benign childhood epilepsy with centrotemporal spikes

This was one of the first types of epilepsy in which family studies were performed, regarding both the incidence of seizures in relatives, and the incidence of centrotemporal foci on EEGs. Two studies have shown that the occurrence of the same type of epilepsy in siblings is 10–15% [6, 15]; the occurrence of the same type of EEG abnormality, however, is higher than this, between 30% and 40%, with the highest frequency between the ages of six and ten years [5, 15]. Both groups of authors conclude that the EEG pattern is inherited as an autosomal dominant trait, with age-dependent penetrance.

5.3.2   Childhood epilepsy with occipital paroxysms

This is a benign and specific type of epilepsy, affecting children particularly aged 7–8 years, and with a good prognosis. Gastaut [28] observed a family history in about half of his patients and Beaumanoir [29] in about one-third of her patients. The complete genetic data was not presented, and in any case would be difficult to interpret with such small numbers. However it does appear that this type of epilepsy has a specific genetic predisposition that is probably distinct from that for other types.

5.3.3   Benign neonatal convulsions

Plouin [30] reviewed the literature and concluded that there were two types of benign neonatal convulsions. The first type occurs around the fifth day of life; no cause can be found, there is no family history and outcome is favourable. The second type occurs earlier and is associated with a constant family history showing autosomal dominant inheritance. About 10–20% of individuals with the dominant form develop fits later in childhood, but these rarely lead to serious epilepsy.

5.3.4   Benign myoclonic epilepsy in infancy, childhood absence epilepsy, juvenile absence epilepsy, juvenile myoclonic epilepsy, epilepsy with grand mal seizures on awakening

These five clinical syndromes are considered together because they are probably all manifestations of generalized idiopathic epilepsy, with a similar genetic predisposition, but with varying age of onset producing different clinical pictures. Many patients with one of the last four clinical pictures also develop one of the other types of epilepsy [14, 31]. The main evidence for a common genetic predisposition comes from two studies: that of Doose *et al.* [14] on spike-wave absences and that of Tsuboi and Christian [32] on juvenile myoclonic epilepsy. The evidence for benign myoclonic epilepsy of infancy belonging to the same group is less strong, as so few patients have been described, but Dravet *et al.* [33] consider this syndrome to belong to the same category.

Doose *et al.* [14] studied the families of 252 index patients who had absence epilepsy and 3 Hz spike-waves on their EEGs. Six per cent of parents and 7% of siblings had convulsions, which consisted of grand mal seizures (in 38%), absences (in 9%), astatic fits (in 1%), myoclonic fits (in 1%), focal seizures (in 2%) and other fits, including febrile convulsions, in 56%. These findings demonstrate that, given a common genetic predisposition, other factors act to determine what type of epilepsy (if any) develops. The same spike-wave pattern found in the index patients was observed in up to 20% of siblings, and was related to age.

Tsuboi and Christian [32] had similar findings in their study of 319 index patients with juvenile myoclonic epilepsy. Of the first degree relatives, 15% had specific spike wave patterns on their EEGs and 4–5% of parents, siblings and offspring suffered from epilepsy. These convulsions took the form of juvenile myoclonic epilepsy (in 15%), grand mal seizures on awakening (in 17%) and juvenile absence epilepsy (in 14%), with other types making up the remainder. Delgado-Escueta and Enrile-Bacsal [31] also found a variety of clinical types of epilepsy in the first degree relatives of their 43 index patients. Thus all these types of epilepsy may arise from the same genetic predisposition.

5.3.5 West syndrome (infantile spasms)

In about two-thirds of cases, infantile spasms have a known aetiology and their risk of recurrence in sibs depends upon this. For example, infections would rarely produce infantile spasms in a second child. On the other hand tuberous sclerosis is an autosomal dominant condition, usually caused by a new mutation. If however a parent is affected then the risk of recurrence is 1 in 2. A number of metabolic disorders, such as phenylketonuria, can produce infantile spasms, and as these conditions are often autosomal recessive, there is a 1 in 4 risk of recurrence. The Aicardi syndrome is an example of a developmental anomaly affecting the retinae and corpus callosum; it is probably an X-linked dominant condition in which nearly all affected males die *in utero*. All patients are female, and as there is no recurrence risk for siblings, they are thought to be new mutations. Another cerebral malformation syndrome, lissencephaly, may be associated with infantile spasms; this disorder is autosomal recessive and there are easily recognizable dysmorphic features. There is one family described with infantile spasms and mental retardation inherited as an X-linked recessive [34].

Empiric risks of recurrence for siblings have to be used when no cause can be found for the infantile spasms in the index patient. These risks are low, namely 1–3% [35–37].

5.3.6   Myoclonic astatic epilepsy of early childhood

Doose [16] considered that this clinical type of epilepsy was distinct from the idiopathic generalized epilepsy, with clinical picture varying according to age of onset, which was described earlier. Doose studied the families of 100 index patients, among whom there were twice as many males as females. He found a greater incidence of affected relatives with the same type of epilepsy than in any other type of epilepsy. Of the 154 siblings 16% had epilepsy as did 5% of 198 parents. An abnormal EEG was found in 46% of siblings. When giving genetic counselling to families it should be borne in mind that, unlike most idiopathic epilepsies, this type may have an unfavourable course, particularly if the epilepsy starts early in life. Neurological signs with dementia may develop [16].

5.3.7   Early myoclonic encephalopathy

Aicardi reviewed 25 cases occurring in 28 families [38] and Bundey and Griffiths [39] observed two further families. In the Aicardi series, the total number of siblings is not given, but is likely to have been about 50. On this assumption, the combined data give 11 affected siblings out of 54 and one instance of parental consanguinity. These data would fit autosomal recessive inheritance. Aicardi points out that specific metabolic disorders (such as hyperglycinemia, D-glyceric acidemia and propionic acidemia) can cause this clinical syndrome and so should be searched for in all cases.

5.3.8   Severe myoclonic epilepsy in infants

Although an appreciable minority of patients have relatives with epilepsy [40] the data are incomplete and the mode of inheritance, or empirical risks of recurrence, are not known.

5.3.9   Epilepsy with continuous spikes and waves during slow sleep

This is a rare disorder with a poor prognosis. There is no reported occurrence in siblings.

5.3.10   Landau-Kleffner syndrome

This is an uncommon and acute disorder of language, accompanied by epilepsy in about two-thirds of cases, and by multifocal spikes and waves on the EEG in all cases. It may be due to an encephalopathy. There is no reported recurrence of the Landau-Kleffner syndrome in relatives, but the relatives of those patients with epilepsy can have an increased risk of epilepsy [41]. Presumably an inherited tendency to convulse determines whether or not a patient receiving the cerebral insult which causes the Landau-Kleffner syndrome will also develop epilepsy.

5.3.11 Progressive myoclonic epilepsies of childhood and adolescence

There are two main types [41a]. Lafora body disease is a rare disorder in which myoclonic epilepsy develops at around the age of 15 and is accompanied by progressive dementia and death within about ten years. Inclusion bodies (Lafora bodies) are seen in a variety of tissues. It is an autosomal recessive disease and is probably genetically heterogenous. For example, Kraus-Ruppert *et al.* [42] described two brothers, with onset at 20 years and a milder, more protracted illness, who had Lafora bodies at autopsy; a further family with a mild disorder was described by Sukuki *et al.* [43].

There is a form of progressive myoclonic epilepsy which is less severe and which has a slightly earlier age of onset; no Lafora bodies are found in tissues. This is particularly common in the countries bordering the Baltic Sea, leading to a suggestion that it be termed 'Baltic myoclonus' [44]. In Finland 1 in 20 000 may be affected [45]. This type of myoclonic epilepsy is also an autosomal recessive condition, as the Finnish study [45] observed an equal sex ratio of patients, a proportion of affected siblings equalling 0.26, and healthy parents but a parental consanguinity rate of 22%. It is an important condition to recognize as it responds well to sodium valproate but neurological deterioration, which may occur naturally is more marked following treatment with phenytoin [44].

5.4 EMPIRICAL RISKS USED IN GENETIC COUNSELLING

5.4.1 Risks for siblings

A summary of these is presented in Table 5.4. Sometimes, when advising relatives on recurrence risks, it is not possible to determine the precise type of epilepsy in the index patient. If this is not known, the empirical risk of recurrence for siblings, of recurrent, non-febrile seizures is about 4% [46]. The total risk for epilepsy in siblings, including single and febrile convulsions, lies between 9% and 11%. These risks are largely those for epilepsy developing in childhood. Longer follow-up periods are likely to give even higher figures.

5.4.2 Risks for offspring

It is not so easy to obtain figures for the offspring of index patients, because they are a generation younger and therefore not so readily observed. Moreover the precise type of epilepsy in the index patient may well not be known by the

The Genetic Basis of the Epilepsies

Table 5.4   Risks to siblings of epilepsy (excluding febrile or non-recurrent seizures)

Clinical type of epilepsy	Risks for same type of epilepsy (%)
Febrile convulsions [19, 21, 22]	10–20
Begign childhood epilepsy with centrotemporal spikes [6, 15]	10–15
Benign familial neonatal convulsions [30]	50
Generalized idiopathic epilepsy (includes the absence and grand mal epilepsies) [4, 14, 32]	4–8
Idiopathic infantile spasms [35–37]	1–3
Myoclonic astatic epilepsy of early childhood [7, 16]	12–16*
Early myoclonic encephalopathy [38]†	~ 25
Progressive myoclonic epilepsies of childhood and adolescence [45]†	25
Symptomatic epilepsy [23]	2
Other types of epilepsy, or type of epilepsy not known [46]	4

* This figure includes febrile convulsions as these may be the first manifestation of myoclonic astatic epilepsy.
† These syndromes are heterogenous.

time he/she is an adult and asks for genetic advice concerning risks for children. However, the above study from Rochester [46] and two others [47, 48] have specifically addressed this problem. It has been shown that if one parent has epilepsy, the risk for each offspring developing epilepsy is about 4%. Janz and Beck-Mannagetta [47] observed that amongst 768 offspring who had one epileptic parent, there were 26 (3.4%) who had afebrile recurrent seizures. This proportion was likely to increase, as most of the offspring were still children. It is likely that very long term follow-up studies would show even more substantial risk in the siblings of affected children, as the cumulative risk to the eighth decade of life of more than one non-febrile seizure has been shown to be more than 3% (Chapter 1). Tsuboi and Endo [48] and Annegers *et al.* [46] have calculated from their observed data on 698 and 113 offspring respectively that the cumulative risk for recurrent epilepsy to the age of 20 is 4.2 and 4.1%. Figure 1.2 indicates that the cumulative risk for the population as a whole is 1.0% by this age. The total risk of convulsions of any sort, including isolated seizures and febrile convulsions, is 11–13%. These risks apply if the affected parent has focal or generalized epilepsy, but are only just increased over the population risk if the parent has symptomatic epilepsy. It is interesting that Tsuboi and Endo [48] found specific spike and wave abnormalities in the EEGs of 25–37% of the offspring of epileptic parents, suggesting that many of the parents were transmitting an autosomal dominant trait to half of their children.

If both parents are epileptic, the risks are probably similar to those for families in which two first degree relatives are epileptic [4, 46], namely between 10% and 13%.

REFERENCES

1. Vogel, F. (1970) The genetic basis of the normal human electroencephalogram (EEG). *Hum. Genet.*, **10**, 91–114.
2. Vogel, F. and Motulsky, A. G. (1979) *Human Genetics: Problems and Approaches.* Springer-Verlag, Berlin.
3. Juel-Nielsen, N. and Harvald, B. (1958) The electroencephalogram in uniovular twins brought up apart. *Acta Genet. Stat. Med.*, **8**, 57–64.
4. Metrakos, J. D. and Metrakos, K. (1966) Childhood epilepsy of sub-cortical ('centrencephalic') origin. *Clin. Paediatr.*, **5**, 536–42.
5. Bray, P. F. and Wiser, W. C. (1964) Evidence for a genetic aetiology of temporal-central abnormalities in focal epilepsy. *N. Engl. J. Med.*, **271**, 926–33.
6. Bray, P. F. and Wiser, W. C. (1965) Hereditary characteristics of familial temporal-central focal epilepsy. *Pediatrics*, **36**, 207–11.
7. Doose, H., Gerken, H., Leonhardt, R., *et al.* (1970) Centrecephalic myoclonic-astatic petit mal. *Neuropädiatrie*, **2**, 59–78.
8. Doose, H., Gerken, H., Hien-Völpel, K. F. and Völzke, E. (1969) Genetics of photosensitive epilepsy. *Neuropädiatrie*, **1**, 56–73.
9. Doose, H. and Gerken, H. (1973) On the genetics of EEG-anomalies in childhood. IV Photoconvulsive reaction. *Neuropädiatrie*, **4**, 162–71.
10. Gerken, H. and Doose, H. (1972) On the genetics of EEG-anomalies in childhood. II Occipital 2–4/s rhythm. *Neuropädiatrie*, **3**, 437–54.
11. Lennox, W. G. (1951) The heredity of epilepsy as told by relatives and twins. *JAMA*, **146**, 529–36.
12. Gedda, L. and Tatarelli, R. (1971) Essential isochronic epilepsy in MZ twin pairs. *Acta Genet. Med. Gemellol.*, **20**, 380–3.
13. Smith, C. (1970) Heritability of liability and concordance in monozygous twins. *Ann. Hum. Genet.*, **34**, 85–91.
14. Doose, H., Gerken, H., Horstmann, T. and Völzke, E. (1973) Genetic factors in spike-wave absences. *Epilepsia*, **14**, 57–75.
15. Heijbel, J., Blom, S. and Rasmuson, M. (1975) Benign epilepsy of childhood with centrotemporal EEG foci: a genetic study. *Epilepsia*, **16**, 285–93.
16. Doose, H. (1985) Myoclonic astatic epilepsy of early childhood, in *Epileptic Syndromes in Infancy, Childhood and Adolescence* (eds J. Roger *et al.*), John Libbey, London and Paris, pp. 78–88.
17. Gerken, H., Kiefer, R., Doose, H. and Völzke, E. (1977) Genetic factors in childhood epilepsy with focal sharp waves. I Clinical data and familial morbidity for seizures. *Neuropädiatrie*, **8**, 3–9.
18. Gastaut, H. (1985) Benign epilepsy of childhood with occipital paroxysms, in *Epileptic Syndromes in Infancy, Childhood and Adolescence* (eds J Roger *et al.*), John Libbey, London and Paris, pp. 159–70.
19. Tsuboi, T. (1982) Febrile convulsions, In *Genetic Basis of the Epilepsies* (eds V. E. Anderson *et al.*), Raven Press, New York pp. 123–34.

20. Van den Berg, B. (1974) Studies on convulsive disorders in young children. IV Incidence of convulsions among siblings. *Dev. Med. Child Neurol.*, **16**, 457–64.
21. Fukuyama, Y., Kagawa, K. and Tanaka, K. (1979) A genetic study of febrile convulsions. *Eur. Neurol.*, **18**, 166–82.
22. Hauser, W. A., Annegers, J. F., Anderson, V. E. and Kurland, L. T. (1985) The risk of seizure disorders among relatives of children with febrile convulsions. *Neurology*, **35**, 1268–73.
23. Rimoin, D. L. and Metrakos, J. D. (1961) The genetics of convulsive disorders in the families of hemiplegics, in *Proceedings of the 2nd International Congress of Human Genetics 1961 III*, Instituto G. Mendel, Rome, pp. 1655–8.
24. Jeavons, P. M. and Harding, G. F. A. (1975) Photosensitive epilepsy: a review of the literature and a study of 460 patients, in *Clinics in Developmental Medicine*, **56**, 1–121. Spastics International Publications and William Heinemann Medical Books, London.
25. Daly, R. F. and Forster, F. M. (1975) Inheritance of reading epilepsy. *Neurology*, **25**, 1051–4.
26. Dreifuss, F. E., Martinez-Lage, M., Roger, J., *et al.* (1985) Proposal for classification of epilepsies and epileptic syndromes. *Epilepsia*, **26**, 268–78.
27. Roger, J., Dravet, C., Bureau, M., *et al.* (eds) (1985) *Epileptic Syndromes in Infancy, Childhood and Adolescence*, John Libbey, London and Paris.
28. Gastaut, H. (1982) A new type of epilepsy: benign partial epilepsy of childhood with occipital spike waves. *Clin. Electroenceph.*, **13**, 13–22.
29. Beaumanoir, A. (1983) Infantile epilepsy with occipital focus and good prognosis. *Eur. Neurol.*, **22**, 43–52.
30. Plouin, P. (1985) Benign neonatal convulsions, in *Epileptic Syndromes in Infancy, Childhood and Adolescence* (eds J. Roger *et al.*), John Libbey, London and Paris, pp. 2–9.
31. Delgado-Escueta, A. V. and Enrile-Bacsal, F. (1984) Juvenile myoclonic epilepsy of Janz. *Neurology*, **34**, 285–94.
32. Tsuboi, T. and Christian, W. (1973) On the genetics of the primary generalized epilepsy with sporadic myoclonias of impulsive petit mal type. *Hum. Genet.*, **19**, 155–82.
33. Dravet, C., Bureau, M. and Roger, J. (1985) Benign myoclonic epilepsy in infants, in *Epileptic Syndromes in Infancy, Childhood and Adolescence* (eds J. Roger *et al.*), John Libbey, London and Paris, pp. 51–7.
34. Feinberg, A. P. and Leahy, W. R. (1977) Infantile spasms: a case report of sex-linked inheritance. *Dev. Med. Child Neurol.*, **19**, 524–6.
35. Bundey, S. and Carter, C. O. (1974) Recurrence risks in severe undiagnosed mental deficiency. *J. Ment. Def. Res.*, **18**, 115–34.
36. Fleiszar, K. A., Daniel, W. L. and Imrey, P. B. (1977) Genetic study of infantile spasms with hypsarrhythania. *Epilepsia*, **18**, 55–62.
37. Riikonen, R. and Donner, M. (1979) Incidence and aetiology of infantile spasms from 1960 to 1976: a population study in Finland. *Devel. Med. Child Neurol.*, **21**, 333–43.
38. Aicardi, J. (1985) Early myoclonic encephalopathy, in *Epileptic Syndromes in Infancy, Childhood and Adolescence* (eds J. Roger *et al.*), John Libbey, London and Paris, pp. 12–21.

39. Bundey, S. and Griffiths, M. (1977) Recurrence risks in families of children with symmetrical spasticity. *Dev. Med. Child Neurol.*, **19**, 179–91.

40. Dravet, C., Bureau, M. and Roger, J. (1985) Severe myoclonic epilepsy in infants, in *Epileptic Syndromes in Infancy, Childhood and Adolescence* (eds J Roger *et al.*), John Libbey, London and Paris, pp. 58–67.

41. Beaumanoir A. (1985) The Landau-Kleffner Syndrome, in *Epileptic Syndromes in Infancy, Childhood and Adolescence* (eds J Roger *et al.*), John Libbey, London and Paris, pp. 181–91.

41a. Berkovic, S. F., Andermann, F., Carpenter, S. and Wolfe, L. S. (1986) Progressive myoclonus epilepsies: specific causes and diagnosis. *New Engl. J. Med.*, **315**, 296–305.

42. Kraus-Ruppert, R., Ostertag, B., and Häfner, H. (1970) A study of the late form (type Lundborg) of progressive myoclonic epilepsy. *J. Neurol. Sci.*, **11**, 1–15.

43. Sukuki, K., David, E. and Kutschuman, B. (1971) Presenile dementia with 'Lafora-like' intraneuronal inclusions. *Arch. Neurol.*, **25**, 69–80.

44. Eldridge, R., Iivanainen, M., Stern, R., *et al.* (1983) 'Baltic' myoclonus epilepsy: hereditary disorder of childhood made worse by phenytoin. *Lancet* **ii**, 838–42.

45. Norio, R. and Koskiniemi, M. (1979) Progressive myoclonus epilepsy: genetic and nosological aspects with special reference to 107 Finnish patients. *Clin. Genet.*, **15**, 382-98.

46. Annegers, J. F., Hauser, W. A., Anderson, V. E. and Kurland, L. T. (1982) The risks of seizure disorders among relatives of patients with childhood onset epilepsy. *Neurology*, **32**, 174–9.

47. Janz, D. and Beck-Mannagetta, G. (1982) Epilepsy and neonatal seizures in the offspring of parents with epilepsy, in *Genetic Basis of the Epilepsies* (eds V. E. Anderson *et al.*), Raven Press, New York, pp. 135–43.

48. Tsuboi, T. and Endo, S. (1977) Incidence of seizures and EEG abnormalities among offspring of epileptic parents. *Hum. Genet.*, **36**, 173–89.

CHAPTER SIX

The First Seizure, and the Diagnosis of Epilepsy

Patients commonly present to neurologists after a first seizure. Community surveys have estimated that up to 5.9% [1, 2] of the population will experience at least one non-febrile seizure at some stage of their life. Most patients with seizures are referred to hospital for help with management after the first seizure [3]. Questions that are often raised by the patients themselves include the following. How many patients go on to have subsequent seizures, and by the definition outlined in Chapter 1 become 'epileptic'? (i.e. have more than one non-febrile seizure). What factors are associated with recurrence? How many subjects have some definite cause established for their first seizure, and what investigations are appropriate? Should anticonvulsants be given to reduce the chances of a subsequent seizure? What is the effect of the first seizure upon the life of the patient? This chapter outlines what information there is in response to these questions.

6.1 THE RISK OF RECURRENCE AFTER AN INITIAL SEIZURE

Anthony Hopkins and Andrea Garman

The risk of seizure recurrence after the first seizure has been addressed in eight previous studies (Table 6.1). The recurrence rates obtained range from 27% to 71%. Broadly speaking, three of these studies [4, 6, 9] found that only about a third of the patients presenting with a single seizure had a second seizure, and a further group [5, 7, 10, 11] found that about two-thirds had a second seizure.

Differences in method that may at least in part account for these different results include (1) the size of the sample; (2) the seizure types studied; (3) the time elapsed between the first seizure and the study entry point; (4) differences in exclusions made for allegedly 'provoked and symptomatic seizures'; (5) anticonvulsant treatment, and (6) length of follow-up. The studies are briefly reviewed below.

In 1959 Thomas [4] reported a recurrence of seizures in 27% of 48 patients evaluated in his EEG laboratory for a single convulsive seizure. No patients

Table 6.1   Studies of recurrence rates after the first seizure

	No. of patients	Recurrence (%)	Mean age in years (range)	Mean follow up in months (range)
Thomas (1959) [4]	48	27	(2–66)	(42–102)
Johnson *et al.* (1972) [5]	77	64	23.2 (17–48)	36
Saunders and Marshall (1975) [6]	39	33	36 (15–57)	26 (10–48)
Blom *et al.* (1978) [7]	74	58	(0–15)	36
Cleland *et al.* (1982) [8]	70	39	36 (16–65)	57 (36–120)
Hauser *et al.* (1982) [9]	244	27	(0–40)	22 (6–55)
Elwes *et al.* (1985) [10]	133	71	21 (2–74)	15 (1–69)
Annegers *et al.* (1986) [11]	424	56	(0–55+)	60
Lühdorf *et al.* (1986) [11a]	151	67	>60	12
Royal College of Physicians Study [12]	408	see Fig. 6.1	(16–79)	(1–30)

were excluded from the study on the grounds that the cause of the seizure, such as alcohol, was known.

Johnson *et al.* [5] studied 77 men enlisted in the Navy who were admitted to hospital after a single convulsion, seizure or unexplained loss of consciousness. Of these men 64% had subsequent seizures within the next three years. These workers were only interested in those patients for whom there could be found no organic causes for their presenting symptoms at first evaluation. They also excluded any patient with chronic alcoholism. No anticonvulsant medication was given to these patients.

In a study of 39 patients with a single seizure of any kind referred to an EEG laboratory, Saunders and Marshall [6] reported a recurrence rate of 33%. Follow-up varied from ten months to four years. The interval between the attack and the EEG varied between three weeks and five months. They excluded any seizures thought to be related to drug withdrawal, alcohol intake, head injury, and heart disease.

Blom *et al.* [7] reported that 58% of a group of 74 children identified at the time of the first seizure had a recurrence within three years. No patients were excluded on the grounds that the cause of the seizure was known. Some seizures in association with fever were included.

Cleland *et al.* [8] studied retrospectively 70 adult patients of whom 39% had subsequent seizures. Follow-up ranged from three to ten years. These patients were seen between two and ten weeks after a witnessed major convulsion. They excluded patients whose seizures had been associated with head injury or intoxication by drugs, or who had already been started on anticonvulsants at the time of the first neurological consultation.

Hauser *et al.* [9] studied 244 children and adults seen after their first seizure and made no exclusion for seizure type. Of these patients 27% recurred in the next three years. They excluded a group of patients with 'acute symptomatic seizures' such as those seizures occurring in the first week after the onset of an acute neurological event such as a stroke, cranial trauma, and a central nervous system infection. They also excluded seizures occurring concurrently with an acute systemic metabolic disturbance such as uraemia, hyponatraemia or hypoglycaemia. Febrile convulsions and alcohol withdrawal seizures were also excluded. About two-thirds of these patients were on anticonvulsants, though compliance during the study period was not monitored by blood levels.

Elwes *et al.* [10] studied 133 children and adults. A recurrence rate of 71% was obtained after three or four years. This study was unusual in so far as a proportion of the patients were identified retrospectively, having already relapsed. This must account in part for their very high relapse rate. They excluded seizures related to alcohol withdrawal, drugs, acute metabolic disturbance or fever. No patient was given anticonvulsants after the first seizure.

Annegers and colleagues (including Hauser) [11] followed up 424 patients with initial seizures identified through the medical record linkage system for residents of Rochester, Minnesota, for the period of 1935–79. In so far as this is a community-based survey, the results are perhaps of greater interest than the others listed above. Exclusions were similar to those of Hauser's study [9]. The risks of recurrence were 9% by one month, 21% by three months, 30% by six months, 36% by one year, 48% by three years and 56% by five years. Both this study, and that of Hauser and colleagues [9] used appropriate methods for analysing losses to follow up when estimating risk.

6.2   FACTORS THAT INCREASE THE PROBABILITY OF RECURRENCE

Anthony Hopkins and Andrea Garman

The sample size of the studies of first seizure patients already mentioned have all been too small to study in depth factors which are associated with recurrence, and to provide sound prognostic guidance. Even the larger studies [9, 11] found that low recurrence rates precluded detection of any but the most potent risk factors. Neither of these studies showed any effect of age or sex upon the rate of recurrence.

6.2.1 Prior neurological insult, and seizure type

Hauser *et al.* [9] found that patients with a history of prior neurological insult, for example, stroke, head trauma, or central nervous system infection had a significantly higher risk of recurrence. The rate of recurrence for the group of patients without a history of prior neurological insult was 14% at 12 months and 17% at 20 months, compared to a rate of recurrence of 28% at 12 months and 34% at 20 months in the group with a positive history. It must be remembered that other workers, for example, Johnson *et al.* [5], excluded such patients from their studies.

Annegers *et al.* [11] found that risk of recurrence varied with the aetiologic classification of the initial seizure. 'Remote symptomatic' seizures, comparable to the group of prior neurological insult described above, carried a risk of recurrence of 56% by one year and 77% by five years, compared to those whose seizures were classed as 'idiopathic' (26% by one year, 45% by five years). The small group of patients with a perinatal insult evidenced by cerebral palsy or mental retardation had a particularly high relapse rate – 92% by one year.

Annegers and colleagues [11] classified as 'idiopathic' those patients who had no remote neurological insult, or deficit from birth to which the epilepsy could be reasonably attributed. However, even in this group there were some with neurological signs – so it is clear that the epilepsy was not 'idiopathic' in the sense of being primary generalized epilepsy. Among 'idiopathic' cases with abnormal findings, on examination the risk of recurrence was 41% by one year and 72% by five years, compared with 24% and 43% by one and five years amongst patients with normal findings on examination ($p<0.002$). This difference had not emerged in the earlier, smaller study by Hauser and colleagues [9], nor did that study reveal any influence on prognosis of seizure type. However, in the study of Blom *et al.* [7], it was noted that all children with initial complex partial seizures had a further seizure, and among the 'remote symptomatic' subjects of Annegers *et al.* those with an initial partial seizure had a relative risk of 1.8 (95% confidence limits 1.1–3.0) of recurrence compared with subjects whose initial seizure had been generalized.

6.2.2 Family history

Hauser and colleagues [9] found that patients with initial 'idiopathic' seizures who had a sibling with a history of seizures had a higher risk of recurrence, and of earlier recurrence than those without an affected sibling. Of the other studies listed in Table 6.1, only that of Blom's group [7] evaluated family history as a possible risk factor for recurrence, and found no effect.

6.2.3 Time of occurrence of the initial seizure

The ongoing Royal College of Physicians study [12] has shown that first seizures occurring between the hours of midnight and 09.00 hours are more likely to be followed by recurrence.

6.2.4 The interval since the initial seizure

A good part of the differences in recurrence rate can be accounted for by differences in the intervals after which those who have had an initial seizure attend a neurologist. Annegers *et al.* [11] found that 9% of their subjects had recurrences by one month and 14% by two months. They point out the potential for a marked underestimation of total cumulative risk in studies based upon referrals with 'lagged' times of ascertainment (e.g. [8]). This is confirmed by the Royal College of Physicians study [12], illustrated in Fig. 6.1, which shows the markedly higher relapse rate of those subjects seen within one week of their initial seizure compared with those seen subsequently. Those who had already relapsed in the interval between one week and, say, two months (when they were first seen) were no longer eligible for recruitment into the study. Their withdrawal presumably leaves a group with an intrinsically lesser risk of relapse. A family of probabilities can be constructed from data analogous to that shown in Fig. 6.1 for the interval after the first seizure that has already been reached without recurrence to that interval.

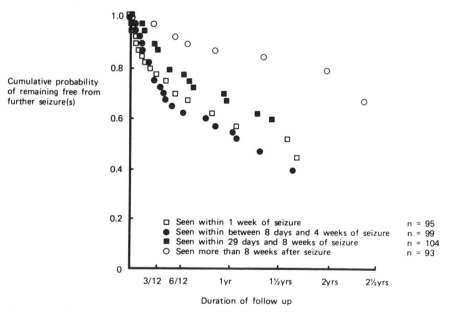

Figure 6.1 Probability of relapse following a first untreated seizure. Note the lesser probability of relapse for those recruited into the study after a long interval.

6.2.5   Electroencephalographic (EEG) abnormalities

Thomas [4] reported that nearly all of his group of 13 patients who had a relapse after the first seizure had an abnormal EEG, although it is not clear what type of abnormality was associated with recurrence. Saunders and Mashall [6] in contrast found that the EEG was not a useful predictive factor.

Annegers and colleagues [11] reported that among subjects with an initial 'idiopathic' seizure, EEG patterns of generalized spike and wave, focal spikes and slowing, and non-specific slowing were associated with one year recurrence risks of 25%, 25% and 29% respectively, all higher than the one year rate of 16% for similar subjects with normal EEGs. Cleland and colleagues [8] also found that an abnormal EEG (regardless of type of abnormality) was significantly associated with an increased risk of recurrence after the first seizure. Thirty-nine per cent of those whose seizures remained isolated and 68% of those who had recurrent seizures had an abnormal EEG – either non-specific abnormalities, focal slowing over the temporal lobe, or generalized slow activity.

Hauser and colleagues [9] found that only generalized spike and wave discharges were associated with higher rates of recurrence, 50% at 24 months compared to 14% with normal EEGs. The presence of a spike wave pattern at the time of evaluation for the initial seizures was also associated with an increased recurrence in the study of naval personnel by Johnson *et al.* [5]. Hauser and colleagues [9] found that there was no significant increase in risk of recurrence in patients with a focal EEG abnormality, or photoconvulsive response. However Blom [7] noticed seizure recurrence in all children with central spikes. No EEG abnormality has yet emerged as being associated with recurrence in the Royal College of Physicians Study [12].

6.2.6   Abnormalities on the CT scan

None of the studies listed in Table 6.1 have looked at the association between an abnormal CT scan and risk of recurrence, though the ongoing Royal College of Physicians study will be looking at this. However, two studies have examined the diagnostic value of the CT scan in the assessment of single seizures. Russo and Goldstein [13] found that nearly half of their group of 62 first seizure patients had abnormal CT scans. The majority of these patients (69%) also had abnormal findings on neurological examination – either a focal neurological deficit or dementia. Generalized atrophy was the only abnormality found in the nine patients with abnormal CT scans and no abnormalities on clinical neurological examinations. They concluded that the CT scan was only useful and essential in first seizure patients with abnormal clinical findings. In contrast, Ramirez-Lassepas *et al.* [14] scanned 148 first seizure patients and found 14 patients with a structural lesion, who had no abnormalities on neurological examination. They concluded that the CT scan was of major value in ascertaining the cause of first seizure in adults.

Other investigations in many centres traditionally include a chest and skull radiograph, a full blood picture, VDRL (test for syphilis), serum calcium, blood sugar, electrolytes and urea. It does not seem likely that any of these will be useful in predicting the likelihood of recurrence after an initial seizure, though they may be useful in identifying a cause (Chapter 4), or in distinguishing a seizure from other causes of disturbed consciousness, a problem which is considered below in section 6.3. In the interesting study by Day and colleagues [15] of the evaluation of the outcome of 189 emergency room patients with transient loss of consciousness, a skull radiograph was never helpful in reaching a diagnosis, and the history and physical examination were sufficient for diagnosis in 85% of cases.

6.3   THE DIFFERENTIAL DIAGNOSIS OF AN INITIAL OR EPILEPTIC SEIZURE

Anthony Hopkins

The distinction between an initial seizure due to a paroxysmal neuronal discharge, and some other event disturbing consciousness is primarily a clinical one, based upon the description of the experience given by the subject himself, and, most usefully, a witness of the event. Although many patients expect it, there is no 'proof' of the diagnosis of epilepsy. Although the EEG may provide useful ancillary information, it may be normal in patients who have had undoubted convulsive seizures [3], or 'abnormal' (if the limits of normality are not carefully defined), in normal subjects. These difficulties are fully reviewed by Binnie in Chapter 7.

The differential diagnosis of isolated and recurrent seizures are not distinct, and both aspects are now discussed.

6.3.1   Syncope

The commonest cause of loss of consciousness in early adult life must be syncope, based upon routine outpatient clinical experience, though I know of no community-based epidemiological survey to substantiate this. The survey of emergency room visits by 189 patients for episodes of transient loss of conciousness by Day and colleagues [15] showed the following figures:

Vasovagal or psychogenic syncope	40%
Seizures (including 4 patients whose seizure was the first manifestation of a tumour)	29%
Migraine	2%
Transient ischaemic event	1%

Cardiac causes	8%
Alcohol	5%
Hypoglycaemia	1%
Illicit drugs	1%
Unknown	25%

The word 'syncope' is derived from the Greek, and means 'a cutting short' [16]. The impairment of consciousness, and the symptoms preceding it are due to transient failure of *global* cerebral perfusion (from whatever cause) as opposed to a transient *focal* failure of perfusion such as occurs in the transient ischaemic attacks of cerebrovascular disease. Causes of syncope include the sudden cardiac slowing or standstill associated with emotional factors, such as the sight of blood or fear of venepuncture, or transient cardiac tachyarrhythmias, or bradyarrhythmias (Stokes-Adams attacks). Inadequate cardiac output for cerebral perfusion may also arise as a result of aortic stenosis, or subaortic obstructive cardiomyopathy, particularly on effort, when there is associated vasodilatation in skeletal musculature. An atrial myxoma may produce the same effect by limiting left ventricular filling.

Even if the cardiac output is near normal, syncope may arise as a result of peripheral vasodilatation, and/or postural hypotension. Prolonged maintenance of the erect posture at school assembly, or on parade in the Armed Forces, is one common cause of this variant, as is the sudden assumption of the erect posture after prolonged lying or sitting. It is very unusual, though not unknown, for syncope to occur in the supine position, except in patients with cardiac arrhythmia.

Some patients have some degree of failure of baroreceptor mechanisms, for example in diabetes [17]. There may be a failure of autonomic control, for example in cases of autonomic neuropathy, or primary autonomic failure as in the Shy-Drager syndrome [18]. Commonly hypotension attributable to medication, particularly with antihypertensive agents and antidepressants, is identified as a factor precipitating postural syncope.

Another common story is of a man who gets up at night to pass urine, and loses consciousness during or immediately after this. Injuries may result from striking the head on the lavatory bowl, bath or basin. Although there are postural elements in this – the act of getting up from a warm bed to a standing position – a factor of some importance is undoubtedly the reflex vasodilatation that occurs during the act of micturition.

Finally there are reflex causes of syncope. The carotid sinus may be particularly sensitive to external pressure [19], so that syncope may result from turning the head within (at least apocryphally) a tight collar. The incidence of carotid sinus sensitivity is higher in older subjects, those with hypertension, and with coronary artery disease. Hypersensitivity of the sinus is of two types – depression of sinus activity, and varying degrees of atroventricular (AV) block. Methyl dopa and propranolol may both induce sinus hypersensitivity. Vigorous coughing, by raising atrial pressure, may also result in reflex cardiac slowing – so-called cough syncope [20].

Some syncopal attacks are of such abrupt onset that the subject can himself give no useful account of what has transpired. This is particularly likely in cases of micturition and cough syncope. In these cases, the diagnosis must rest upon the circumstances of the episodes. In other cases of syncope, particularly those which arise from postural hypotension and/or emotional factors (such as a medical student watching an operation for the first time), the sufferer will give a clear account of pre-syncopal warning symptoms, which are associated with failing cerebral perfusion. A sense of unease or anxiety is accompanied by nausea. The intense cutaneous peripheral vasoconstriction reflex that accompanies falling blood pressure is perceived as a sense of coldness. There may be associated pilo-erection (goose-pimples) and sweating – the so-called 'cold sweat'. Tinnitus occurs, and the voices of bystanders sound far away. The failure of retinal perfusion results in a 'greying-out' or 'blacking-out' of vision, at a time when consciousness is still reasonably well preserved. A bystander will notice an air of unease and distraction, associated with pallor, and a cold moist skin. He may find the pulse extremely slow or imperceptible. If the subject is allowed to complete his faint, he will fall limply to the floor. Assumption of the horizontal posture aids the hypotensive cerebral circulation, and full consciousness, without significant confusion, is resumed within a minute or so.

If such a story is obtained, there is little chance of confusion between a seizure (that may for the purposes of this discussion be classed as an epileptic seizure, even if the first of its type), and syncope. The difficulties principally arise in a misunderstanding of the nature of the pre-syncopal symptoms. If a subject is unwise enough to say that 'voices sounded distorted and far away', an inexperienced physician may interpret this as a sense of unreality, and make an unthinking diagnosis of a complex partial seizure. The other principal difficulty is that if the fainting subject is supported in the sitting position, cerebral hypoperfusion may be such that 'one or two generalized myoclonic jerks appear which are not reflected in the EEG. Then suddenly the patient develops an intense generalized tonic spasm in extension, with opisthotonus, looking exactly like decerebrate rigidity or a tonic cerebellar fit. These tonic contractions may be stronger on one side that the other, and therefore cause lateral deviation of the head' [16]. This quotation comes from the classic paper from Gastaut's laboratory, in which syncope was induced in susceptible subjects by ocular compression during EEG monitoring. From this description of what are now called 'anoxic seizures' [21] it is clear that it is no use asking a witness whether the patient was 'stiff' and 'limp', nor even whether he was jerking or not, as the bystander may well confuse the initial myoclonic jerks of an anoxic seizure with the clonic phase of an epileptic seizure.

In short, in the absence of ECG or EEG monitoring of seizures, not available in everyday clinical practice and certainly not available to help in the diagnosis of an isolated event, the distinction between syncope and a first or epileptic seizure depends upon the circumstances in which the episode occurs, the nature of the subjective perceptions before the episode, and the account of any bystander [22].

If a firm conclusion cannot be reached on the basis of the history, and examination, further investigation may be justified, using ambulatory EEG or ECG (Holter) monitoring. Of the two, the latter is easiest to arrange. It might be thought that the limited number of EEG channels that can be accommodated on a cassette recorder, the low signal strength and the number of artefacts would make interpretation of ambulatory EEG records more difficult than ECG records. Furthermore, EEG cassette records are at present less capable of automatic analysis, though 'page scanning' of the type provided by Oxford Instruments is reasonably satisfactory. In practice, these drawbacks are more apparent than real, as simultaneous cassette recording and cable telemetry have shown a high concordance of diagnostic yield, even if only three channels are available for the cassette recording [23].

The proportion of episodes of disturbed consciousness that prove to have a cardiac rather than a cerebral cause is dependent upon patient selection in the departments from which reports have been made (see [22] for review and references). Before proceeding to ambulatory ECG monitoring, a standard ECG is of course essential, as a defect in atrioventricular conduction or evidence of inferior wall myocardial infarction raises the possibility of Stokes-Adams attacks. Pre-excitation syndromes characterized by a short P–R interval, or a prolonged Q–T interval, will warn of the possibility of tachyarrhythmias.

Circulatory abnormalities responsible for syncope have recently been shown to include 'excessive vagal tone' as judged by prolonged AV nodal effective and functional refractory periods, and AV Wenkebach block at low (<120) atrial pacing rates. The interest in this observation is that some patients, who suffered recurrent syncope without predisposing cause, greatly benefited from an anticholinergic agent, propantheline bromide [24].

The interpretation of data obtained by ambulatory ECG is often not easy, as benign complex arrhythmias and conduction defects occur in symptomless healthy people. Conversely, sampling errors are such that patients who have at other times a significant arrhythmia responsible for disturbance of consciousness may fail to produce evidence of this in a 24 hour recording. Furthermore, Blumhardt and colleagues [25] and Devinsky and colleagues [26] and Smaje and colleagues [26a] have shown how ECG abnormalities may occur during undoubted temporal lobe seizures. In the majority of cases in the first study, cardiac acceleration preceded the appearance of the EEG seizure discharge by several seconds, although the authors indicate that this could have been due to the limited electrode montage available for cassette recording. The commonest irregularity found was repeated sinus acceleration and deceleration during the seizure discharge, though an increased number of ventricular extrasystoles, and bradycardia, were also seen. In the study of Devinsky and colleagues [26], five of their six patients presented with atypical anginal pain as a cardiac manifestation of complex partial seizures. One patient had a cluster of symptoms suggesting a phaeochromocytoma, and tachy- and bradyarrhythmias were also seen. It is clear that clinicians must be cautious in concluding from ECG monitoring alone that cardiac arrhythmias, even when they coincide with symptoms, are the primary cause of a patient's complaints.

The practical value of extensive investigation is best illustrated by the work of Kapoor and colleagues [27]. Of their 210 patients admitted to the wards, the cause of disturbed consciousness was evident from the initial history and examination in 89. Of the remaining 121 patients, a definitive diagnosis was made in only 13, at an average cost per patient of $2463 in 1982.

A further study of syncope in the elderly by Kapoor and colleagues [28] showed that, not surprisingly, a cardiovascular cause was twice as common (34%) as a cause of syncope in a group of 210 patients with an average age of 71, than in a younger group of 190 patients where the average age was 39.

6.3.2   Panic attacks

Attacks of panic disorder may be manifested by the sudden onset of intense apprehension, fear or terror, associated with feeling of impending doom, dizziness, parasthesiae, and a sense of unreality [29, 30]. These descriptions are not far removed from perceptions reported by those with complex partial seizures. Furthermore, panic attacks may occur on waking, reminiscent of some seizures. An important point is that hyperventilation can induce *focal* neurological symptoms, such as a hemisensory disturbance, or blurring of vision [31] which adds to the difficulty of distinguishing these from complex partial seizures. The distinction rests primarily upon the disturbance of consciousness in seizures. In practice, once the differential diagnosis is thought of, a distinction is usually fairly easy. The symptoms of panic disorder may be considerably relieved by a beta-adrenergic blocker.

6.3.3   Pseudoseizures

Up to 20% of those referred for the evaluation of intractable epilepsy eventually prove to have pseudoseizures ([32]; pp. 539–42). The problem seldom arises in relation to the diagnosis of a first seizure. Helpful diagnostic criteria listed by Krumholz and Niedermeyer [32] include these points. Pseudoseizures are more often precipitated by stressful circumstances, occur in the presence of others, and may occur in response to suggestion. Motor activity is composed of purposeful, asynchronous and integrated motor activity, and may include writhing or thrashing about. Responsiveness and awareness may be retained during 'major' seizures. There is no postictal confusion. The serum prolactin does not become elevated postictally [33]. Although it is said [32] that subjects are rarely injured or incontinent, my experience is that if true epilepsy coexists, patients are often incontinent during their simulated as well as their true seizures. Epilepsy was coexistent in 37% of the series of Krumholz and Niedermeyer [32], though uncommonly active at the same time. It was present in only 5% of the patients reported by Lesser and colleagues [34]. The personality of those with pseudoseizures, as judged by the Minnesota Multiphasic Personality Inventory, is not significantly different from the personality of those with epilepsy [35].

Although the differential diagnosis is usually between tonic-clonic seizures and pseudoseizures, some behavioural disturbances, including acts of aggression followed by amnesia, may be misinterpreted by the unwary as types of complex partial seizures.

The ictal EEG is the most important technique for establishing that seizures are not truly epileptic. However, the interictal EEG may be abnormal in patients with pseudoseizures, partly because of the coexistence of, or previous existence of epilepsy, and partly because of the mental retardation that is found in some cases prone to pseudoseizures.

6.3.4 Migraine

The periodic disturbances of neurological function associated with classical migraine may be confused with epilepsy. Distinguishing factors include the common occipital cortical disturbances in migrainous episodes (teichopsia). Seizures arising occipitally are distinctly uncommon. The slow evolution over a period of many minutes of classical migrainous symptoms is unlike that of a seizure discharge. Epilepsy and migraine may coexist, as noted by Gowers [36].

6.3.5 Transient ischaemic attacks

Transient ischaemic attacks in the territory of the carotid circulation may produce transient arrest of speech (aphasia), and loss of function of one hand or one side of the body. The clinical distinction is that ischaemic events are *negative* phenomena; epileptic events in the same territory have the positive effects of jactitation, for example.

Episodes of transient global amnesia [37] almost certainly have a vascular basis, but the distinction between such an episode and a complex partial seizure may be very difficult. During an episode of global amnesia, the subject may appear confused, and will, by definition, be amnesic for the events thereafter. Episodes of transient global amnesia tend to be non-recurrent; this, their long duration (1–4 hours) and the presence of vascular disease may aid the distinction from a complex partial seizure.

6.3.6   Periodic pain syndromes

Pain may be a feature of some epileptic seizures [38]. As abdominal discomfort is a frequent initial symptom of many complex partial seizures, it has been proposed that periodic abdominal pain alone may be an epileptic manifestation. A review by Mitchell and colleagues [39] has stressed just how rarely this is the case.

6.3.7   Breath-holding attacks

These usually begin before the age of 18 months, and are unusual after the age of three years. They are of two types – cyanotic, and pallid (p. 483). Cyanotic episodes are more commonly caused by anger or frustration, the child stopping breathing in expiration, then becoming limp, cyanosed and unconscious. If prolonged, there follows an opisthotonic phase, sometimes followed by a few clonic jerks. Pallid episodes usually follow a minor injury, often to the head. Apnoea, pallor and loss of consciousness are associated with cardiac asystole [40], but clonic jerks do not usually appear.

6.3.8   Night terrors and nightmares

Night terrors are abrupt arousals during stage 3–4 of non-rapid eye movement sleep (NREM), and usually occur in childhood (p. 483). A sudden cry wakens the parents, who find the child looking terrified with widely dilated pupils, sweating, and with a tachycardia. The child is confused but rapidly settles with reassurance, and is amnesic for the event the next day [41]. An awareness of this syndrome, or perhaps better still having seen one's own child in a night terror, is sufficient to distinguish such an episode from a seizure. Nightmares affect all ages. They are awakenings from REM sleep, with good recall of the unpleasant dream. They may occur as a result of treatment with adrenergic blocking drugs, reserpine or on withdrawal from alcohol and some hypnotics [41].

6.3.9   Narcolepsy–cataplexy syndrome

The characteristic irresistible desire to sleep, and the sudden paralysis arising as a result of some sudden surprise, anger or laughter are not likely to be mistaken for seizures. Less common and less well known are the vivid hypnagogic hallucinations – 'the sensory errors of half sleep' [41] – that affect about one-third of those with this syndrome, and which may superficially suggest the dreamy state of complex partial seizures.

6.3.10 Hypoglycaemia

Except in the rare cases of insulinoma, hypoglycaemia sufficient to cause neurological symptoms is only likely to arise in diabetics receiving insulin therapy. Definite diagnostic problems do arise however, as hypoglycaemia may precipitate seizures in patients with an otherwise quiescent seizure focus [42]. Seizures were the presenting symptom in only nine of the 125 'neurological' instances of hypoglycaemia collected by Malouf and Brust [43], but a history of pre-existing epilepsy or alcoholism was common. However, in one study quoted by these authors, none of the 70 patients with epilepsy had seizures induced by an insulin injection that reduced the blood sugar to a median of 40 mg/100 ml.

In concluding this section on the differential diagnosis of seizures, I stress again the cardinal importance of an account from a witness of the event under review. A surprising number of patients arrive unaccompanied to their first consultation for a 'blackout' or 'turn'. If there were any witness present at the time, then that observer should be seen before embarking upon any investigations.

6.4 THE USE OF ANTICONVULSANTS AFTER AN INITIAL SEIZURE

Anthony Hopkins

The studies reviewed earlier in this chapter underline the high probability of recurrence in the early weeks after an initial seizure. Elwes and colleagues [10] and others have commented upon the possibility that early treatment might prevent the establishment of recurrent seizures. Over a century ago Gowers [44] commented that 'when one attack has occurred, whether in apparent consequence of an immediate excitant or not, others usually follow without any immediately traceable cause. The effect of a convulsion on the nerve centres is such as to render the occurrence of another more easy, to intensify the predisposition that already exists. Thus every fit may be said to be, in part, the result of those which have preceded it, the cause of those which follow it.' Nonetheless, the present consensus view seems to be that a single seizure does not often warrant treatment. There are a number of reasons for this. First, many patients, and their physicians, have a healthy respect for the unwanted effects of anticonvulsant drugs, not least the potential teratogenic effect in women of childbearing age (Chapter 12) and the mild sedative effect that seems more prominent than many research studies would suggest (Chapter 9). In children, the known effects of phenytoin, including coarsening of facial appearance, hirsutism and gum hypertrophy are all features that militate against the unnecessary prescription of this drug.

Another drawback is that physicians are concerned that, if an anticonvulsant is started, then a decision will subsequently have to be made to stop it, with all the uncertainties that that entails – not least the possibility of a withdrawal seizure.

Goodridge and Shorvon [45] reviewed the medical records of 6000 patients in the community. They found that one-third of those who had had one or more seizures had received anticonvulsants after the first. Personal difficulties in recruiting patients for a randomized trial suggest that the current practice of primary care physicians is to prescribe immediate anticonvulsants more often than this. This may be the correct decision, but there is no evidence to support this. Hauser and colleagues [9] found no difference in prognosis between those treated and untreated after an initial seizure. However, patients given treatment were probably judged by clinicians to be at a higher risk of recurrence. Patients were more likely to be treated if the clinical examination or the EEG were abnormal, or if there had been a history of prior neurological insult. Hauser's group pointed out that, even in those treated, blood levels of anticonvulsants were seldom monitored, and available information about adequacy of dosage and compliance was limited.

There has been no prospective investigation of the value of anticonvulsants in the management of an initial seizure, and there is certainly a need for a proper controlled trial. In order to be 90% sure of detecting a reduction in relapse rate from 40% to 25%, approximately 500 patients would be required in each arm of the trial. Numbers treated before neurological referral and the ethical difficulties of randomly allocating women of childbearing age to anticonvulsant treatment of uncertain benefit caused a personal attempt to founder. Another problem was that, when an explanation of the trial was given before randomization, many of those who held driving licences chose to opt for treatment, even though the benefits are not proven.

The problem of whether or not to treat a first seizure has been reviewed recently [46–48]. Until more information is available, few would quarrel with the conclusion of Hachinski that the certainty of the diagnosis, the occupation and attitude of the patient and the nature of the lesion responsible (if any) will all influence the decision [48].

6.5 SOCIAL CONSEQUENCES OF A SEIZURE

Anthony Hopkins

A seizure is an alarming event both for the subjects, who recognize their vulnerability to recurrence, and for relatives or onlookers, who often feel the patient might have died in the attack. The social implications of the first seizure are considerable – those whose jobs involve driving, flying or working potentially dangerous machinery are particularly affected. The fear of a second attack may alter relationships in their family and the question 'Is he/

she an epileptic?' is in the forefront of the minds of the patient, and relations. Chapter 17 reviews these aspects at length, but all physicians must bear these justifiable anxieties in mind during the course of a consultation that is seemingly routine, but of inestimable importance to the patient.

REFERENCES

1. Research Committee of the College of General Practitioners (1960) A survey of the epilepsies in General Practice. *Br. Med. J.*, **2**, 416–22.
2. Hauser, W. A. and Kurland, L. T. (1975) The epidemiology of epilepsy in Rochester, Minnesota, 1935 through 1967. *Epilepsia*, **16**, 1–66.
3. Hopkins, A. and Scambler, G. (1977) How doctors deal with epilepsy. *Lancet*, **i**, 183–6.
4. Thomas, M. H. (1959) The single seizure: its study and management. *J.A.M.A.*, **169**, 457–9.
5. Johnson, L. C., De Bolt, W. L. and Long, M. T. (1972) Diagnostic factors in adult males following initial seizures. A three year follow up. *Arch. Neurol.*, **27**, 193–7.
6. Saunders, M. and Marshall, C. (1975) Isolated seizures: An EEG and clinical assessment. *Epilepsia*, **16**, 731–3.
7. Blom, S., Heijbel, J. and Bergfors, P. G. (1978) Incidence of epilepsy in children: A follow-up study three years after the first seizure. *Epilepsia*, **19**, 343–50.
8. Cleland, P. G., Mosquera, I., Steward, W. P. and Foster, J.B. (1981) Prognosis of isolated seizures in adult life. *Br. Med. J.*, **283**, 1364.
9. Hauser, W. A., Anderson, V.E., Loewenson, R. B. and McRoberts, S. M. (1982) Seizure recurrence after a first unprovoked seizure. *N. Engl. J. Med.*, **307,** 522–8.
10. Elwes, R. D. C., Chesterman, P. and Reynolds, E. H. (1985) Prognosis after a first untreated tonic-clonic seizure. *Lancet*, **ii**, 752–3.
11. Annegers, J. F., Shirts, S. B., Hauser, W. A. and Kurland, L. T. (1986) Risk of recurrence after an initial unprovoked seizure. *Epilepsia*, **27**, 43–50.
11a. Lühdorf, K., Jensen, L. K. and Plesner, A. M. (1986) Epilepsy in the elderly: prognosis. *Acta Neurol. Scand.*, **74**, 409–15.
12. Hopkins, A., Garman, A. and Clarke, C. R. A. C. (work in progress).
13. Russo, L. S. and Goldstein, K. H. (1983) The diagnostic assessment of single seizures. Is cranial computed tomography necessary? *Arch. Neurol.*, **40**, 744–6.
14. Ramirez-Lessepas, M., Golla, R. J., Morilo, L. R. and Gumrit, R. J. (1983) Value of computed tomographic score in the evaluation of adult patients after their first seizure. *Ann. Neurol.*, **15**, 536–43.
15. Day, S. C., Cook, E. F., Funkenstein, H. and Goldman, L. (1982) Evaluation and outcome of emergency room patients with transient loss of consciousness. *Am. J. Med.*, **73**, 15–23.
16. Gastaut, H. and Fischer-Williams, M. (1957) Electroencephalographic study of syncope: its differentiation from epilepsy. *Lancet*, **ii**, 1018–25.
17. Scharpey-Schafer, E. P. and Taylor, P. J. (1960) Absent circulatory reflexes in diabetic neuritis. *Lancet*, **i**, 559–63.
18. Bannister, R. G. (1983) *Autonomic failure: A Textbook of Clinical Disorders of the Autonomic Nervous Sytem*, Oxford University Press, UK.

19. Schweitzer, P. and Teicholz, L. E. (1985) Carotid sinus massage: its diagnostic and therapeutic value in arrthymias. *Am. J. Med.*, **78**, 645–54.

20. Scharpey-Schafer, E. P. (1953) The mechanism of syncope after coughing. *Br. Med. J.*, **2**, 860–4.

21. Gastaut, H. (1973) *Dictionary of Epilepsy. Part I. Definitions*, World Health Organisation, Geneva.

22. Critchley, E. M. R. and Wright, J. S. (1983) Evaluation of syncope. *Br. Med. J.*, **1**, 500–1.

23. Ebersole, J. S. and Bridgers, S. L. (1985) Direct comparison of 3- and 8-channel ambulatory cassette EEG with intensive inpatient monitoring. *Neurology*, **35**, 846–54.

24. McLaren, C. J., Gersh, B. J., Osborn, M. J. *et al.* (1986) Increased vagal tone as an isolated finding in patients undergoing electrophysiological testing for recurrent syncope; response to long term anticholinergic agents. *Br. Heart. J.*, **55**, 53–7.

25. Blumhardt, L. D., Smith, P. E. M. and Owen, L. (1986) Electrocardiographic accompaniments of temporal lobe epileptic seizures. *Lancet*, **i**, 1051–6.

26. Devinsky, O., Price, B. H. and Cohen, S. I. (1986) Cardiac manifestations of complex partial seizures. *Am. J. Med.*, **80**, 195–202.

26a. Smaje, J. C., Davidson, C., Teasdale, G. M. (1987) Sino-atrial arrest due to temporal lobe seizures. *J. Neurol. Neurosurg. Psychiatr.*, **50**, 112–13.

27. Kapoor, W. N., Karp, L. and Maher, Y. (1982) Syncope of unknown origin. The need for a more cost effective approach to its diagnostic evaluation. *JAMA*, **247**, 2687–91.

28. Kapoor, W. N., Snustad, D. and Peterson, J., *et al.* (1986) Syncope in the elderly. *Am. J. Med.*, **80**, 419–28.

29. Hibbert, G. A. (1984) Hyperventilation as a cause of panic attacks. *Br. Med. J.*, **288**, 263–4.

30. Porter, R. J. (1984) *Epilepsy: 100 Elementary Principles*, W.B. Saunders, Philadelphia.

31. Coyle, P. K. and Sterman, A. B. (1986) Focal neurologic symptoms in panic attacks. *Am. J. Psychiat.*, **143**, 648–9.

32. Krumholz, A. and Niedermeyer, E. (1983) Psychogenic seizures: a clinical study with follow up data. *Neurology*, **33**, 498–502.

33. Trimble, M. R. (1983) Serum prolactin in epilepsy and hysteria. *Br. Med. J.*, **2**, 1682.

34. Lesser, R. P., Lueders, H. and Dinner, D. S. (1983) Evidence for epilepsy is rare in patients with psychogenic seizures. *Neurology*, **33**, 502–4.

35. Vanderzant, C. W., Giordani, B., Berent, B., *et al.* (1986) Personality of patients wih pseudoseizures. *Neurology*, **36**, 664–8.

36. Gowers, W. R. (1907) *The Borderland of Epilepsy; faints, vagal attacks, vertigo, migraine, sleep symptoms and their treatment*. P. Blakiston Son & Co., Philadelphia.

37. Fisher, C. M. and Adams, R. D. (1964) Transient global amnesia. *Acta Neurol. Scand.*, **40**, (Suppl. 9), 1–83.

38. Young, G. B. and Blume, W. T. (1983) Painful epileptic seizures. *Brain*, **106**, 537–54.

39. Mitchell, W. G., Greenwood, R. S. and Messenheimer, J. A. (1983) Cyclic vomiting as the major symptom of simple partial seizures. *Arch. Neurol.*, **40**, 251–2.

40. Stephenson, J. B. P. (1978) Reflex anoxic seizures ('white breath-holding attacks'): non-epileptic vagal attacks. *Arch. Dis. Child.*, **53**, 193–200.
41. Parkes, J. D. (1985) *Sleep and its Disorders*, W. B. Saunders, London.
42. Aird, R. B., Masland, R. L. and Woodbury, D. M. (1984) *The Epilepsies: A Critical Review*, Raven Press, New York.
43. Malouf, R. and Brust, J. C. M. (1985) Hypoglycaemia: causes, neurological manifestations, and outcome. *Ann. Neurol.*, **17**, 421–30.
44. Gowers, W. (1901) *Epilepsy and Other Chronic Convulsive Diseases*, Churchill, London.
45. Goodridge, D. M. G. and Shorvon, S. D. (1983) Epileptic seizures in a population of 6000. I. Demography, diagnosis and classification of seizures, and role of the hospital services. *Br. Med. J.*, **287**, 641–4.
46. Hauser, W. A. (1986) Should people be treated after a first seizure? *Arch. Neurol.*, **43**, 1287–88.
47. Hart, R. G. and Easton, J. D. (1986) Seizure recurrence after a first, unprovoked seizure. *Arch. Neurol.*, **43**, 1287–90.
48. Hachinski, V. (1986) Management of a first seizure. *Arch. Neurol.*, **43**, 1290.

CHAPTER SEVEN

Electroencephalography and Epilepsy

Colin D. Binnie

As should be evident from Chapter 3 the EEG (electroencephalogram) has played a crucial role in formulating present concepts of epilepsy and in classifications of epileptic seizures and syndromes. Unfortunately this fact has given rise to various expectations or assumptions which are either false or subject to important qualifications, notably:

(1) That during an epileptic seizure the EEG invariably exhibits spikes or spike wave complexes.
(2) That the interictal EEG can be used to prove or exclude the diagnosis of epilepsy.
(3) That the amount of interictal epileptiform EEG activity is closely related to the severity of the epilepsy and to the frequency of seizures, and is reduced by effective antiepileptic medication.
(4) That the interictal EEG is predictive of prognosis in epilepsy.

Because epilepsy is a disorder of cerebral function and EEG a functional investigation, epilepsy is sometimes regarded as a test case for assessing the clinical value of the EEG [1]. The failure to fulfil expectations similar to those listed above may then be cited as evidence that it is not a very useful investigation [2]. It must be admitted that electroencephalographers have contributed to this misunderstanding by failing to acknowledge the limitations of the EEG or to emphasize its important applications.

7.1 'EPILEPTIFORM ACTIVITY'

During an epileptic seizure by definition abnormal cerebral electrical activity is present. This can be recorded with suitably placed depth electrodes and often in the scalp EEG also. This activity characteristically involves rapid and brief changes of electrical potential producing spiky wave-forms, usually followed by slower potentials. Activity of similar morphology often occurs in interictal records of people with epilepsy. According to the Terminology Committee of the International Federation of the Society for Electro-encephalography and Clinical Neurophysiology [3] the most characteristic wave-forms are defined as follows:

Epileptiform pattern. Interpretive term. Applies to distinctive waves or complexes, distinguished from background activity, and resembling those recorded in a proportion of human subjects suffering from epileptic disorders and in animals rendered epileptic experimentally. Epileptiform patterns include spikes and sharp waves, occurring singly or in bursts lasting at most a few seconds. The Committee comments that: (1) Term refers to interictal paroxysmal activity and not to seizure patterns. (However, this recommendation ignores common usage, as many European workers employ the term to include ictal phenomena and 'seizure patterns' is often used to describe interictal discharges in North America.) (2) Probability of association with clinical epileptic disorders is variable.

Seizure pattern, EEG. Phenomenon consisting of repetitive EEG discharges with relatively abrupt onset and termination and characteristic pattern of evolution, lasting at least several seconds. The component waves or complexes vary in form, frequency and topography. They are generally rhythmic and frequently display increasing amplitude and decreasing frequency during the same episode. When focal in onset, they tend to spread subsequently to other areas. Comment: EEG seizure patterns unaccompanied by clinical epileptic manifestations detected by the recordist and/or reported by the patient should be referred to as 'subclinical'. (cf. epileptiform pattern.)

Paroxysm. Phenomenon with abrupt onset, rapid attainment of a maximum and sudden termination, distinguished from background activity. Comment: commonly used to refer to epileptiform patterns and seizure patterns. (cf. epileptiform pattern; seizure pattern, EEG.)

Spike. A transient, clearly distinguished from background activity, with pointed peak at conventional paper speeds and a duration from 20 to under 70 ms, i.e., $\frac{1}{50}-\frac{1}{14}$ s, approximately. Main component is generally negative relative to other areas. Amplitude is variable. Comments: (1) EEG spikes should be differentiated from sharp waves, i.e. transients having similar characteristics but longer durations. However, it is well to keep in mind that this distinction is largely arbitrary and serves primarily descriptive purposes. Practically, in inkwritten EEG records taken at 3 cm/s, spikes occupy 2 mm or less of paper width and sharp waves more than 2 mm. (2) EEG spikes should be held in clear contradistinction to the brief unit spikes recorded from single cells with microelectrode techniques. (cf. sharp wave.)

Sharp wave. A transient, clearly distinguished from background activity, with pointed peak at conventional paper speeds and duration of 70–200 ms i.e. over $\frac{1}{14}-\frac{1}{5}$ s approximately. Main component is generally negative relative to other areas. Amplitude is variable. Comments: (1) Term does not apply to (i) distinctive physiological events such as vertex sharp transients, lambda waves and positive occipital sharp transients of sleep, (ii) sharp transients poorly distinguished from background activity and sharp-appearing individual waves of EEG rhythms. (2) Sharp waves should be differentiated from spikes, i.e. transients having similar characteristics but shorter duration. However, it is well to keep in mind that this distinction is largely arbitrary and serves primarily descriptive purposes. Practically, in inkwritten EEG records taken at 3 cm/s, sharp waves occupy more than 2 mm of paper width and spikes 2 mm or less. (cf. spike.)

Spike-and-slow-wave complex. A pattern consisting of a spike followed by a slow wave. Comment: hyphenation facilitates use of term in plural form: spike-and-slow-wave complexes or spike-and-slow-waves.

Sharp-and-slow-wave complex. A sequence of a sharp wave and a slow wave. Comment: hyphenation facilitates use of term in plural form: sharp-and-slow-wave complexes or sharp-and-slow-waves.

3 Hz spike-and-slow-waves. Characteristic paroxysm consisting of a regular sequence of spike-and-slow-wave complexes which: (1) repeat at 3–3.5 Hz (measured during the first few seconds of the paroxysm), (2) are bilateral in their onset and termination, generalized and usually of maximal amplitude over the frontal areas, (3) are approximately synchronous and symmetrical on the two sides of the head throughout the paroxysm. Amplitude is variable but can reach values of 1000 μV (1 mV).

6 Hz spike-and-slow-waves. Spike-and-slow-wave complexes at 4–7 Hz, but mostly at 6 Hz, occurring generally in brief bursts bilaterally synchronously, symmetrically or asymmetrically, and either confined to or of larger amplitude over the posterior or anterior regions of the head. Amplitude is variable but generally smaller than that of spike-and-slow-wave complexes repeating at slower rates. Comment: The clinical significance of this pattern, if any, is controversial.

Multiple spike complex. A sequence of two or more spikes. Preferred to synonym: polyspike complex.

Multiple spike-and-slow-wave complex. A sequence of two or more spikes associated with one or more slow waves. Preferred to synonym: polyspike-and-slow-wave complex.

Hypsarrhythmia. Pattern consisting of high voltage arrhythmic slow waves interspersed with spike discharges, without consistent synchrony between the two sides of the head or different areas on the same side.

It will be noted that these definitions are far from rigorous as they do not clearly define how spikes and sharp waves should be distinguished from the background, and indeed imply that the definition of a spike itself depends upon the background against which it arises (Fig. 7.1).

Similar discharges may not only occur in the interictal records of patients with epilepsy, as noted above, but are found in some persons without a seizure disorder. Spikes, sharp waves and spike wave complexes can occur in a variety of primary and secondary cerebral disorders, without evidence of epileptic seizures. There are also several normal EEG phenomena, commonly seen in normal subjects, which have spiky wave-forms meeting the criteria set out above, but which are in various ways readily distinguishable from those seen

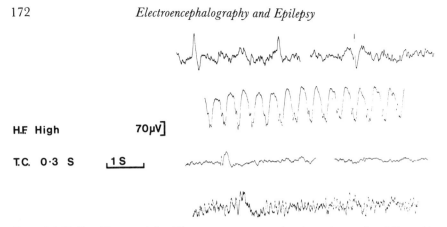

Figure 7.1 Epileptiform activity. The two upper examples show clear spikes followed by slow waves, and the next spike-wave activity, although in this instance the spikes are rather inconspicuous. The remaining examples illustrate the effect of ongoing activity on the visibility of these discharges and may highlight the lack of an objective definition. (Reproduced with permission from Binnie *et al.* [4]).

in epilepsy. Moreover scalp EEG changes during epileptic seizures do not necessarily have a spiky wave-form, but may consist simply of new rhythmic activities not previously present in the EEG (Fig. 7.2) or even a change, usually a reduction, in amplitude of ongoing activity (Fig. 7.3). Considerable conceptual and terminological difficulties therefore arise in finding an acceptable generic term for pathological EEG discharges. Such considerations have led electroencephalographers to adopt a variety of terms. The name 'epileptic

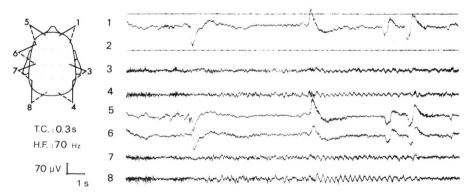

Figure 7.2 Appearance of new, rhythmic, but non-spiky, activity during a complex partial seizure. Channel 2 is a time-marker used to synchronize the EEG record with a video image. Seizure onset corresponded to the EMG artifact to the left of the figure; the most marked EEG change is rhythmic theta activity at the back of the head starting some 12 s after the first clinical events.

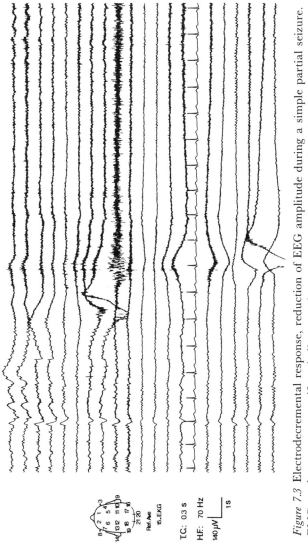

Figure 7.3 Electrodecremental response, reduction of EEG amplitude during a simple partial seizure. EMG and movement artifact indicates seizure onset; patient experienced epigastric sensation, derealization, and a 'funny feeling in the head'.

activity' is rightly criticized as it implies that the discharges are diagnostic of epilepsy, which is not the case. 'Seizure discharges', favoured by many North American electroencephalographers, appears even less acceptable, as these phenomena may be interictal even in persons with epilepsy. The phrase 'paroxysmal activity' is widely used in Europe but is also inappropriate, as many normal EEG phenomena other than those in question are paroxysmal, i.e. transient in nature, for instance K-complexes and lambda-waves. The term 'irritative activity', employed particularly in the Netherlands, is merely a euphemism in that, if it means anything at all, it implies epileptogenesis. This indeed is the heart of the problem, for the only reason for seeking a suitable generic term for such EEG activity is its known, although not invariable, association with epilepsy. In the present text the phrase 'epileptiform activity' will be used which at least recognizes this concept and also stresses the fact that, except in the case of discharges occurring during a seizure (which may correctly be called 'epileptic'), this activity is defined by its morphology.

7.2 EPILEPTIFORM ACTIVITY IN NON-EPILEPTIC SUBJECTS

As indicated above various normal EEG phenomenon are spiky in nature. Failure to distinguish these from abnormal wave-forms has caused considerable confusion, leading to inflated estimates of the incidence of epileptiform activity in normal subjects. These spiky normal activities were recently reviewed by Riley [5] and by Naquet [6]; the following are some of the principal sources of confusion:

7.2.1 Positive spikes

Positive spikes have a characteristic arcuate wave form (one phase being sharp, and the other rounded) and a frequency close to 6 or 14 Hz (Fig. 7.4). They produce a diffuse electrical field and are therefore most easily recognized when common reference methods of derivation are employed. Typically the spiky phase is surface-positive with a potential maximum in one or other posterior temporal region. Positive spikes occur during drowsiness in some 20% of adolescents and young adults. Their incidence may be slightly increased in various disorders (of which epilepsy is not one), but the association with any particular disease state is so weak as to be of negligible diagnostic value. Their clinical significance may be likened to that of left-handedness or red hair, both of which are statistically associated with various disorders but of little significance in any given patient.

7.2.2 '6 Hz spike wave phantom'

A phenomenon probably related to positive spikes, and indeed sometimes coexisting with them, consists of low voltage spike wave activity at about

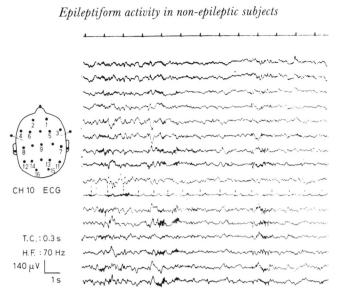

Figure 7.4 Positive spikes, seen chiefly on channels 12, 14, and 16 recording from the left posterior temporal-occipital region.

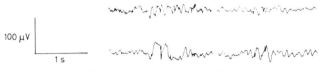

Figure 7.5 6 per second spike-wave.

6 Hz sharing the other features of positive spikes (Fig. 7.5). This too is of no diagnostic significance in relation to epilepsy.

7.2.3 Benign epileptiform transients of sleep (BETS)

BETS, sometimes descriptively termed 'short sharp spikes', occur over the temporal regions during sleep in some 40% of normal subjects (Fig. 7.6). They are characterized by their stereotyped very sharp wave form. Using depth-recordings, Westmoreland *et al.* [7] have shown that when BETS occur in a patient who does in fact have a partial epilepsy, the BETS are totally independent of the pathological epileptogenic focus.

7.2.4 Mid-temporal rhythmic discharge

Mid-temporal rhythmic discharge is, as the name suggests, a rhythmic activity at about 6 Hz seen over the temporal regions, often occurring in runs of many minutes duration and inflenced very little by arousal or sleep (Fig. 7.7). This phenomenon may be present in repeated tracings from the same

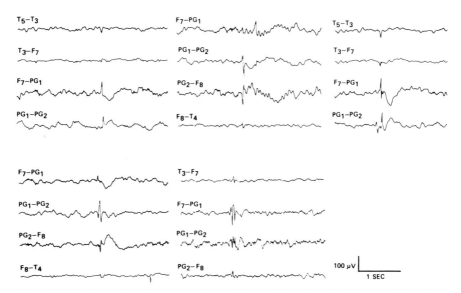

Figure 7.6 Benign epileptiform transients of sleep. (Reproduced with permission from White *et al.* [8].)

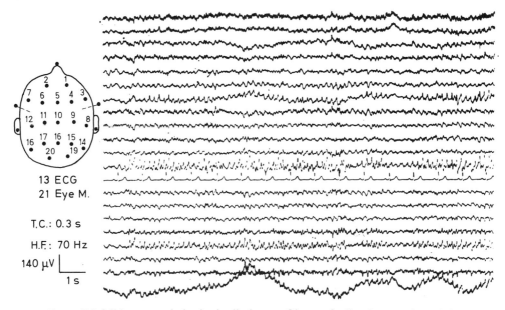

Figure 7.7 Mid-temporal rhythmic discharge. Chance finding in a patient claiming amnesia after a driving offence; no evidence of epilepsy.

subject over many years. It is not influenced by antiepileptic drugs nor can any change in awareness or psychological function be demonstrated during the discharge. The phenomenon is rare and its incidence increased in various groups of patients, some of whom may have epilepsy [9, 10]. It is however of no diagnostic significance and the supposed relationship to temporal lobe epilepsy which gave rise to the earlier name of 'psychomotor variant' [11] is weak.

A similar rhythmic sharp wave activity, 'subclinical rhythmic EEG discharge of adults' (or SREDA) occurs in the parietotemporo-occipital regions. The subjects are generally elderly with various complaints, but rarely epilepsy [12, 13].

7.2.5 Photosensitivity

A generalized discharge of spikes or spike wave activity, consistently elicited by intermittent photic stimulation (IPS), (Fig. 7.8) is termed a photoconvulsive response (PCR) and was described in detail by Bickford *et al.* [14]. If the criterion is added to their account that the discharge should continue for at least some hundred milliseconds after the termination of the stimulus train,

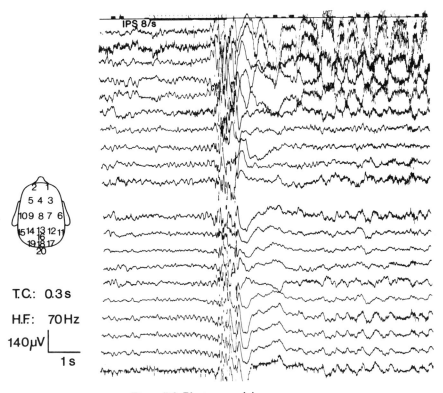

Figure 7.8 Photoconvulsive response.

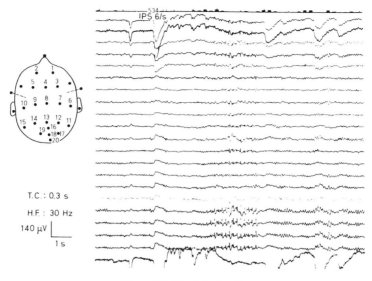

Figure 7.9 Occipital spikes.

then this phenomenon is strongly associated with epilepsy [15] (see also Section 7.5 below). However the term photosensitivity is used, particularly in the German literature, to include a range of more or less unusual responses to IPS which do not have this clinical significance. These include occipital spikes, supra- and subharmonic components of photic following and bursts of slow activity confined to the back of the head (Fig. 7.9). These phenomena may be genetically determined [16] but are only weakly associated with epilepsy and indeed may occur in 15% of normal children. Also open to misinterpretation is the photomyoclonic response, an EMG phenomenon due to reflex contraction of scalp and facial muscles in response to photic stimulation (Fig. 7.10). With a high stimulus intensity this may be elicited in 50% of normal subjects [14]. Its occurrence is moreover favoured by a high level of muscle tone, demonstrable by asking the subject to grimace. This may account for reports that photomyoclonus is more common in psychiatric patients.

7.2.6 'Instability' to hyperventilation

Voluntary hyperventilation is performed routinely for 3–5 minutes during clinical EEG investigation. This produces slowing of cerebral activity in young subjects. If the $p\text{CO}_2$ falls by 15 mm Hg, frontal delta activity will usually appear (Fig. 7.11). In practice this is usually achieved by persons up to the age of 20 or by well motivated subjects up to 30 years. In older subjects the changes in $p\text{CO}_2$ and EEG response are less marked. This normal response is often reported by inexperienced electroencephalographers as evidence of 'electro-

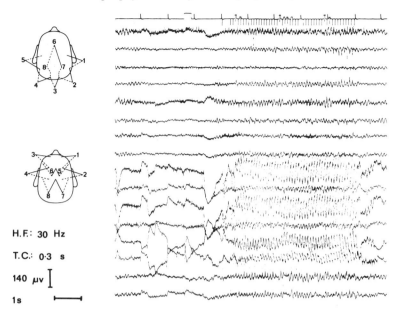

Figure 7.10 Photomyoclonus. EMG activity maximal at front of head and synchronous with flashes.

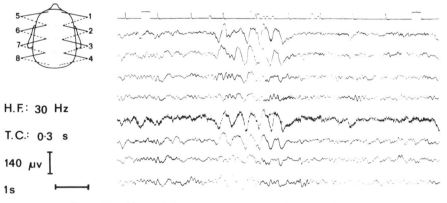

Figure 7.11 Normal slow wave response to hyperventilation.

cortical instability', which all too frequently leads to the administration of antiepileptic drugs to young persons who are not suffering from epilepsy.

7.2.7 Incidence of epileptiform activity in normals

The physiological basis of normal spiky phenomena is largely unknown. However, as Stevens [17] points out, in a readable and thought-provoking review, depth recordings in various species, including man, suggest that spikes represent a normal means of transmitting signals of high biological import- ance, for instance, during orgasm, suckling and aggression.

There are other phenomena which, though usually seen in patients, are unrelated to epilepsy. These phenomena are characterized by morphological and topographical features so distinctive that there is rarely any excuse for confusing them with activities related to epilepsy. There have been com- paratively few studies of the incidence of epileptiform activity in healthy subjects which have specifically excluded these normal phenomena. It is interesting to note that when epileptiform activity in a strict sense is found in a supposedly healthy volunteer, further enquiry usually reveals a history of seizures or other cerebral disorder [18–20]. The most extensive study in adults is that of Robin and coworkers [19] who investigated more than 7000 air force personnel. Of these, 140 exhibited epileptiform EEG activity. However, further enquiry showed that half of these had in fact suffered epileptic seizures and of the remainder all but 15 had been excluded from flying duties on neuropsychiatric grounds, excluding the EEG. We may conclude that the incidence of epileptiform activity in healthy subjects is of the order of 2 per 1000 and is thus similar to that of undiagnosed epilepsy itself [21].

7.3   DIAGNOSTIC EEG INVESTIGATION IN EPILEPSY

As in other diseases of the brain, so also in those producing seizures, the EEG may reflect the underlying cerebral pathology, but, in general, neuroradiologi- cal imaging techniques provide more useful information concerning structural abnormalities. The present text will consider only the specific diagnostic role of the EEG in the investigation of seizures, that is, for the purpose of establishing the diagnosis or determining the type of epilepsy. Except in patients with extremely frequent seizures, in status epilepticus, or with attacks which can be precipitated by physical means, EEG diagnosis must be based on interictal recordings. A study by Ajmone Marsan and Zivin [22] of repeated EEG recordings in patients with epilepsy showed that some 35% consistently exhibited interictal epileptiform EEG activity in waking records. Conversely 15% were equally consistent in never demonstrating interictal discharges in the waking EEG even when this was repeated a dozen times or more. The remaining 50% exhibited interictal epileptiform activity in some records and not in others. An analysis of some 6000 consecutive referrals to the EEG department of the Instituut voor Epilepsiebestrijding closely supports these figures. The implications for the diagnostic investigation of epilepsy are represented in Table 7.1.

A routine waking EEG of some 30–60 min duration which includes hyperventilation and photic stimulation will demonstrate epileptiform activity in approximately 50 out of 100 patients with epilepsy. These 50 will comprise 35 who consistently show interictal discharges and 15 of those who

Table 7.1   Diagnostic EEG investigation of epilepsy: EEG findings on investigation of 100 typical subjects with epilepsy

	Interictal epileptiform activity (EA) found in waking			EA found (cumulative)
	Never	Sometimes	Always	
	15	50	35	
Wake EEG recorded	15	50	35	
EA found	—	15	35	50*
Sleep EEG recorded	15	35	0	
EA found	5	25	—	80
Repeated wake and sleep EEGs recorded	10	10	0	
EA found	2	10	—	92

*Some of these patients will nevertheless require sleep recording for other, specific purposes, e.g. focus localization or investigation of nocturnal attacks of uncertain origin.

sometimes do and sometimes do not. Simply repeating the EEG in those where epileptiform activity has not been demonstrated will produce a further yield of positive findings, and with multiple recordings epileptiform activity will eventually be demonstrated in 85% of subjects. However the yield can be increased and fewer recordings are required if use is made of the activating effect of sleep on the EEG. The profound effect of the sleep–wake cycle on the EEG in epilepsy is well established and many patients show a marked increase in epileptiform discharges during sleep. However the yield in clinical practice of diagnostically useful information from sleep recording is difficult to determine. The overwhelming majority of published studies confound the effects of sleep recording with those of simply repeating the EEG. Light sleep and drowsiness produce a marked increase in the incidence of abnormalities, particularly of focal epileptiform EEG discharges. Departments where routine waking EEGs are short and hurried, affording the patient little opportunity to relax or become drowsy, will tend to report a lower incidence of epileptiform activity in waking and a greater yield of diagnostically useful information in sleep. Conversely, centres of excellence which can permit themselves a more leisurely approach to routine recording will paradoxically find a smaller yield of new information from sleep. This probably accounts for the findings of Gloor and colleagues [23] who, in contrast to many other authors, reported sleep recording to be of little diagnostic value in epilepsy.

There is also a certain lack of agreement concerning the optimal technique for inducing sleep during working hours in the EEG laboratory. Hypnotic drugs such as quinalbarbitone are most often used, but specific activating effects have been claimed for promethazine and thiopentone. This last is of course administered intravenously, which saves time but may cause the patient to pass very rapidly through light drowsiness and stage I sleep, in which the yield of diagnostically useful information, particularly in the partial epilepsies, is greatest. Prolonged deprivation of sleep is known to aggravate epilepsy in many patients and can induce seizures in persons not ordinarily suffering from epilepsy [24]. It may therefore be reasonable to expect that sleep deprivation will not only provide a convenient means of causing the patient to fall into natural sleep during the working hours of the EEG laboratory, but will also have an activating effect in its own right.

Most studies have confounded the effects of repeated EEG investigation of sleep, and of sleep deprivation, on the incidence of epileptiform activity. Only one study [25] employed a randomized design to compare in the same subjects routine recording, drug-induced sleep and sleep deprivation, and differentiated between the incidence of discharges in waking and in the various stages of sleep. No evidence of specific activating effects of sleep deprivation *per se* was demonstrable. It should be added, however, that the study included neither children nor persons with primary generalized epilepsy, and in both groups sleep deprivation has been claimed to have a particularly marked activating effect.

Drug-induced sleep recording may not only be of value as a means of demonstrating epileptiform discharges. Asymmetries of barbiturate-induced beta activity or of sleep spindles may reflect underlying pathology. Despite some claims to the contrary this appears to be of lateralizing significance in patients with partial epilepsies [26]. Some drugs, notably the benzodiazepines, have a differential suppressant effect on generalized and focal discharges. Consequently, in patients with focal epileptiform activity which undergoes rapid secondary generalization, the use of diazepam for sleep recording may help to unmask the focal components, due to the activating effects of sleep on the one hand, and the suppression of the secondary generalized discharges on the other [26].

The overall yield of diagnostically useful EEG information in persons with epilepsy is difficult to assess. Departments with a specialized interest in epilepsy receive a disproportionate number of patients presenting diagnostic problems and conversely those receiving less selected material may not follow optimal practice or be interested in analysing and publishing their results. It appears that a waking EEG of 30 min duration (i.e. 30 min recording, not 30 min devoted to the total investigation) and including periods of hyperventilation and photic stimulation will demonstrate epileptiform activity in some 50% of persons with epilepsy. In perhaps a third of these, some further EEG investigation will be required in connection particularly with the classification of the epilepsy or epileptic syndrome. For instance, if generalized but asymmetrical spike-wave discharges are demonstrated whilst awake, it may be reasonable to obtain a sleep recording to determine whether or not focal epileptiform activity can also be found. Where a focus has indeed been demonstrated in the waking state in a patient who might possibly prove a candidate for neurosurgical treatment, a sleep recording will again be required to determine whether or not other foci are demonstrable. In these, and in the 50% of patients in whom the waking record was negative, a sleep recording should be obtained. It is sometimes difficult to convince colleagues of the importance of, as they see it, repeating a negative investigation; however, if there were grounds for obtaining a diagnostic EEG in the first place there will also be a case for obtaining a sleep record if the wake tracing is negative. In most departments sleep will be induced by drugs as discussed above, although some centres resort directly to sleep deprivation, as means of obtaining a sleep recording. Focal epileptiform discharges will most usually be activated during light sleep (stages I and II) whereas generalized epileptiform activity is more likely to appear in the deeper stages. Patients with secondary generalized epilepsy in particular tend to exhibit characteristic generalized multiple spike and slow wave discharges in deeper sleep (Fig. 7.12).

The possible significance of localized depression of barbiturate-induced fast activity or sleep spindles as evidence of underlying epileptogenic pathology has been noted above. A further finding, albeit of limited diagnostic value, is the occurrence in many patients with epilepsy of atypical spiky K-complexes [27]. Indeed, there appears to be a continuum between the classical K-complex, the leading component of which is a single sharp wave, and responses to arousal consisting of polyspike-wave activity. The literature is curiously deficient on the precise morphology and topography of the sleep EEG in normal subjects, chiefly because the bulk of recording in healthy volunteers takes place in sleep laboratories, using only the one or two EEG channels (together with polygraphy) required for sleep staging. It remains unclear whether a spiky K-complex is supportive of a diagnosis of epilepsy or is to be categorized with the various spiky but normal phenomena of sleep mentioned above.

If a waking EEG and drug-induced sleep recording have still failed to make any contribution to diagnosis, a further tracing will generally be obtained after sleep deprivation, although as indicated above, there is little evidence that sleep deprivation as such has a specific activating effect on the EEG of persons with epilepsy.

In specialized epileptological practice, use of this diagnostic programme (Table 7.1) will result in epileptiform discharges being demonstrated in some 90% of patients with epilepsy. Such findings may not only provide support for the diagnosis but can also give some indication of the type of epilepsy.

7.4 THE EEG AND CLASSIFICATION OF THE EPILEPSIES

Routinely using EEG and clinical information for classifying the epilepsies (see Chapter 3) leads rapidly to a realization of the limitations of the current classifications.

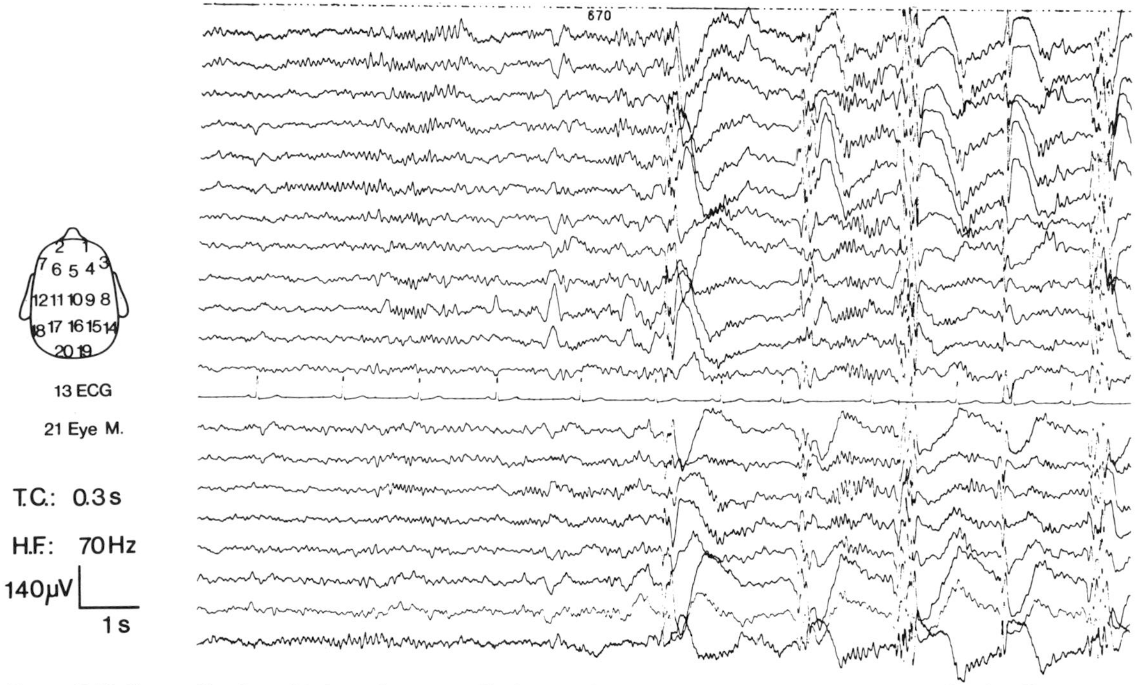
670
13 ECG
21 Eye M.
T.C.: 0.3 s
H.F.: 70 Hz
140μV
1 s

Figure 7.12 Generalized multiple spike-wave discharges in sleep EEG of secondary generalized epilepsy.

7.4.1   Primary generalized epilepsy

The interictal EEG in primary generalized epilepsy is characterized by normal background activity (unless modified by drugs or the effects of head injuries suffered during seizures) and the occurrence of generalized symmetrical spike-wave activity. In patients with absence seizures, this is typically rhythmic with a frequency of 2.5–4 Hz, it usually occurs spontaneously in the course of a 30 min recording and can in any event be elicited by hyperventilation. In patients with only tonic-clonic convulsions the waking record is less likely to show epileptiform discharges although these may be seen in sleep. Again patients may display spike-wave activity but faster and less regular than that associated with absence seizures. Other types of primary generalized epilepsy, notably those with myoclonic seizures, will generally produce more complex interictal discharges of polyspike wave activity, typically symmetrical. Some 30% of patients with primary generalized epilepsy, particularly those with myoclonic attacks, are photosensitive (see below).

Unfortunately the picture is often less simple than that outlined above. Generalized spike wave activity in patients with absence attacks may be somewhat asymmetrical, particularly over the frontal regions, or of atypical irregular wave form and variable frequency. Some patients with a diagnosis of primary generalized epilepsy exhibit background EEG abnormalities, or jagged temporal theta waves, affording room for discussion as to whether or not these should be classified as focal epileptiform discharges.

7.4.2   Partial epilepsy

Partial epilepsies are typically associated with focal interictal discharges, most commonly over the temporal regions and usually comprising sharp waves, spike-wave complexes or short runs of spike-wave activity. Such activities tend to increase in light sleep. There may be other generalized or localized abnormalities reflecting the underlying pathology, possibly a loss of fast activity or an excess of theta or even delta activity surrounding the focal discharge. A particularly distinctive picture is that associated with benign epilepsy of childhood, characterized by high voltage, sharply focal spikes located in the central or centrotemporal region of one or both hemispheres. The very frequent occurrence of these discharges may cause some alarm, unnecessarily, for this is a benign condition which readily responds to therapy. Many siblings of patients with this type of epilepsy show the same EEG phenomena without apparently suffering any seizures.

The picture in many patients with a clinical diagnosis of partial epilepsy is more complex. There may be more than one focus of epileptiform discharges. If the foci are bilaterally symmetrical and discharge synchronously, perhaps more frequently on one side than the other, one may speculate on the possibility of there being a mirror focus, generated in the homologous region of

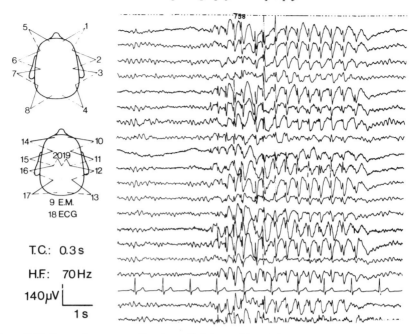

Figure 7.13 Secondary generalization of left frontal focal discharge, seen most clearly on channels 5, 14, and 15. Seizures began consistently with paraesthesia in right hand.

the contralateral hemisphere by direct projection from the primary site of epileptogenesis (pp. 56–57). The existence of mirror foci in man has however never been proven. Often this explanation does not seem acceptable: the foci may be independent, and the patient may in some instances have multiple seizure patterns shown by ictal recordings to arise from the different foci. More often it appears that the habitual seizures arise consistently from only one focus, but this may not be easy to identify from the interictal EEG. Focal discharges frequently become secondarily generalized (Fig. 7.13). In many instances this is easily recognized, in others only close inspection of the tracing will reveal that a seemingly generalized discharge has a consistent focal beginning. The EEG phenomenon of secondary generalization invites confusion with secondary generalized epilepsy, a term which employs the word, secondary, to signify symptomatic. A new draft international classification of the epilepsies [28] which has been proposed, and is reviewed in Chapter 3, happily abandons this confusing terminology.

7.4.3 Symptomatic generalized epilepsy

Secondary generalized epilepsy is typically characterized by a diffuse generalized abnormality of background activity which may range in severity from mild to gross. Multiple polymorphic foci of epileptiform discharges are

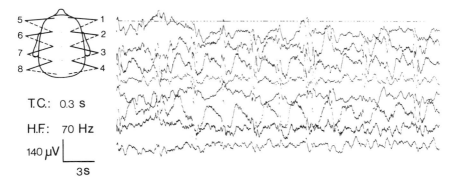

Figure 7.14 Slow spike wave activity in Lennox–Gastaut syndrome.

seen and these often exhibit secondary generalization. Two specific EEG patterns in secondary generalized epilepsy may be noted: the chaotic high voltage hypsarrhythmic EEG of infantile spasms, and the slow generalized spike wave activity associated with the Lennox-Gastaut syndrome (Fig. 7.14).

There is an area of uncertainty in distinguishing between partial and secondary generalized epilepsies. Patients with multiple but discrete foci and corresponding seizure types may present problems of classification, as may those with diffuse severe brain damage displaying a single seizure pattern arising from one focus.

7.5   ACTIVATION PROCEDURES

The use of sleep recording to increase the yield of diagnostically useful information in epilepsy has been considered above. Two other activating procedures, hyperventilation and photic stimulation, are routinely employed and other methods less commonly, such as the use of convulsant drugs.

7.5.1   Hyperventilation

Some three minutes vigorous hyperventilation is performed during routine diagnostic EEG investigation of patients up to the age of 65 years unless there is some contraindication, such as cerebrovascular or pulmonary disease. Slowing of background activity may be observed in normal subjects. Up to the age of some 30 years, or older, if hyperventilation is performed effectively, bilateral frontal delta activity appears. This change is generally attributed, despite some evidence to the contrary, to reduced cerebral perfusion in response to hypocapnia. In various cerebral disorders EEG abnormalities may be increased or appear *de novo*, and in particular epileptiform activity is often activated. The most striking example is provided by generalized spike-wave activity in persons with absence seizures. This is so consistently elicited by adequate hyperventilation that the lack of this response may lead the diagnosis of uncontrolled absence seizures to be questioned. Other generalized, and also focal, discharges may be enhanced, generally less dramatically than by sleep recording. A marked but qualitatively normal response, including frontal delta activity, does not constitute supportive evidence either of epilepsy or of subclinical 'cerebral hyperexitability' (see Section 7.2.6). Indeed even abnormal delta activity can hardly be regarded as supportive of epilepsy if not associated with spikes or occurring during a seizure.

7.5.2 Photic stimulation

Photic stimulation similarly forms a part of routine EEG examination. The aspect which is most relevant in the context of diagnostic investigation of possible epilepsy is the eliciting of a photoconvulsive response. As previously indicated in Section 7.2.5 above, this phenomenon, if strictly defined, is virtually confined to persons with epilepsy and their close relatives. Approximately 5% of people with epilepsy exhibit a photoconvulsive response, particularly those with primary generalized epilepsy or with a family history of the disorder. Photosensitivity is twice as common in females as in males; it is most frequently detected at about the age of 12 years, the incidence declining sharply after adolescence. Sixty per cent of photosensitive patients have experienced seizures precipitated by environmental visual stimuli, as for instance sunlight reflected on water or seen through moving foliage, discotheque lighting, and most importantly in Western Europe, television. Fifty per cent of photosensitive patients with epilepsy have no spontaneous seizures, all their attacks being apparently triggered by visual stimuli. Thus, although photosensitive epilepsy is comparatively rare, its recognition may be of considerable importance for the management of the individual patient, whose seizures may be greatly reduced or eliminated simply by avoidance of the provocative stimuli. A detailed analysis of the problem in the EEG laboratory may therefore be justified. Procedures for routine and special investigation of photosensitivity are discussed in detail by Binnie *et al.* [4].

Some 30% of photosensitive patients also exhibit epileptiform EEG discharges when viewing black and white grating patterns, and some report seizures induced by environmental patterns of this type. Pattern sensitivity can readily be investigated in the EEG laboratory by presenting the appropriate stimuli [29]. Where television epilepsy is in question, a normally functioning black and white TV monitor can be used as a provocative test. In advising about measures to avoid seizures it should be noted that two mechanisms are involved in television epilepsy [30]. Some patients who are sensitive to photic stimulation at 50 flashes/s (the flicker rate of European TV) exhibit discharges when watching TV, often at a distance of several metres from the screen; they are to some extent protected by viewing in a well-lit environment. Others exhibit discharges in response to television only at a very short viewing distance. They usually are not photosensitive to frequencies as high as 50 flashes/s but are pattern sensitive, apparently responding to the linear pattern of the raster. In contrast with the first group these patients become more sensitive to TV in a well lit environment and are best advised to maintain a distance of 2 m or more from the television [31]. Alternatively, they should obtain a screen so small that the raster pattern cannot be resolved.

A further clinically important aspect of photosensitivity is the fact that some patients, perhaps as many as 25% [32], make use of their photosensitivity to elicit EEG discharges or indeed seizures in themselves. Self-induced seizures are often resistant to therapy and it is clinically important to recognize the problem. Although some mentally subnormal patients induce seizures by staring at the sun or bright lights and waving one hand with the fingers spread in front of the eyes, most patients use a more subtle technique of slow eye closure with rapid blinking [33] which may most readily be demonstrated by a period of EEG and video monitoring (see below) [34].

7.5.3 Chemical activation

Various chemical methods of EEG activation have been advocated from time to time. These range from methohexitone, said to have some direct epilepto-genic action in addition to inducing sleep, to frank convulsants such as pentylenetetrazol. During recording with depth electrodes from patients with seizures of clearly focal origin, it has been shown [35] that seizures induced by pentylenetetrazol may be totally different both clinically and electrographically from those occurring spontaneously. For this and other reasons the technique has rightly fallen into disuse.

More general reviews of both standard and unorthodox methods of EEG activation are available [4, 36].

7.6 EPILEPSY MONITORING

As indicated above, conventional EEG investigation provides evidence supportive of a diagnosis of epilepsy and contributes to the classification in some 90% of patients. In many of the remaining 10% a confident clinical diagnosis is in any event possible, but in some there remains considerable uncertainty and additional diagnostic evidence would be of value. In a second important category of patients, typically comprising some 15% of referrals to specialist epileptological practice, there are attacks resembling seizures but which are not of epileptic origin. In both groups the diagnosis may be established by detailed clinical and electrophysiological observation of the seizures themselves. Except in patients with very frequent attacks, as for instance absences which may occur hundreds of times a day, or attacks which may be reliably precipitated by hyperventilation or other means, a prolonged period of observation may be required to obtain the necessary information. For this

Table 7.2 Main features of current monitoring technologies

Features	Hard-wired EEG machine	EEG monitoring technologies			
		Cable telemetry	Radio telemetry	Cassette (normal tape speed)	Cassette (low tape speed)
Technical quality	+++	+++	+	++	–
Range	3 m	50 m	500 m free field. Variable in building	Unlimited	Unlimited
Cost	Nil extra for hardware, labour intensive	+	+++	++	+++
Applications					
Intensive diagnosis	++	+++	+	+	–
Seizure frequency	+	++	++	–	+++
Precipitants	+	++	+++	++	+++
Effects of normal activity in natural environment	–	–	+	++	+++

purpose registration with a conventional EEG recorder from a patient lying immobile in bed or in a chair is hardly suitable if the investigation is expected to last more than a few hours. It is usual to employ some form of EEG telemetry (Table 7.2) for longer recordings or to investigate patients during various activities.

Recent reviews of the various technologies are available [37–39]. Many early monitoring studies were performed using radio transmission of the EEG signals, but this gave rise to considerable practical difficulties and many workers now prefer where possible to record the EEG through a flexible cable of some 50 m length which allows the patient considerable freedom of movement within the confines of a ward or EEG department.

An alternative and popular technology is the use of miniaturized cassette recorders of up to eight channels and capable of recording continuously for 24 hours. These systems push present tape recording technology to its limits. They are not very reliable and suffer from a limited range of amplitude and frequency response. They nevertheless provide the only readily available means of recording from patients in their natural environments, and are ideal for studying the occurrence of known EEG phenomena under particular circumstances, for instance to determine the incidence of absence seizures in a child at school. For many purposes careful documentation, or preferably video recording, of behaviour is desirable and for this purpose admission to an observation unit is preferable to ambulatory cassette monitoring in out-patients. Fully equipped monitoring units incorporate sophisticated video recording facilities with remotely controlled cameras, some of them equipped with infrared-sensitive tubes for registration at night. Various methods may be employed for correlating the EEG and behavioural information, of which the simplest and most popular is a simultaneous 'split screen' registration of the patient and his EEG as a single video picture. Some examples are given in Chapter 3.

The clinical applications of intensive epilepsy monitoring are summarized in Table 7.3.

In most units the most important single indication is the differential diagnosis of epileptic and non-epileptic seizures, the latter most often being pseudoseizures, which may of course also occur in persons with epilepsy. Reliable documentation of the clinical manifestations often leads to a strong suspicion of pseudoseizures, but in many instances the ictal EEG findings are conclusive, and sometimes surprising.

As was pointed out above (Section 7.1) the scalp EEG during an epileptic seizure does not necessarily exhibit activity generally regarded as epilepti-form. Changes may consist of the appearance of frequencies not previously present or simply a change in amplitude of ongoing activity (Figs 7.2 and 7.3).

Certain seizure types are generally not accompanied by any ictal EEG change, although epileptiform activity may be found in depth recordings. The most noted example is provided by simple partial seizures with psychic

Table 7.3 Indications for epilepsy monitoring

Differential diagnosis
 Pseudoseizures
 Enuresis
 Nocturnal restlessness/apnoea
 Cardiac disorder/syncope
 Diurnal sleepiness
 Episodic behavioural disturbance
 Metabolic: hypoglycaemia, etc.
 Hyperventilation

EEG correlates of known seizures
 Classification
 Focus localization

Clinical correlates of EEG discharge
 Transitory cognitive impairment

Seizure frequency

Seizure precipitants
 Reflex epilepsy
 Self-induction
 Situational factors

symptomatology [40] or, less consistently, with viscerosensory symptoms or focal motor phenomena. It is therefore by no means the case that the absence of ictal epileptiform activity or indeed of any change in the scalp EEG excludes the possibility that a seizure is epileptic in nature, rather it is essential that the clinical manifestations be taken into account. The absence of ictal EEG change is however conclusive evidence of a non-epileptic origin in attacks simulating absences, tonic-clonic convulsions, and complex partial seizures with automatism, as these seizure types are invariably accompanied by ictal EEG changes. The implications are obvious: EEG monitoring is rarely of value for establishing a diagnosis of pseudoseizures unless it includes accurate documentation, preferably by video recording, of behaviour.

Other diagnostic problems which may be resolved by monitoring include bizarre nocturnal events particularly those occurring in children and the differential diagnosis between attacks of cerebral and cardiac origin; these last certainly require simultaneous ECG monitoring.

In patients where the diagnosis of epilepsy is already established, intensive monitoring may be required for seizure classification. The instance most frequently cited is that of the differential diagnosis between absences and brief complex partial seizures, which of course respond selectively to different types of medication (pp. 237–40). The case may in fact have been over-stated, as a study of diagnostic monitoring in therapy-resistant patients presenting this differential diagnosis [41] served only to highlight the ambiguities inherent in the International Classification of Epileptic Seizures. Many patients' attacks could not with confidence be classified. These responded most frequently to combinations of drugs ordinarily used for partial seizures, such as phenytoin or carbamazepine, with those more appropriate for absences, as sodium valproate and ethosuximide. This experience is supported by the findings of Stefan [42] and of Hendriksen [43].

A small but important group of patients with established epilepsy requiring monitoring are those with partial seizures undergoing evaluation for possible neurosurgical treatment (pp. 287–291). There is little uniformity in practice between various centres in the use made of monitoring for this purpose. Some groups employ extremely conservative criteria based on the clinical manifestations, neuroradiology and meticulous interictal scalp EEG investigation augmented by sphenoidal recording [44]. Such an approach achieves an impressive success rate, but presumably excludes from the possibility of treatment patients who fail to meet these criteria, for instance by virtue of multiple or ill-defined foci in the interictal EEG. Some workers such as Engel [45] require ictal recording with depth electrodes in virtually all patients being assessed for surgery. An intermediate position is represented by Olivier and coworkers [46], who until recently employed traditional conservative criteria [47] supplemented by ictal scalp recordings; depth registration was undertaken in only 12–15% of patients. More recently this group has made more use of ictal depth registrations and find this offers the possibility of identifying the trigger focus and offering surgical help to patients previously regarded as inoperable. Comparisons of scalp and depth records [48] highlight the limited reliability of the scalp EEG, including ictal recordings, for localizing the focal origin of seizures. Electrocorticography and depth recording are considered further below.

The numbers of ictal events may be difficult to determine when the frequency is extremely high, as in many patients with absence seizures, or when they are not readily detectable by the patient or other observers. Monitoring is useful in such instances to establish seizure frequency, and to assess response to therapy [49]. Where the ictal EEG phenomena are easily detected, as in absence seizures, it may be sufficient for this purpose to count the spike-wave discharges. In patients with subtle clinical and EEG manifestations of partial seizures, meticulous inspection of the entire video tapes and EEG records may be required. Sometimes indeed the clinical ictal manifestations may fall within the patient's normal behavioural repertoire and, if not recognized by the subject himself as involuntary, can be identified only on the grounds that a particular act, as for instance turning the head slightly to one side and smiling, is consistently accompanied by an epileptiform discharge.

The principle of attempting to detect subtle clinical correlates of EEG discharges may be extended further by the use of psychological testing during monitoring. It has been known almost since the beginning of clinical electroencephalography that psychological testing during subclinical discharges often reveals transitory cognitive impairment (TCI) [50]. Over the years some 40 studies have documented this phenomenon. Generalized regular spike-wave discharges of more than 3 s duration are most likely to produce demonstrable TCI whereas asymmetrical, irregular or short discharges do so less readily. The chances of demonstrating any cognitive disturbance are also dependent upon the psychological test used. Simple repetitious tasks such as tapping and counting or simple reaction time are known to be relatively insensitive to the effects of subclinical discharges. By contrast, tasks involving memory and/or language are much more readily disrupted, particularly when the level of difficulty ensures that the subject is extended. Investigating TCI presents some practical problems: attention frequently suppresses discharges so that the paroxysms may occur less than once in 5 min. The tasks used for most studies of this phenomenon are so very boring that subjects are rarely prepared to persist with them for more than a few tens of minutes. Consequently, the chances of sufficient discharges occurring during testing to permit any reliable assessment are poor. Research studies have overcome this difficulty by employing only patients with a very high discharge rate but it is desirable also as a routine clinical service to be able to assess any patient who exhibits subclinical discharges in the waking state. For this purpose, use may be made of continuous tasks presented as television games which will hold the subject's attention for an hour or more [51]. Using such a task it is possible to test most patients with reasonably frequent subclinical discharges as a routine clinical service. Moreover the tasks described by Aarts *et al.* [51] were sufficiently sensitive to demonstrate cognitive impairment during focal discharges, and to show that discharges over the dominant hemisphere selectively disrupted performance of a verbal task whereas non-dominant discharges had more effect on a task involving topographic material.

The clinical relevance of TCI may be questioned. A change in cognitive function accompanied by an EEG discharge fulfils most contemporary definitions of an epileptic seizure (p. 1). Apart from the semantic question as to whether this phenomenon should therefore be regarded as a seizure, there is the practical question of whether or not TCI adversely effects the performance of patients in the world outside the EEG laboratory, their educational potential, their ability to concentrate on their work, etc. At an anecdotal level, patients are reported in whom subclinical discharges, occurring in the absence of known epileptic seizures, were associated with TCI in the laboratory and problems at work or school. In some such subjects medication to suppress the discharges was followed by a clear improvement in psychosocial function. How many patients with subclinical discharges might benefit from such therapy is however uncertain. 'Cosmetic' treatment of the EEG cannot be justified, unless there is clear evidence of TCI and a probability that this is adversely affecting psychosocial function.

Monitoring may be of value for investigating various forms of sensory precipitated epilepsy, as has already been noted in the context of self-induced seizures. Patients with the more recherché forms of reflex epilepsy may have reported their history accurately to many physicians before the significance of the precipitating sensory factor is appreciated. Conclusive diagnosis of reflex epilepsy generally requires EEG and behavioural documentation of an induced seizure. Reflex epilepsies triggered by elementary stimuli as flicker, touch, startle, etc., may be investigated during routine EEG recording. Those produced by cognitive or situational factors such as reading, eating and mental tasks, etc., often require prolonged exposure in the appropriate environment. Investigation will be assisted by use of monitoring facilities.

Finally it may be noted that there exist many specific problems not readily categorized in the scheme above which may be usefully addressed by combined studies of EEG, behaviour, psychological function and antiepileptic drug levels. These last may be estimated at hourly intervals by means of an indwelling catheter flushed at regular intervals with heparinized saline to maintain patency [52].

7.7   EEG, TREATMENT AND PROGNOSIS

The introduction questioned the proposition that the amount of interictal epileptiform activity reflected the severity of epilepsy, the effect of treatment, or the prognosis. In some specific situations, such relationships are indeed found. The amount of generalized spike-wave activity correlates closely with the frequency of absence seizures and is dramatically reduced by effective medication. In mentally subnormal patients with epilepsy, marked EEG abnormality, including the presence of large amounts of epileptiform activity, implies a poor prognosis for remission. These are, however, special cases. The generalized spike-wave discharge in a patient with absences generally indicates a clinical event (p. 191) and counting these discharges is therefore tantamount to counting seizures. The EEG abnormalities in the subnormal patient with epilepsy largely reflect the severity of the brain damage, which is the determinant of prognosis.

In routine EEG practice there is in general little correlation between discharge rate and reported seizure frequency, either within or between patients [53]. EEG spike counts do not often prove useful as outcome variables in antiepileptic drug trials [54, 55]. The presence of continuing discharges in patients who have become seizure-free on medication is predictive of relapse after drug withdrawal in children [56, 57] but not in adults [58].

7.8   CONCLUSION

As was noted in the introduction, epilepsy is sometimes regarded as a test case for assessing the clinical usefulness of EEG. It is however also true that epilepsy provides some excellent examples of the ways in which clinical EEG can be misused. Little useful contribution is made by the recording of routine EEGs without any specific question, in the belief that EEG forms part of the 'standard work-up' of people with epilepsy. Conversely, there are many problems in epileptology to which the EEG makes a unique and indispensable contribution. In many instances the investigations required are long, complex and of a non-routine nature, specifically designed to address a particular issue. It may justifiably be considered that such investigations cannot be performed under the conditions existing in most routine EEG departments. However referral policy can often be adapted to reduce the demand for inappropriate and unrewarding investigations in order to free the capacity required for flexible, problem-orientated EEG investigation of persons with epilepsy.

REFERENCES

1. Matthews, W. B. (1964) The use and abuse of electroencephalography. *Lancet*, **ii**, 577–9.
2. Hopkins, A. and Scambler, G. (1977) How doctors deal with epilepsy. *Lancet*, **i**, 183–6.
3. Chatrian, G. E., Bergamini, L., Dondey, M. *et al.* (1974) A glossary of terms most commonly used by clinical electroencephalographers. *Electroenceph. Clin. Neurophysiol.*, **37**, 538–48.
4. Binnie, C. D., Rowan, A. J. and Gutter, T. (1982) *A Manual of EEG Technology*, Cambridge University Press, UK.
5. Riley, T. L. (1983) Normal variants in EEG that are mistaken as epileptic patterns, in *Pseudoepilepsy* (ed. M. Gross), D. C. Heath, Lexington, pp. 25–7.
6. Naquet, R. (1983) The clinical significance of EEG in epilepsy, in *Epilepsy: An Update on Research and Therapy* (eds G. Nistico *et al.*), Alan R. Liss Inc., New York, pp. 147–64.
7. Westmoreland, B. F., Reiher, J. and Klass, D. W. (1979) Recording small sharp spikes with depth electroencephalography. *Epilepsia*, **20**, 599–606.
8. White, J. C., Langston, J. W., Pedley, T. A. (1977) Benign epileptiform transients of sleep: clarification of the small sharp spike controversy. *Neurology*, **27**, 1061–8.
9. Hughes, J. R. and Cayaffa, J. J. (1973) Is the 'psychomotor variant' – 'rhythmic mid-temporal discharge' an ictal pattern? *Clin. Electroenceph.*, **4**, 42–9.
10. Lipman, I. J. and Hughes, J. R. (1969) Rhythmic mid-temporal discharges. An electro-clinical study. *Electroenceph. Clin. Neurophysiol.*, **27**, 43–7.
11. Gibbs, F. A. and Gibbs, E. L. (1953) *Atlas of Electroencephalography, Vol. 2: Epilepsy*, Addison-Wesley Press, Cambridge, USA, p. 422.
12. Naquet, R., Louard, C. and Rhodes, J. (1961) A propos de certaines dècharges paroxystiques. Leur activation par l'hypoxie. *Rev. Neurol. (Paris)*, **105**, 203–7.
13. Westmoreland, B. F. and Klass, D. W. (1981) A distinctive rhythmic EEG discharge of adults. *Electroenceph. Clin. Neurophysiol.*, **51**, 186–91.
14. Bickford, R. G., Sem-Jacobsen, C. W., White, P. T. and Daly, D. (1952) Some observations on the mechanism of photic and photo-metrazol activation. *Electroenceph. Clin. Neurophysiol.*, **4**, 275–82.

15. Reilly, E. L. and Peters, J. F. (1973) Relationship of some varieties of electro-encephalographic photosensitivity to clinical convulsive disorders. *Neurology (Minneap.)*, **23**, 1050–7.

16. Doose, H. and Gerken, H. (1973) On the genetics of EEG-anomalies in childhood: IV. photoconvulsive reaction. *Neuropaediatrie*, **4**, 162–71.

17. Stevens, J. R. (1977) The EEG spike: signal of information transmission. *Ann. Neurol.*, **1**, 309–14.

18. Binnie, C. D., Batchelor, B. G., Bowring, P. A. *et al.* (1978) Computer-assisted interpretation of clinical EEGs. *Electroenceph. Clin. Neurophysiol.*, **44**, 575–85.

19. Robin, J. J., Tolan, G. D. and Arnold, J. W. (1978) Ten-year experience with abnormal EEGs in asymptomatic adult males. *Aviat. Space Environ. Med.*, **49**, 732–6.

20. Roubicek, J., Volavka, J. and Matousek, M. (1967) Elektroencefalogram u normalni populace. *Cesk. Psychiatr.*, **63**, 14–19.

21. Zielinski, J. J. (1974) Epileptics not in treatment. *Epilepsia*, **15**, 203–10.

22. Ajmone Marsan, C. and Zivin, L. S. (1970) Factors related to the occurrence of typical paroxysmal abnormalities in the EEG records of epileptic patients. *Epilepsia*, **11**, 361–81.

23. Gloor, P., Tsai, C., Haddad, F. and Jasper, H. H. (1957) The lack of necessity for sleep in the EEG or ECG diagnosis of temporal seizures. *Electroenceph. Clin. Neurophysiol.*, **9**, 379–80.

24. Bennett, D. R. (1962) Sleep deprivation and major motor convulsions. *Neurology (Minneap.)*, **13**, 953–8.

25. Veldhuizen, R., Binnie, C. D. and Beintema, D. J. (1983) The effect of sleep deprivation on the EEG in epilepsy. *Electroenceph. Clin. Neurophysiol.* **55**, 505–12.

26. Gotman, J., Gloor, P., Quesney, L. F. and Olivier, A. (1982) Correlations between EEG changes induced by diazepam and the localization of epileptic spikes and seizures. *Electroenceph. Clin. Neurophysiol.*, **54**, 614–21.

27. Niedermeyer, E. (1965) Sleep electroencephalograms in petit mal. *Arch. Neurol.*, **12**, 625–30.

28. Dreifuss, F. E., Martinez-Lage, M., Roger, J. *et al.* (1985) Proposal for classification of epilepsies and epileptic syndromes. *Epilepsia*, **26**, 268–78.

29. Darby, C. E., Wilkins, A. J., Binnie, C. D. and De Korte, R. A. (1980) Routine testing for pattern sensitivity. *J. Electrophysiol. Technol.*, **6**, 202–10.

30. Wilkins, A. J., Darby, C. E., Binnie, C. D. *et al.* (1979) Television epilepsy: the role of pattern. *Electroenceph. Clin. Neurophysiol.*, **47**, 163–71.

31. Binnie, C. D., Darby, C. E., De Korte, R. A. *et al.* (1980) EEG sensitivity to television: effects of ambient lighting. *Electroenceph. Clin. Neurophysiol.*, **50**, 329–31.

32. Binnie, C. D., Darby, C. E., De Korte, R. A. and Wilkins, A. J. (1980) Self-induction of epileptic seizures by eyeclosure: incidence and recognition. *J. Neurol. Neurosurg. Psychiatr.*, **43**, 386–9.

33. Green, J. B. (1966) Self-induced seizures: clinical and electroencephalographic studies. *Arch. Neurol.*, **15**, 579–86.

34. Darby, C. E., De Korte, R. A., Binnie, C. D. and Wilkins, A. J. (1980) The self-induction of epileptic seizures by eyeclosure. *Epilepsia*, **21**, 31–42.

35. Wieser, H. G., Bancaud, J., Talairach, J. *et al.* (1979) Comparative value of spontaneous and chemically and electrically induced seizures in establishing the lateralization of temporal lobe seizures. *Epilepsia*, **20**, 47–59.

36. Naquet, R. (1976) Activation and provocation methods in clinical electro-encephalography, in *Handbook of Electroencephalography and Clinical Neurophysiology* **3D** (ed. A. Rémond), Elsevier, Amsterdam, pp. 1–174.

37. Binnie, C. D. (1983) Telemetric EEG monitoring in epilepsy, in *Recent Advances in Epilepsy*, I (eds T. A. Pedley and B. S. Meldrum), Churchill Livingstone, Edinburgh, pp. 155–78.

38. Ebersole, J. S. (1986) EEG: telemetered and ambulatory cassette – review of current systems and techniques, in *Advances in Neurology: International Conference on Neurodiagnostic Monitoring* (ed. R. J. Gumnit), Raven Press, New York, in press.

39. Gotman, J., Ives, J. R. and Gloor, P. (eds) (1985) Long-term monitoring in epilepsy. *Electroenceph. Clin. Neurophysiol.*, **Suppl. 37**.

40. Wieser, H. G. (1979) 'Psychische Anfälle' und deren stereo-elek-troenzephalographisches Korrelat. *EEG EMG*, **10**, 197–206.

41. Binnie, C. D. and Van der Wens, P. (1986) Diagnostic re-evaluation by intensive monitoring of intractable absence seizures, in *Intractable Epilepsy: Experimental and Clinical Aspects* (eds D. Schmidt and P. Morselli), Raven Press, New York, pp. 99–107.

42. Stefan, H. (1986) Absence seizures – long term therapeutic monitoring, in *Intractable Epilepsy: Experimental and Clinical Aspects* (eds D. Schmidt and P. Mor-selli), Raven Press, New York.

43. Hendriksen, O. (1986) Absence seizures – multiple and reduction of multiple drug therapy, in *Intractable Epilepsy: Experimental and Clinical Aspects* (eds D. Schmidt and P. Morselli), Raven Press, New York.

44. Polkey, C. E. (1981) Selection of patients with chronic drug-resistant epilepsy for resective surgery: 5 years' experience. *J. Roy. Soc. Med.*, **74**, 574–9.

45. Engel, J., Rausch, R., Lieb, J. P. *et al.* (1981) Correlation of criteria used for localizing epileptic foci in patients considered for surgical therapy of epilepsy. *Ann. Neurol.*, **9**, 215–24.

46. Olivier, A., Gloor, P., Quesney, L. F. and Andermann, F. (1983) The indications for and the role of depth electrode recording in epilepsy. *Appl. Neurophysiol.*, **46**, 33–6.

47. Bloom, D., Jasper, H. and Rasmussen, T. (1959) Surgical therapy in patients with temporal lobe seizures and bilateral EEG abnormality. *Epilepsia*, **1**, 351–65.

48. Lieb, J. P., Walsh, G. O., Babb, T. L. *et al.* (1976) Comparison of EEG seizure patterns recorded with surface and depth electrodes in patients with temporal lobe epilepsy. *Epilepsia*, **17**, 137–60.

49. Browne, T. R., Penry, J. K., Porter, R. J. and Dreifuss, F. E. (1974) A comparison of clinical estimates of absence seizure frequency with estimates based on pro-longed telemetered EEGs. *Neurology (Minneap.)*, **24**, 381–2.

50. Schwab, R. S. (1939) A method of measuring consciousness in petit mal epilepsy. *J. Nerv. Ment. Dis.*, **89**, 690–1.

51. Aarts, J. H. P., Binnie, C. D., Smit, A. M. and Wilkins, A. J. (1984) Selective cognitive impairment during focal and generalized epileptiform EEG activity. *Brain*, **107**, 293–308.

52. Meinardi, H., Binnie, C. D. and Meijer, J. W. A. (1985) Assessment of effect of antiepileptic drugs, in *Long-Term Monitoring in Epilepsy* (eds J. Gotman *et al.*). *Electroenceph. Clin. Neurophysiol.*, **Suppl. 37**, pp. 201–14.

53. Binnie, C. D. (1986) The interictal EEG, in *What is Epilepsy?* (eds M. R. Trimble and E. H. Reynolds), Churchill Livingstone, London, pp. 116–25.
54. Gram, L., Drachmann Bentsen, K., Parnas, J. and Flachs, H. (1982) Controlled trials in epilepsy: a review. *Epilepsia*, **23**, 491–519.
55. Van Wieringen, A., Binnie, C. D., De Boer, P. T. E. *et al.* (1985) Visual and spectral analysis of EEGs during anti-epileptic drug trials. *Electroenceph. Clin. Neurophysiol.* **61**, S214.
56. Emerson, R., D'Souza, B. J., Vining, E. P. (1981) Stopping medication in children with epilepsy: predictors of outcome. *N. Engl. J. Med.*, **304**, 1125–9.
57. Todt, H. (1981) Zur Spaetprognose kindlicher Epilepsien: Ergebnisse einer prospektiven Laengsschnittstudie. *Deutsch. Gesundheitswes.*, **36**, 2011–16.
58. Overweg, J. (1985) *Anti-epileptic Drug Withdrawal in Seizure-free Patients:* Thesis, University of Amsterdam, The Netherlands.

CHAPTER EIGHT

Imaging in the Investigation of Epilepsy

Simon Shorvon

Diagnostic imaging in neurology has been revolutionized in the past two decades. Advances in this period have been unparalleled in any previous epoch. As epilepsy is often based in abnormal function, rather than structure, the impact of these changes may have been less dramatic than in some other fields. However, improvements in diagnostic techniques, particularly for the non-invasive detection of underlying structural abnormalities, have significantly altered the approach to clinical investigation. Newer techniques are currently being developed, and the prospects for further improvement seem bright.

8.1   PLAIN RADIOLOGY

With the development of advanced imaging techniques such as computerized tomography (CT) or magnetic resonance imaging (MRI, NMR), the value of plain skull radiology tends to be forgotten, yet it still has a definite place [1]. Although for much of the imaging necessary in epilepsy it is inferior to newer techniques in both sensitivity and specificity, it is cheap, widely available and relatively innocuous, although it should not be forgotten that the radiation dose from a full skull series of radiographs is approximately equivalent to that necessary for a CT scan. Moreover for the visualization of some bony structures plain skull radiology is still superior. It should probably be carried out in most cases of epilepsy, and all cases in which more sophisticated radiology is not judged necessary. A lateral view should be routinely obtained; an AP view, Townes view, basal views, or special views such as of the petrous bone or pituitary fossa, or tomography may be required. A number of changes on the plain skull radiograph in epilepsy should be sought.

(a)   Bony changes

Bony changes on skull radiology in patients with epilepsy may be subdivided into six categories:

(1)   Signs of raised intracranial pressure: This may cause erosive changes of the pituitary fossa, thinning of the inner table, a copper beaten vault appearance in children, and if present before their fusion, widening of the skull sutures and macrocephaly. However, the changes of raised intracranial

pressure are now seen in only a small minority of patients with epilepsy due to an intracranial mass lesion.

(2) New bone formation: Localized thickening of the inner table and sclerosis of the diploe are seen at the site of a meningioma in about one-third of cases at the time of diagnosis, often in association with the other radiological signs of meningioma. This is a highly characteristic appearance, and only sclerosing secondary deposits from carcinoma of prostate or breast are likely to cause confusion in this clinical setting. A thickened skull vault is a frequent non-specific finding in chronic epilepsy. The cause of this is obscure.

(3) Bony erosion: This is an unusual finding as an association with epilepsy. If present, it is usually caused by metastases. More rarely, primary tumours of bone, infections with *Echinococcus*, metabolic diseases such as hyperparathyroidism, or pressure from surrounding masses such as a meningioma, aneurysm, or porencephalic cyst may cause localized erosion. Occasionally, a meningioma may cause a purely lytic appearance.

(4) Cranial hemiatrophy: If the underlying cerebral structures develop less on one side during the first years of life, the skull overlying the atrophic areas may be thickened and flattened; the base may also be elevated and the sinuses enlarged. Less severe changes may occur following damage in later childhood. These may be important factors when assessing a patient with epilepsy, as they may indicate a childhood origin of the pathological process causing the seizures.

(5) Pathological vascular markings: A meningioma is the commonest cause of these. The abnormal vascular markings are largely due to the dilated middle meningeal vessels supplying the tumour, but changes in the diploic vessels and the emissary venous vessels may also be seen. The changes may be bilateral in parasagittal lesions. Meningiomas are also associated with hyperostosis and intracranial calcification. Angiomatous malformations may also result in increased meningeal vascular markings in the skull vault which are usually less localized than with meningiomas; they may be bilateral, and there may also be enlarged emissary venous markings.

(6) Congenital cranial abnormalities: Some of the rare congenital or hereditary diseases associated with mental retardation and epilepsy have characteristic radiological appearances. These include specific changes such as those of meningocoele or encephalocoele platybasia, or less specific changes such as microcephaly. In most cases of epilepsy due to congenital causes, however, plain skull radiology is normal.

(b) Abnormal calcification

Many of the structural conditions causing epilepsy show variable degrees of pathological calcification.

(1) Amongst the cerebral tumours, about 5% of gliomas show calcification on radiology, about 15% of meningiomas, and higher proportions of the

benign tumours such as hamartomas. Calcification is more frequent in the more slowly growing gliomas. Serpiginous calcification is said to be a characteristic finding in oligodendroglioma. Other rarer tumours may be calcified. The position of the calcification may be diagnostic. Cranio-pharyngiomas, for example, have demonstrable calcification in 75% of childhood cases, in the form of flecks, or cystic, linear or curvilinear shadowing of variable density in the frontal areas, with characteristic changes of the dorsum sella.

(2) In arteriovenous malformations, calcification is seen in about 15% of cases, usually as flecks of calcium or as curvilinear shadowing in vessel walls. In about 60% of cases of Sturge-Weber syndrome, unilateral calcification is seen, typically with a characteristic appearance of sinuous parallel lines ('tram lines') several millimetres thick (Fig. 8.1). The calcification is in the atrophic cortex underlying the superficial angioma; these changes are most common in the occipital or parietal region. There may also be more extensive underlying cerebral calcification, but this is usually better seen on CT. Curvilinear calcification is also occasionally seen in aneurysms (the calcium is usually in the vessel walls) and other vascular conditions. Intracerebral haematomas may also eventually calcify.

(3) Several of the infectious diseases causing epilepsy may be associated with pathological intracranial calcification. Cysticercosis is the most import-ant. Epilepsy may occur in up to 90% of cerebral cases, and may be the only clinical manifestation. In certain parts of the world, such as India, this parasitic disease is amongst the commonest causes of epilepsy. On plain radiology, calcified cysts may sometimes, but not invariably, be seen in muscle – most often in the thigh – as well as in cerebral tissue. In muscle the cysts may be multiple, elongated and 1–2 cm long. On the skull radiograph, calcification may occasionally be seen in the extracranial soft tissues. Intracranial calcifica-tion is less common (about 14% in one series). The calcification is usually multiple, pin-point or nodular. Each nodule represents a dead larva, and may be up to 6 mm or 7 mm in size; the densities are often widely scattered. In the UK, cysticercosis often presents in its racemose form, causing obstructive hypdrocephalus, occasionally with radiological signs of raised intracranial pressure. However, epilepsy is an unusual manifestation of this form of the disease.

Tuberculomas calcify poorly (less than 1% are detectable on plain radi-ology) and the nodular calcification has no specific features. In India, the tuberculoma is the commonest of intracranial mass lesions, and epilepsy is frequently the presenting symptom. They may be seen without other clinical evidence of TB (tuberculosis), although chest radiological changes are usual. Congenital toxoplasmosis may cause linear shadows or flecks of subependymal or basal ganglia calcification in about 40% of cases, and the appearances may be diagnostic. The CT may show associated gross cerebral atrophy. There may be associated radiological evidence of hydrocephalus and

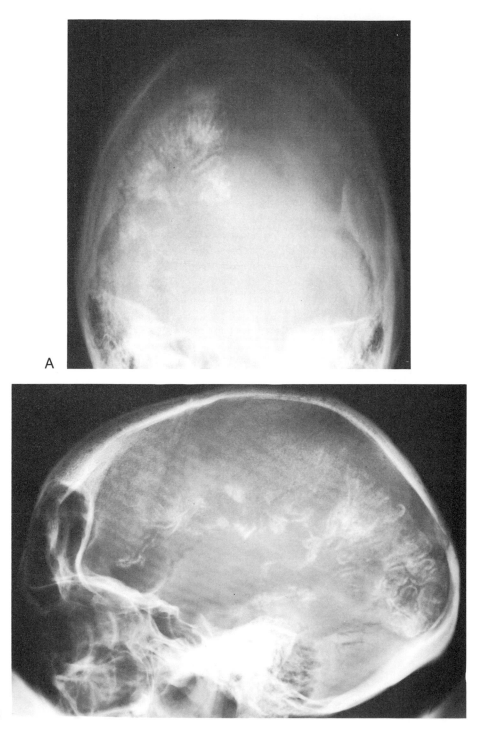

A

B

microcephaly. Intrauterine cytomegalovirus infection may also show micro-cephaly and intracranial nodular calcification, occasionally outlining the dilated ventricular system bilaterally and symmetrically. Paragonamiasis calcifies in about 50% of cases typically with lobulated aggregates of calcium ('soap bubbles') and this is an important cause of epilepsy in China and the Far East. Less commonly other parasitic diseases may also cause seizures and intracranial calcification; these include schistosomiasis, amoebiasis, and trichinosis. Calcification may also be seen in old abscess cavities, but is not present in acute cerebral abscess.

(4) Congenital anomalies of the brain may produce abnormal calcification, associated typically with a clinical picture of mental retardation, variable focal neurological signs and with early onset epilepsy. Hypocalcaemic and hypercalcaemic syndromes may both show intracranial calcification; and calcification of the basal ganglia is one of the characteristic radiological features, for instance, of Albright's pseudohypoparathyroidism. The dys-plastic lesions of tuberous sclerosis become progressively calcified throughout childhood and early adult life, and are frequently demonstrable on plain skull radiology as nodular or curvilinear shadows situated around the ventricles and basal ganglia, or less commonly as linear or dense shadowing. Occasion-ally, obstructive hydrocephalus may be seen. The lesions may undergo malignant change and the presence of signs of raised intracranial pressure is strongly suggestive of this. Other radiological changes include mesodermal dysplasia of bone, nodular sclerosis and periosteal cyst formation in the hands and feet, bony erosion from subungal fibromata, renal hamartoma, and rarely a honeycomb pulmonary infiltration or cyst formation. In tuberous sclerosis, however, there may be no clinical or plain radiological findings, and cases have been described in which small lesions seen on CT were the only clinical or radiographic signs. Thus, for genetic counselling purposes, clinical examina-tion and plain radiology may not be sufficient.

All forms of pathological calcification are seen better on CT than on plain radiology, and the yield of positive cases using CT is higher in every category.

8.2 COMPUTERIZED TOMOGRAPHY (CT)

Since its introduction into clinical practice in the early 1970s, computerized tomography has transformed the practice of neuroradiology and clinical neurology. Moreover, over this short period, substantial technical advances have been made, and the resolution and definition of the modern scanners are

Figure 8.1 (A) AP and (B) lateral skull radiograph of an adult patient with longstand-ing epilepsy due to Sturge-Weber syndrome. The radiograph shows the characteristic 'tramline calcification' of the cortex underlying the meningeal arteriovenous malformation.

far in advance of those used even a few years ago. The impact of CT on the determination of aetiology in patients with epilepsy has been impressive.

8.2.1 Technique

The scan is made by passing a fine beam of X-rays through the head to a series of detectors regularly spaced around the head. The intensity of the X-ray beam, after it has passed through the head, is measured circumferentially, and sets of readings are taken in a continuous series as the beam is rotated around the head in each section. This results in a very large number of measurements of absorption of photons directed at various angles; these measurements are then analysed by computer, and manipulated to provide values of X-ray absorption for points throughout the field irradiated. These points are actually small blocks or volume elements – voxels. This matrix of points is then displayed as a two dimensional image, the voxel being represented by a point, the pixel. The final display is usually a horizontal slice through the cranium, although a scan in any orientation is possible. A series of such images at different sections through the cranium is usually made. Tissues of different radiodensity are distinguished in this way, and with modern scans, the sensitivity is such that grey matter is easily distinguished from white matter. Fat, cerebrospinal fluid (CSF), cyst fluid and vasogenic oedema are all less dense than cerebral tissue, and with high resolution scans can usually be differentiated from each other. Haemorrhage, calcification and bone are more dense than cerebral tissue and again are usually easily distinguished. Repeat scanning following the intravenous injection of radio-opaque contrast medium causes an increase in radiodensity in some lesions, especially vascular structures or lesions in which the blood–brain barrier has been breached. With modern scanners, the larger individual cerebral arteries can be identified.

8.2.2 Scanning in patients with epilepsy

In epilepsy, the scanner has been used largely for the detection of structural lesions and for the determination of cerebral atrophy. The first reports were presented at the 21st European Congress of Electroencephalography and Epilepsy in 1975; the importance of CT in epilepsy was thenceforward established. At this conference were reported the results of CT in a total of 1702 patients from seven research groups [2–8]. CT abnormalities were found in 46% of these selected patients. The commonest abnormality was atrophy. Tumours were found in about 10% of cases. Gastaut [2] in his summary of the meeting concluded that CT 'is by far the best method for detecting cerebral lesions responsible for epilepsy and for determining their nature and exact location'. This statement still stands, although with the advent of MRI (magnetic resonance imaging) the relative indications for CT and MRI have yet to be determined. In subsequent years, CT has been carried out in more restricted groups of patients, and its relative usefulness has been more refined. Yang *et al.* [9] reported the results of scanning in 256 children with epilepsy, and found abnormalities in 33% overall. The proportion of patients with abnormal scans was greater in those with focal clinical or EEG signs, those with partial seizures, particularly simple partial seizures, and those with neonatal seizures or seizures which began in the neonatal period (Table 8.1).

Table 8.1 CT Findings in 256 children with seizure disorders (from Yang *et al.* [9]

	Percent with abnormal CT
Generalized seizures with normal neurological and EEG examinations	2.5
Children with normal neurological and EEG examinations (excluding neonates)	5
Idiopathic generalized seizures	8
Partial seizures with complex symptomatology	30
Generalized seizures of known aetiology	40
Partial seizures with elementary symptomatology	52
Focal slowing on EEG	63
Abnormal neurological examination	64
Neonates with seizures	68

The proportion of abnormalities is higher in those with late onset epilepsy, vascular disease, tumour and atrophy being the most common abnormal findings [10]. The proportion and type of CT abnormality varies in different seizure types (Table 8.2). The lowest yield of abnormalities is found in primary generalized seizures (absence or tonic-clonic), and the highest yield in simple and complex partial seizures.

The indications for CT scanning in epilepsy have been the subject of some debate. Young *et al.* [16], scanning 220 adult patients presenting at a neurological clinic, found abnormalities in 24% of the patients overall. In this series the scans were abnormal in over half of the patients in whom there were either focal clinical and or focal EEG findings, but in only 6% of cases in the absence of focal findings. The authors concluded that CT should be reserved for patients with focal findings. This view has been challenged. There is little doubt that if this policy is adopted, occasional treatable cerebral lesions will be missed. Available investigative facilities vary for economic reasons, but as CT remains the non-invasive investigation of choice for the detection of structural lesions, it should be available in developed countries for patients in whom there is a possibility of treatable cerebral disease.

The range of CT abnormalities found in several large series is shown in

Table 8.2 The proportion of normal scans, tumours and atrophy found on CT scans according to seizure type

	n.	Normal %	Tumour %	Atrophy %
Primary generalized epilepsy				
Angeleri *et al.* [8]	9	100	0	0
Gastaut and Gastaut [11]	80	89	0	11
Moseley and Bull [3]	ns	100	0	0
Secondary generalized epilepsy (West syndrome)				
Gastaut and Gastaut [11]	30	23	1	66*
Secondary generalized epilepsy (Lennox-Gastaut syndrome)				
Gastaut and Gastaut [11]	90	48	2	47
Generalized epilepsy (all types or unspecified)				
Scollo-Lavizzari *et al.* [7]	68	66	9	ns
Van Gall *et al.* [5]	148	50	10	28
Cala *et al.* [12]	ns	42	8	30
McGahan *et al.* [13]	93	67	4	23
Yang *et al.* [9]	138	81	ns	ns
Dellaportas *et al.* [14]	53	72	2	26
Simple partial seizures				
Gastaut and Gastaut [11]	69	33	38	29
McGahan *et al.* [13]	12	42	8	33
Yang *et al.* [9]	34	48	ns	ns
Complex partial seizures				
Gastaut and Gastaut [11]	84	40	14	45
McGahan *et al.* [13]	28	67	0	33
Yang *et al.* [9]	46	30	ns	ns
Benign rolandic epilepsy				
Gastaut and Gastaut [11]	20	100	0	0
Partial epilepsy (all types or unspecified)				
Bogdanoff *et al.* [15]	50	65	4	30
Caille *et al.* [6]	66	53	12	32
Gastaut and Gastaut [11]	308	ns	24	ns
Cala *et al.* [12]	ns	39	24	29
McGahan *et al.* [13]	54	49	4	30
Dellaportas *et al.* [14]	47	58	4	38

Criteria of patient selection vary, n=number of patients; ns=not stated.
*Atrophy/malformations.

Table 8.3. Cerebral tumours are demonstrated in about 10–20% of patients presenting over the age of 40 with newly diagnosed epilepsy, but in less than 5% of children.

Table 8.3   The CT abnormalities found in five series of patients with epilepsy

	Cala[a] et al. [12] n = 367 (%)	McGahan[b] et al. [13] 150 (%)	Dellaportas[c] et al. [14] 127 (%)	Yang[d] et al. [9] 256 (%)	Bogdanoff[e] et al. [15] 50 (%)
Normal	47	60	65	68	65
Diffuse atrophy	18	13	18	12	10
Focal atrophy	4	9	12	8	4
Porencephaly	0	3	1	1	12
Hydrocephalus	3	3	0	1	2
Hemiatrophy	0	0	0	2	0
AVM/aneurysm	2	4	1	0	0
Infarction	5	4	0	0	0
Neoplasm	14	4	4	2	4
Calcification	5	0	0	3	0
Other (misc.)	1	0	0	5	2

[a] Unselected cases.
[b] Consecutive cases.
[c] New adult referrals.
[d] Consecutive children.
[e] Unselected focal epilepsy.

8.2.3   CT and the EEG

It is important to recognize that the EEG and the CT scan are complementary and not competitive investigations (p. 180). The value of the CT scan is the detection and identification of structural abnormalities easily and without risk. In this regard, CT is clearly superior to the EEG. Much of the debate about the relative place of the two investigations has mistakenly concentrated on this usage. Although the EEG does usually show focal abnormalities in the presence of structural lesions, it seldom defines a specific cause. There is, moreover, a significant false positive and false negative rate. The EEG is a test of function and the epileptic seizure is a functional abnormality. It is in this regard that the EEG has a fundamental importance. It is invaluable in the typing of seizures, the quantification of seizure activity, monitoring of progress, monitoring in the acute situation, in the localization of seizure discharges, and in the differential diagnosis of seizures. For these purposes, the CT scan has little place. As Gastaut [2] noted in his early work with CT, 'the EEG remains the only paraclinical method capable of recognizing the epileptic characteristics of a cerebral condition, whether it is of a functional nature or due to a lesion'. Indeed, since the introduction of CT scanning, in one survey the number of EEG requests was found to have increased, the author attributing this to the increased interest in epilepsy and its full assessment [7]. An interesting attempt to correlate EEG and CT findings has been made by Gastaut and Michel [18], in which the radiological features associated with specific EEG patterns are discussed.

8.2.4   The CT characteristics of specific cerebral lesions in epilepsy

(a)   Cerebral tumour

It has been estimated that, when requested for diagnostic reasons in epilepsy, the CT scan detects about 95% of cerebral tumours. This is superior to all other non-invasive methods, with the possible exception of MRI. The attenuation of tumour varies considerably, and may be of high, equal or low density when compared with cerebral tissue. In addition, abnormal densities due to oedema, calcification, cysts or haemorrhages may be seen. Cerebral tumours may often show enhancement with marked contrast. The tumours may cause deformity or displacement of normal structures, sometimes to an extraordinary extent. Dilatation of part or all of the ventricular system due to obstruction may be seen. Bony changes or soft tissue masses outside cerebral structures are also well shown on CT. The appearances are such that a diagnosis of tumour by CT can often be made with considerable certainty, and in a proportion of cases the pathological nature of the tumour can also be determined with a fair degree of confidence.

The commonest primary tumour diagnosed by CT in epileptic patients is a glioma. Although the diagnosis of glioma is often clear, histological grading on CT is less accurate. The more malignant gliomas are often variable in density and enhancement, and are surrounded by oedema; the lower grade gliomas are often hypodense with no enhancement or oedema. Calcification is commoner in the less malignant tumours. It is a characteristic feature of an oligodendroglioma, which may cause epilepsy for many years before the tumour is diagnosed. Haemorrhage, necrosis, and cyst formation are also commonly seen in primary gliomas, especially the malignant astrocytomas. None of these features however are histologically specific. Tumours may show ring enhancement; this is usually irregular, and hence can usually but not always be distinguished from the enhancement around an acute cerebral abscess. Metastatic tumours account for many cases of late onset epilepsy, and again are often diagnosed by CT. They are usually better defined than primary gliomas, and are surrounded by extensive vasogenic oedema of the white matter. Metastases may be multiple and may show necrotic centres. Calcification is rare. There is however no absolutely reliable way of distinguishing a metastasis from a glioma by CT.

Epilepsy is the commonest presenting symptom of meningioma. These tumours have highly characteristic CT appearances and CT is superior to all other investigations including MRI in their detection. They occur peripherally, are usually regular and well demarcated, with variable and sometimes extensive oedema and variable attenuation characteristics. They usually show very marked and uniform contrast enhancement. Bony thickening may be seen, and occasionally calcification or cyst formation. Other benign cerebral tumours well demonstrated by CT are also important in the causation of epilepsy. The commonest of these are hamartomas in the temporal lobe. These frequently cause temporal lobe epilepsies – indeed this is usually the only clinical feature of these small tumours – and are often amenable to surgical treatment. They usually appear on CT as small, regular high density lesions which do not enhance. On CT grounds, such tumours cannot be differentiated from low grade gliomas. The dysplastic lesions of tuberous sclerosis (epiloia) are well shown by CT, which may be abnormal in the absence of any clinical signs. The tubers are often seen on CT in early childhood, and are almost invariably present by early adult life. Typically they are seen as multiple small, partly calcified, lesions of varying sizes, located periventrically and elsewhere; they may enhance (Fig. 8.2). Other abnormali-

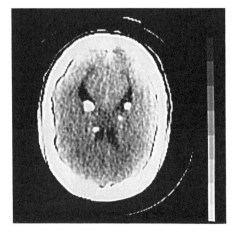

Figure 8.2 CT scan of an adolescent with longstanding epilepsy and mild mental retardation, showing multiple paraventricular high density lesions due to tuberous sclerosis.

ties in tuberose sclerosis include ventricular dilatation, less well defined calcification and cerebral asymmetries. In adult life, the periventricular lesions may show gliomatous changes.

(b) Cerebral infection

Pyogenic abscesses frequently cause seizures. CT is the method of choice for the diagnosis of acute abscess, and the appearances may be diagnostic. The lesions appear as irregular low attenuation areas with mass effect. The abscess wall shows dramatic enhancement as a regular thin smooth ring. There is usually extensive surrounding oedema. A focal cerebritis is the earliest stage in the formation of an abscess, and at this stage the wall may not have had time to form. Ring enhancement may, therefore, be absent, which may cause diagnostic errors. A tuberculous granuloma may have various forms. It may mimic a pyogenic abscess, although usually the centre is less hypodense, and the walls less regular. It may appear as a solid enhancing mass. There is often basal meningeal enhancement caused by the granulomatous meningitis. Chronic tuberculomata may show as non-specific high density nodules, in any cerebral site; they are often multiple (Fig. 8.3). Associated hydrocephalus is frequently present in cerebral tuberculosis. Other forms of cerebral abscess are also well shown on CT.

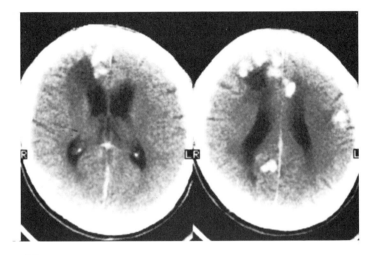

Figure 8.3 CT scan of a 20-year-old Indian patient presenting with focal epilepsy and with a past history of tuberculous meningitis. The scan shows multiple tuberculomata which enhance and also associated areas of infarction.

Herpes simplex encephalitis commonly results in epilepsy, both in the acute stage of the illness and as a permanent late complication. In the acute stages, CT typically shows bilateral temporal low attenuation, with mass effect, oedema, sometimes with haemorrhage and variable enhancement. Subsequent atrophy or cyst formation develops in the areas of destruction. Other encephalitic illnesses also show on CT as ill-defined areas of low attenuation, usually with associated oedema. The CT is also the most useful diagnostic test in cerebral cysticercosis. The lesions are usually multiple and widely distributed in the subependymal and cerebral tissue. They initially take the form of small low density areas, which may then develop calcification, sometimes ring calcification, with surrounding low density due to an inflammatory reaction. Finally the lesions appear as flecks of calcification. At this last stage, the parasite is dead, but the calcified cyst may still be epileptogenic. The belief, however, that epilepsy occurs only at the stage of calcification, many years after the primary infection, is incorrect. There is frequently associated hydrocephalus, which may be due to obstruction by cysts, or a communicating hydrocephalus secondary to an inflammatory arachnoid response. The common racemose form of cysticercosis results in hydrocephalus, and a posterior fossa mass may be seen on CT. This form of the disease does not, however, usually cause epilepsy. Toxoplasmosis may show on CT as nodules or flecks of calcification, and if congenital, hydrocephalus and cerebral malformations may also be seen (Fig. 8.4). Meningitis may cause epilepsy, usually due to associated vascular changes; CT may show abnormal basal meningeal enhancement and vascular lesions due to arteritis.

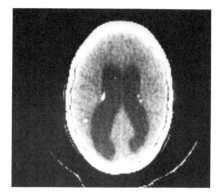

Figure 8.4 CT scan of an adolescent with a longstanding epilepsy and mental retardation due to congenital toxoplasmosis. The scan shows calcified periventricular lesions and hydrocephalus.

(c) Degenerative cerebrovascular disease

The demonstration of cerebral infarction on CT depends on the timing of the scan and the size and site of the lesion. In the 24 hours following an infarct, the scan may be normal. The typical changes then develop if the infarct is large enough. There is a zone of low attenuation, often affecting white and grey matter and sometimes wedge-shaped in the territory of the affected artery. There may be associated oedema in acute infarction. As time passes, the CT changes may lessen or shrink. In a significant proportion of cases, the scan may become normal. By the third week after infarction, 80% of the lesions show enhancement, and at this time the mass effect is usually maximal. However, by the third month enhancement is very unusual. By contrast, enhancement in acute cerebral infarcts may on occasions be marked, and differentiation from cerebral neoplasia may be difficult. Infarcts may be multiple and may vary in size (Fig. 8.5). A mature infarct may be manifest as focal atrophy on the CT scan. Lacunar infarction may also be demonstrated, although as with the cerebral infarcts, these show a tendency to disappear with time. Watershed infarction has a typical distribution and pattern, and may be

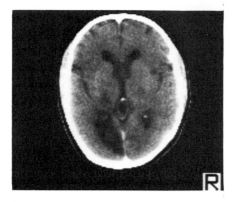

Figure 8.5 CT scan of a 50-year-old man with mitral stenosis who presented with a single generalized seizure. The scan shows a cortical infarct and an additional left capsular infarct due to cerebral embolism.

caused by systemic hypotension. Patchy areas of low attenuation in the deep white matter around the lateral ventricles are seen in patients with degenerative vascular disease, particularly in hypertensive patients; this may be the only sign of vascular disease.

In summary, although the CT scan has proved a major advance in the noninvasive detection of degenerative cerebrovascular disease, in a significant proportion of cases the scan may be normal, and the abnormalities may change over time. It is not at all unusual to receive reports of CT scans that are normal in patients whose arteriograms show gross vascular disease.

CT scanning has shown that frank infarction in association with neonatal seizures is probably commoner than previously realized. It may be demonstrated in the absence of focal clinical features [19]. Cerebral infarction is the most common specific CT change in late onset epilepsy. Indeed it has been only since the introduction of CT that the importance of degenerative vascular disease as a cause of late onset epilepsy has been easily clinically illustrated. In one series of cases, with controls, lacunar infarction was found to be an important CT marker of presumably more widespread vascular disease in late onset epilepsy (Table 8.4) [10].

(d) Post-traumatic epilepsy

CT abnormalities were found in 69% of one series of 100 cases of post-traumatic epilepsy presenting for investigation [20]. The abnormalities included generalized atrophy in 18%, hydrocephalus (ventricular enlargement) in 5%, focal abnormalities in 41%, and other miscellaneous changes in a further 5%. The changes correlated well with focal EEG abnormalities, but, as with all structural lesions, EEG abnormalities were of less localizing value. The commonest focal abnormality was low attenuation in the inferior frontal

Table 8.4 CT scan findings in 79 patients with late onset epilepsy and matched controls

	Patients	Controls
Ischaemic lesions: Total	13	2
Lacunar infarction alone	3	0
Cerebral infarction alone	1	1
White matter low attenuation alone	3	1
Combinations of the above	6	0
Atrophy: Total	37	35
Grade Mild	27	24
Severe	10	11
Distribution: Generalized	17	17
Focal	3	2
Central	7	9
Peripheral	10	7

From a prospective series of 74 patients presenting with late onset epilepsy and 74 age- and sex-matched controls without epilepsy or overt cerebral disease (Shorvon *et al.* [10]).

white matter, sometimes extending to the overlying cortex and sometimes associated with frank focal atrophy. Focal lesions were common in those with a history of prolonged unconsciousness or prolonged post-traumatic amnesia. As in the case of tumours and vascular disease, the presence of focal features in the seizures did not correlate well with the occurrence of focal CT findings.

(e) Cerebral haemorrhage and haematoma

Recent haemorrhage is easily demonstrated by CT as dense uniform high attenuation (50–90 Hounsfield units) often with a thin surrounding rim of low attenuation. Intracerebral, subdural and extradural blood can be confidently diagnosed in the majority of cases. Blood in the ventricular system is also easily seen, outlining the ventricles; a fluid level may sometimes be demonstrated. As the intracerebral haematoma matures it may become isodense with cerebral tissue; it eventually forms a scar or cyst.

Subdural and extradural haemorrhage show high attenuation for about seven days, and then become isodense and hypodense after several weeks. An extradural haematoma is often concave outwards. Subdural blood may be less localized. When isodense, it shows up only by obliteration of the sulci, and by mass effect.

Cerebral haemorrhage is an important finding in neonatal seizures, occurring in 32% of the series of Yang *et al.* [9], but is an unusual finding in adult patients presenting for investigation of their epilepsy, possibly because the CT characteristics of haemorrhage have often disappeared before consequent epilepsy develops.

(f) Cerebral arteriovenous malformation

These are well shown on CT, and the appearances may be diagnostic. The unenhanced scan may show an area of low attenuation, often with associated atrophy and calcification. There is dramatic and often uniform enhancement with contrast. Small temporal lobe angiomas are a well recognized cause of temporal lobe epilepsy, and may be difficult to visualize on CT due to their size and to bony artefact. Specially angled views of the temporal lobes may be helpful in such cases and for other temporal lobe lesions.

In Sturge-Weber syndrome, the CT appearances are diagnostic. High attenuation due to cortical calcification is usually massive, and more extensive than the calcification seen on plain radiology. There is associated cerebral hemiatrophy without mass effect. No angioma is usually seen on CT, but there may be enhancement of the area by contrast.

(g) Generalized cerebral atrophy on CT and its relation to epilepsy

Generalized cerebral atrophy may be predominantly central, with ventricular enlargement, predominantly cortical with sulcal atrophy or both central and cortical. Atrophy was soon recognized as a common finding in patients with epilepsy (see Table 8.1), and accounts for at least one-half of the 'abnormalities' seen on CT in people with epilepsy in most series. Only more recently however has it been established that similar atrophy is to be found in control scans of seemingly healthy subjects. In the only series of patients with late onset epilepsy in which CT scans were matched with controls, the frequency, severity and type of atrophic changes in the epileptic patients were very similar to those in the control population (Table 8.4). There was therefore only a weak relationship to the presence of overt cerebrovascular disease. Furthermore, CT 'atrophy' may change over time in any one patient either spontaneously, or in response to metabolic or toxic effects, for example with the use of alcohol in alcoholic patients [21]. Many reports of CT atrophy in patients with epilepsy are therefore of uncertain significance. It is important to emphasize this, as the erroneous assumption that atrophy represents a significant structural change in individual patients may unfairly prejudice their clinical and psychosocial management.

(h) Focal atrophy in epilepsy

Focal atrophic lesions and porencephaly are an important finding in epilepsy. They may be due to perinatal damage, genetic or congenital diseases, or to the final result of vascular or encephalitic damage. Such lesions are well demonstrated on CT, which is again the investigation of choice. Focal atrophy is often present in the absence of any focal clinical deficit. The EEG may show attenuation of electrical activity over larger lesions, or other focal changes, but these are seldom specific, and the EEG is often normal over smaller atrophic lesions.

(i) Other congenital lesions and epilepsy

CT is the investigation of choice in most of the other rare structural cerebral abnormalities which result in epilepsy, which are usually of childhood onset and accompanied by mental retardation and variable focal neurological deficits. The commonest of these is agenesis of the corpus callosum. This accounted for 13% of Gastaut's series of infantile spasms investigated by CT [11], and about 1% of the scans of children referred to a children's hospital with epilepsy [9]. The CT appearances are diagnostic. These include widely spaced ventricles, a misplaced third ventricle, and dilatation of the trigone and occipital horns (Fig. 8.6).

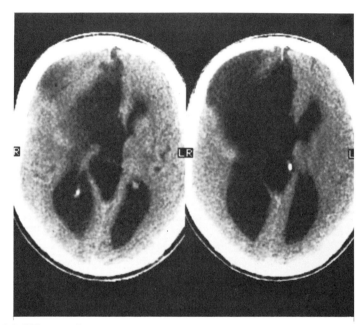

Figure 8.6 CT scan of a 40-year-old man with epilepsy since the age of 20 with mild intellectual dullness but no other abnormal neurological signs. It shows agenesis of the corpus collosum with associated porencephaly.

Cerebral hemiatrophy is an important CT finding in epilepsy, and various other abnormalities of cerebral development (e.g. schizencephaly, congenital hydrocephalus, anencephaly) often have diagnostic CT appearances. A thickened skull and a small anterior or middle fossa are commonly seen on CT in relation to overlying focal congenital cerebral atrophy.

(j) The CT scan in temporal lobe epilepsy

Imaging of the temporal lobe is particularly important because of the possibility of resective surgery in cases of intractable temporal lobe epilepsy.

CT scanners are now effective in demonstrating small hamartomas, gliomas, angiomas, focal atrophy or enlargement of the temporal horn. In virtually all clinical settings, CT has replaced air encephalography for the demonstration of atrophic lesions, although this is still one of the few indications for this latter investigation. The mesial temporal lobe may be relatively obscured by bone in some CT scans, and in one UK centre at least, scanning with the head tilted at a more acute angle is advocated as a method of improving sensitivity, sometimes with intraventricular contrast injection although interpretation of the images may be difficult. All cases should have contrast enhancement to demonstrate small arteriovenous malformations. Small tumours detected only on CT and otherwise clinically unsuspected have been found in up to 15% of patients undergoing temporal lobectomy (p. 120). It is therefore essential to scan any patient with temporal lobe epilepsy in whom temporal lobe resection is a possible treatment option. In general, however, the number of surgically correctable lesions detected by CT in the absence of any clinical suspicion is small [22].

(k)   The CT scan in other epileptic syndromes [11]

In the benign rolandic epilepsies of childhood, CT is invariably normal. Although this is clinically and electroencephalographically a syndrome with a focal origin, CT is clearly unnecessary. CT is also almost always normal in the true, strictly defined, primary generalized epilepsies. In other patients with tonic-clonic seizures, however, without the well-defined EEG criteria of the primary generalized epilepsies, CT may be abnormal in up to 10% of patients, and one should not assume, as is frequently done, that any patient with seemingly primary generalized seizures has one of the primary generalized epilepsies. CT is abnormal in about three-quarters of patients with infantile spasms. The abnormalities seen include focal atrophy, porencephaly, abnormal calcification, generalized atrophy, tumours, agenesis of the corpus callosum, and the dysplastic lesions of tuberous sclerosis. The prognosis of infantile spasms is worse in patients with lesions demonstrated on CT. In about 50% of infants with the features of the Lennox-Gastaut syndrome, a similar range of abnormalities is found. In the progressive familial myoclonic epilepsies, the CT does usually not provide useful diagnostic information.

Finally, an epileptic seizure itself may occasionally cause reversable CT abnormalities. These are usually areas of hypodensity but contrast enhancement has also been reported. The frequency of such changes, their mechanism and their pathological basis are completely obscure [23].

8.3   CEREBRAL ANGIOGRAPHY

The need for angiography in epilepsy has been dramatically reduced by the introduction of CT. At the National Hospital, Queen Square, London, for instance, in spite of an increased patient load, the number of angiograms carried out in recent years is now one-third of the yearly total of the early 1970s. The main indications for cerebral angiography in current practice in epilepsy are:

(1) To delineate vascular abnormalities for diagnostic purposes. In epilepsy, these include the identification of arteriovenous malformations (especially small temporal lobe angiomas), aneurysm, intracranial infarction, degenerative arterial disease, venous thrombosis or thrombophlebitis, and congenital vascular anomalies.

(2) To determine the vascularity, vascular supply, extent and site of intracranial masses (e.g. tumours, angiomas, abscess) as part of the investigation necessary prior to intracranial surgery. The dependence on angiography in this setting varies from centre to centre, but a neurosurgeon may well be keen to see the site of normal and abnormal vessels preoperatively.

(3) To identify the pathological nature of an intracranial lesion by its vascular characteristics (e.g. meningioma, granuloma, abscess), although this function has now also been largely superceded by CT. About 5% of intracranial tumours are undetected on CT at the time of presentation, and these may occasionally show angiographic abnormalities. More often, the CT features may be ambiguous, and angiography may increase diagnostic specificity. Extracerebral lesions such as bilateral subdural haematomas, small extradural haematomas or epidural abscesses, may also be better demonstrated by angiography or MRI rather than by CT.

(4) The carotid amytal test is also an important pre-surgical investigation in temporal lobe epilepsy.

8.4 AIR ENCEPHALOGRAPHY

Prior to CT, this was widely used in epilepsy, and particularly as the most reliable method of demonstrating atrophic lesions. The indications for this unpleasant examination have now been almost abolished where advanced CT is available. At the National Hospital, Queen Square, London, for instance, there is now no air encephalographic apparatus in use. In some centres, there is still some neurosurgical preference for air encephalography for the demonstration of mild ventricular asymmetry, especially of the temporal horns in temporal lobe epilepsy, for studies of lesions in the region of the third ventricle, or for some types of hydrocephalus. With modern CT, however, in epilepsy, the indications for air encephalography are now negligible.

The extent to which CT has superceded other invasive investigations is shown by Tatler and Moseley [24], who reported that in 81 cases in which invasive investigation was carried out in spite of normal CT, a positive finding was demonstrated in only one instance.

8.5 POSITRON EMISSION TOMOGRAPHY (PET)

There have already been a number of publications concerning the use of PET in epilepsy, though little information of clinical value has been so far produced. For clinical purposes, this technique has at present few applications, and whether this situation will change in the next few years is difficult to say. As a research tool, however, PET is already providing useful information.

8.5.1 Technique

Short-lived isotopes which emit positrons such as ^{18}F, ^{13}N, ^{15}O and ^{14}C can be incorporated into a variety of substances, which are then taken up by brain tissue. The positrons are then emitted intracerebrally, and after emission collide with electrons. Each collision produces two photons which are propelled in exactly opposite directions through cerebral tissue from the point of the collision. These two photons are then identified by two detectors placed at opposite sides of the head The detectors are programmed to register only simultaneous events (coincident detection) and so record only that photon activity originating in the area of study. If detectors are arranged circumferentially around the head, sufficient coincidence data can be collected to allow computation of photon emission from all points between the detectors. At present, the spatial resolution is about 8 mm. The mathematical reconstructions of the image are essentially similar to those of CT, the image being displayed as a two dimensional cut, usually, as with CT, as horizontal sections at varying levels through the cranium. Because the positron emitting isotopes have a very short half-life, they have to be produced within seconds of their use, and this requires an on-site cyclotron. The technology is therefore expensive and complex. In epilepsy studies to date, three main isotopes have been utilized, ^{18}F-labelled 2-fluorodeoxyglucose, ^{13}N-labelled NH$_3$, and ^{15}O-labelled compounds. These are either inhaled or injected intravenously or intra-arterially into the subject already positioned in the scanner. Using ^{15}O labels, regional blood flow, oxygen extraction and utilization can be measured, and using ^{18}F-labelled 2-fluorodeoxyglucose, glucose metabolism can be derived from the proton activity [25–31].

8.5.2 PET in patients with epilepsy

(a) Temporal lobe epilepsy and complex partial seizures
In interictal studies with PET, focal glucose hypometabolism in the abnormal temporal lobe has been a relatively consistent finding. It has been claimed that this finding is of some usefulness in the selection of patients for temporal lobe surgery [32–34]. The size and shape of the hypometabolic zone is variable. In one study, a correlation was found between the degree of cell loss on pathological examination of the surgically removed temporal lobe, and the

degree of hypometabolism [35]. The size of the surgical lesion is always smaller than the size of the zone of hypometabolism. This presumably reflects the complex physiology of the epileptic focus [36]. No correlation has been found between the degree of hypometabolism and the amount of EEG spike activity from depth electrode recordings; indeed in individual cases widely disparate findings have been recorded. Although PET is now part of the schedule of investigation in patients being considered for temporal lobectomy in some centres, there is controversy about its real value, and most surgical units proceed to surgery without recourse to PET. The UCLA [34] group claim that PET reduces the need for depth electrode studies in about one-third of patients, but as that unit has in the past used depth electrode studies more extensively than others, it is still difficult to generalize from their experience. In other studies, no correlation between the degree of hypometabolism and other clinical parameters was found. In interictal studies of temporal lobe epilepsy with ^{15}O-labelled compounds, hypometabolism was found in the affected temporal lobe, but in addition more general hypometabolism and particularly cerebellar hypometabolism has been found [37]. The significance of these findings is totally unclear.

Ictal studies of complex partial seizures have also been reported, although major methodological criticisms may be levelled against some of these. In general the results of these studies have shown (not surprisingly) hypermetabolism at the focus, which in the interictal period is hypometabolic. In future studies, it might prove possible to follow the spread of the ictal discharges.

(b) Generalized seizures

^{18}Fluorine-labelled glucose studies have also been reported in patients with generalized absence and tonic-clonic seizures, and both ictal and interictal scans have been reported [38]. Ictal scans during hyperventilation-induced absence attacks produced a diffuse increase in glucose utilization, and very high values were obtained. One patient has been scanned during absence status, and here there appeared to be generalized hypometabolism. Interictal scans are reported to be normal in the generalized epilepsies.

(c) Structural cerebral lesions

PET has been used extensively to study cerebral tumours, cerebral infarction and other structural lesions, some of which have been associated with epilepsy, but none of these studies have added any specific information about the epilepsy *per se*.

Major limitations of PET at present are inadequate spatial and temporal resolution. Spatial resolution is improving with the newer machines, and anatomical detail should improve. From the point of view of studies in epilepsy, structures such as the hippocampus and amygdala should soon be reliably identifiable. In the imaging of seizures, inadequate temporal resolution is a major drawback. [18]Fluorine-labelled glucose studies particularly are slow, as it is currently necessary to obtain steady state conditions which may take 20–40 min. ^{15}O-labelled studies are quicker, but even so, the changes caused by electrophysiological events lasting a few milliseconds are well outside the temporal resolution of the currently available technologies. The other limitations are of course financial and technical. Whether an investigation which requires an on-site cyclotron and considerable technical backup will ever gain much clinical popularity is doubtful, and it seems very unlikely that this technique will become rapidly widely available for routine clinical purposes.

What the future holds for PET in epilepsy research in humans is uncertain. Further work on different epileptic seizure types and aetiologies continues [39] using the techniques described above, but whether results in this area will prove of fundamental importance is doubtful. A much more interesting area of future work is that which involves the administration of positron-labelled pharmaceuticals, ligands and other neurochemicals, and the *in vivo* study of their regional metabolism. Such studies might provide insights into the neurochemistry of the living epileptic brain, the effects of seizures and the effects of drugs.

8.6 NUCLEAR MAGNETIC RESONANCE IMAGING (MRI, NMR, NMRI)

The first experimental MRI image was published in 1973, and since that time there has been an explosive development in this field. MRI became clinically available in the last few years, and already its impact in neurology has been widely felt. There seems no doubt that this imaging method will play an increasingly important part in the investigations of cerebral disease. Experience in epilepsy is small to date, but the applications are likely to be numerous.

8.6.1 Technique [39, 40, 41]

In clinical practice, MRI is largely devoted to the imaging of radiowave emissions from hydrogen atoms [40, 41]. The technique depends on the fact that atoms with an odd number of protons or neutrons, spin (or rather behave as if they spin) and in doing so generate a magnetic field. If placed in a powerful external field, the atoms then align themselves along the lines of magnetic force, like compass needles. If a deflecting force is applied to the atoms, they move out of alignment, and when this force is removed they will swing back. If the force is applied in pulses close to the needle's natural frequency, the needle will absorb energy, and the amplitude of the swing will increase (resonance). In practice, the magnetic displacement can be achieved by passing a radiowave pulse through the field. In rotating back (precessing) to align themselves along the magnetic field, the atoms emit a radiowave. The precession depends on the frequency and direction of the pulsed radiowave. The precession in a longitudinal plane is due to the interaction between the proton and the surrounding nuclei (the lattice) – a process called spin–lattice relaxation. This occurs exponentially, with decay time T_1. The precession in a transverse plane is due to energy exchanges between neighbouring protons – the spin–spin relaxation – and also occurs exponentially. The combined time decay of the spin–spin and spin–lattice relaxation is known as T_2.

In clinical imaging, spatial resolution of the MRI image is achieved by applying a magnetic field the strength of which is progressively increased, resulting in resonant frequencies which vary in a gradient throughout the object being imaged. In practice, a magnetic gradient is applied simultaneously with the pulse, and those spins which are at the same frequency of the pulse respond, which because of the gradient represents only a thin slice of tissue. This is repeated with differing gradients, and the MRI characteristics of each part under study can be identified. The information from each individual recording is computed much as with CT, and an image is produced in which data from a small volume of tissue (voxel) is represented by a point value (pixel). Because water has a high concentration of mobile hydrogen atoms, T_1 and T_2 depend largely on the water content of the tissue. Tissues of differing chemical constitutions will have differing T_1 and T_2 values, and tissue differentiation is possible. Varying the times between pulses and the directions of the pulse will allow further differentiation, and two particular methods are in common use currently. The Spin–Echo sequence, in which a 180° pulse is given between initial excitation and recording, is dependent mainly on T_2. The Inversion Recovery Sequence, in which the magnetism is first inverted by a 180° pulse, is mainly dependent on T_1. The images produced depend on the timing of the pulse sequences, and the characteristics of the sequences themselves, and these may have to be individualized for different purposes.

In clinical practice, MRI machines consist of a large magnet producing a uniform magnetic field, into the centre of which the patient is placed. Additional magnetic pulses are applied by means of smaller coils placed around the part to be imaged. High voltages are not required and there are no sophisticated moving parts, which are advantages over CT. Routine imaging of the brain currently takes about 20 min, and there are no serious biological ill effects known to be due to this procedure, nor do the problems of X-ray exposure apply. Many patients find the machines claustrophobic.

8.6.2 Comparative value of MRI and CT

In normal brain, the inversion recovery sequences show differentiation between white and grey matter, and anatomical detail which is superior to CT in many instances. Spaces containing CSF, and oedema, are well shown. Bone is inert (as there is not much free water present), and bony structures or margins are therefore poorly shown, but equally there are no problems due to bony artefact as occurs in CT scanning. Similarly, calcification may not be seen with MRI. At present the spatial resolution of MRI is less than that of the modern CT scanner, but MRI images in many planes may be easily constructed and displayed. From the clinical point of view therefore, CT and MRI have differing strengths and weaknesses. For many (perhaps most) applications, however, MRI will produce more useful information than CT. Imaging of the posterior fossa, the temporal lobes and the spinal cord is particularly superior, due to the lack of bony artefact (Fig. 8.7). Pathological changes which are better shown on MRI include demyelination, cerebral infarction and some

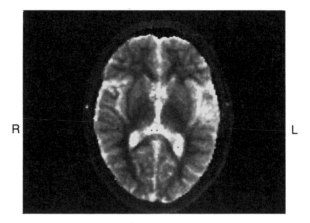

R   L

Figure 8.7 MRI scan of a 25-year-old patient with longstanding temporal lobe epilepsy due to unilateral left temporal atrophy.

types of cerebral tumour. Blood flow is also better shown on MRI. CT is still superior in demonstrating calcified or bony lesions and meningiomas. The limits of normality of MRI have not yet been fully established, and the significance of the disparity between the extent of abnormal signals in some lesions (particularly tumours) between MRI and CT has not been fully evaluated. The actual quantification of T_1 and T_2 measurements is easy to achieve and the clinical possibilities of this have yet to be explored. The imaging of phosphorus in this manner will allow the regional energy status of the brain to be quantified and this method is potentially of great value.

8.6.3 MRI and epilepsy [42–48]

The impact of MRI on epilepsy has not yet been fully defined. Preliminary studies demonstrating the value of MRI in defining structural brain lesions have been carried out, some comparing MRI with CT [42–49], and it seems clear that in the detection of most structural lesions and tumours, MRI is superior to CT (Fig. 8.8). MRI is also superior in the detection of vascular disease, many white matter disorders and demyelinating disease. A comparison of PET, MRI and CT scanning by the Bethesda group showed that MRI was more sensitive than CT scanning at revealing spin–echo 'lesions'

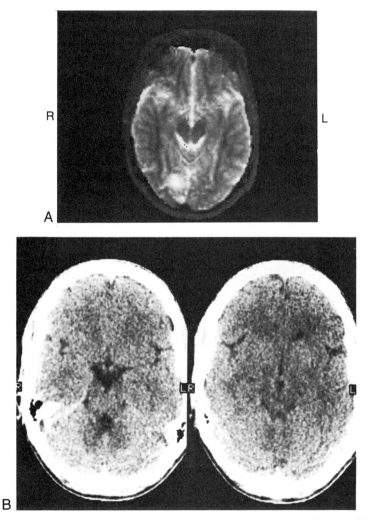

Figure 8.8 (A) MRI and (B) CT scan on a 20-year-old patient with a five year history of focal epilepsy. The CT is normal but the MRI shows an occipital lesion due to a glioma.

accompanying areas of hypometabolism seen on the PET scan [46]. Abnormalities imaged on MRI often appear larger than those on CT, and the implications of this to clinical – particularly surgical practice have yet to be fully explored. Apart from its value in imaging, the use of MRI spectroscopy in epilepsy has enormous potential. Prospects look exciting for the study of epilepsy; and the use of quantified data, the study of regional energy requirements, the relevance of changes in blood flow in epilepsy, and the better definition of disease processes are all areas of promise.

I would like to gratefully acknowledge the assistance of Dr G. L. V. Tatler in the provision of the illustrations in this chapter.

REFERENCES

1. Bull, J. W. D. and Zilkha, K. J. (1968) Rationalizing requests for X-ray films in neurology. *Br. Med. J.*, **2**, 569–70.
2. Gastaut, H. (1976) Conclusions: Computerized transverse axial tomography in epilepsy. *Epilepsia*, **17**, 337–8.
3. Moseley, I. F. and Bull, J. W. D. (1976) Summary: Computerized transverse axial tomography in epilepsy. *Epilepsia*, **17**, 339.
4. Collard, M., Dupont, H. and Noel, G. (1976) Summary: Computerized transverse axial tomography in epilepsy. *Epilepsia*, **17**, 339–40.
5. Van Gall, M., Becker, H. and Hacker, H. (1976) Summary: Computerized transverse axial tomography in epilepsy. *Epilepsia*, **17**, 340–1.
6. Caille, J. M., Cohadon, F., Loiseau, P. and Constant, P. H. (1976) Summary: Computerized transverse axial tomography in epilepsy. *Epilepsia*, **17**, 341.
7. Scollo-Lavizzari, G., Eichhorn, K. and Wuthrich, R. (1976) Summary: Computerized transverse axial tomography in epilepsy. *Epilepsia*, **17**, 341–2.
8. Angeleri, F., Amici, F., Marchesi, G. F. *et al.* (1976) Summary: Computerized transverse axial tomography in epilepsy. *Epilepsia*, **17**, 342.
9. Yang, P. J., Berger, M. D., Cohen, M. E. and Duffner, P. K. (1979) Computed tomography and childhood seizure disorders. *Neurology*, **29**, 1084–8.
10. Shorvon, S. D., Gilliatt, R. W., Cox, T. C. S. and Yu, Y. L. (1984) Evidence of vascular disease from CT scanning in late onset epilepsy. *J. Neurol. Neurosurg. Psychiatr.*, **47**, 225–30.
11. Gastaut, H. and Gastaut, J. L. (1977) Computerized axial tomography in epilepsy, in *Epilepsy, the Eighth International Symposium* (ed. J. K. Penry), Raven Press, New York, pp. 5–15.
12. Cala, L. A., Mastaglia, F. L. and Woodings, T. L. (1977) Computerized tomography of the cranium in patients with epilepsy: a preliminary report. *Clin. Exp. Neurol.*, **14**, 237–44.
13. McGahan, J. P., Dublin, A. B. and Hill, R. P. (1979) The evaluation of seizure disorders by computerized tomography. *J. Neurosurg.*, **50**, 328–32.
14. Dellaportas, C. I., Dawson, J. M. and Reynolds, E. H. (1982) Computerized tomography (CT) in new referrals with epilepsy. *Br. J. Clin. Pract.*, Suppl., **18**, 201–3.
15. Bogdanoff, B. M., Stafford, C. R., Green, L. *et al.* (1975) Computerized transaxial tomography in the evaluation of patients with focal epilepsy. *Neurology*, **25**, 1013–17.
16. Young, A. C., Borg Constanzi, J., Mohr, P. D. and Forbes, W. (1982) Is routine computerized axial tomography in epilepsy worthwhile? *Lancet*, **ii**, 1446–7.

17. Critchley, E. M. R. (1978) Electroencephalography today. *J. R. Soc. Med.*, **71**, 473–6.
18. Gastaut, H. and Michel, B. (1978) The impact of cranial computerized tomography on electroencephalography. *Contemp. Clin. Neurophysiol..* (Suppl. **34**), 123–32.
19. Levy, S. R., Abrams, I. F., Marshall, P. C. and Rosquete, E. E. (1985) Seizures and cerebral infarction in the full term neonate. *Ann. Neurol.*, **17**, 366–70.
20. Moseley, I. F. and Ruiz, J. S. (1983) Computerized tomography in post-traumatic epilepsy, in *Research Progress in Epilepsy* (ed. F. C. Rose), Pitman, London, pp. 293–300.
21. Ron, M., Acker, W., Shaw, G. K. and Lishman, W. A. (1982) CT changes in chronic alcoholics: a survey and follow up study. *Brain*, **105**, 497–514.
22. Jabbari, B., Huott, A. D., Di Chiro, G. *et al.* (1980) Surgically correctable lesions solely detected by CT scan in adult-onset chronic epilepsy. *Ann. Neurol.*, **7**, 344–7.
23. Sethi, P. K., Kumar, B. R., Madan, V. S. and Mohan, V. (1985) Appearing and disappearing CT scan abnormalities and seizures. *J. Neurol. Neurosurg. Psychiatr.*, **48**, 866–9.
24. Tatler, G. L. V. and Moseley, I. F. (1982) Use of invasive neuroradiological investigation in patients with normal computerized tomography. *Br. Med. J.*, **285**, 1026–8.
25. Mazziotta, J. C. and Engel, J. (1985) Advanced neuro-imaging techniques in the study of human epilepsy: PET, SPECT and NMR-CT, in *Recent Advances in Epilepsy*, Vol. 2 (eds T. A. Pedley and B. S. Meldrum), Churchill Livingstone, Edinburgh, pp. 65–99.
26. Engel, J., Kuhl, D. E. and Phelps, M. E. (1983) Functional imaging of the epileptic brain with positron computed tomography, in *Research Progress in Epilepsy* (ed. F. C. Rose), Pitman, London, pp. 301–14.
27. Phelps, M. E., Schelbert, H. and Mazziotta, J. C. (1983) Positron computed tomography in the study of myocardial and cerebral function. *Ann. Intern. Med.*, **98**, 339–59.
28. Kuhl, D. E., Engel, J. E., Phelps, M. E. and Selin, C. (1980) Epileptic patterns of local cerebral metabolism and perfusion in humans determined by emission computed tomography of ^{18}FDG and ^{13}NH$_3$. *Ann. Neurol.*, **8**, 348–60.
29. Engel, J. (1984) The use of PET scanning in epilepsy. *Ann. Neurol.*, **15** (Suppl.), 5180–91.
30. Engel, J., Kuhl, D. E. and Phelps, M. E. (1983) Regional brain metabolism during seizures in humans. *Adv. Neurol.*, **34**, 141–8.
31. Engel, J., Kuhl, D. E. and Phelps, M. E. (1982) Patterns of human local cerebral glucose metabolism during epileptic seizures. *Science*, **218**, 64–6.
32. Engel, J., Kuhl, D. E., Phelps, M. E. and Crandell, P. H. (1982) Comparative localization of the epileptic foci in partial epilepsy by PET and EEG. *Ann. Neurol.*, **12**, 529–37.
33. Engel, J., Kuhl, D. E., Phelps, M. E. and Mazziotta, J. C. (1982) Interictal cerebral glucose metabolism in partial epilepsy and its relation to EEG changes. *Ann. Neurol.*, **12**, 510–17.
34. Engel, J., Rausch, R., Lieb, J. P. *et al.* (1981) Correlation of criteria used for localizing epileptic foci in patients considered for surgical therapy of epilepsy. *Ann. Neurol.*, **9**, 215–24.
35. Engel, J., Brown, W. J., Kuhl, D. E. *et al.* (1982) Pathological findings underlying

focal temporal lobe hypometabolism in partial epilepsy. *Ann. Neurol.*, **12**, 518–28.

36. Theodore, W. H., Newmark, M. E., Sato, S. *et al.* (1983) [^{18}F] fluorodeoxyglucose positron emission computed tomography in refractory complex partial seizures. *Ann. Neurol.*, **14**, 419–28.

37. Bernardi, S., Trimble, M. T., Frackowiak, R. S. *et al.* (1983) An interictal study of partial epilepsy using positron emission tomography and the oxygen-15 inhalation technique. *J. Neurol. Neurosurg. Psychiatr.*, **46**, 473–7.

38. Theodore, W. H., Brooks, R., Margolin, R. *et al.* (1985) Positron emission tomography in generalized seizures. *Neurology*, **35**, 684–90.

39. Ackermann, R. F., Engel, J. and Phelps, M. E. (1986) Identification of seizure mediating brain structures with the deoxyglucose method: studies of human epilespy with positron emission tomography and animal seizure models with contact autoradiography, in *Basic Mechanisms of the Epilepsies* (eds A. V. Delgado-Escueta *et al.*) Raven Press, New York, pp. 921–34.

40. Pykett, I. L., Newhouse, J. H., Buoanno, F. S. *et al.* (1982) Principles of nuclear magnetic resonance imaging. *Radiology*, **143**, 157–68.

41. Ormerod, I. E. C. and Johnson, G. (1985) Nuclear magnetic resonance imaging of the central nervous system. *J. Electrophysiol. Technol.*, **11**, 119–40.

42. McLaughan, R. S., Nicholson, R. L., Blume, W. T. *et al.* (1985) Magnetic resonance imaging (MRI) in temporal lobe epilepsy (TLE) – pathological correlations (abstract). *Epilepsia*, **26**, 543.

43. Bergen, D., Morrell, F., Bleck, T. P. *et al.* (1985) Tissue histology in patients with abnormal MRI scans (abstract). *Epilepsia*, **26**, 543–4.

44. Oldendorf, W. H. (1984) The use and promise of nuclear magnetic resonance imaging in epilepsy. *Epilepsia*, **25** (Suppl.), S105–17.

45. Bydder, G. M., Steiner, R. E., Young, I. R. *et al.* (1982) Clinical NMR imaging of the brain: 140 cases. *Am. J. Radiol.*, **139**, 215–36.

46. Theodore, W. H., Dorwart, R., Holmes, M. *et al.* (1986) Neuroimaging in refractory partial seizures. *Neurology*, **36**, 750–9.

47. Latack, J. T., Abou-Khalil, B. W., Siegel, G. J., Sackellares, J. C., Gabrielsen, T. O. and Aisen, A. M. (1986) Patients with partial seizures: evaluation by MR, CT and PET imaging. Radiology, **159**, 159–63.

48. Sperling, M. R., Wilson, G., Engel, J., Babb, T. L., Phelps, M. and Bradley, W. (1986) Magnetic resonance imaging in intractable partial epilepsy: correlative studies. *Ann. Neurol.*, **20**, 57–62.

49 Ormson, M. J., Kispert, D. B., Sharbrough, F. W. *et al.* (1960) Cryptic structural lesions in refractory partial epilepsy: MR imaging and CT studies. *Radiology*, **160**, 215–19.

FURTHER READING

Gadian, D. G. (1982) *Nuclear Magnetic Resonance and Its Applications to Living Systems*, Clarendon Press, Oxford.

Sutton, D. (ed.) (1980) *A Textbook of Radiology and Imaging, Vol. 2*, Churchill Livingstone, Edinburgh.

Du Boulay, G. H. (1964) *The Skull*, Butterworth, London.

Du Boulay, G. H. and Moseley, I. F. (eds) (1977) *Computerised Axial Scanning* (1st European Seminar), Springer-Verlag, Berlin.

CHAPTER NINE

The Treatment of Epilepsy by Drugs

Simon Shorvon

The drug treatment of epilepsy has been greatly improved in recent decades, partly because of the introduction of new compounds, but perhaps more because of a greater understanding of clinical pharmacokinetics and clinical therapeutics. Several reference works concerned with the chemical, pharmacological and clinical aspects of the anticonvulsant drugs have been published in recent years [1–9, 13].

9.1 PHARMACOKINETICS [1–4, 13]

The rational use of a drug depends on its pharmacokinetic properties. A basic understanding of simple pharmacokinetic principles is essential for the practising physician.

9.1.1 Drug absorption

Oral absorption depends on a number of factors, such as the constitution of the tablet or capsule, gastrointestinal physiology, absorption kinetics and first pass metabolism. It varies considerably from individual to individual, and in any one individual over time. *Bioavailability* is a measure of the proportion of an oral dose that is available for utilization by the body. A useful clinical measure of absorption is the time it takes for a drug once administered to achieve peak serum level (T_{max}). This reflects the balance between absorption and elimination. Absorption is the major factor in determining T_{max} for most drugs.

9.1.2 Drug elimination

The elimination of a drug depends on its biotransformation (metabolism) and excretion. The rate of elimination is the major determinant of the duration of action of most anticonvulsant drugs, and is useful for calculating dosages and dosing intervals. A measure of this is the *biological half-life* which is defined as the period of time in which – after absorption – half the drug is eliminated from the body. This depends on any of the factors that influence either metabolism or elimination. There may be marked individual variation. The *clearance* of a drug is a measure of the amount of drug excreted in a unit time, and is related to its half-life.

9.1.3   Drug distribution

The distribution of a drug after ingestion may be complex, but two particular points are of common practical importance. First, it should be realized that in plasma, only the unbound fraction is active and available for pharmacological action. The total plasma concentration of a drug is the sum of this unbound fraction, and of the fraction bound to plasma proteins. Many anticonvulsants are very strongly protein-bound and any change in the properties that determine protein binding will alter the balance between the bound and unbound fractions. When this happens, the total plasma concentration may prove a misleading guide to the available amount of active drug. The second common problem concerns the distribution of a lipid-soluble drug in the fat stores. While this may be constant at normal doses for many anticonvulsant drugs, at high doses the stores may become saturated. Small dosage increments of the drug may then lead to disproportionately large increases in serum concentration. This consideration is important when using large doses of intravenous drugs in the treatment of status epilepticus.

9.1.4   Measurements of anticonvulsant concentration in the serum – 'serum levels'

The ability to measure anticonvulsant drug serum levels is an essential tool in anticonvulsant prescribing. It provides a window onto the vagaries of absorption, elimination and distribution. An intelligent appraisal of drug serum levels is a powerful method of monitoring drug activity. The serum level reflects the balance of these pharmacological properties, and as each is dependent on many individual factors, it is of no surprise that the levels show considerable inter-individual and intra-individual variation. In most clinical situations, the *steady state serum level* is the most useful measure, and this is achieved when the balance of the pharmacological processes reaches equilibrium. The time taken to reach a steady state after the introduction of a new drug by repeated oral administration is known as T_{ss}. In practice, this time is most dependent on factors concerned with elimination – biotransformation and excretion. Steady state levels may also alter as individual patient factors alter. An important example is the induction of hepatic metabolism by the drug itself, or by other medication.

The total serum level is a measure of the combined concentrations of the drug bound to plasma proteins and the free (unbound) drug. Although only the unbound drug is actively available to the body for tissue uptake or metabolism, the total level – which usually bears a consistent relationship to the unbound level – is a sufficient measure for the great majority of clinical purposes. In recent years, it has become possible to measure the free fraction directly, and in some situations this has proved advantageous. For some drugs, salivary levels may also be measured, and these are equivalent to the free fraction.

Various techniques for drug level measurement are used, including gas–liquid chromatography, enzyme immunoassay and EMIT. Whichever method is used, the laboratory should participate in a quality control scheme.

9.1.5 The concept of the optimum range

Following the widespread usage of anticonvulsant serum levels, it became apparent that both anticonvulsant efficacy and toxicity were correlated to anticonvulsant serum levels for some drugs in some patients. The concept has arisen – on shaky experimental evidence – of a range of levels within which anticonvulsant action is maximized and toxicity is minimized. In spite of theoretical objections, this concept has gained wide currency. The usefulness in practice of this concept varies with different drugs and in different clinical circumstances: there is certainly no 'optimum range' for every contingency. With phenytoin, for instance, many patients (perhaps up to half) are perfectly well controlled at serum levels below the 'optimum' range, and in such cases it would be quite wrong to increase the dosage simply because the drug levels were 'suboptimum'. The range is most useful in monitoring phenytoin, carbamazepine, ethosuximide and phenobarbitone dosage, and is of little help with valproate, primidone or the benzodiazepine drugs. With these last three drugs, brain levels, pharmaceutical action and the degree of receptor binding are not well correlated with serum levels. The main importance of the range lies in the definition of an upper limit to treatment, above which toxicity may develop and additional response is unlikely and not in its ability to predict the response to treatment in any individual patient.

In Tables 9.1 and 9.2 are listed some pharmacokinetic properties of the commonly used anticonvulsant drugs, and in Table 9.3 comments about the serum level monitoring of the five commonly monitored drugs. In Table 9.4 are summarized factors which influence anticonvulsant serum levels.

9.1.6 Interactions between drugs

Anticonvulsant drugs are likely to be taken for many years, often in combination with other anticonvulsant or other drugs. With the introduction of monitoring of serum levels, it has become clear that many interactions between these drugs occur, and that these are sometimes of great clinical importance. There are a number of common mechanisms underlying interactions between anticonvulsants.

(1) *Hepatic enzyme induction.* Many anticonvulsant drugs induce hepatic

Table 9.1   Pharmacological characteristics of ten commonly used anticonvulsant drugs

	Acetazolamide	Carbamazepine	Clonazepam	Clobazam
Chemical structure	Sulphonamide	Tricyclic	Benzo-diazepine	Benzo-diazepine
Bioavailability	Good	Variable, often poor	Good	Good
Time to peak serum level (T_{max})	2–3 h	Very variable, mean 6–12 h	1–4 h	1–2 h
Time to steady state (T_{ss}) (after oral administration)	48 h	2–10 d	5–14 d	7 d
% Protein bound	80–95	75	80	—
Elimination half-life of parent drug (adults on chronic therapy)	48 h	10–30 h	15–50 h	10–55 h
Elimination half-life of active metabolites	—	—	—	35–133 h (desmethyl-clobazam)
Enzyme inducer	No	Yes	No	?
Active metabolites	None	Carbamazepine-10,11-epoxide	None	Desmethyl-clobazam
% Excreted unchanged	100	<20	<5	<5

*May occasionally be much longer.

enzymes. This induction may increase the clearance of both the inducing drug and other drugs. This effect is particularly important when drugs share similar enzymic pathways. Phenytoin, carbamazepine and the barbiturate drugs are all potent hepatic enzyme inducers. The increased hydroxylation and hence inactivation of the low oestrogen dosage contraceptive pill by phenytoin is an example of this effect.

(2) *Competitive metabolic inhibition.* If metabolic pathways are shared by several drugs, competitive inhibition of metabolism may occur, resulting in reduced drug clearance. This is an important consideration with many anticonvulsants which share the non-specific cytochrome P450 hepatic enzyme system. The inhibition of phenytoin metabolism by sulthiame is an example of this effect.

(3) *Competition for plasma protein binding.* Highly protein-bound drugs may compete with other drugs for protein binding sites. Combination therapy may result in reduced binding, and an increase in the free fraction and drug clearance. The combination of phenytoin and valproate is an example, and in this case, total phenytoin measurements may prove a misleading guide to the concentration of the free fraction.

(4) *Effects on absorption.* Other drugs may interfere with the absorption of

Ethosuximide	Methsuximide	Phenytoin	Phenobarbitone	Primidone	Valproate
Succinimide	Succinimide	Hydantoin	Barbiturate	Barbiturate	Fatty acid
Good	Good	Variable	Good	Good	Good
1–7 h	1–4 h	4–12 h	2–12 h	2–5 h	1–2 h
6–14 d (adults) 3–6 d (children)	14–21 d (N-desmethyl-methsuximide	14–28 d	14–28 d	14–28 d (derived phenobarbitone)	3–6 d
Minimal	60 (N-desmethyl-methsuximide)	70–95	50	<20	90
20–70 h	2 h	10–34 h*	40–160 h	5–18 h (Prim)	6–18 h
—	38 h (N-desmethyl-methsuximide)	—	—	40–160 h (Phenob) 15–30 h (PEMA)	—
Yes	—	Yes	Yes	Yes	No
None	N-desmethyl-methsuximide	None	None	Phenobarbitone ? PEMA	None
<20	<5	<10	30	15–70	5

some anticonvulsant drugs by a number of mechanisms. The effect of antacids on phenytoin absorption is an example of this interaction.

(5) *Specific pharmacological effects.* In some cases, the effects of an interaction are not necessarily due to altered serum levels, but to more complex pharmacological reactions. These are often not fully understood. One example is the stupor induced by combined medication with valproate and phenobarbitone. The toxic effects of the drugs are enhanced by combined anticonvulsant therapy, but there is little evidence that anticonvulsant efficacy is ever consistently additive. Certainly the view that drug combinations commonly potentiate anticonvulsant action is now not widely held.

The degree of interaction may depend on the levels of the drugs, the enzyme saturation (in those drugs with saturatable metabolism), and individual patient factors which may be genetic or constitutional. The effects are usually complex and often unpredictable. There is almost always considerable interindividual variation in the degree of any interaction, and often intraindividual variation over time. Because these drug interactions are common and unpredictable, the intelligent use of serum anticonvulsant levels has proved of great value. Unnecessary anticonvulsant combination therapy should also clearly be avoided.

Table 9.2 Therapeutic aspects of ten commonly used anticonvulsant drugs

	Acetazolamide	Carbamazepine	Clonazepam	Clobazam
Examples of proprietary names (UK, US)	Diamox	Tegretol	Rivotril Clonopin	Frisium
Usual formulations*	caps/tabs 250 mg	tabs 100 mg, 200, 400 mg syrup 100 mg/ 5 ml	tabs 0.5 mg, 2 mg inj. 1 mg/ml	tabs 10 mg
Usual oral daily maintenance dose				
Adult	250–750 mg	400–1800 mg	1–10 mg	10–30 mg
Child	8–30 mg/kg	100–200 mg (<1 yr) 200–400 mg (1–5 yr) 400–600 mg (6–10 yr) 600–1000 mg (10–15 yr)	250 μg (<1 yr) 500 μg–1 mg (1–5 yr) 1–6 mg (6–12 yr)	5 mg
Usual regimen	Twice a day	Two–four times a day	Once or twice daily	Once a day
First line indication	—	Tonic-clonic Partial tonic	Myoclonic Atonic	—

*UK formulations
†Sustained release

9.1.7 Anticonvulsant toxicity

Patients may have to take anticonvulsant drugs for many years, often in substantial doses and sometimes in combination, and their toxicity is an important clinical consideration. Many chronic side effects remained unrecognized for decades (Fig. 9.1). Even today there is still considerable uncertainty about some aspects of toxicity. The long established drugs such as phenytoin have been more intensively studied than the newer or second line drugs, and it is possible that important toxic effects of these latter drugs are as yet undetected. The recognition of cerebral or neurological toxic effects in particular may be difficult in an epileptic patient, who may have underlying brain damage and in whom overt or subclinical seizure activity may produce similar symptoms.

The toxic effects of the anticonvulsants may be divided into acute (dose-related) effects, hypersensitivity reactions, and chronic toxic effects. Both the acute dose-related side effects, which are encephalopathic in nature, and the

Ethosuximide	Methsuximide	Phenytoin	Phenobarbitone	Primidone	Valproate
Emeside Zarontin	Celontin	Epanutin Dilantin	Luminal Eskabarb Phenobarbital Gardenal	Mysoline Midone	Epilim Depakine Depomide
tabs/caps 250 mg elixir 250 mg/ 5 ml	caps 300 mg	tabs/caps 25, 50, 100 mg susp. 30 mg/ml inj. 50 mg/ml	tabs 15, 30, 60 mg caps (s/r)† 60 mg susp. 30 mg/10 ml inj. 200 mg/ml	tabs 250 mg susp. 250 mg/ 5 ml	tabs 200, 500 mg elixir 200 mg/ 5 ml
500–1500 mg 250 mg (1–6 yr) 500–1000 mg (6–12 yr)	600–1200 mg 150–450 mg	200–500 mg 5–8 mg/kg	60–180 mg 5–10 mg/kg	250–1000 mg 20–30 mg/kg	600–2500 mg 20 mg/kg (up to 4 yr) 30–50 mg/kg (over 4 yr)
Twice a day	Twice a day	Once or twice a day	Once or twice a day	Once or twice a day	Once–three times a day
Typical absence Atonic	—	Tonic-clonic Partial tonic	Tonic-clonic Partial tonic	Tonic-clonic Partial tonic	Tonic-clonic Generalized absence Myoclonic Atonic

hypersensitivity reactions are usually easily recognized, but the chronic toxic effects may take many forms, may be unpredictable, variable and insidious in their development and may be very difficult to detect. Almost without exception, the chronic effects, although not immediately dose-related, are more prevalent at higher doses, after prolonged treatment and in those patients on combination drug therapy. Because of this, drug therapy should be minimized as much as possible, and carefully monitored, with serum level measurements where appropriate. Some effects need no active treatment (e.g. mildly abnormal biochemical or haematological findings); others may be offset by specific therapy (e.g. folate or calcium supplementation) or by simple measures (e.g. meticulous dental hygiene to prevent gingival hypertrophy); others can be reversed only by stopping the anticonvulsant concerned. Careful surveillance of drug therapy is imperative, and a high index of suspicion must be maintained if the many and varied toxic side effects are to be detected or avoided. In this chapter, the frequent, important or serious toxic effects of the commonly used anticonvulsant drugs only will be described.

Table 9.3 Serum level monitoring of anticonvulsant drugs

	Carbamazepine	Ethosuximide	Phenobarbitone	Phenytoin
Value of monitoring	very useful	very useful	useful	essential
'Therapeutic' range μmol/l	15–50	300–700	40–180	30–80
μg/ml	3.5–11.5	40–100	9–40	7–20
Timing of specimen	Sometimes important	Important	Unimportant	Unimportant
Comments	Efficacy and toxicity related to level. Monitoring of the epoxide may also be useful.	Efficacy and toxicity related to level.	Wide individual variations in tolerance to high levels. Doubtful relationship between efficacy and level.	Efficacy and toxicity related to level. Non-linear kinetics. Narrow therapeutic index.

(For primidone – measure phenobarbitone levels, primidone levels of no routine value. Measurement of valproate probably also not generally useful as there is no clear relationship between efficacy and blood levels.)
Serum level monitoring for other drugs is not routinely available.

Table 9.4   Factors influencing anticonvulsant drug serum levels

---

Drug factors:
Chemical constitution
Bioavailability and drug formulation
Drug interactions
Timing of blood sampling and dosage schedules

Patient factors:
Genetic or constitutional factors (may vary with age)
Absorption (may be influenced by gastrointestinal disease/function)
Metabolism (may be influenced by hepatic disease)
Distribution (may be influenced by serum proteins, body weight, pregnancy)
Excretion (may be influenced by renal disease/function)
Compliance

9.2   PRINCIPLES OF DRUG TREATMENT [1–4, 6–8, 13]

9.2.1   The choice of anticonvulsant drug

In spite of their wide variety, the causes, the severity, the clinical features, and the pathophysiology of epilepsy have little influence on the choice of anti-epileptic drug. This choice depends largely on seizure type (Table 9.5).

(1) *Generalized absence seizures (petit mal).* Treatment should be initiated with either ethosuximide or sodium valproate. Second line drugs include clonazepam, acetozolamide and methsuximide. Other drugs such as phenobarbitone and phenytoin may exacerbate absence seizures.

(2) *Generalized tonic-clonic seizures (grand mal).* The drugs of first choice are carbamazepine and phenytoin, followed by primidone, phenobarbitone and sodium valproate. The relative value of sodium valproate is controversial; it is most effective if the seizures form part of the spectrum of the primary generalized epilepsies, if the EEG shows 3 Hz spike wave discharges or if there is photosensitivity. In other generalized tonic-clonic seizures carbamazepine or phenytoin are probably to be preferred. Phenobarbitone and primidone are also effective, but their toxicity may preclude their use as early first line drugs, especially in children. There is some evidence that they may be particularly effective in late onset epilepsy. Second line drugs include clonazepam, clobazam, acetazolamide and methsuximide.

(3) *Atonic, tonic or atypical absence seizures.* These seizures, which are much less common than other seizure types, are difficult to control. Phenytoin and phenobarbitone are the drugs of first choice for tonic seizures, and sodium valproate, clobazam and clonazepam for atonic attacks. If these drugs fail to control the seizures, the addition of any of the other first or second line drugs may be tried.

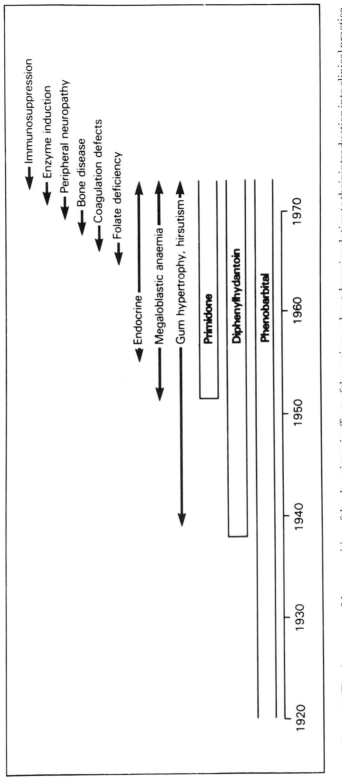

Figure 9.1 The time course of the recognition of the chronic toxic effects of the anticonvulsant drugs in relation to their introduction into clinical practice, demonstrating the marked delay in the detection of many important effects. (Reproduced with permission from Reynolds [5].)

Table 9.5 First and second line anticonvulsant drug therapy

Generalized tonic-clonic seizures:
First line drugs — Carbamazepine, phenobarbitone/primidone, phenytoin, sodium valproate
Second line drugs — Acetazolamide, clobazam, clonazepam, methsuximide

Generalized absence seizures:
First line drugs — Ethosuximide, sodium valproate
Second line drugs — Acetazolamide, clonazepam, methsuximide

Tonic seizures:
First line drugs — Carbamazepine, phenobarbitone, phenytoin
Second line drugs — Clobazam, clonazepam, methsuximide, sodium valproate

Atonic and atypical absence seizures:
First line drugs — Clobazam, clonazepam, sodium valproate
Second line drugs — Acetazolamide, carbamazepine, methsuximide, nitrazepam, phenytoin, phenobarbitone/primidone

Myoclonic seizures:
First line drugs — Clonazepam, ethosuximide, sodium valproate
Second line drugs — Acetazolamide, clobazam, clonazepam, methsuximide, nitrazepam, phenytoin

Partial seizures (simple and complex and including secondarily generalized seizures):
First line drugs — Carbamazepine, phenytoin, phenobarbitone/primidone
Second line drugs — Clobazam, clonazepam, sodium valproate

This list is based on the author's personal practice, and as the exact indications for individual drugs are often controversial, the list is admittedly arbitrary. (Indications for individual drugs are given in the text.)

(4) *Myoclonic seizures.* If these form part of the spectrum of primary generalized epilepsy, sodium valproate is the drug of choice. In the other myoclonic epilepsies, treatment is often unsatisfactory. Sodium valproate, ethosuximide, and clonazepam are the drugs of first choice and acetazolamide, clobazam, phenytoin, phenobarbitone, methsuximide, nitrazepam and carbamazepine may also be tried.

(5) *Simple partial, complex partial and secondarily generalized seizures.* Carbamazepine or phenytoin are the drugs of first choice for these seizure types. Sodium valproate is probably less effective, and both phenobarbitone and primidone although effective are not usually used as early first line drugs because of their toxicity. Second line drugs include the benzodiazepine drugs and acetazolamide.

The stratagems for treatment depend on the usefulness of anticonvulsant serum level measurements (Table 9.3).

(1) *For phenytoin, carbamazepine, phenobarbitone or ethosuximide.* In previously untreated patients, treatment should be initiated with a single drug at low dosage, and after an appropriate time has elapsed (Table 9.1) to ensure a steady state level, the serum anticonvulsant level should be measured. If levels are low, and if seizures recur, the dose should be increased and levels monitored to obtain high therapeutic levels. If seizures are suppressed in the presence of low levels no dosage increases are indicated. If seizures recur in spite of optimum levels of a single drug, this drug should be substituted with another first line medication and the same procedure followed. Combination therapy should be instituted only if single drug treatment with each of the first line drugs has failed; this is discussed in more detail below. Once a regime has been established which provides complete control, serum anticonvulsant level measurements should be occasionally monitored. In chronic uncontrolled patients, the drug should be tried at a dose which produces levels which are high in the therapeutic range. Only then can its full potential be assessed.

(2) *For sodium valproate and the benzodiazepine drugs.* Serum level monitoring is of less use in treatment with these drugs (although it is helpful in detecting non-compliance). The general policies outlined above should be followed, but the maximum doses chosen are those that produce no clinical toxicity.

(3) *For other drugs.* Serum level monitoring of other anticonvulsant drugs is not generally available. The general policies outlined above should be used, and the maximum doses chosen are those limited by toxicity.

It is essential to counsel the patient about the importance of good compliance with the treatment regimen. Compliance may also be improved by simplification of the drug regimen (to a once or twice daily regime), regular serum level measurement, frequent consultations and by the use of a weekly pill box. Patients with active seizures should also be encouraged to keep a seizure calendar to aid accurate assessment of anticonvulsant efficacy.

9.2.2 Anticonvulsant treatment in the previously untreated patient [6–11]

The diagnosis of epilepsy has many profound implications to the sufferer, not least of which is the fact that medication may have to be taken every day for many years. The drugs may cause toxic side effects, require continual medical supervision, and may have complex psychosocial consequences. The decision to initiate drug treatment is not therefore one to be taken lightly. This decision depends on a number of clinical factors:

(1) The diagnosis of epilepsy must be certain. There is little place for a 'trial of anticonvulsant therapy' in possible epilepsy. To overlook non-epileptic

causes of paroxysmal attacks of altered awareness (e.g. cardiac syncope, hypoglycaemia, transient cerebral ischaemic attacks discussed in Chapter 6) may have serious medical results. Diagnosis may sometimes be difficult, and should be kept under constant review.

(2) Estimates of the chances of seizure recurrence must be made, and the extent to which anticonvulsant therapy will improve these chances. Studies in this area have however been contradictory. After a first isolated epileptic seizure, estimates of recurrence have varied from 27–82% (p. 152) [8]. The higher figures have been noted in community-based and prospective studies, and are more representative of an unselected epileptic population. In all studies, the risks of recurrence have been found to be highest in the days or weeks after the first attack. In about 30% of those cases that recur the second attack will have occurred within three months of the first and in almost all cases within two years. After two or more attacks, the risks of recurrence are greater, but here data is more sparse. It is probable however that the more attacks experienced the more likely is the epilepsy to persist. These recurrence risks are influenced by various clinical factors. Higher rates are found in progressive or structural cerebral disease, patients with spike-wave discharges or frequent focal spiking on EEG, partial seizures, neurological signs, mental retardation or psychiatric handicap. Epidemiological studies have shown however that the overall prognosis of newly diagnosed patients is nevertheless good. Community-based studies have shown that in about 70% of patients developing epilepsy, prolonged remission is achieved. In about one-half of cases the epilepsy is short-lived, the total number of seizures experienced small, and drug treatment will be taken for a relatively short time [8]. In these investigations, the majority of patients are treated, and whether treatment influences this generally satisfactory outcome is not clear. Remarkably, there is no comprehensive data concerning the prognosis of untreated patients, and the natural history of untreated epilepsy is totally obscure.

The efficacy of anticonvulsant therapy after a first seizure has not been studied. After two or more attacks, monotherapy with first line anticonvulsant drugs will provide complete seizure control in between 50–90% of cases, and the use of serum level monitoring to optimize therapy where necessary further improves the outcome. These results are considerably better than those in chronic patients, and most previously untreated patients initiated on anti-convulsant therapy can expect a complete or substantial suppression of seizures, at least in the early stages of their epilepsy. The effect of treatment on the longer term outlook is less clear, and the exact role of anticonvulsant medication at this stage is uncertain. The traditional view is that the drugs act by simply suppressing seizures, and have no more fundamental influence on the final outcome of the epilepsy. More recently, however, the possibility has been raised that the early suppression of seizures may also lessen the longer term propensity to attacks and that to some extent early treatment is thus 'curative'. If this is the case, there are obvious implications to the management of early epilepsy.

(3) The potential toxic side effects of chronic anticonvulsant therapy must be considered.

(4) Individual factors are often very important in the decision to initiate therapy. The implications of further seizures or drug therapy may vary depending on employment, social and domestic circumstances, psychological factors, the requirement for driving and so on. The attitude of the patient and his relatives to treatment is an essential factor; if compliance is poor, attempted treatment is likely to be counterproductive.

(5) In a proportion of cases, clearly identified precipitating factors exist for the seizures, which may modify the need for therapy. Common examples include febrile convulsions in children, or seizures induced by alcohol, drugs or photosensitivity in adults (see Chapter 6).

It should be clear from the above points, that in any patient, the decision to start therapy may be difficult to make, and depends on a variety of unquantifiable factors. General guidelines can be however drawn:

(1) After a single seizure, treatment should usually be recommended if the seizure occurred on the basis of progressive or structural brain disease, or if the EEG shows clear paroxysmal spike-wave activity, as the chances of recurrence are high, particularly if the first attack was very recent. Conversely, if a single seizure has occurred without obvious reason, the risk of recurrence is lower (although still substantial) and it may be best to delay therapy.

(2) After two or more seizures, even if no cause is found, therapy is usually recommended unless there has been a long gap, say more than 12 months, between attacks.

Both the above recommendations are entirely arbitrary, as there are no studies comparing treatment with no treatment in these early stages. Such studies are urgently needed.

(3) If precipitating factors are identifiable, the need for regular anticonvulsant therapy may be modified. After uncomplicated febrile seizures in children, continuous anticonvulsant therapy is usually avoided. In adults with alcohol or drug-induced seizures anticonvulsant treatment may actually increase the chances of further seizures when the drugs are withdrawn.

With other common precipitants such as stress, fatigue or photosensitivity, advice is less easy, but it may be best to avoid medication if only a few attacks have occurred and the precipitating circumstances can be henceforth avoided.

(4) The attitude of the patient to treatment is a very important consideration. If compliance is likely to be poor, therapy should usually be avoided, and there is a considerable risk from withdrawal seizures if anticonvulsants are taken intermittently.

In all cases, it is essential here to inform and involve the patients. Counselling should be given concerning the function of medication, the length of time that treatment is needed, its potential hazards, the importance of regular compliance, the use of serum level monitoring, the social and psychological implications of therapy, the interactions with alcohol or the contraceptive pill and so on. Sadly, however, treatment is often started without much thought, in response to an immediate crisis. Explanations are forgotten, and the patients are frequently confused. The result is inadequate compliance, treatment failure, disillusion and an erosion of the patient's trust.

If drug treatment is initiated, monotherapy with anticonvulsant suitable to the seizure type should be used according to the principles outlined in section 9.2.1.

9.2.3 The treatment of patients with uncontrolled seizures

These patients feature prominently in hospital-based neurology clinics, but form a minority of all patients with a history of epilepsy. Drug treatment may be difficult and is less satisfactory than for newly diagnosed patients, but a number of general principles can be applied:

(1) The diagnosis of epilepsy should be reassessed in all patients with resistant seizures, before assuming the seizures to be intractable. Even in specialist epilepsy clinics, the seizures in up to 20% of such cases may prove to be non-epileptic in origin.

(2) The cause of the epilepsy should again be considered, and progressive cerebral disease excluded.

(3) A complete treatment history should be taken, an essential step which is often overlooked. In most chronic cases, the previous response to an individual drug is a useful guide to any future response. Information should be obtained regarding the drugs previously taken, the duration of therapy, the maximum dosage and serum levels, and compliance.

(4) Drug changes should be made in a planned and coherent fashion.

  (i) First line drugs which have not received an adequate previous trial should be introduced for a trial of treatment, under close supervision and with serum level monitoring where appropriate.

 (ii) Second line drugs should then be considered.

(iii) Anticonvulsants which, on historical grounds, have provided no benefit should be withdrawn.

The aim of these manipulations should be single drug therapy or combination therapy with no more than two drugs; it is seldom necessary to use more complicated anticonvulsant regimes. The drugs chosen should be those which have been shown conclusively to provide a measure of control, and minimum toxicity. These drug changes may take months to complete, will often require close supervision, preferably by a single experienced physician, and may place a strain on medical resources. Nevertheless, it is only in this way that severe epileptics will obtain optimum anticonvulsant medication. A reduction in total medication will paradoxically improve seizure control in a substantial proportion of cases, and toxicity – frequently previously unrecognized – is often markedly reduced. There are no clear cut ways of predicting response to the reduction of therapy; the EEG, for instance, is of little use.

(5) The withdrawal of individual drugs from a patient with active epilepsy may be difficult to achieve. Both the barbiturate and the benzodiazepine drugs require staged withdrawal over a long period of time to avoid the precipitation of withdrawal seizures, and their withdrawal is sometimes accompanied by other physical and psychological withdrawal symptoms. Withdrawal of the other anticonvulsant drugs has been little studied, but it seems likely that more rapid withdrawal is possible, as the tendency for withdrawal symptoms and seizures is less marked.

(6) It is important to realize that there are limits to anticonvulsant treatment. The seizures in some patients – albeit a small but chronic group – will not be fully controlled with presently available anticonvulsant drugs. In such cases, it is best to reduce medication where possible to minimize toxicity, while providing partial control. Very occasionally, some patients with chronic active epilepsy may in fact be best managed by the total withdrawal of medication, although this is a hazardous course of action as status epilepticus may be induced. Close supervision is essential. This course of action should be only considered in those with partial seizures, in which there is no risk of physical injury.

9.2.4 The drug treatment of ongoing seizures

In known epileptics, no emergency drug treatment is usually necessary after a single epileptic attack. If a series of attacks occurs, or if a single attack is usually followed by a cluster of attacks, the administration of 10–20 mg of diazepam will frequently prevent further seizures. Oral diazepam is absorbed too slowly in most situations, and rectal or intravenous administration is usually required. A useful proprietary rectal solution of diazepam is available (available in the UK as Stesolid), which is easy to use and may often be administered by parents or relatives. Alternatively, the intravenous preparation may be successfully instilled rectally via a soft plastic cannula. Wax suppositories of diazepam or intramuscular diazepam should not be used for the acute treatment of seizures, for absorption is slow and erratic with both methods of administration. Intramuscular paraldehyde (5–20 ml) is also effective when diazepam has failed to control the seizures or is contraindicated.

Status epilepticus is frequently preceded by increasing serial seizures. It is an important but little realized principle that the propitious use of rectal (or intravenous) diazepam in serial seizures will markedly cut down this risk.

Patients and their relatives should be told what action to take during a seizure. In a convulsive attack, it is important to emphasize that no attempt should be made to put anything into the mouth or to force the teeth open (in the mistaken belief that this will protect the tongue), or to restrain the convulsive movements. The patient should be moved only to keep him from a dangerous place (e.g. near a fire or road). After the convulsive movements have finished, he should be placed in the coma position, and his airway checked. In the immediate postictal phase, the patient may be confused and need reassurance and sympathy, but the minimum amount of fuss. Transfer to a hospital is only necessary if the fit is atypical, prolonged or is repeated, or if injury or anoxia has occurred. Minor fits, similarly, need very little active management, and in an automatism the minimum amount of restraint to prevent further injury only should be applied. The patient should however be observed until the postictal confusion is completely resolved.

9.2.5   The treatment of patients whose seizures are in remission [7, 8]

In this group, the question of either withdrawal or reduction of anticonvulsant medication is often raised, but informed advice is difficult to give. Unnecessary treatment should be avoided, but in no individual case can the safety of drug reduction be guaranteed. A number of clinical factors may influence the decision:

(1) *Overall risks of relapse after withdrawal of medication.* In hospital-based studies of withdrawal of medication after two or three years of freedom from seizures, relapse following withdrawal has been recorded in between 15–70% of cases in different series. As many patients in remission will have stopped attending specialist outpatient clinics, these studies are of highly selected groups. Many patients discontinue therapy on their own initiative. In community-based surveys, it is clear that a higher proportion of patients do successfully withdraw therapy.

In all studies, the longer the seizure-free period prior to withdrawal of medication, the less likely was subsequent relapse found to occur.

(2) *Risks of relapse during withdrawal of therapy.* The risks of relapse are at their greatest during withdrawal, when about 50% of relapses occur, or soon afterwards. The longer is the period free from seizures without medication, the less likely is subsequent relapse.

(3) *Factors influencing the risks of withdrawal.* A number of prognostic factors have been identified. Relapse after withdrawal of medication is more likely in the presence of identified cerebral disease, neurological signs, psychiatric disturbances, or persisting paroxysmal EEG abnormalities – at least in children (p. 195) – and with partial or mixed seizure types. Certain childhood syndromes carry a good prognosis after cessation of seizures. These include primary generalized absence seizures (petit mal), benign rolandic epilepsy and febrile convulsions. An important factor, often overlooked, is the previous

pattern of seizures. If the epilepsy was active for a relatively short time, if only a few seizures had occurred, or if there had been previous periods of prolonged remission, the chances of relapse are probably substantially reduced.

(4) *Speed of withdrawal of medication.* The rate of withdrawal is said to be important, and some authors recommend staged withdrawal of therapy over a very long period (months or years). This cautious approach derives from experience with barbiturate withdrawal, and whether it is really necessary for other non-sedative drugs is doubtful though this is one of the variables currently being explored in the MRC trial in the UK.

(5) *Individual factors.* These include the attitude of the patient towards medication, the social and medical effects of further seizures, the patient's employment, the requirement for a driving licence, and so on.

The above considerations apply similarly to the reduction of therapy rather than its complete discontinuation. In a few cases, even a small reduction in medication may result in further seizures. Furthermore, full control may not be achieved subsequently, even if the previous drug regimen is restored.

Practice regarding the withdrawal (or reduction) of therapy varies considerably. In general terms, reduction of treatment is often attempted sooner in children than in adults, perhaps because of the more severe social consequences of seizures in adults, but different physicians have widely differing opinions. The points outlined above should be considered in every individual case, and recommendations applicable to all individual cases are difficult to make. A few broad guidelines can however be given:

(1) Withdrawal may usually be considered after two or more years of freedom from seizures. If prognostic factors are unfavourable, however, the risks of recurrence even after this period are higher. The longer the seizure-free period the less likely is subsequent recurrence to occur. If the period of active epilepsy prior to the remission was short, however, withdrawal of medication may be attempted earlier. After a single attack, for instance, six months may suffice, although there is as yet no good evidence on this point.

(2) Withdrawal should usually be carried out gradually and in stages. For the barbiturate or benzodiazepine drugs this may require a period of many months. A withdrawal rate of 30 mg a month for phenobarbitone is commonly recommended. For the other anticonvulsants, faster withdrawal may be possible, and weekly reductions of 50 mg of phenytoin, 100 mg of carbamazepine or 200 mg of sodium valproate are often used. The patient should be carefully supervized over this period, in case bursts of seizures occur.

(3) The risks of recurrence should be very clearly explained to the patient, and the possible medical and social implications made explicit, particularly in regard to the laws about driving (Chapter 20). These should be balanced against the toxicity of the medication prescribed.

(4) Only one drug at a time should be reduced or withdrawn.

9.3 THE FIRST LINE ANTICONVULSANT DRUGS
[1, 2, 4, 5, 9, 13]

The drug treatment of epilepsy has changed considerably during this century, but the commonly used drugs have been available for considerable periods of time (Tables 9.6 and 9.7). Prescribing habits in epilepsy are conservative, and once a satisfactory regime is achieved, patients may take the same anticonvulsant drug for many years. Although a wide variety of drugs are said to have anticonvulsant action, only a relatively small number are commonly used. In

Table 9.6 Anticonvulsant drug therapy in 1901. From Gowers 1881 [10] and 1901 [11].

1. Drugs of definite benefit*	2. Drugs of doubtful benefit
Bromide of ammonium	Camphor
potassium	Aconite
sodium	Hydrocyanic acid
lithium	Iodide of potassium
strontium	Mistletoe
Digitalis	Turpentine
Belladonna	Cocculus Indicus
Atropine	Chloral
Stramonium	Nitrate of silver
Cannabis indica	Sulphate of copper
Gelsemium sempervirens	Benzoate of soda
Opium	Nitroglycerine
Zinc	Piscidia Erythrina
Borax	Codeia
Iron	Calabar bean
Wildersmith	Ergot
Hyoscine	Sclerotic acid
Strophanthus	Nitrite of amyl
Bromine and Sesame oil	Bromide of aluminium
	Osmic acid
	Curara
	Hydrastin
	Chinolin
	Resorcin
	Antipyrine
	Acetanilide
	Bromide of Rubidium
	Bromalin

* Of these Gowers recognized the prime position of Bromide.

Table 9.7 Contemporary anticonvulsant drug therapy (with date of first clinical report)

Acetylurea:	Pheneturide 1949
Barbiturates:	Phenobarbitone 1912
	Methylphenobarbitone 1932
	Primidone 1952
	Dimethoxy-methylphenobarbitone 1975
Benzodiazepines:	Nitrazepam 1963
	Diazepam 1965
	Oxazepam 1968
	Clonazepam 1976
	Clobazam 1980
Dipropylacetate:	Sodium valproate 1961
Hydantoins:	Phenytoin 1938
	Ethotoin 1956
	Methoin 1956
	Deltoin 1966
	Albutoin 1967
Iminostilbene:	Carbamazepine 1962
Proprionamide:	Beclamide 1956
Oxazolidinediones:	Troxidone 1945
	Paramethadione 1954
Succinimides:	Phensuximide 1951
	Methsuximide 1951
	Ethosuximide 1958
Sulphonamides:	Acetazolamide 1955
	Sulthiame 1960

(c.f. Table 9.1)

this section, the seven first line oral anticonvulsants will be described. Less commonly used drugs and new anticonvulsants are described on page 281, and the drugs used in the treatment of status epilepticus in Chapter 14.

9.3.1 Carbamazepine

This drug was introduced into clinical practice in 1962, and has been increasingly recognized as a major first line drug in the treatment of epilepsy. It is chemically related to the tricyclic antidepressants, and is a neutral compound which is poorly soluble in water. Its mechanism of action is unclear, but it shares many physiological properties with phenytoin, including an action in limiting high frequency sustained repetitive neuronal firing. It also affects several neurotransmitter systems.

(a) Indications

Carbamazepine is a drug of first choice in tonic-clonic, tonic and partial (simple and complex) seizures, and may be used in all other seizure types except generalized absence seizures (petit mal). Its efficacy in tonic-clonic and partial seizures is equivalent to that of phenytoin and superior to that of phenobarbitone and its toxicity significantly less. It is useful in children and adults and in epilepsy of differing aetiologies. It is the least toxic of all the major anticonvulsant drugs. Very occasionally, however, seizures may be exacerbated by carbamazepine.

(b) Clinical therapeutics

In the UK the drug is available as 100 mg, 200 mg and 400 mg tablets and as a syrup. In most adults it is best given on a twice daily regimen. A three times daily regimen is occasionally needed if serum levels vary excessively throughout the day, or if dose-related time-locked side effects are noted after a single dose. These include transient unsteadiness or diplopia, which are fairly common after a single high dose. In children, a three or occasionally four times a day regime is needed because of their faster metabolism. The usual adult maintenance dose is between 600–1200 mg daily, although higher doses (up to 2000 mg/day) are sometimes required. Measurements of serum drug level are very useful in monitoring the dose. Estimations of 'trough' levels are often helpful. In routine practice, it is vital to introduce the drug slowly over two or three weeks, as too high an initial dose may cause drowsiness, nausea or dizziness. A gradual initiation of therapy will avoid these effects. In general, carbamazepine is one of the best tolerated of the antiepileptic drugs and produces few troublesome side effects. There is no parenteral preparation of carbamazepine.

Carbamazepine levels are relatively stable throughout pregnancy and dose changes are usually unnecessary. A mother taking carbamazepine at normal doses may safely breast feed an infant.

(c) Clinical pharmacology

The absorption of the drug is slow, irregular and incomplete after oral administration. Bioavailability is between 75–85%. Peak serum levels in adults are usually reached within 6–12 hours, although there is considerable variation; in some studies, peaks up to 32 hours after ingestion have been reported. The size of the administered dose may influence absorption, and in a minority of patients this may be clinically relevant. In such cases, it may be necessary to administer doses on a three times a day basis because of reduced absorption and delayed peak levels. Administration with food may also speed absorption. Absorption is faster in children (peak levels within 4–8 hours) and in neonates (peak levels within 3–6 hours).

The drug is about 70–75% bound to plasma proteins at all normal clinical concentrations. The CSF and salivary levels are similar to the unbound levels in plasma, and levels in milk are about 60–70% those in maternal plasma. Brain concentrations are similar to plasma concentrations.

There are a number of metabolic pathways for carbamazepine, the most important being the epoxidation to 10,11-carbamazepine epoxide. This compound has anticonvulsant action itself, equivalent to that of carbamazepine. This 10,11-epoxide is metabolized mostly to 10,11-dihydroxy carbamazepine. About 2% of the parent drug is excreted unchanged in the urine. Carbamazepine induces its own metabolism. The half-life after chronic administration is between 5–26 hours compared with a half-life of 18–55 hours on initiation of therapy. This process of autoinduction reaches completion within 20–30 days in volunteers, but is possibly shorter in patients already taking inducing drugs. The time to achieve steady state values is also shorter in such patients (2–3 days) than in patients not previously taking drugs (7–8 days). The initial dosage in this latter group of patients should therefore be lower than in patients already taking other anticonvulsant drugs. Only about 2% of the drug is excreted unchanged in the urine. The relationship between oral dose and serum level is linear. Increments in dosage produce a more predictable response than is the case with phenytoin. The pharmacokinetic properties of carbamazepine make the drug altogether more easy to use than phenytoin.

Carbamazepine levels may be markedly depressed by concomitant medication with phenytoin or barbiturate anticonvulsant drugs. The total dose necessary to produce adequate serum levels may be very much higher than that needed when the drug is taken alone. Indeed, on occasions, therapeutic levels are impossible to achieve in combination regimens.

As the 10,11-epoxide has an anticonvulsant action equivalent to that of carbamazepine, its pharmacokinetic characteristics are clinically significant. It is present in plasma at a concentration of about 10% of that of carbamazepine, is about 30% protein bound, and enters brain and CSF readily. Its metabolism is also self-induced. The ratio between carbamazepine and its epoxide varies when other interacting drugs are present. The relationship between oral dose and serum level, as with carbamazepine, varies widely between individuals. It has been suggested that some of the dose-related side effects of carbamazepine are in fact due to the epoxide, and it is sometimes worth measuring serum epoxide levels.

(d) Drug interactions

A number of clinically important interactions of carbamazepine are recognized. Carbamazepine levels are often lowered by simultaneous medication with other drugs. This effect is common when carbamazepine is used in combination with phenytoin; indeed, as already mentioned, it may sometimes be impossible to obtain satisfactory levels of carbamazepine in the presence of phenytoin. In clinical practice, this effect may require the withdrawal of phenytoin. In many situations, carbamazepine monotherapy is superior to combination therapy with phenytoin for this reason. Combined medication with phenobarbitone may have a similar but usually less significant effect. Carbamazepine may itself decrease the clearance of phenytoin, and possibly also that of phenobarbitone, and increase the clearance of ethosuximide and sodium valproate, but these effects are usually of little clinical significance. Carbamazepine may reduce effective warfarin levels. Occasionally it may induce oestrogen metabolism sufficiently to render unreliable the low-dose oestrogen contraceptive pill, but this effect is less common than with phenytoin. Erythromycin, and dextro-propoxyphene may increase carbamazepine levels due to hepatic enzyme inhibition, but the most dramatic reported example of such inhibition is the several fold increase in carbamazepine levels due to co-medication with imidazole drugs such as denzimol. Other drugs which have been reported to elevate carbamazepine levels include isoniazid, viloxazine, cimetidine, verapamil, and diltiazem.

9.3.2 Clonazepam

The first reports of the use of this benzodiazepine drug in epilepsy were made in 1970, and since then there have been a number of clinical and pharmacological studies. It is now probably the most widely used benzodiazepine drug for long term oral anticonvulsant therapy. The mechanism of action of the drug is uncertain, but it possibly acts by effects on GABA-mediated synapses, or on serotonin or glycine or dopaminergic metabolism.

(a) Indications

Clonazepam is a drug of early choice for the treatment of all types of myoclonic seizures, although nowadays sodium valproate is usually preferred. It may also be tried in other types of seizure including absence seizures. It seems to have more application in paediatric than in adult practice. It has two major drawbacks which limit its usefulness; the first is pronounced sedation that may occur at even moderate doses, and the second is the tendency – common to all benzodiazepine drugs – for tolerance to develop to its anticonvulsant effects. Serum level monitoring is not yet routinely available. Clonazepam is also a useful intravenous preparation in status epilepticus, with properties equivalent to those of diazepam, although it is doubtful whether it has any significant advantages over diazepam.

(b) Clinical therapeutics

Clonazepam is available as 0.5 mg and 2 mg tablets in the UK and as an intravenous preparation. The usual adult maintenance dose varies from 3–8 mg/day, although much higher and lower doses are sometimes used. In children up to one year of age a dose of 0.5–1 mg/day is usual, at age 1–5 years 1 mg–3 mg/day, and at age 6–12 years 3–6 mg/day. The drug should be introduced slowly over several weeks to minimize the development of drowsiness. The final dose chosen is often dictated by the sedative effects of the drug. It is usually given on a once (at night) or twice daily regime, as fluctuations in serum level probably do not influence the drug's efficacy. Withdrawal seizures may be precipitated by abrupt cessation of therapy. As with other benzodiazepine and barbiturate drugs, cautious and slow staged withdrawal is usually advised; a reduction of 0.25 mg a week is suggested. Intravenous clonazepam may be used at a dose of 1 mg given over 30 seconds, which may be repeated. However, there is a significant risk of respiratory depression or cardiovascular collapse, and cardiorespiratory function must be monitored, and facilities for resuscitation must be available.

(c) Clinical pharmacology
Clonazepam is well absorbed and peak levels usually appear within four hours of taking an oral dose. It is metabolized into several compounds, some with anticonvulsant activity, but the active metabolites are present in small concentrations only, and do not contribute significantly to the efficacy of the drug. Less than 1% of the drug is excreted unchanged in the urine. The half-life of clonazepam is between 15–50 hours, and steady state levels are reached within 5–8 days. The serum concentrations in different individuals at any given dose of clonazepam are very variable. The drug is about 80% protein bound, and probably does not induce liver enzymes to a significant extent. There are no potent drug interactions. Tolerance to the anticonvulsant effects – but unfortunately not to drowsiness – is a common phenomenon, usually occurring within 1–6 months of the onset of therapy. This is only partly reversed by an increase in dose.

9.3.3 Ethosuximide

This drug was introduced into clinical practice in 1958, and was quickly recognized to be highly effective against petit mal (typical absence) seizures. Of the series of succinimide compounds introduced at that time, only ethosuximide has maintained a position as a first line drug. The mechanism of action of ethosuximide is uncertain, but depression of repetitive transmission, inhibition of the presynaptic membrane ATPase and inhibition of cortical excitatory pathways have all been demonstrated experimentally.

(a) Clinical therapeutics
Serum and salivary levels for the drug are easily determined. Considerable individual variation exists in the relation between dose and serum level. In general, children require a higher dose per kilogram than adults. The drug's efficacy is highly correlated to serum level and a well-established therapeutic range exists for this drug 300–700 μmol/l (40–100 μg/ml) and levels of less than 300 μmol/l (40 μg/ml) seldom control absence seizures. In view of this

and of the inter-individual relation between dose and serum level, plasma level monitoring is well worthwhile.

The drug is available as a capsule of 250 mg and a suspension. The usual adult dosage range is 500–1500 mg/day. It should be introduced over two weeks, and administered in a twice daily regimen.

(b) Clinical pharmacology

Ethosuximide is well absorbed with almost complete bioavailability. Peak serum levels are usually achieved within three hours (range 1–7 hours) of oral administration. Steady state levels are reached within ten days of continuous therapy in adults, and within six days in children. The drug is only minimally bound to protein, so that salivary and breast milk levels are soon equivalent to those of serum. The half-life of the compound is usually between 20–70 hours, but is very variable, particularly in children. The drug is hydroxylated and methylated in the liver. The major metabolite is 2-(-1-hydroxyethyl)-2-methylsuccinimide. About 20% of the drug is excreted in urine unchanged. None of the metabolites of the drug have significant antiepileptic activity.

(c) Drug interactions

As the drug is not protein bound and as its metabolic pathway differs from that of other drugs, there are no common significant drug interactions. Enzyme induction does not occur on administration of ethosuximide.

9.3.4 Phenobarbitone

This drug was introduced into clinical practice in 1912, and its anticonvulsant action was appreciated widely after the First World War. It still retains its place as a major first line anticonvulsant drug. It is a weak acid, which is poorly soluble in water. Its exact mechanism of action is unknown, but it both inhibits the spread of the epileptic discharge and also raises the threshold to induced experimental seizures. It may act at three levels – postsynaptically by modifying neurotransmitter action, presynaptically by reducing calcium entry, and by blocking the release of neurotransmitter, and non-synaptically by reducing sodium and potassium conductances and by blocking receptor sites.

(a) Indications

Phenobarbitone is a first line drug for the treatment of tonic-clonic and tonic seizures, and is also useful in all other seizure types, with the exception of generalized absence seizures which may be exacerbated by barbiturate therapy. Its anticonvulsant efficacy is equivalent to that of phenytoin, but because of its sedative effects, its withdrawal effects, its potential as a drug of abuse and its danger in overdose, its use is now often restricted to patients who have not responded to other first line drugs. Phenobarbitone is relatively contraindicated in children because it frequently causes paradoxical excitement and hyperactivity. It is effective in epilepsies of all aetiologies, and like phenytoin may be particularly effective in symptomatic cases. It is usually well tolerated in the elderly, and there is an impression that it may be superior to other anticonvulsants in the older patient.

(b) Clinical therapeutics

In the UK, phenobarbitone is available as 15 mg, 30 mg, 60 mg and 100 mg tablets, as an elixir, Spansule and injection. The usual adult maintenance dose varies between 30–150 mg/day, although occasionally higher doses are required. It may be given on a once daily regimen, usually best taken on retiring. At higher doses, twice daily regimens are frequently given, although this is probably unnecessary in the great majority of cases. It may be given intramuscularly at a dose of 200 mg repeated six hourly if necessary to a maximum of 600 mg/day. Where therapeutic levels need to be obtained quickly, an oral loading dose of two times the maintenance dose can be given for four days running. Steady state levels will then be achieved within 36 hours. This rapid induction of therapy, however, may produce marked drowsiness, which may persist for several weeks. In some countries phenobarbitone is a controlled drug, and epileptic patients taking this medication are advised to carry some form of confirmation of their medical need for its prescription. Serum level monitoring is of less use than with phenytoin, for instance, as the therapeutic ranges can be misleading. Many patients are well controlled at low serum levels, and toxic side effects may occur with levels usually considered therapeutic. Conversely, patients are sometimes seen with very high levels and no obvious side effects. Nevertheless, it is usual to avoid high levels, so that regular serum level measurements are recommended in any patient on chronic phenobarbitone therapy.

Phenobarbitone levels in pregnancy have not been extensively studied, but the dosage requirements of the drug are usually slightly increased. At high maternal levels, breast feeding may produce drowsiness in the infant, but this is unusual. Provided the infant is carefully monitored there is no contraindication to breast feeding in most clinical situations. If artificially fed, the infant may show withdrawal symptoms of 'jitteriness' and occasionally seizures (p. 386).

(c) Clinical pharmacology

Phenobarbitone is said to be well absorbed from the gastrointestinal tract, although evidence on this point is conflicting. At normal dosage, peak levels are obtained usually within 2–12 hours of oral administration, and absorption is complete. The drug may be given by intramuscular injection, and in adults the serum levels obtained, and the time to peak levels, are much the same as after oral administration. In neonates however, absorption is slower and irregular. The drug is also absorbed after rectal administration.

Phenobarbitone is about 50% bound to plasma proteins, and alterations in plasma proteins in clinical practice do not have a significant effect on serum levels. Brain concentrations are approximately equivalent to serum concentrations, and salivary and CSF levels are approximately equivalent to free plasma concentrations.

Phenobarbitone is metabolized in the liver by the oxidase enzyme system, largely to a parahydroxylated metabolite which is subsequently conjugated and excreted as a glucuronide or sulphate derivative. These metabolites have no significant anticonvulsant activity. About 30% of the drug is excreted unchanged. The elimination half-life of the drug in adults is usually between 40–160 hours (median 4–5 days), but there is great inter-individual variability. After initiation of a normal oral dose, the steady state is not usually reached for 2–4 weeks. The elimination half-life in children is shorter (30–80 hours) and the dose requirements higher; children between the ages of 1–14 years require a dose of 2–3 times that of the adult dose (on a mg/kg basis). Steady state levels are usually reached in about 10 days. In neonates, the half-life is longer than in children or adults (61–175 hours). Due to the long half-life and slow metabolism, a single daily dosage regimen is sufficient in most clinical circumstances, and as blood levels are stable throughout the day, the interpretation of the plasma levels need not take the time of administration into account. There is a wide inter-individual variation in the relation between oral dose and serum level. Over the normal dosage range, the relation between oral dose and serum level is probably linear, although evidence for this is conflicting. Drug interactions may also have an important effect on serum levels.

(d) Drug interactions

Detailed studies of drug interactions with phenobarbitone are surprisingly few. Nevertheless as the barbiturate drugs induce hepatic microsomal enzymes, albeit to a lesser extent than phenytoin, increased clearance of other compounds metabolized in the liver might be expected. Compounds affected include other anticonvulsant drugs, warfarin, antibiotics such as griseofulvin, doxycycline and chloramphenicol, and the contraceptive pill. The interactions with other anticonvulsants are generally small, a particular exception being that with sodium valproate; this combination may result in marked somnolence, which may even progress to coma. The mechanism of this effect is uncertain, but may relate to sodium valproate-induced hyperammonaemia. Phenytoin given with phenobarbitone may increase phenobarbitone levels, and conversely the addition of phenobarbitone may lower phenytoin levels. As the drug is only moderately protein bound, it is unlikely to displace or be displaced to any significant degree by other protein bound drugs.

### 9.3.5	Phenytoin

This drug was introduced in 1938 – a year of Jubilee for epileptics according to Lennox. Since then it has remained the most widely used of all antiepileptic drugs. It is furthermore the drug which has been most intensively studied, and is often the yardstick against which other compounds are measured.

### (a)	Indications

It is a drug of first choice in tonic-clonic, tonic, atonic and partial seizures (both complex and simple), and may be used in myoclonic seizures also. It is contraindicated in generalized absence seizures, but is occasionally helpful in atypical absence seizures. It may be used in epilepsy of all aetiologies, and at all ages, but is perhaps best avoided as a drug of first choice in young women, because of risk of cosmetic side effects and its teratogenicity. There is some anecdotal evidence that the drug is more useful in symptomatic epilepsies than the newer first line drugs. It is also of proven value in cryptogenic late onset seizures. It is a difficult drug to use due to the non-linear relation between dose and serum level, and the narrow therapeutic index, between effective and toxic effects. Measurements of serum levels are essential in monitoring therapy. Phenytoin may also be administered intravenously in status epilepticus (p. 428).

### (b)	Clinical therapeutics

Phenytoin is available in the UK in 50 mg and 100 mg tablets and as 25 mg, 50 mg and 100 mg capsules. Phenytoin may be given in a once daily regimen to most adults. It is usually most convenient to take this at night. In some patients, particularly at higher doses, a twice daily regimen is advisable. In children, because of their faster metabolism of the drugs, phenytoin is best given twice daily. There is no need for the dose to be divided into a three or even four times a day regimen, a practice which simply increases the chances of accidental non-compliance.

The usual maintenance dose is between 200–400 mg/day in adults, and between 5–8 mg/kg/day in children, but both lower and higher doses are needed in some patients. Serum level measurements are invaluable in monitoring the dose of phenytoin. A therapeutic dose should normally be introduced in stages over several weeks to minimize initial side effects. If a rapid effect is needed, an oral loading dose of 1000 mg for an adult may be given over a 24 hour period, or the drug may be given by slow intravenous injection at a dose of 15–18 mg/kg in an adult or 5 mg/kg in a child, at a rate not exceeding 50 mg/min. ECG monitoring should be carried out and resuscitation facilities must be available. Intramuscular phenytoin is very poorly absorbed, and this route of administration is not recommended in any clinical circumstance.

Phenytoin is a difficult drug to use during pregnancy, as the levels may fall sharply in the later stages, and the ratio of free-to-total phenytoin may also alter pp. 385–86. Frequent serum level estimations may be necessary, and measurements of the free phenytoin levels are advisable in some patients. After delivery, phenytoin levels may rise rapidly to pre-pregnant levels and, unless the dose is altered to take this into account, toxicity may be precipitated. Breast feeding by a mother taking normal doses of phenytoin may be safely carried out. Vitamin K should be given immediately after delivery to infants born to mothers treated with phenytoin, as phenytoin can induce the infantile hepatic enzyme system to an extent that may compromise vitamin K-dependent coagulation mechanisms, resulting in neonatal haemorrhage (p. 386).

(c) Clinical pharmacology

Phenytoin is a weak acid which is relatively insoluble in water at physiological pH. The mechanism of its anticonvulsant actions is uncertain. It stabilizes neuronal (and other) membranes, perhaps due to its ability to prevent the influx of sodium ions during depolarization – lowering intraneuronal sodium concentrations – and this may in turn be due to the displacement of calcium from binding sites on the membrane surface. It decreases post-tetanic potentiation, perhaps due to a decrease in neurotransmitter release due to the interference with the entry of calcium into the presynaptic terminal. It also partially blocks axonal conduction of nervous impulses, especially during high firing rates.

Because of its poor solubility and acidity, the absorption of phenytoin is variable and affected by a number of different factors. The proportion absorbed varies widely in different individuals. Oral absorption takes place mainly in the small intestine. The proportion absorbed may be altered by disorders of the biliary circulation, certain foods, certain drugs (including antacids) and nasogastric feeding. Pregnancy also reduces absorption, and absorption of the drug in neonates and infants is particularly unpredictable. Absorption is non-linear; in adults peak levels are usually reached between four and eight hours after oral dosage. The different generic forms of phenytoin previously available have shown marked differences in bioavailability, and this has had serious clinical consequences. With modern formulations, however, this appears to be less of a problem.

Intramuscular absorption of the drug is slow and incomplete, and the drug may crystallize at the injection site. The serum levels achieved are low and variable, and although peak levels are usually reached by 24 hours, absorption may continue slowly for many days. In a personally observed case, levels continued to rise for one week after a single large intramuscular injection. The dosage necessary to switch from oral to intramuscular administration is also entirely unpredictable.

Phenytoin is about 90% bound to plasma proteins (range from 70–95%), and the proportion bound does not significantly vary within the normal ranges of plasma concentrations. Peak brain concentrations are achieved one hour after an intravenous injection. The concentration in brain is up to three times that in plasma, due to protein and lipid binding. The concentration of the drug in CSF and saliva is equivalent to the concentrations of free drug in plasma. The concentrations in breast milk are 0.15–0.55 those in maternal blood. The serum concentration in cord blood and in neonates is equivalent to the maternal serum levels.

The predominant metabolic transformation of phenytoin is parahydroxylation to 5-(*p*-hydroxyphenyl)-5-phenylhydantoin (*p*-HPPH), which is then largely conjugated to HPPH-glucuronide. The enzymes responsible are those of the hepatic cytochrome oxidase system. Other pathways account for a small proportion of metabolism only. The parahydroxylation of phenytoin is the rate limiting step, and this enzyme system is easily saturated. For most subjects, the maximum rate of elimination of phenytoin is 4–12 mg/kg/day, and at higher dosages, a small increase will produce large rises in serum level. Phenytoin in chronic therapy induces its own metabolism, by increasing hepatic enzyme activity, as do a number of other drugs and anticonvulsants. The elimination half-life is age dependent, being between 10–34 hours in adults, 5–18 hours in young children, and 10–140 hours in neonates. None of the metabolites have significant anticonvulsant action. Less than 5% of the drug is excreted unchanged in the urine.

These various metabolic and pharmacokinetic parameters conspire to make phenytoin a difficult drug to handle in clinical practice (Fig. 9.2). With the introduction of serum level measurements, however, the vagaries of metabolism of the drug can be negotiated. Because of the variability in absorption and metabolism, the dosage to provide equivalent serum levels in different individuals may vary considerably. Neonates have unpredictable requirements; young children require relatively more than adults. There is little correlation between dosage requirements and weight, but there are ethnic and genetic differences. In order to maintain steady serum levels, the dosage may need to be increased in pregnancy, especially in the third trimester, and then lowered sharply in the puerperium. Concomitant drug therapy may also alter phenytoin levels due to metabolic interaction and to effects on protein binding. Steady state levels of phenytoin are reached after a very variable period – usually between 2–4 weeks, but occasionally as long as ten weeks – after the initiation of therapy at a normal therapeutic doses; the interpretation of serum levels must take this into account. After an oral loading dose, therapeutic levels are achieved within 24 hours and steady state levels within three days, but transient side effects are common. After an intravenous loading dose, therapeutic levels are reached within 30–45 min.

The relation between oral dose of phenytoin and serum level in clinical practice is complex. Phenytoin often exhibits Michaelis-Menten kinetics, and over the therapeutic ranges, small increments in dosage may produce large increases in serum level. In the example shown in Fig. 9.3, for instance, an

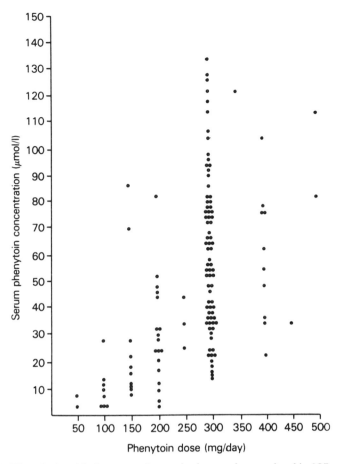

Figure 9.2 The relationship between phenytoin dose and serum level in 137 patients on chronic phenytoin therapy (often in combination with other anticonvulsant drugs excepting sulthiame), demonstrating the marked interindividual variation. (Reproduced with permission from Richens in Laidlaw and Richens [3].) ($1 \mu g/ml = 4 \mu mol/l$)

increase in dosage from 200 mg to 300 mg raises the serum level from subtherapeutic to supratherapeutic values and precipitates toxicity. This effect is very variable, both in different subjects and in the same subject in different conditions, and again serum level monitoring is vital when dose changes are implemented. The fact that phenytoin is available in 100 mg, 50 mg and 25 mg strengths reflects the sensitivity of the relation between oral dose and serum level.

(d) Drug interactions
The interactions of other drugs with phenytoin have been intensively studied. Many drugs have been shown to increase phenytoin levels due to interference

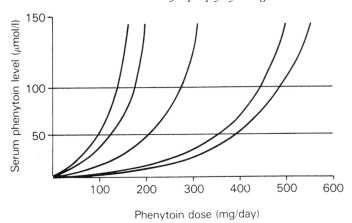

Figure 9.3 The relationship between phenytoin dose and serum level in five patients in steady state concentrations at several different doses, demonstrating the non-linear dose/serum level relationship and its marked individual variation. The area between the horizontal lines indicates the 'therapeutic range' of serum levels. (Reproduced with permission from Richens and Dunlop (1975) [12].) (1 μg/ml=4 μmol/l)

at a metabolic level. Others have been shown to lower the levels by displacing phenytoin from protein binding sites, or less often by inducing phenytoin metabolism. Other drugs may interfere with phenytoin absorption. A selection of the known interactions are shown in Table 9.8. Because of these effects and non-linear pharmacokinetics, frequent monitoring of phenytoin levels is often advisable, particularly if the phenytoin metabolism is nearing saturation levels.

The most important interactions in clinical practice are those with other anticonvulsant drugs. A marked increase in levels is produced by simultaneous medication with sulthiame. This is a consistent and important effect. Phenobarbitone, primidone and carbamazepine may increase or reduce phenytoin levels to a variable degree, which may occasionally be clinically significant. This variability is due to the complexity of the interactive mechanisms, some acting to increase and some to decrease phenytoin levels. Moreover, in any individual these mechanisms may change over time. The effect of sodium valproate on phenytoin levels is an example, varying probably because of changes in protein binding. It may therefore be better in some patients to monitor free rather than total levels. Indeed effects that are clearly predictable, such as an increase in levels with sulthiame, are unusual.

Phenytoin may also affect the metabolism of other anticonvulsants. Levels of carbamazepine are commonly reduced and this may seriously compromise the efficacy of carbamazepine in combination regimens. Phenytoin may also accelerate the metabolism of primidone to phenobarbitone, and markedly increase the ratio of serum phenobarbitone:primidone in primidone-treated patients.

Table 9.8 Phenytoin drug interactions

Anticonvulsants		Non-anticonvulsants	
Drugs shown to reduce phenytoin levels			
Diazepam	Antacids		
Clonazepam	Diazoxide		
Carbamazepine	Oxacillin		
Phenobarbitone	Pyridoxine		
Primidone	Tolbutamide		
Sodium valproate	Folate		
Drugs shown to raise phenytoin levels			
Ethosuximide		Calcium carbimide	Methylphenidate
Methoin		Chloramphenicol	Nortriptyline
Methsuximide		Chlorpheniramine	Phenylbutazone
Phenylacetylurea		Chlorpromazine	Phenyramidol
Pheneturide		Clofibrate	Prochlorperazine
Sulthiame		Disulfiram	Propoxyphene
		Frusemide	Propranolol
		Halothane	Sulphonamides
		Impiramine	Warfarin
		Isoniazid	
Drugs levels of which are lowered by phenytoin			
Carbamazepine		Antipyrine	Metyrapone
Clonazepam		Chlorpromazine	Nortryptyline
Primidone		Cortisol	Phenazone
(but phenobarbitone		Contraceptive pill	Phenylbutazone
levels are raised)		Dexamethasone	Pyridoxine
		Dicoumarol	Quinine
		Digitoxin	Vitamin D
		Doxycycline	Warfarin

Other important interactions have been observed with antibiotics. Isoniazid is a powerful inhibitor of phenytoin metabolism; the extent of this effect may depend on the patient's acetylator status. Chloramphenicol may also markedly increase phenytoin levels in some patients, as may some sulphonamide drugs. Dextropropoxyphene may also markedly inhibit phenytoin metabolism. Aspirin may increase phenytoin clearance, although this latter effect is usually not of great significance. Phenytoin may also enhance the metabolic degradation of the contraceptive pill, leading to contraceptive failure. This is a particular problem in contraceptive pills containing low levels of oestrogen. Breakthrough bleeding is a useful indicator of contraceptive unreliability in these circumstances. The prescription of a higher oestrogen dose pill may be all that is necessary to increase contraceptive protection, but patients should be warned that the risk of pregnancy is higher than is usual on the pill.

9.3.6 Primidone

Primidone was introduced into clinical practice in 1952 and has been widely used since then as a first line antiepileptic drug. It is a neutral, poorly soluble substance, which is rapidly converted into phenobarbitone and phenylethylmalonamide in the body. Controversy exists as to whether primidone adds any anticonvulsant effect to that of the derived phenobarbitone. Animal experimentation suggests that there is a true difference, although this has not been conclusively shown in man. Indeed, this would be difficult to show, due to the complexity of the drug's metabolism. Whatever the answer is, any differences in efficacy between the two drugs are slight, and the major *in vivo* anticonvulsant effect of the drug is undoubtedly due to the derived phenobarbitone. The mechanism of the anticonvulsant actions of primidone (or phenylethylmalonamide) – if any – is not known.

(a) Indications
Indications for the use of primidone in epilepsy are identical to those for phenobarbitone. The efficacy and chronic toxicity of the two drugs are approximately equal.

(b) Clinical therapeutics
The drug is available as 250 mg tablets. The usual adult maintenance dose is 500–1500 mg/day. The drug is usually given in a once or twice daily regimen. The drug is not available in injectable or rectal forms. On beginning therapy with primidone, some patients develop a remarkable idiosyncratic reaction, comprising dizziness, nausea, drowsiness and general debility. This may occur within hours of the first dose, and last for at least 24 hours after a single dose. This reaction is common, but is usually mild and tolerable. Occasionally it is severe. Because of this, it is always advisable to initiate therapy with 62.5 mg or 125 mg of the drug, taken at night, and to warn the patient of the possible effects. The side effects usually diminish with repeated doses, and within several days of continuous therapy the drug no longer produces these symptoms. The cause of this curious response is unclear.

Assessment of the effects of primidone is complicated by the fact that primidone and its metabolites, phenobarbitone and phenylethylmalonamide, each have differing metabolic properties, half-lives and pharmacological actions. As primidone itself has a short half-life, there is a wide diurnal variation in its serum level. There is little to be gained from monitoring its serum level, however, and it is usual to monitor the dose of the drug according to the levels of the derived phenobarbitone.

Considerations about the use of phenobarbitone in pregnancy and while breast feeding (p. 386) apply also to primidone.

(c) Clinical pharmacology

Primidone is well absorbed orally, and has a bioavailability of almost 100%. Peak levels are obtained about three hours after a single oral dose, although there is considerable individual variation. On chronic therapy, peak levels are probably achieved more slowly. There may be some differences in the time to peak absorption in different manufactured products, although this has not been systematically studied, and is probably of little clinical significance. Absorption is generally reliable, and there are no known factors of clinical importance which inhibit full absorption.

The drug is only slightly bound to plasma proteins (perhaps up to 20% bound), although there is wide individual variation. The concentrations of primidone in CSF, saliva, serum and brain are roughly equivalent; the drug is also distributed into breast milk and across the placenta. It is very rapidly oxidized to phenobarbitone and phenylethylmalonamide, in all probability in the liver. The proportion metabolized varies from individual to individual, and differs in chronic and acute administration. A large percentage of the drug is excreted by the kidney unchanged. The elimination half-life of primidone is of the order of 5–18 hours, and of the derived phenobarbitone 46–136 hours. There is a relatively linear relationship between primidone and phenobarbitone levels over a normal clinical range, but the relationship varies widely between individuals. The proportion of primidone metabolized to phenobarbitone differs in newly treated and chronic patients, probably due to autoinduction.

(d) Drug interactions

Phenytoin increases the rate of conversion of primidone to phenobarbitone in the body, due to enzyme induction, and the serum phenobarbitone:primidone ratio is raised. Carbamazepine appears to have a variable effect on primidone levels, but simultaneous medication with primidone will often lower the carbamazepine level. A complex interaction with sodium valproate has also been reported. The interactions involving phenobarbitone are described above.

9.3.7 Sodium valproate (valproic acid)

The anticonvulsant properties of sodium valproate (or valproic acid) were first reported in 1961, but it is only in the past 15 years that the drug has attracted wide interest. It is now recognized as an important first line anticonvulsant drug. Valproic acid is a short branched-chain fatty acid, which is only slightly soluble in water. The mechanism underlying the anticonvulsant action of the compound is not clear. It is an inhibitor of the enzymes gamma-aminobutyrate (GABA) transaminase and glutamate decarboxylase, and because of this, administration of the drug results in a marked increase of cerebral GABA levels. GABA is an inhibitory neurotransmitter (Chapter 2), and it is possible that the anticonvulsant action of the drug is due to this increased GABA concentration. However, evidence is conflicting, and this simple explanation does not fit all the available experimental evidence. Other possible mechanisms have been proposed, including a stabilizing membrane action, and a direct potentiation of the GABA receptor resulting in increased neuronal inhibition.

(a) Indications
Sodium valproate is a drug of first choice for the treatment of typical absence seizures, for myoclonic seizures and also for generalized tonic-clonic seizures. It is most efficacious in primary generalized epilepsy, strictly defined. In other primary generalized seizures, its effect is greatest in the presence of photosensitivity, or 3 Hz spike wave EEG patterns. Its efficacy in partial epilepsies is controversial, although in the author's experience it is less useful than other first line drugs in complex and simple partial seizures, and in secondarily generalized seizures. In intractable partial epilepsies it should however be tried as a second line drug, and it may also have some action in other generalized seizure types. It is a relatively easy drug to use in clinical practice. Serum level monitoring is unnecessary (see below) and the common side effects are broadly speaking dose-related. Serious hepatic toxicity is rare, but nevertheless the use of this drug, particularly in children, should be circumspect. It is probably not helpful to monitor liver function routinely in an asymptomatic patient.

(b) Clinical therapeutics
In the UK, sodium valproate is available as 200 mg and 500 mg enteric coated tablets, 100 mg crushable tablets, and as a 200 mg/5 ml liquid and syrup; in some countries tablets of 300 mg are also available. The usual adult maintenance dose is between 600–2000 mg/day, although higher doses may be used. In children up to 20 kg, the usual dose is up to a maximum of 40 mg/kg/day, and in older children a maximum of 30 mg/kg/day. The tablets are best taken after food, although with the enteric coated forms this is not obligatory. The drug is usually given on a twice daily regimen, although some authorities recommend single daily doses and others three or four times a day regimens. Diurnal serum levels fluctuate widely even when doses are given three times a day, but no correlation between serum level and seizure control has been demonstrated. These fluctuations are not of any known clinical significance. Indeed, routine measurement of sodium valproate levels is unhelpful in monitoring efficacy or toxicity, although useful in detecting non-compliance. If serum levels are to be monitored for this reason, the sample timing should be regulated in view of the wide diurnal variaion, and trough levels are usually taken. There is no particular need for a slow staged introduction of the drug, although in routine practice the full dose is usually initiated over several weeks. For a rapid effect, the full maintenance dose may be started immedi-

ately, and there is no need for a larger loading dose. There are no parenteral formulations currently available for general use.

The effects of pregnancy on sodium valproate levels are not clearly established, but strong binding to albumin means that alterations in total plasma level might be expected (p. 393). Breast feeding may be safely carried out by mothers taking sodium valproate.

(c) Clinical pharmacology

Sodium valproate is very well absorbed, and bioavailability after oral dosage is almost complete. Absorption is rapid, and peak levels after a single dose are achieved within 1–2 hours, or 4–8 hours after ingestion of the enteric coated formulation. The degree or rate of absorption is not influenced by age, sex or other clinical considerations.

In normal plasma concentrations, sodium valproate is strongly protein bound (approximately 90% protein bound), but as concentrations rise, the proportion of free fraction increases. The drug is present in breast milk at a concentration less than 10% that of the maternal serum. There is a poor correlation between serum and salivary sodium valproate. The drug is present in CSF at approximately 10% of the plasma concentration. The protein binding is tight, and although other protein bound antiepileptic drugs do not have a significant affect on sodium valproate binding, sodium valproate itself may alter their binding. However, free fatty acids and salicylates are known to lower the protein binding, and increase the free fraction. The free fraction may also be raised several fold in liver disease and renal disease. The drug is extensively metabolized by a variety of pathways with less than 5% excreted unchanged in the urine.

In spite of the minimal effect on protein binding, sodium valproate clearance is markedly increased by concomitant therapy with other anticonvulsants; this is due to enzyme induction. This may result in a considerable reduction of sodium valproate plasma levels. The half-life of the drug in epileptic patients is about nine hours. In infants under two months the half-life is longer, and in hepatic disease the half-life may also be prolonged.

(d) Drug interactions

Drug interactions with valproate are common and often clinically significant. An important effect is an increase of phenobarbitone levels on co-medication with sodium valproate. The mechanism of the frequent and occasionally severe sedative effect of combination therapy with sodium valproate and a barbiturate drug is, however, obscure and is not fully explained by the individual drug levels. Sodium valproate does not induce the hepatic cytochromal enzymes in the same manner as phenytoin, barbiturates or carbamazepine, but it is exclusively metabolized in the liver and may interfere with the metabolism of other drugs. Similarly, many other drugs may alter the clearance of sodium valproate by effects on hepatic enzymes. Sodium valproate is also strongly bound to serum albumin, and many important interactions are due to competitive alterations in plasma binding. Total phenytoin levels may decline if sodium valproate is added, due to its displacement from protein binding sites; the free levels of phenytoin may rise sharply in the early stages of combination therapy, although once a steady state is reached the levels are roughly equivalent to pre-sodium valproate values. The addition of carbamazepine therapy reduces sodium valproate levels, and the addition of sodium valproate increases carbamazepine levels, but these effects are usually not clinically significant. Aspirin may increase sodium valproate levels due to displacement from albumin binding sites. A similar reaction may occur with any other strongly protein-bound drug.

9.3.8   Toxic effects of the first line anticonvulsant drugs

The toxic effects of these drugs may be conveniently described together, as there is often a considerable overlap. This is particularly true of the barbiturate drugs and phenytoin. Many of the effects described are also noted with other less commonly used anticonvulsant drugs, but information on these compounds is often much less detailed. Their specific effects will be described in later sections. Of the first line anticonvulsants, the older drugs have been the most intensively investigated, and there are no doubt adverse effects of the newer compounds which are as yet unrecognized.

(a)   Cerebral side effects

Acute encephalopathic side effects are seen in most patients with each of the anticonvulsant drugs at high doses (intoxication). There is a consistent relationship between the symptoms of intoxication and serum levels of phenytoin, ethosuximide, and carbamazepine. The effects are largely similar for all drugs, differing only in degree; they include drowsiness, dizziness, incoordination, headache, nausea, ataxia and nystagmus. Drowsiness is particularly prominent with sodium valproate, barbiturate and benzodiazepine drugs, ataxia with phenytoin, and diplopia and unsteadiness with carbamazepine. The effects are dose related and reversible.

   More difficult to detect are the mental side effects associated with chronic therapy. These have been generally underrated. Whilst it is recognized that all conventional anticonvulsant drugs may cause mental sedation and confusion at high doses, this is not an all-or-none response, and how much sedation is present at normal doses is difficult to determine. One should always take seriously a patient's complaint of lethargy or intellectual blunting even if doses are small or serum levels satisfactory. It is remarkable how often the extent of such side effects remain unnoticed, to be recognized only in retrospect after the drug is withdrawn. The prevalence and degree of drug-induced effects on memory and other aspects of intellectual function are not fully established. It is often difficult in an individual patient to disentangle the effects of drug toxicity from the effects of the epilepsy and the cerebral pathology causing the epilepsy. Deleterious effects have been particularly ascribed to the hydantoin, barbiturate and benzodiazepine drugs, but these drugs have been the most intensively studied. Irritability, hyperexcitability, aggressive behavioural disturbances and personality changes may be produced occasionally by various anticonvulsants. A particularly severe disturbance is caused by the barbiturate drugs in children. This is sufficiently common to caution their use in routine paediatric practice. Dose-related involuntary movement disorders (asterixis, dystonia, orofacial dyskinesia and chorea) are sometimes produced by phenytoin, carbamazepine, sodium valproate or ethosuximide, but are usually not severe. Tremor is especially seen with sodium valproate therapy, but the mechanism is not known. Severe obtundation progressing to stupor is rarely produced by sodium valproate in combination with phenobarbitone (and perhaps other anticonvulsants). The mechanism of this is not clear but may be related to hyperammonaemia induced by sodium valproate.

It has been claimed that several anticonvulsants, notably carbamazepine, may have a positive psychotropic effect, elevating mood, and the 'speed' of mental function. Similar claims were made for phenytoin when it was first introduced. The observed effects might have been partly due to the benefits of good seizure control, or the replacement of more sedative drugs. Marked depression of mood in some patients is seen with the sedative anticonvulsant drugs, particularly the barbiturates, and this is most noticeable with combination therapy. Psychotic reactions have been reported occasionally with various anticonvulsant drugs.

(b) Other neurological effects

It is common experience that phenytoin frequently produces reversible cerebellar signs at high dosage. More recently it has been suggested that a permanent cerebellar syndrome may also result from chronic therapy. A mild subclinical peripheral neuropathy is also common after prolonged phenytoin therapy, and may occur with other drugs too. Much more rarely, an acute reversible symptomatic neuropathy can be produced by phenytoin in high dosage. Carbamazepine consistently produces reversible double vision, visual blurring or difficulty with focusing at high dosage. These symptoms may be an important indication of drug intoxication. A reversible disorder of taste has been reported with carbamazepine. Dose-related headache seems to be a relatively common complaint of patients on ethosuximide therapy.

Sleep patterns are commonly changed by anticonvulsant therapy, usually only in the short term, and various disturbances of sleep and dreaming may also be experienced.

(c) Hepatic effects

Many anticonvulsant drugs have strong hepatic enzyme inducing properties (e.g. phenytoin, phenobarbitone and carbamazepine), and chronic therapy frequently causes asymptomatic alterations in serum liver enzymes. Such effects are clinically unimportant.

Acute hepatic disturbances have also been recorded with carbamazepine, phenytoin and phenobarbitone but these are extremely rare, and may be part of a generalized hypersensitivity reaction. About 100 cases of acute fatal hepatic failure in association with sodium valproate therapy have been reported, and more with a non-fatal outcome. This is a rare reaction, the mechanism of which is unclear. It has occurred mainly in younger children, usually on multiple drug therapy, within six months of the onset of treatment. It may be related to an already present underlying metabolic abnormality, possibly a deficiency of ornithine carbamoyltransferase. This reaction should be distinguished from the frequent transient and benign rise in liver enzymes caused by sodium valproate (in about 30% of cases) which is of no clinical significance. An acute fatal haemorrhagic pancreatitis has also been reported with sodium valproate therapy. These idiosyncratic reactions to sodium valproate are a serious problem. The physician must monitor carefully all patients taking this drug, though it unfortunately remains true that hepatic failure may occur explosively without warning. Estimations of prothrombin times and fibrinogen levels may be useful.

(d) Metabolic bone disease

Biochemical and radiological features of osteomalacia and rickets have been increasingly reported with long term anticonvulsant therapy with phenytoin and/or barbiturate drugs, due to a drug-induced vitamin D deficiency, although the biochemical mechanism by which this is produced is uncertain. Subclinical changes are common, but frank rickets or osteomalacic myopathy are only occasionally seen, and usually in those already predisposed to metabolic bone disease. Asian immigrants to zones of low solar activity are particularly at risk. Elevation of serum alkaline phosphatase levels is very common on phenytoin, barbiturate and carbamazepine therapy and may be due to liver enzyme induction, as well as vitamin D deficiency. Frank hypocalcaemia is less common, but may itself be a cause of seizures, and should not be attributed to anticonvulsant therapy without further investigation.

(e) Other metabolic and endocrine effects

Carbamazepine has a direct antidiuretic action and may produce dose-related hyponatraemia and water retention. This is particularly likely after a large fluid load – a heavy intake of beer being the commonest culprit. Although symptomatic hyponatraemia is unusual, subclinical biochemical changes are common.

Sodium valproate consistently causes hyperammonaemia, as a dose-related phenomenon, due to inhibition of urea cycle enzymes. The extent of the rise in serum ammonia varies considerably, and is probably dependent on genetic factors. The clinical significance of drug-induced hyperammonaemia is not entirely clear, but has probably been underestimated. It may present as lethargy, loss of appetite, nausea or vomiting. Sodium valproate therapy should probably be discontinued if such symptoms develop. The risk may be particularly great in patients with inherited defects of urea cycle enzymes, which may be symptomatic. Hyperglycinaemia, hyperglycinuria, hyperaminoaciduria and a relative carnitine deficiency have also been reported, but all are probably of little clinical significance. Sodium valproate as a short chain fatty acid has numerous potential metabolic actions due to inhibition of mitochondrial enzymes. Many have not been formally investigated.

Most anticonvulsant drugs do produce chemical alterations in endocrine function, especially of pituitary, thyroid, adrenal and sex hormones. The exact mechanisms are unclear, but may be related to enzyme induction, altered protein binding, direct end-organ effects or to effects on cerebral and pituitary function. The clinical significance of these changes are usually minimal, and symptomatic endocrine dysfunction is very unusual. It has been claimed that hyposexuality and even reduced fertility may be related to the alteration in testosterone binding, seen particularly with phenytoin or barbiturate drugs. Sodium valproate may occasionally cause ammenorrhea or menstrual irregularities. Phenytoin has been shown to induce hyperglycaemia in susceptible patients, particularly when given intravenously. This may prove an important complication in the treatment of diabetic patients.

(f) Haematological effects

Marrow hypoplasia has been reported with most major anticonvulsant drugs as a hypersensitivity phenomenon, often associated with other signs of hypersensitivity, such as rash or fever. These complications are serious, but fortunately are very rare. Phenytoin itself has not been reported to cause total marrow aplasia, although very rarely red blood cell aplasia and severe agranulocytosis has been recorded, but its close chemical relation, meth-phenytoin has been a frequently reported cause of marrow aplasia, and is now seldom used. When carbamazepine was first introduced, a number of cases – some fatal – of marrow aplasia, affecting especially the granulocytic cell lines, were recorded. This effect is however very rare, and routine haematological monitoring is probably unnecessary, though remains recommended by the manufacturer. Severe marrow aplasia has also been rarely reported with ethosuximide, benzodiazepine drugs and sodium valproate.

Mild haematological changes, especially leucopenia or thrombocytopenia, are common on prolonged anticonvulsant therapy and are usually of no clinical significance. Sodium valproate may increase the bleeding time. This may be due to decreased platelet adhesiveness, thrombocytopenia or occasionally to hepatic disturbance. Other anticonvulsant drugs less frequently affect coagulation, although the enzyme inducing drugs (phenytoin, barbiturates and ethosuximide) prescribed to the mother during pregnancy may result in neonatal hypocoagulability due to decreased vitamin K levels (p. 386).

Folate deficiency causing macrocytosis is common on phenytoin therapy, and indeed may be seen in up to one-half of patients on chronic phenytoin therapy. It is also frequently encountered with barbiturate drug treatment. A frank megaloblastic anaemia is much less common, occurring in under 1% of patients on chronic phenytoin or barbiturate treatment. Methsuximide and carbamazepine may also occasionally induce megaloblastic changes. The clinical relevance of the induced folate deficiency is uncertain, but it is possible that it contributes to neuropsychiatric toxicity, particularly depression and mood changes. The megaloblastosis may be reversed by folate therapy, although this is not routinely recommended in the absence of symptoms. It has been suggested that folate may have convulsant properties, although this is seldom clinically relevant. Folic acid therapy may also result in a slight reduction in phenytoin serum levels. Folate therapy is recommended however in the presence of frank megaloblastosis or a megaloblastic anaemia.

Eosinophilia, associated often with rash or fever, occurs as part of a hypersensitivity reaction to many anticonvulsant drugs, and occasionally isolated eosinophilia is also noted.

Phenytoin may occasionally produce a clinical picture resembling that of a lymphoma. Generalized lymphadenopathy, sometimes with hepatosplenomegaly and fever, may develop and lymph node biopsy show appearances of lymphoma or Hodgkin's disease. These changes reverse when the drug is stopped. The mechanism of this remarkable effect is unclear.

(g) Immunological effects

Low IgA levels have been found in 25% of patients receiving phenytoin therapy, and low levels of IgM and IgG less commonly. Alterations of cellular and humoral immune responses have been reported with several drugs but the clinical significance of these changes is uncertain. Phenytoin may also precipitate myasthenia gravis in previously unaffected patients, and exacerbate the condition in affected individuals.

A syndrome similar to lupus erythematosis due to phenytoin, and less commonly to carbamazepine, ethosuximide and phenobarbitone has been reported, sometimes as part of a more generalized hypersensitivity reaction. This is uncommon and unpredictable. In its minor form, antinuclear antibodies and other chemical markers may develop without overt clinical signs. More rarely, a frank lupus-like clinical syndrome is produced, which may be indistinguishable from systemic lupus erythematosis. The condition may be severe or fulminant. Other rare immunological reactions include an autoimmune thrombocytopenic purpura, due to sodium valproate therapy.

(h) Dermatological disorders

Anticonvulsant hypersensitivity most commonly takes the form of an allergic rash. This is seen in between 5% and 10% of patients starting carbamazepine therapy, but is less common with other anticonvulsants. The rash usually develops within months of the initiation of therapy. It is non-specific in appearance, and resolves on discontinuation of treatment. Other haematological, hepatic or immunological manifestations of hypersensitivity may accompany the rash. More serious hypersensitivity reactions include the Stevens–Johnson syndrome, Lyell syndrome, dermatitis bullosa and an exfoliative dermatitis, and these have been observed with many anticonvulsant drugs but are fortunately rare.

(i) Hair and connective tissue changes

Sodium valproate may have a number of curious effects on hair growth. Thinning or curling of hair is not uncommon and may be severe, resulting occasionally in complete alopecia. These changes are sometimes transient, but sometimes require discontinuation of therapy. The mechanism of this effect is unclear, but may be dose related. It usually develops within six months of beginning therapy. Hair loss may also occur with clonazepam therapy.

Coarsening of facial features is a common effect of chronic phenytoin and barbiturate therapy, and may produce marked cosmetic changes. Gum hypertrophy is seen in about one-third of patients receiving phenytoin and also occurs with barbiturate therapy. It is seen especially in patients with poor oral hygiene, and in adolescent patients. The problem is dose related. It may be a severe and embarrassing problem and require expert dental treatment. Less commonly, fibromata may develop in the gums, in breast tissue or subungually. Hirsuitism and acne are common in patients receiving phenytoin or phenobarbitone, although recently the association of acne with anticonvulsant therapy has been challenged. Dupuytren's contracture, and a similar affliction of the plantar fascia has been associated with prolonged phenytoin and phenobarbitone therapy and may be severe. The frozen shoulder syndrome has been attributed to phenobarbitone therapy. Phenytoin may also induce cholasma-like pigmentary changes.

(j) Gastrointestinal symptoms

Mild gastric symptoms are common with the non-enteric coated formulations of sodium valproate, but can be avoided by the use of enteric coated tablets and are seldom a significant clinical problem. Mild nausea, abdominal discomfort or pain, and anorexia may also occur with carbamazepine, phenytoin and succinimide therapy, but these symptoms are usually mild and may be avoided by taking tablets with food.

(k) Miscellaneous

Weight gain is commonly seen due to sodium valproate therapy, and may sometimes be very remarkable. Gains of 20 kg within a few months have been reported. It is a dose-related effect, related presumably to stimulation of appetite and may sometimes warrant discontinuation of treatment.

Renal disturbance is rarely caused by anticonvulsant drugs, except as part of a severe hypersensitivity reaction. In phenytoin hypersensitivity, albuminuria is encountered in about 5% of cases, and functional renal impairment in less than 3%. Lens opacities and chromosomal changes have been reported with carbamazepine, although whether these are true drug-induced effects must be doubtful. It has been suggested, but not substantiated, that phenytoin and the barbiturate drugs may have an oncogenic effect.

Acute hepatic porphyria may be precipitated by all the first line anticonvulsant drugs. This is a particular risk with the barbiturate drugs and phenytoin, and least likely with sodium valproate and clonazepam.

(l) Teratogenecity
This problem is discussed in Chapter 12.

9.4   OTHER ANTICONVULSANT DRUGS [1, 2, 13]

A number of other anticonvulsant drugs are available, but are used only rarely. Details of their clinical pharmacology are often more sparse and evidence of their efficacy more slim than with the widely used compounds.

9.4.1   Other hydantoin drugs

Phenytoin is the only hydantoin drug in common contemporary use. Other chemically related compounds have been marketed, but these are generally more toxic or less efficacious than phenytoin, but do have a place in the treatment of occasional patients.

Methoin has clear anticonvulsant action, which indeed may be superior to that of phenytoin in some patients. The drug is said also to cause less gum hypertrophy or hirsuitism than phenytoin. Its major metabolite 5-ethyl-5-phenylhydantoin has unfortunately been frequently reported to cause marrow aplasia, and this has severely restricted its usefulness. The indications for its use are intractable tonic-clonic or partial seizures, particularly simple partial seizures. The usual maintenance dosage in adults is 200–600 mg, and once daily dosing only is required. Peak plasma concentrations occur within 1–2 hours of absorption; it is rapidly metabolized, and the plasma half-life of the drug is about 7 hours and of 5-ethyl-5-phenylhydantoin 96 hours. Ninety per cent of the drug is present as 5-ethyl-5-phenylhydantoin at steady state levels, and this metabolite is responsible for most of the anticonvulsant efficacy of the drug. The drug is about 30% protein bound. There are a number of drug interactions reported due to induction of metabolism, and there is also considerable autoinduction. The drug has a relatively high toxicity, and there is a particularly high incidence of severe marrow depression. It may also frequently result in other allergic reactions such as serious rashes and hepatitis. The incidence of drowsiness also seems higher than with phenytoin, although the cosmetic side effects may be less common.

Ethotoin has antiepileptic activity, but probably is not as efficacious as that of phenytoin. It may be used for tonic-clonic and partial seizures. It is quickly absorbed, is about 50% protein bound, has no active metabolites and a short half-life. Because of this, four times a day dosage regimens are recommended. The usual adult starting dose is 1000 mg/day, and this is increased over a few weeks to 2000–3000 mg/day. It is significantly less toxic than phenytoin or methoin; side effects include rashes and gastrointestinal symptoms. The drug causes ataxia or drowsiness only at high doses. Other hydantoin drugs which have been previously marketed include deltoin and albutoin.

Phenacemide is a straight chain analogue of 5-phenylhydantoin, and probably has a similar mechanism of action to the hydantoin drugs. Its main indication is for the treatment of complex partial seizures, although it may be tried in all other seizure types. The usual adult maintenance dose is 2000–3000 mg/day given in a thrice daily regimen. It is well absorbed and metabolized to inactive compounds in the liver. It is a toxic drug causing frequent encephalopathic symptoms, and this has severely restricted its use. Haematological effects, including marrow aplasia, rashes, gastrointestinal effects and hepatitis are also relatively common.

9.4.2   Other barbiturate drugs

Methylphenobarbitone was introduced into practice in 1932. It has the same indications as phenobarbitone and is largely metabolized to phenobarbitone after absorption. Anecdotal reports suggest that it causes less sedation or hyperactivity in children than phenobarbitone, but there are no controlled studies of this. Its oral bioavailability is about 50%. The steady state serum concentration of the drug is between 10–15% less than that of the derived phenobarbitone, and serum phenobarbitone plasma measurements should be used to monitor the dose. Doses of about 4 mg/kg produce similar phenobarbitone levels as 2 mg/kg of phenobarbitone. Metharbital (*N*-methylbarbitone) and dimethoxy-methylphenobarbitone have also been marketed. Both are metabolized after several steps to phenobarbitone, and are said to be less sedative than phenobarbitone, although this is based on anecdotal evidence only. None of these drugs has a significant place in current therapy in the UK, although the use of mephobarbital is apparently as common as that of primidone in Australia.

9.4.3   Other succinimide drugs

Of the three succinimide drugs introduced in the 1950s, only ethosuximide is commonly used. *Methsuximide* however still has a place as a second line drug in the treatment of a variety of seizure types.

In view of its structural similarity to ethosuximide, methsuximide was first used in the treatment of refractory petit mal seizures. As adjunctive therapy in uncontrolled cases, it has been said to control seizures completely in up to 30% of cases, and significantly to reduce seizures in up to 66%. In a study of previously untreated patients, however, it did not produce complete control in any, and reduced seizures significantly in only 20% As ethosuximide and sodium valproate are so effective in the treatment of petit mal absence seizures, in modern practice methsuximide has a minor place in the treatment of this seizure type, although this is the one indication approved by the FDA. Subsequent experience with this drug, however, has shown it to have useful effects in refractory complex partial or in atypical absence seizures, and in UK practice this is now its major indication, although the drug can only be obtained by direct approach to the manufacturers. In four reports on complex partial epilepsy, the addition of the drug produced control in up to one-third of patients and a significant reduction in seizures in up to three-quarters. Gratifying results have also been reported in atypical absence seizures, and in epilepsy with slow spike-wave EEG patterns, a situation in which conventional treatment is often totally ineffective. Its mechanism of action is completely obscure.

Methsuximide is a more toxic drug than ethosuximide, and causes drowsiness, ataxia and irritability in a significant minority of patients, although side effects have usually been reported in patients also taking other drugs. A variety of other encephalopathic side effects have been reported less commonly. An allergic rash seems to be relatively common, and cases of systemic lupus erythematosis have occurred. Cases of Stevens–Johnson syndrome have also been reported. Transient leucopenia and other blood dyscrasias may occur. A single case of fatal pancytopenia has been reported.

The usual side effects of the drug can be minimized by starting the drug at low dosage (150 mg/day for an adult) and building the dose up over several weeks to a usual dose of 600–900 mg/day and a maximum of 1200 mg/day in two divided doses. Serum levels of N-desmethylmethsuximide can be measured by gas–liquid chromatography, effective levels lie between 50–150 μmol/l (10–40 μg/ml) although a therapeutic range has not been well established.

Methsuximide is well absorbed orally, metabolized in the liver mainly by N-demethylation. This metabolite accounts probably for most of the anticonvulsant action of the drug *in vivo*. The parent drug and desmethylmethsuximide are subsequently hydroxylated and the hydroxylated metabolites are the main urinary products. The serum half-life of methsuximide itself is short, a mean of 1.4 hours in one study of five patients, but with N-desmethylmethsuximide it is much longer, a mean of 38 hours. Methsuximide co-medication will frequently increase the serum levels of both phenytoin and phenobarbitone, due to competitive inhibition of hepatic enzyme activity. The proportion of N-desmethylmethsuximide is also increased in combination therapy.

Phensuximide is effective in absence seizures, but probably less so than the

other two related compounds. It is well absorbed and is largely metabolized to
N-desmethyl-phensuximide, which is responsible for most of the antiepileptic
action of the drug. The half-lives of the parent drug and its metabolite are both
short. The average dose is 1500 mg/day and it is prescribed in three or four
divided doses. It is a toxic drug, and has a higher incidence of idiosyncratic
reactions than other succinimide drugs. It may cause serious renal damage,
marrow aplasia, and severe dermatological reactions. It also has unusual
encephalopathic effects at high doses, and shares the other common but less
severe side effects of succinimide therapy, such as nausea, drowsiness or
dizziness.

9.4.4 Other benzodiazepine drugs

Many benzodiazepine drugs have powerful antiepileptic action, although
their clinical usefulness is often severely limited by the development of
tolerance. Of these drugs only three – clonazepam, diazepam, and clobazam –
are particularly used in the UK in the treatment of epilepsy. Each has a
differing spectrum of clinical action, and only clonazepam is regularly used as
a first line compound. Other benzodiazepine drugs may occasionally be used
in the treatment of epilepsy, and new benzodiazepines with anticonvulsant
action are being developed.

Diazepam is highly effective as an intravenous or rectal preparation in the
emergency treatment and prophylaxis of epileptic seizures, and febrile convulsions. Because of the development of tolerance however – often within a matter
of days or weeks – it has unfortunately very little application as oral treatment
in chronic epilepsy. It may be used orally as occasional intermittent therapy to
prevent seizures occurring at especially hazardous times, for example prior to
a long journey. In this setting, it is sometimes very efficacious.

The drug is available in 2 mg, 5 mg and 10 mg tablets, and in an injectable
preparation of 5 mg/ml and as a rectal solution (Stesolid) of 2 mg/ml or 4 mg/
ml. Its intravenous use in status epilepticus is discussed in Chapter 14. Neither
the intramuscular or wax suppository preparations of diazepam are well
absorbed, and these methods of administration should not be used.

Peak serum levels are reached within a few minutes of administration of a
rectal solution, and at a dose of 10–20 mg the risk of respiratory depression is
slight. After oral administration, peak levels are reached within 1–3 hours, and
the half-life of the drug is between 10–50 hours. In chronic therapy, however,
levels are difficult to maintain. The drug is demethylated to
desmethyldiazepam and then further metabolized to oxazepam. Both
metabolites have anticonvulsant activity, and both have a longer half-life, and
may contribute to the efficacy of the parent drug. Further hepatic metabolism
occurs and very little of the drug is excreted unchanged. The drug is strongly
protein bound, and rapidly enters brain and lipid stores. There are few
significant interactions with diazepam.

Encephalopathic side effects on oral therapy are frequent, and include dizziness, drowsiness, unsteadiness, change in personality and behaviour, irritability, and sedation. The effects are usually worse on initiation of therapy and tolerance to these quickly develops. The dangerous respiratory and cardiovascular depression common with intravenous therapy is not encountered after oral or rectal administration. Allergic haematological reactions and rash are rarely seen, but marrow aplasia has been reported. There is a danger of habituation to the drug in chronic therapy, but this is slight. The withdrawal of diazepam may produce withdrawal symptoms, including withdrawal seizures, and it is usually recommended that this be carried out in a slow, staged fashion.

Clobazam is a 1,5-benzodiazepine, which has anticonvulsant properties which differ from the other 1,4-benzodiazepine drugs. It was first introduced into the treatment of epilepsy in 1979, having previously been used for its tranquillizing properties and efficacy in treating anxiety. Its mode of action is unknown.

Its main use is as adjunctive treatment in patients with a variety of seizure types resistant to therapy. It has also been successfully used in catamenial epilepsy being given intermittently around the menstrual period (p. 376). The drug is available as 10 mg tablets, and is usually given as a single dose at night, initially at 10 mg which may be increased to 20–40 mg, although there is little evidence to suggest that the higher doses are any more efficacious than 10–20 mg. The effect of therapy is usually apparent immediately, but unfortunately the development of tolerance is a common occurrence, which severely limits the usefulness of the drug. This may develop after weeks or months after the onset of therapy, and is seen at least to some extent in most patients. Nevertheless, a small proportion of patients derive considerable and long lasting benefit from the addition of clobazam to conventional therapy, and for this reason a trial of treatment is often worthwhile. If seizures do recur after an initially good response, it is probaby best to withdraw the drug. The second major difficulty with clobazam in routine clinical practice is the propensity – shared with other benzodiazepine drugs – for rebound seizures and other withdrawal symptoms to occur following abrupt withdrawal, and occasionally the withdrawal syndrome may be very severe. It is probably best to withdraw the drug slowly, at a rate of 10 mg a month, but even then in some patients, withdrawal effects may occur.

The drug is well absorbed, and is largely metabolized to desmethyl-clobazam. The parent drug is four times more potent an anticonvulsant than the metabolite, but as the half-life of the parent drug only is 10–55 hours and the metabolite 35–133 hours, the major part of the anticonvulsant action of the drug *in vivo* is due to desmethylclobazam. On steady state therapy, the levels of the metabolite are considerably higher than that of the parent drug. The serum levels of clobazam tend to fall with concomitant anticonvulsant therapy, and the levels of the metabolite rise. There is a suggestion that the addition of clobazam induces a rise in other anticonvulsant levels, although the extent of this is uncertain, and in practice this effect is not usually of any clinical significance. There is no information concerning the effects of clobazam in pregnancy, although other benzodiazepine drugs have been shown to have teratogenetic effects. The commonest side effect of clobazam therapy is sedation, although this is usually mild. Changes in behaviour may occur, and may occasionally be severe. Irritability, aggression and depression are the commonest effects, and may be more frequent in patients with pre-existing brain damage. Muscle weakness and fatigue are also relatively common complaints. Other side effects are rare.

A number of other benzodiazepine drugs possess antiepileptic activity, although when given orally in chronic therapy this is generally slight, and the drugs are usually given as adjunctive therapy. Commonly used compounds include clorazepate, nitrazepam and lorazepam. Clorazepate, which is metabolized to *N*-desmethyldiazepam, an active metabolite with a longer half-life than diazepam, is particularly used in the treatment of partial seizures, and nitrazepam in the treatment of myoclonic seizures in childhood and in infantile spasms. The toxicity of these drugs is similar to that of other benzodiazepine drugs. Personality change and behaviour disorder may be seen in children.

9.4.5 Sulphonamide drugs

Two sulphonamide drugs have been widely used in the treatment of epilepsy, acetozolamide and sulthiame.

Acetazolamide, an unsubstituted sulphonamide, was introduced into clinical practice as an anticonvulsant in 1952. Its main biochemical action is the inhibition of carbonic anhydrase, an enzyme distributed widely in brain and other tissues. This is probably the mode of anticonvulsant action of the drug. Carbonic anhydrase is found in glial cells and in myelin. Its inhibition in the brain causes a rise in total brain carbon dioxide levels and also a blockade of chloride and bicarbonate membrane transport, which increases the transmembrane chloride gradient. Both effects may contribute to its anti-convulsant action.

The drug is well absorbed orally at conventional dosage, and a peak plasma concentration is reached within 2–3 hours of administration. It is between 80–95% protein bound and is distributed to tissues containing carbonic anhydrase, where it is actively bound to the enzyme. Because of this active binding, drug concentration in the brain is higher than the free plasma levels. It is not metabolized in the liver and is excreted unchanged in the urine. The dissociation constant of the drug–enzyme complex is low, and so the drug is released only slowly into the tissue after binding. This accounts for the long half-life of several days. Steady state serum levels are reached after about 48 hours treatment.

The drug has been used in the treatment of various seizure types, Its initial principal indication was as an adjunctive therapy in refractory absence seizures, although as ethosuximide and sodium valproate are so effective in this seizure type, acetazolamide is seldom so used in current practice. It is now more commonly used in tonic-clonic seizures, both primary and secondarily generalized, in atypical absence seizures, and less often in simple or complex partial seizures. Degrees of seizure suppression in various uncontrolled studies have varied, but some reports show striking efficacy. The drug has usually been tested as adjunctive therapy, and useful action has been reported particularly in combination with carbamazepine, though it is doubtful that this combination has specific properties. It is not clear whether the drug has useful anticonvulsant action in monotherapy. The drug is commonly recommended as intermittent therapy in catamenial epilepsy, in the hope that this will reduce the tendency for tolerance to develop, although there are no well-controlled studies to demonstrate its value in this setting.

The usual dose is 250–750 mg/day. There is little point in giving higher doses as brain carbonic anhydrase is almost completely inhibited at these doses. A therapeutic plasma level of between 35–60 μmol/l (10–14 μg/ml) has been suggested. As the drug is not metabolized in the liver there are no metabolic interactions, although because of its strong protein binding, other agents might be displaced from protein binding sites. An elevation of carbamazepine levels due to the addition of the drug has been reported. As acetazolamide increases the concentration of weak acids in tissues, it may result in increased brain concentrations of other antiepileptic drugs, and this may potentiate both their efficacy and neurological toxicity.

The toxicity of the drug is low. As with other sulphonamides, skin reactions may occur and may be severe, and other hypersensitivity reactions have also been reported. Reversible nausea and other gastrointestinal disturbances may occur. Urinary calculi may develop due to the reduction in urinary citrate excretion. The drug is contraindicated in the porphyrias, and in hepatic failure as it impairs ammonia excretion. At high doses, acetazolamide produces a unique reversible syndrome due to carbonic anhydrase inhibition, comprising facial parasthesiae, numbness of the fingers and toes, nausea, perspiration and hyperpnoea.

Sulthiame is a sulphonamide drug, without antibacterial action, once widely used in the treatment of epilepsy, but now rarely prescribed and no longer available in the UK. Its mechanism of action is unknown. It is a carbonic anhydrase inhibitor, but is only one-sixteenth as potent as acetalozamide. Its anticonvulsant action, if any, is probably not related to this property. It was first introduced for the treatment of partial seizures, especially temporal lobe epilepsy, but has been reported to benefit myoclonic and other seizure types also. It was available in 50 mg and 200 mg tablets. Adult maintenance doses are usually between 200–1000 mg/day. The drug is well absorbed, protein bound and between 30–70% is eliminated unchanged in the urine. Sulthiame when used with phenytoin causes a considerable increase in phenytoin serum levels, probably due to inhibition of phenytoin metabolism. It has been suggested that its anticonvulsant action is solely due to this effect. This seems unlikely in the author's experience, but it is clear that the drug's activity is only slight in comparison to other major antiepileptic drugs, and its place in current therapy is therefore small. The rise in phenytoin levels produced by the addition of sulthiame therapy may result in severe phenytoin toxicity. Sulthiame itself, however, is a relatively non-toxic drug. It may cause hyperpnoea and parasthesiae of the fingers and toes, which are dose-related reversible side effects. It may also cause mental effects including catatonia. It has been reported to cause renal tubular acidosis.

9.4.6   Oxalolidinedione drugs

Two oxalolidinedione drugs have been used in the treatment of epilepsy, but the mechanism of action of these compounds is uncertain.

Trimethadione (troxidone) has been the most widely used. Its main indication is for the treatment of generalized absence seizures intractable to other medication. It has also been used in myoclonic or atonic seizures or intractable seizures of other types. It is highly effective in absence seizures, but because of its toxicity its use is restricted to the rare patient in whom sodium valproate or ethosuximide proves ineffective. The usual maintenance dose is 750–1250 mg/day in adults and 20–50 mg/kg/day in children. The drug is absorbed rapidly and completely, with peak plasma levels achieved within 30 min of oral dosing. It is not protein bound. It is rapidly metabolized to dimethadione, which has equal anticonvulsant action. The metabolism of dimethadione is much slower than that of the parent drug. The plasma dimethadione concentration is twenty-fold that of trimethadione, and the metabolite is therefore responsible for most of the activity of the drug. The half-life of dimethadione is 10 days or more. Therapeutic levels may therefore take weeks or months to be achieved. There is little variation in daily plasma levels, and once daily dosing may be appropriate. The drug does not induce liver enzymes. The drug is toxic, and for this reason finds little place in routine therapy today. Haematological side effects are frequently seen and include neutropenia, thrombocytopenia or pancytopenia. These may be serious and occasionally fatal. Frequent examinations of the blood are necessary. Neurotoxic effects are frequent, and include drowsiness and behaviour change. Other common side effects include day blindness, due to retinal changes, which occurs in 30% of subjects, skin rashes and gastrointestinal symptoms. A nephrotic syndrome, myasthenic syndrome, lupoid reactions, and hair loss have all been reported. The drug is severely teratogenetic, and over one-third of children born to mothers taking this drug may be born with malformations (p. 393).

Paramethadione (paradione) has also been used in the treatment of absence seizures. Its clinical pharmacology is very similar to that of trimethadione. It is probaby less effective however and may be less toxic. It is rapidly absorbed and peak serum levels are achieved within an hour. Like trimethadione, it is largely dealkylated in the liver. The *N*-desmethyl metabolite is the active agent, which is very slowly excreted in the urine. The drug is available in 300 mg capsules.

9.4.7   Miscellaneous drugs

Beclamide is a propionamide derivative which was introduced in 1953. There are reports of efficacy in grand mal and psychomotor epilepsy, in epilepsy in mentally defective patients with behavioural disorders and in childhood epilepsy. All these reports are uncontrolled. Oral absorption is good; the drug is extensively metabolized and less than 1% is excreted unchanged. The drug and its metabolites are almost completely eliminated from the body within 48 hours. It induces hepatic enzyme activity, and so drug interactions should be anticipated. However, detailed pharmacokinetic properties of the drug have not been studied. The drug is available in 500 mg tablets. The usual adult maintenance dose is 500–1000 mg three or four times a day. In children up to five years, the dose is 0.75–1 g/day and between 6–12 years 1.5 g/day in divided doses. It is apparently remarkably free of toxic side effects. It has no sedative action, although it may cause dizziness and nervousness. Rashes, renal and minor gastrointestinal side effects have also been reported.

Paraldehyde is a polymer of acetaldehyde which is poorly water soluble. It has been used since 1882 as intramuscular emergency treatment for acute epilepsy and intravenously for status epilepticus. It is not nowadays routinely given orally or rectally. Its effectiveness is undoubted in the emergency setting, and it has the significant advantage of causing little respiratory or cardiovascular depression. It is an unpleasant drug, however, which decomposes when diluted or on exposure to light. It reacts with plastic tubing or syringes, and has a pungent clinging odour. It should be carefully stored and used within 24 hours of exposure. It is normally given as a deep intramuscular injection, 5–10 ml into each buttock in an emergency setting, often as a preliminary to more definitive treatment or in the home prior to transfer to hospital care. Care should be taken to ensure that decomposition has not occurred, that the injection site is well removed from the course of the sciatic nerve and contact with plastic should be minimized. Recorded toxic effects include bronchial constriction, pulmonary oedema, nephritis, rash, hepatitis, and cardiac failure. The intramuscular injection is very painful, and sterile abscesses may result. Inadvertent injection near the sciatic nerve may cause a severe causalgic syndrome. Patients frequently cough on administration, but as respiratory depression is rare, it is a safe drug to use in situations in which facilities for resuscitation are inadequate. It causes drowsiness but not marked sedation.

Peak plasma levels are reached within 20–60 min of intramuscular injection; the drug is inactivated in the liver and 20–30% is exhaled unchanged in the lungs. The elimination half-life is about 7 hours. Paraldehyde may cross the placenta, causing neonatal resiratory embarrassment.

Corticosteroid drugs, either prednisolone, dexamethasone or ACTH, are occasionally used in epilepsy. Steroid therapy is the treatment of choice for infantile spasms, with often an immediate response. Whether steroid therapy significantly affects long term prognosis is however controversial (pp. 344–46). In epilepsia partialis continua, and in severe serial partial epilepsy, steroids may again produce a remarkable improvement in seizure frequency, although the mechanism of this is uncertain, as is the effect on long term outcome. Dosage is arbitrary. In infantile spasms 20 units of ACTH may be given daily, and if there is no response, this may be increased to 30 or 40 units. Maintenance doses of prednisolone depend on response. In adult patients, an initial dose of 30 mg of prednisolone a day may be used, and lower maintenance doses depending on response.

Pyridoxine deficiency may very occasionally result in neonatal seizures or infantile spasms, and a trial of *pyridoxine* is worthwhile in all infantile seizures of unknown cause.

9.5 NEW ANTICONVULSANT DRUGS [14]

The testing of potential new anticonvulsant drugs at the scientific level, the animal experimental level and the clinical trial stage has been considerably standardized over recent years, and comprehensive guidelines have been established. Critics of this approach claim that this method is too bureaucratic and rigid, and inhibits free development. The programme of development is certainly very time consuming. It may take a decade or so for a compound to proceed through the testing procedures, and become generally available for clinical use. Nevertheless, there are at present a large number of compounds in various stages of development, and perhaps more drugs at an advanced stage of clinical testing than at any previous time. Interest in this area has been stimulated by a comprehensive developmental scheme. Amongst these compounds are new GABA agonists such as gamma vinyl GABA [15] gabapentin, stiripentol and progabide; the sulphonamide drug zonisamide; the imidazole derivatives denzimol and nafimidone; the new benzodiazepines oxazepam and midazolam; the carbamazepine derivative oxcarbazepine; a cinnarizine derivative fluzarizine; several new barbiturate drugs and other unrelated drugs such as cinromide, flupirtine phenyl propanediol dicarbamate, pentylaminoacetamide, ralitoline, mexilitine and fluzinamide. How many of these compounds will fulfill their experimental promise is yet to be seen, but current prospects for the introduction of effective new anticonvulsant compounds are bright.

REFERENCES

1. Woodbury, D. M., Penry, J. K. and Pippenger, C. E. (eds) (1982) *Antiepileptic Drugs*, 2nd edn, Raven Press, New York.
2. Eadie, M. J. and Tyrer, J. H. (1980) *Anticonvulsant Therapy*, 2nd edn, Churchill Livingstone, Edinburgh, London and New York.
3. Laidlaw, J. and Richens, A. (1982) *A Textbook of Epilepsy*, 2nd edn, Churchill Livingstone, Edinburgh, London and New York.
4. Browne, T. R. and Feldman, R. G. (eds) (1983) *Epilepsy Diagnosis and Management*. Little, Brown and Co., Boston.
5. Reynolds, E. H. (1975) Chronic antiepileptic toxicity: a review. *Epilepsia*, **16**, 315–52.
6. Reynolds, E. H. and Shorvon, S. D. (1981) Monotherapy or polytherapy for epilepsy. *Epilepsia*, **22**, 1–10.
7. Reynolds, E. H. and Chadwick, D. (1985) When to start and when to stop anticonvulsant treatment. *Br. Med. J.*
8. Shorvon, S. D. (1984) The temporal aspects of prognosis in epilepsy. *J. Neurol. Neurosurg. Psychiatr.*, **47**, 1157–65.
9. Schmidt, D. (1982) *Adverse Effects of Antiepileptic Drugs*, Raven Press, New York.
10. Gowers, W. G. (1881) *Epilepsy and Other Chronic Convulsive Disorders*, 1st edn, Churchill, London.
11. Gowers, W. G. (1901) *Epilepsy and Other Chronic Convulsive Disorders*, 2nd edn, Churchill, London.
12. Richens, A. L. and Dunlop, A. (1975) Serum phenytoin levels in the management of epilepsy. *Lancet*, **ii**, 247–9.
13. Frey, H. H. and Janz, D. (eds) (1985) *Antiepileptic Drugs*, Springer-Verlag, Berlin.
14. Meldrum, B. S. and Porter, R. J. (eds) (1986) *Current Problems in Epilepsy, 4: New anticonvulsant drugs*. John Libbey, London.
15. Browne, T. R., Mattson, R. H., Penry, J. K. *et al.* (1987) Vigabatrin for refractory complex partial seizures: Multicenter single-blind study with long-term follow-up. *Neurology*, **37**, 184–9.

CHAPTER TEN

The Management of Epilepsy Uncontrolled by Anticonvulsant Drugs – surgery and other treatments

10.1 THE SURGICAL MANAGEMENT OF EPILEPSY

Anthony Hopkins

Many patients with intractable epilepsy sooner or later think what an excellent idea it would be if the 'bad part' of their brain, responsible for their epilepsy, could be cut out, leaving them free from seizures. Unfortunately, all too often, such patients are not suitable for surgery, most often because seizures arise from a number of different sites, or because the lesion is not so confined that it cannot be excised without leaving significant disability. The same idea does not seem to occur so frequently to the physicians looking after patients with intractable epilepsy, and many units specializing in the management of intractable epilepsy feel that neurologists do not refer patients for surgery often enough, or soon enough. This chapter reviews the selection and preoperative investigation of patients for surgery for epilepsy, the types of operation, and the outcome. This field has been the subject of a number of recent reviews by centres very active in surgery for epilepsy [1–5], but I attempt here a synthesis from the perspective of the neurologist rather than the surgeon or neurophysiologist.

10.1.1 The types of surgery available

This chapter is not concerned with lesions such as tumours causing epilepsy, which require surgery in their own right – for example, an astrocytoma or a sphenoidal wing meningioma presenting with seizures. The presence of such gross lesions causing epilepsy naturally led to the idea that the removal of smaller discrete cortical epileptogenic foci might be worthwhile for the control of seizures. The arch-proponents of this view were the Montreal school. A vast amount of clinical and neurophysiological data were obtained by Penfield and Jasper [6]. Three main threads of experience emerged – that discrete focal superficial epileptogenic lesions accessible to surgery were uncommon, that electrocorticographic recording showed discharges arising over a much wider area of cortex than appeared abnormal on inspection, and finally that most epileptogenic foci lay in one or other temporal lobe. Over the next 30 years surgeons have concentrated their attention on the temporal lobes. This chapter is therefore largely devoted to temporal lobe surgery, though the indications for and results of other surgical operations, such as stereotactic or other procedures designed to interrupt the pathways along which seizures propagate, are reviewed in section 10.3 (pp 324–27).

10.1.2   The numbers of patients who might benefit from temporal lobe surgery

The prevalence of active epilepsy is between 3 and 6 per 1000 (Chapter 1), and probably 70–80% of adults with epilepsy have partial and secondarily generalized seizures [7]. Delgado-Escueta and Walsh [1] estimate that 30–45% of patients with partial epilepsies are intractable. Using the highest and lowest of each of these figures, it may be estimated that between 0.6 and 2 per 1000 have poorly controlled partial epilepsies. Even the lower figure of 0.6 per 1000 must be a gross overestimate of the numbers of those with uncontrolled partial epilepsies in the community in whom life is so seriously disrupted that surgery should be considered. There is no reliable estimate of a need for surgery that is being unmet. Although no surgeon doubts that suitable patients are not being proposed for surgery, active centres may have already exhausted the backlog of suitable cases in their immediate area, rather in the same way as the early operations for rheumatic heart disease soon exhausted the supply of local patients appropriate for surgery. The preoperative assessment of suitable patients with epilepsy is sufficiently complex and expensive that there are good arguments for concentrating the necessary skills and technology in a comparatively small number of centres – perhaps one centre per 10–20 million, undertaking up to 200 assessments and 100 operations per year.

10.1.3   When should epilepsy be considered 'intractable', and surgery considered?

The wide availability of estimation of concentrations of anticonvulsants in the serum makes a decision about when to increase or abandon a drug rather easier than fifteen years ago. Formerly, a drug such as phenytoin might be abandoned if it failed to control seizures in an oral dose of, say, 600 mg/day. It is now recognized that variations in intestinal absorption and rate of hydroxylation may result in low serum levels in spite of high oral dosage. The 'definition' of therapeutic ranges of serum concentrations of anticonvulsant drugs may, however, be counterproductive. The upper end of the therapeutic range is that level at which toxic effects become quite likely, but some patients will benefit from, and not suffer side effects, with serum concentrations of phenytoin and carbamazepine above the usually accepted upper limit. It is therefore right to press both phenytoin and carbamazepine – superior drugs to phenobarbitone and primidone in the management of partial epilepsies [8] –

until unwanted effects are just beginning to occur, which may not arise until levels of 100–105 μmol/l (20–21 μg/ml) of phenytoin, and 55 μmol/l (13 μg/ml) of carbamazepine are obtained.

If phenytoin or carbamazepine fail to control partial and secondarily generalized tonic-clonic seizures, or result in unacceptable unwanted effects, then the first step adopted by many workers will be to phase out the first of these drugs that has been tried and phase in the second. A very small proportion of patients will be additionally benefited by the substitution of one of these drugs for the other, and many clinicians would go on to add, rather than substitute the second drug. In the multicentre trial of assessment of anticonvulsant drugs in the partial and secondarily generalized epilepsies [8], 82 out of an initial 622 patients whose first drug failed, either because of continued seizures or concomitant side effects, had seizures that were so frequent or severe that they were given a combination of two drugs (two out of carbamazepine, phenytoin, phenobarbitone and primidone). Although 32 out of these 82 had fewer seizures over the next year, only 9 (16% of those previously uncontrolled) became seizure-free. Scores for side effects in this trial were also higher in those taking two drugs. In short, if one first line anticonvulsant drug fails, the chances of achieving remission with a change of drug or combination of drugs are not very good, and yet most neurologists and their patients feel that a successive trial of drugs is indicated. It must be remembered that, even if total remission is not achieved with any drug, a reduction in frequency and severity of seizures may make life distinctly more pleasant for the patient.

Other drugs that may occasionally produce worthwhile remissions in the partial epilepsies when the first line drugs have failed include sodium valproate, clobazam and clonazepam (see Chapter 9).

The principal question in this section – when should epilepsy be considered intractable, and surgery considered – depends very largely on the patient's perspective and not on objective measures of seizure disability. Some patients will put up with several complex partial seizures a week, and a few convulsive seizures a year, because the occurrence of these does not interfere greatly within the social structure within which they have learnt to operate. Many of these patients have an understandable and deeply rooted fear of 'brain surgery', and, though it may be proper to raise the question with them if preliminary investigation suggests that they might be suitable candidates, no wise physician would press for surgery in the face of fears that he felt he could not easily dispel.

It should be noted that youth itself is not necessarily a bar to surgery. Meyer and colleagues [8a] have shown that the operative results in 50 young people (mean age 15) compared very favourably with published results in adults.

'Intractability' of epilepsy implies that the known spontaneous natural history of the disorder and the known effects of pharmacological treatment indicate that seizures will continue without remission in the foreseeable future.

No surgeon would consider temporal lobe surgery in the first year or two after onset, as it would take at least that time to evaluate the disorder, and the effects of each of the first line and supplementary anticonvulsant drugs in turn. Rodin, in Chapter 11, outlines the clinical factors which imply a poor prognosis for remission of epilepsy, and Schmidt [9] has examined with particular care the prognosis of chronic epilepsy with complex partial seizures in response to anticonvulsant medication in high dose. The most striking differences between those who achieved and did not achieve a remission was a markedly lower number of seizures in the 12 months before institution of high dose treatment in the patients who became free from seizures, as compared to those patients with an unchanged or increased frequency of seizures. In other words, the more troublesome the epilepsy before high dose treatment, the more difficult it was to control. Those patients who became seizure-free were more likely to have complex partial seizures without automatisms. Conversely, a poor prognosis for seizure control with very energetic medical treatment emerged for those who, in addition to having a high seizure frequency, also had clusters of seizures, a history of more than one complex partial seizure a day (a very similar variable), onset of complex partial seizures with an aura, and a history of severe depression or paranoid psychosis. It is noteworthy that those patients who had complex partial seizures without automatisms responded better to drug therapy. Other workers [4, 10] suggest that complex partial seizures with an initial motionless stare do benefit more from temporal lobe surgery than patients with automatisms (but see p. 290). Thus the very patients who might most seriously be considered for temporal lobe surgery are those who stand the best chance of remission with high dose treatment.

10.1.4 Other preconditions for temporal lobe surgery

Apart from the patient's acceptance of the idea of surgery, and intractability as defined by energetic treatment with high dose anticonvulsant drugs for two to three years, what other factors must be considered in the choice of patients for temporal lobe surgery? The criteria have emerged over the years, based largely on the work of Walker [11], Falconer [12] and the UCLA group [13]. They include:

(1) identification of a favourable seizure type by videotelemetry;
(2) identification of seizure onset consistently within one temporal lobe of the brain;
(3) the absence of evidence of a diffuse cerebral disorder as indicated by:
   (i) low intelligence (IQ <75),
   (ii) bilateral clinical neurological deficits,
   (iii) diffuse EEG abnormalities, and
   (iv) severe psychological abnormality, particularly psychosis.

(a) Identification of a favourable seizure type by videotelemetry

Workers, particularly at the UCLA centre [13] and Zurich [14] have shown the importance of a careful clinical analysis of the seizure. The random occurrence of seizures means that video recording is usually necessary, not least so that it can be seen that all seizures suffered by the patient are of similar type. The seizures can also be repeatedly reviewed. A combination of clinical observation and the analysis of depth electrode encephalography (stereo-encephalography – SEEG, p. 289) allows a correlation between the clinical manifestations and the origin of the seizure discharge. Some workers believe that two types of complex partial seizures can be distinguished [4, 10] (but see p. 290). The first group (Type I complex partial seizures), with SEEG evidence of onset in hippocampus or amygdalar structures, are characterized by an initial motionless state, during which the patient is unresponsive to stimuli. Chewing, swallowing or lip-smacking movements commonly follow. Although quasi-purposeful automatisms may occur subsequently, they are not features of the onset of the attack. The patient may experience abdominal, olfactory or gustatory perceptions, or *déjà vu* before the motionless stare, but there is no initial symptom implicating activity in cerebral cortex outside the medial anterior temporal lobe.

Some type II complex partial seizures have, with the benefit of SEEG, been shown to have clinical and electrophysiological evidence of onset outside the temporal lobe [10]. Videotelemetry shows postural, adversive or focal muscular contractions or quasi-purposive automatisms at the onset of impaired consciousness. Patients may experience epigastric discomfort or *déjà vu* before disturbance of consciousness, as the discharge invades the island of Reil and hippocampus. Some Type II complex partial seizures begin in the frontal lobe [10, 15], particularly Brodmann's area 8 and 4 or supplementary motor cortex. Less frequently the discharge may spread into the temporal lobe from the sensorimotor cortex. Williamson and colleagues [15] have recently written at length about complex partial seizures of frontal lobe origin. Although SEEG studies showed that secondary spread to medial temporal structures may only occasionally occur, clinical features included many classed as 'psychomotor' and tacitly previously accepted as being of temporal lobe origin. Particularly characteristic were brief frequent attacks, complex motor automatisms with kicking and thrashing around, sexual automatisms, vocalizations and frequent complex partial status epilepticus.

(b) Electrophysiological identification of seizure onset consistently within one temporal lobe

A vast amount has been written in the neurophysiological literature about the methodology necessary for firm confirmation that the seizure discharge begins within the temporal lobe, and always the same temporal lobe.

The possibilities are:

(1) reliance on scalp recording,

(2) the use of special leads in the nasopharynx or sphenoidal regions,
(3) chronic epi- or subdural recordings preoperatively,
(4) stereoencephalography,
(5) electrocorticography.

In the early days of epilepsy surgery, scalp recording was the procedure most often used. A number of scalp recordings were taken preoperatively, with or without activation by sleep or methohexitone, and patients with a persistent and consistent anterior temporal spike discharge on one side alone were chosen for surgery, if their epilepsy proved intractable. It has, however, to be acknowledged that the scalp localizations vary in the same patient in different recordings, and the EEG localizations of frontal and temporal discharges may overlap – a distinction that, from the work just discussed, appears to be crucial. It is noteworthy, however, that a recent study from a small institution just 'taking up' temporal lobe surgery, without the facilities for videotelemetry and SEEG, reported that 14 of 24 patients (58%) chosen for surgery were rendered seizure-free, and a further six patients showed a worthwhile improvement [16]. Such a study may, of course, be biased by the selection of the patients in whom the interictal and EEG abnormality is most clearcut, leading to the rejection of patients who might have benefited, and been selected if fuller investigations had been carried out.

The use of scalp recordings can be extended to recording seizures themselves and not just interictal events. The use of cassette recorders or wired telemetry allows the patient to mark an event, such as an aura, allowing the immediately preceding and subsequent EEG to be written out. Rasmussen [17] reported that about 60% of the attacks recorded with scalp and sphenoidal electrodes provided useful localizing information. In about 25% of the recorded attacks, the onset in the EEG record consists of either a generalized onset or a bilaterally symmetrical suppression of activity. In these, and in the remaining 15% in which artefacts during the attack obscure the EEG, no useful information as to the localization of seizure onset is obtained. The Montreal group [18] and the UCLA group [13] believe that it is in these patients that SEEG is useful.

The drawbacks to reliance on scalp recordings alone have been analysed by Quesney and Gloor [18]. Firstly, the mesial surface of the brain, and the inferomesial surfaces of both cerebral hemispheres and the depths of sulci are not adequately explored by scalp electrodes. A scalp electrode may record a 'focal' discharge over one temporal lobe, propagated from some inaccessible primary focus elsewhere, or alternatively the scalp EEG may miss the deeply seated hippocampal focus, ideally suited to surgical excision, but show widespread abnormalities propagated from this focus over the frontotemporal convexity – making the subject appear apparently unsuited to surgery.

The localizing accuracy of ictal and interictal EEG might be improved by the use of electrodes which lie closer to some parts of the brain that are relatively inaccessible to scalp electrodes. Nasopharyngeal and sphenoidal electrodes may be useful in the analysis of discharges arising from the medial temporal lobe, and nasoethmoidal or supraorbital electrodes may record discharges from the orbital surface of the frontal lobe [18].

The efficacy of nasopharyngeal electrodes has been examined by Sperling and Engel [19]. They found that these electrodes may at times be uncomfortable for patients and prone to artefact. In 23 EEGs showing abnormalities at the nasopharyngeal electrodes, spikes or sharp waves were also seen at the anterior temporal or ear electrodes. The same group however, has shown in simultaneous recordings a marked advantage of sphenoidal electrodes – bare wires inserted through a 1.5 inch 22 gauge hypodermic needle immediately below the zygomatic arch [20].

Depth electroencephalography with stereotactically placed electrodes (SEEG) was introduced in the early 1960s by Talairach and Bancaud, and is now practised in several centres, though it is clear that a considerable investment of expertise is required. Useful reviews include those of Engel *et al.* [13] Spencer and colleagues [21, 22], Wieser [14], and Quesney and Gloor [18]. The great advantage of the method is that it is possible to record directly the onset of seizure discharges from implanted electrodes over a period of days or weeks. Unsuspected multiple foci of seizure discharge may be detected. Conversely it may be shown in patients in whom it has previously been thought, on the basis of scalp recordings, that they have bilateral epileptogenic areas, or widespread discharges over one hemisphere, that all seizures begin in one locus in the temporal lobe, so that surgery can, after all, be offered to the patient.

Quesney and Gloor [18] underline one disadvantage of SEEG. Whereas a scalp electrode may detect a spike discharge arising at a considerable distance, with poor localization of the origin of the discharge ('blurred vision'), a depth electrode suffers from 'tunnel vision', in so far as the recording of a spike or discharge is critically dependent upon the precise location of the electrode. The reduction in gain necessary to avoid overloading the amplifiers if the electrode is closely placed to an active spike generator means that other generators, not very far distant, may be missed.

Another difficulty is the enormous amount of information generated by long term recording from a number of depth electrodes. However, computer recognition of seizure discharges may help. For example, Darcey and Williamson [23] have devised integrated relative energy measures of the ictal and preictal EEG, defining the origin of the seizure discharge as that locus to exhibit first statistically significant deviations from the preictal energy levels.

It should be stressed that, in the centres quoted, the decision to operate is made on SEEG recorded seizure discharges. Bilateral independent interictal spikes are often recorded – invariably in Engel's study [24] – and the seizure discharge does not always begin in the lobe with the most interictal spikes.

Views differ about the value of classification of complex seizure type in indicating the need for SEEG. Some workers take the view that if the seizures begin with an initial motionless stare, and if scalp sphenoidal ictal EEGs clearly show a consistent focal seizure discharge – often an initial low voltage fast rhythm seen at one scalp sphenoidal electrode – then SEEG is not required, as these features predict strongly that the seizure origin is focal, and the site of origin can be identified [4, 10]. On the other hand, if the clinical nature of the seizures suggest an extratemporal origin, or if scalp and sphenoidal EEGs show bilateral ictal paryoxysms in the medial temporal regions with only a suggestion of one-sided predominance, then SEEG may discover some patients who will benefit from surgery. The results of the Oregon group are rather different. Brey and Laxer [25] evaluated for surgery 46 patients with complex partial seizures. The seizure focus was ultimately found to be temporal in 41 and frontal in five. Although all five patients with frontal foci had type II complex partial seizures, patients with temporal foci, confirmed at electrocorticography, were equally distributed between types, and a satisfactory surgical result was equally likely to be obtained in those with either type I or type II seizures. These authors also found that a subpial resection of the extratemporal focus identified in five patients with type II complex partial seizures produced a good or excellent outcome. On the basis of these results, Brey and Laxer are understandably keen that the clinical identification of a type II seizure is not seen as a contraindication to epilepsy surgery.

Some quantitative idea of the value of SEEG can be obtained from Spencer's review [21]. She estimates that depth recordings enabled up to 36% of patients to be operated upon who otherwise would have been diagnosed as having non-focal epilepsy. On the other hand, such recordings prevented surgery that probably would have been useless in a further 18%, by demonstrating multiple independent foci.

An alternative to depth recording is the placement of an array of electrodes epidurally [26] under general anaesthesia. The sensorimotor region is identified by recording somatosensory cortical evoked responses from some of the array of up to 48 electrodes. Speech arrest on stimulation of some of the electrodes can outline the speech area if the dominant hemisphere is under examination. The epileptogenic focus is localized by recordings after operative placement of the epidural electrodes, during spontaneously occurring seizures. If the observations identify the boundaries of a single epileptic focus, correlated with video recording of seizures, then this is excised at a second craniotomy. If not, a second craniotomy is necessary to remove the surface electrode array. Either procedure is usually undertaken within a few days, to minimize the chance of infection.

A modification with a smaller array has been used by Goldring [26] for the assessment of patients with complex partial seizures. His observations suggest that it may be unnecessary to penetrate the brain with depth electrodes in order to localize medial temporal foci as, in those cases in which he proceeded to lobectomy, pathological changes were found in every case and, in the majority of cases, epidural recordings could distinguish between a focus in the hippocampus and one in the lateral temporal cortex.

Subdural strip electrodes were first described by Penfield and Jasper, and their use has been revived by the Seattle group [27]. Four 5 mm stainless steel discs are attached to a strip of silastic at intervals of about 1 cm, and between four and eight strips are inserted through burrholes, being pushed gently over the surface of brain with an 'introducer'. Strips have been left in place for up to three weeks, to allow continuous monitoring of seizures and seizure discharges. Strips of electrodes can be passed beneath the temporal lobe, and provide excellent recording from the uncus, most of the amydala, and the hippocampus. Wyler and colleagues [27] point out that the area of cortex studied in this way can be much greater than by probe depth electrodes, and this technique may be useful for determining if a focus is present. Moreover the exact location of the focus may still be confirmed by depth electrodes.

(c) The absence of evidence of other unfavourable factors

Clinical experience in the earlier days of temporal lobe surgery showed that evidence of diffuse cerebral disorder, as witnessed by bilateral clinical neurological deficits, and a diffuse EEG abnormality, were correlated with an unfavourable outcome. An intelligence quotient of less than 75 on the Wechsler Adult Intelligence Scale may also reasonably be taken as supportive evidence for a diffuse neurological disorder. Prior evidence of psychosis is also associated with a poor outcome, and is a contraindication to surgery [3].

10.1.5 Other preoperative investigations

(a) Preoperative localization of language and memory

A careful neuropsychological assessment before operation will help assess damage to language, cognitive function and memory caused by the epileptogenic lesion, and the likely further contribution of the surgical excision (pp. 293–96). Milner [28] found that a performance intelligence quotient on the Wechsler Adult Intelligence Scale (WAIS) more than seven points higher than the verbal quotient, was in favour of a dominant hemisphere lesion. Conversely, a verbal quotient more than two points higher than the performance quotient was in favour of a non-dominant lesion. Frontal damage, supportive of an extratemporal origin to the seizures, can be ascertained by the Wisconsin card sorting test.

The hemispheric localization of language can more reliably be ascertained by the Wada test [29]. Sodium amylobarbitone is injected into one internal carotid artery through a brachial or femoral catheter under EEG control. Effective suppression of the hemisphere is judged by high amplitude 1.5–3 cy/s activity over that hemisphere alone. During this transient suppression, tests of language function and memory can be performed.

(b) Imaging

High definition cranial CT scanning is of course an essential prerequisite of evaluation for surgery. Rich and colleagues [30] have called attention to the probability that very dense and hypodense lesions seen on the scan are in all probability oligodendrogliomas, although often thought by referring neurologists to be hamartomas or old small infarcts.

Conversely to what might be thought, dilatation of the temporal horn does not correlate well with the side of the focus responsible for intractable epilepsy. This has been shown for both CT and MRI studies. Further information about the comparative benefits of CT and MRI is given in Chapter 8.

Wyler and Bolender [31] have shown that careful measurements of the distance between the edge of the mesial temporal structures and the central reference line on a cut at the level of the cerebral peduncles could identify patients with chronic herniation of mesial temporal structures over the free edge of the tentorium, a group very likely to have mesial temporal sclerosis, and thus an excellent response to surgery.

(c) Positron emission tomography

Positron emission tomography is not yet widely available, but the UCLA experience has shown that areas of focal decreased metabolism can be detected using (^{18}F)2-fluoro-2-deoxy glucose in patients with partial epilepsy, even though other imaging methods are normal [33]. Surprisingly, studies indicate that the mesial temporal structures show less hypometabolism than the lateral temporal cortex, possibly because the lateral cortex is partly disconnected from deeper structures, and partly because the technique can only show the combined effect of both neural loss and increased firing rates, which may average out [34].

10.1.6   The results of operation

(a) Surgical mortality and morbidity on the temporal lobe

The relative youth of the patients chosen for surgery, and the advance in anaesthetic and surgical techniques means that most centres can report a 'negligible' mortality [5]. Morbidity, either from surgery or from procedures before operation such as the implantation of depth or epidural electrodes, is also slight, but does occur. For example, in one recent series [35] two of 21 patients who had depth electrodes inserted developed significant complications – a small haemorrhage in the mesial temporal regions, and an abscess. The effect of surgery on memory is considered on p. 294. Operations on the dominant hemisphere do threaten language. Although some centres operate under general anaesthesia, limiting excision of the dominant temporal lobe to a line 5 cm posteriorly from the tip, others rely on intraoperative mapping of language. The presence of repeated errors in naming evoked by stimulation at currents just below the threshold for after-discharge indicates a site to be avoided as essential for language. Ojemann [36] has found essential language areas on occasion less than 4 cm from the temporal tip, usually in the superior temporal gyrus, but occasionally in the middle gyrus. Conversely, large resections, extending 8–9 cm from the temporal tip, can be carried out if stimulation shows that language localization is unusually posterior. In a recent series, three out of 23 patients had a transient post-operative dysphasia [35].

(b) The type of operation

The excision of the anterior temporal lobe in one block, as first practised by the Maudsley group ([12] for references) had the great advantage of allowing histological analysis of the seizure focus (pp. 312–22). Some surgeons remove the defined area with suction, but the majority are refining their procedures so that the minimal area of brain in excess of that which is abnormal is removed. Microsurgical, selective amygdalohippocampectomy has given excellent results in the hands of the Zurich group [14, 37]. Ojemann [36] has described how the operation can be 'tailored' to fit the preoperative and intraoperative EEG findings. A fairly extensive surgical removal is necessary for seizures arising in the posterior temporal neocortex, and this may well be followed by a contralateral defect of the upper visual fields. Opercular foci have proved difficult to excise without leaving some neurological deficit.

The Yale group has described a technique whereby access to the posterior medial temporal structures can be gained through the temporal horn after resection of the anterior 4.5 cm of the temporal lobe, and the lateral cortex gently elevated, exposing the medial temporal structures which are resected in a second block [38].

Other surgical complications, fortunately seldom seen, include damage to the anterior choroidal artery resulting in infarction of part of the internal capsule and hemiparesis, and damage to the third nerve deep to the temporal lobe, resulting in diplopia.

(c) Control of seizures

The manner in which patients are selected will undoubtedly influence the results obtained. Some centres tackling only 'easy' patients, with consistent foci clearly defined by scalp recordings [16], may achieve results as good or better than those centres which try to extend the benefits of surgery to patients with less clearly defined origins to their seizures, who require extensive investigation with implanted depth electrodes. A number of surgical series are reviewed in [1] and [13]. In general, various centres report a 60–80% success rate, in that seizures are either totally abolished (perhaps 50%) or very significantly reduced in frequency (perhaps 30%).

(d) Postoperative changes other than control of seizures

Improvements have been described in cognitive function, psychiatric morbidity and social function. These beneficial effects were particularly stressed by the Maudsley group nearly 20 years ago [12] and many of their observations have since been substantiated and extended. The effects on memory first analysed in detail in Montreal [28] are more complex.

(i)   Cognitive function

Rausch and Crandall [39] found that improvement in cognitive function was largely linked to the effects of temporal lobectomy in controlling the seizures. Patients who had right-sided surgery improved in terms of verbal intellectual scores, whereas patients after left-sided surgery improved with regard to perceptual intellectual scores. The mean increase on the full scale (WAIS) of the patients who improved after surgery was 8.4 IQ points. The authors adduce convincing reasons for believing that this was more than a practice effect on repetition of the WAIS.

It should be noted, however, that the more recent experience from the Maudsley group showed an improvement in only two of 32 patients after temporal lobe surgery, in whom good seizure control occurred, and nine patients showed a decline of intellectual performance, though this was only of practical importance in three [40]. Finally, a detailed study from the Yale group records that significant improvement in verbal and performance IQ scores occurred only in those with good postoperative seizure control, whose operations had been undertaken on the non-dominant temporal lobe.

(ii)   Memory

A number of studies, pioneered by the Montreal group [28], have shown that defects of verbal memory are likely to follow dominant temporal lobectomy, and memory for visual material is likely to be impaired following non-dominant temporal lobectomy. In practice, a disturbance of verbal memory is of potentially much greater importance, especially to a subject in a professional occupation. Bilateral temporal lobe lesions result in gross memory deficits [28]. However, Rausch and Crandall [39] observed that rote verbal memory improved in some patients after non-dominant temporal lobectomy. This aspect has been further analysed by Novelly and colleagues at Yale [41] who observed not only this change, but also the reciprocal effect – that is to say, those patients who had a dominant temporal lobectomy showed a significant improvement in immediate and delayed visual and pictorial memory. The Yale group writes that these results imply that uncontrolled seizures before operation interfere with the memory functions of the temporal lobe contralateral to the epileptogenic focus.

Although the mesial temporal structures, particularly the hippocampus, are important for memory, Ojemann and Dodrill have evidence that the lateral temporal cortex also has a role in memory mechanisms [42]. Intraoperative cortical stimulation and testing of memory allows the cortical contribution to memory to be mapped, and the excision tailored, to some extent, to reduce the memory loss. If preoperative assessment of memory function by intracarotid amylobarbitone perfusion of the side of the proposed resection showed a deficit, then the operation would be tailored to remove the uncus and amygdala, sparing part of the hippocampus and, as far as possible, the relevant lateral cortex. As these workers point out, however, every limitation on resection of the focus reduces, to some extent, the chances of obtaining good seizure control.

(iii) Personality
Some patients with temporal lobe epilepsy have severe behavioural disorders, with aggression a major feature. It was soon realized that an abnormal personality might show a striking improvement after excision of the medial temporal structures, particularly the amygdala [43] or after stereoctactic amydalotomy [44]. The paper by Lindsay and colleagues [45] contains an account of a biography of a patient with temporal lobe epilepsy dating from childhood whose lobectomy was, with the benefit of hindsight, too long delayed. The improvement in quality of life due to improvement in personality is moving. Other adolescents were similarly benefited, suggesting that the operation should more readily be offered to this age group [8a]. However patients with psychosis and temporal lobe epilepsy are in general not benefited.

An attempt to analyse the behavioural changes associated with temporal lobe epilepsy and lobectomy has been made by Fedio and Martin [46]. Patients with left temporal lobe epilepsy reported 'ruminative-intellectual interests in religiosity, metaphysical elements and personal destiny, paranoid concern and hypergraphic tendencies'. Such patients amplified their own negative qualities ('tarnishers'). Conversely, patients with right temporal lobe epilepsy, with more emotional concerns, tended to minimize undesirable attributes ('polishers'). After operation, comparison with non-operated controls suggested an improved self image, as reported by patients on a behavioural inventory. None the less, the patient's 'style' continued. Left lobectomy patients continuing to rate themselves unduly harshly, as 'tarnished'.

(iv) Social function
Socioeconomic changes following temporal lobe surgery were reported by Taylor and Falconer in 1968 [12], and others, and analysed again recently by the Yale group [47]. As would be expected, a substantial reduction in seizures after surgery is associated with maintaining or assuming employment. As many patients came to temporal lobe surgery because of impending loss of work due to seizures, maintenance of employment can also be seen as success for operative intervention. There are certainly exceptions to this overall intuitively expected result – patients with excellent seizure control failing to gain work. Some such patients have a history of previous psychiatric disorder

and social impairment. Augustine and colleagues [47] found that a long period of preoperative unemployment was an unfavourable predictor for postoperative assumption of work. They also found that patients with a markedly lower performance IQ than a verbal IQ, and patients whose temporal lobectomy was on the non-dominant side were more likely to be unemployed, suggesting that these points may be salient factors detracting from general occupational adjustment. These authors indicate some 'non-medical' variables that make work in this field difficult – the local society within which each subject operates may be variously prejudiced against epilepsy. Furthermore, 'it takes considerable effort to surrender a disability income once it has been granted'. All their subjects in receipt of welfare payments had expressed fear of losing their entitlement if operation rendered them seizure-free.

(e)   The prognostic value of the pathological findings

The pathological findings in patients with temporal lobe epilepsy are reviewed on pp. 312–22. In a number of surgical series the presence of mesial temporal sclerosis has been associated with a good outcome for control of seizures (for references see [48]). The worst prognosis, in many series, is if the excised portion of the temporal lobe is normal, presumably because operative excision has 'missed' the seizure focus.

The Seattle group [48] found that 75% of the group of patients with mesial temporal sclerosis had operative evidence of chronic herniation of the mesial temporal structures. As this can be demonstrated preoperatively by CT scanning [32], Turner and Wyler [48] suggest that improved preoperative identification of patients with subtle structural damage to the mesial temporal lobe should, in association with EEG evidence, increase the chances of identifying patients with good prognosis for seizure control.

Duncan and Sagar [49] have reported that certain clinical features predict the operative finding of Ammon's horn sclerosis – defined as severe loss of pyramidal neurones in the H_1 zone, particularly the $H_{1/2}$ border, and endfolium. Ammon's horn sclerosis is likely if convulsions occurred in early childhood, if the initial convulsion was prolonged, and if partial seizures begin in the next few years. If Ammon's horn sclerosis is found, then the outcome after surgery is likely to be good, particularly, according to these workers, if seizures commence with a rising sensation in the epigastrium.

10.1.7   Conclusion

The success of temporal lobe surgery when patients are suitably chosen and investigated should encourage its wider use. We could probably bring the benefits to a larger number of those with intractable seizures of temporal lobe origin by reviewing, on an outpatient basis, some of the predictors of a favourable outcome noted above; and others recently listed by the Seattle group. Using multiple regression analysis, Dodrill and colleagues [50] showed that using four non-EEG factors (WAIS Digit Symbol score, Marching test using the preferred hand, and scores on the MMPI Hysteria and Personality Scales) a favourable or unfavourable outcome could be predicted in 71% of patients. Addition of four EEG factors, three of which refer to simple scalp recordings, increased the probability of a correct prediction to 80%. A careful assessment of verbal and non-verbal memory, and the patient's cognitive function and employment status should reduce the chances of unwanted effects of surgery upon social and intellectual function.

Since this chapter was prepared a full monograph on the surgical treatment of the epilepsies has appeared [51].

References

1. Delgado-Escueta, A. V. and Walsh, G. O. (1983) The selection process for surgery of intractable complex partial seizures: surface EEG and depth electrography, in *Epilepsy* (eds A. A. Ward, J. K. Penry and D. Purpura), Raven Press, New York, pp. 295–326.
2. Aird, R. B., Masland, R. L. and Woodbury, D. M. (1984) *The Epilepsies: A Critical Review*, Raven Press, New York.
3. Crandall, P. H., Cahan, L. D., Sutherling, W. *et al*. (1985) Surgery for intractable complex partial seizures, in *The Epilepsies* (eds R. J. Porter and P. L. Morselli), Butterworths, London, pp. 307–21.
4. Delgado-Escueta, A. V. and Walsh, G. O. (1985) Type I complex partial seizures of hippocampal origin: excellent results of temporal lobectomy. *Neurology*, **35**, 143–54.
5. Delgado-Escueta, A. V., Treiman, D. M. and Walsh, G. O. (1983) The treatable epilepsies. *N. Engl. J. Med.*, **308**, 1576–84.
6. Penfield, W. and Jasper, H. (1954) *Epilepsy and the Functional Anatomy of the Human Brain*, Little, Brown and Co., Boston.
7. Hopkins, A. P. and Scambler, G. (1977) How doctors deal with epilepsy. *Lancet*, **i**, 183–6.
8. Mattson, R. H., Cramer, J. A., Collins, J. F. *et al*. (1985) Comparison of carbamazepine, phenobarbital, phenytoin and primidone in partial and secondarily generalized tonic-clonic seizures. *N. Engl. J. Med.*, **313**, 145–51.
8a Meyer, F. B., Marsh, R., Laws, E. R. *et al*. (1986) Temporal lobectomy in children with epilepsy. *J. Neurosurg.*, **64**, 371–6.
9. Schmidt, D. (1984) Prognosis of chronic epilepsy with complex partial seizures. *J. Neurol. Neurosurg. Psychiatr.*, **47**, 1274–8.
10. Walsh, G. O. and Delgado-Escueta, A. V. (1984) Type II complex partial seizures: poor results of anterior temporal lobectomy. *Neurology*, **34**, 1–13.
11. Walker, A. E. (1974) Surgery for epilepsy, in *The Epilepsies* (*Handbook of Clinical Neurology*, Vol. 15) (eds O. Magnus and A. M. Lorentz de Haas), North Holland, Amsterdam, pp. 739–58.
12. Taylor, D. C. and Falconer, M. A. (1968) Clinical, socioeconomic, and psychological changes after temporal lobectomy for epilepsy. *Br. J. Psychiatr.*, **114**, 1247–61.
13. Engel, J. Jr., Crandall, P. H. and Rausch, R. (1983) The partial epilepsies, in *The*

Clinical Neurosciences (eds R. N. Rosenberg *et al.*), **2**, Churchill Livingstone, New York, pp. 1349–80.

14. Wieser, H. G. (1983) *Electroclinical Features of the Psychomotor Seizure*, Gustav Fischer, Butterworths, Stuttgart and New York.

15. Williamson, P. D., Spencer, D. D., Spencer, S. S. *et al.* (1985) Complex partial seizures of frontal lobe origin. *Ann. Neurol.*, **18**, 497–504.

16. Carey, P., O'Moore, B., Sheahan, K. and Staunton, H. (1985) Experience of temporal lobectomy as a treatment modality for epilepsy, using interictal EEG data alone to localise the epileptogenic focus. *Ir. Med. J.*, **78**, 74–7.

17. Rasmussen, T. B. (1983) Surgical treatment of complex partial seizures: results, lessons, and problems. *Epilepsia*, **24** (Suppl. 1), S65–76.

18. Quesney, L. F. and Gloor, P. (1985) in Long-Term Monitoring in Epilepsy (eds J. Gotman *et al.*). *Electroenceph. Clin. Neurophysiol.*, **Suppl. 37**.

19. Sperling, M. R. and Engel, J. (1985) Electroencephalographic recording from the temporal lobes: a comparison of ear, anterior temporal and nasopharyngeal electrodes. *Ann. Neurol.*, **17**, 510–13.

20. Sperling, M. R., Mendius, J. R. and Engel, J. (1986) Mesial temporal spikes: a simultaneous comparison of sphenoidal, nasopharyngeal and ear electrodes. *Epilepsia*, **27**, 81–86.

21. Spencer, S. S. (1981) Depth electroencephalography in selection of patients with refractory epilepsy for surgery. *Ann. Neurol.*, **9**, 207–14.

22. Spencer, S. S., Spencer, D. D., Williamson, P. D. and Mattson, R. H. (1982) The localising value of depth electroencephalography in 32 patients with refractory epilepsy. *Ann. Neurol.*, **12**, 248–53.

23. Darcey, T. M. and Williamson, P. D. (1985) Spatio-temporal EEG measures and their application to human intracranially recorded epileptic seizures. *Electroenceph. Clin. Neurophysiol.*, **61**, 573–87.

24. Engel, J., Rausch, R., Lieb, J. P. *et al.* (1981) Correlation of criteria used for localising epileptic foci in patients considered for surgical therapy of epilepsy. *Ann. Neurol.*, **9**, 215–24.

25. Brey, R. and Laxer, K. D. (1985) Type I/II complex seizures: no correlation with surgical outcome. *Epilepsia*, **26**, 657–60.

26. Goldring, S. and Gregorie, E. M. (1984) Surgical management of epilepsy using epidural recordings to localise the seizure focus. *J. Neurosurg.*, **60**, 457–66.

27. Wyler, A. R., Ojeman, G. A., Lettich, E. and Ward, A. A. (1984) Subdural strip elecrodes for localising epileptogenic foci. *J. Neurosurg.*, **60**, 1195–200.

28. Milner, B. (1975) Psychological aspects of focal epilepsy and its neurosurgical management, in *Neurosurgical Management of the Epilepsies* (*Advances in Neurology*, Vol. 8) (eds D. P. Purpura *et al.*), Raven Press, New York, pp. 229–312.

29. Blume, W. T., Grabow, J. D., Darley, F. L. and Aronson, A. E. (1973) Intracarotid amobarbital test of language and memory before temporal lobectomy for seizure control. *Neurology*, **23**, 812–19.

30. Rich, K. M., Goldring, S. and Gado, M. (1985) Computed tomography in chronic seizure disorder caused by glioma. *Arch. Neurol.*, **42**, 26–7.

31. McLachlan, R. S., Nicholson, R. L., Black, S. *et al.* (1985) Nuclear magnetic resonance imaging; a new approach to the investigation of refractory temporal lobe epilepsy. *Epilepsia*, **26**, 555–62.

32. Wyler, A. R. and Bolender, N. F. (1983) Preoperative CT diagnosis of mesial temporal sclerosis for surgical treatment of epilepsy. *Ann. Neurol.*, **13**, 59–64.

33. Kuhl, D. E., Engel, J. and Phelps, M. E. (1983) Emission computed tomography in the study of human epilepsy, in *Epilepsy* (eds A. A. Ward, J. K. Penry and D. Purpura), Raven Press, New York, pp. 327–40.

34. Abou-Khalil, B. W., Siegel, G. J., Hichwa, R. D. *et al.* (1985) Topography of glucose hypometabolism in epilepsy of medial temporal origin. *Ann. Neurol.*, **18**, 151–2.

35. King, D. W., Flanigan, I., Gallagher, B. B. *et al.* (1986) Temporal lobectomy for partial complex seizures; evaluation, results, and one year follow up. *Neurology*, **36**, 334–9.

36. Ojemann, G. A. (1983) Neurosurgical management of epilepsy: a personal perspective in 1983. *Appl. Neurophysiol.*, **46**, 11–18.

37. Wieser, H. G. and Yasargil, M. G. (1982) Die 'Selektiv Amygdala – Hippokampektanie'. Als chirugische Behandlung du medio-basal Limbischen Epilepsie. *Neurochirugi.*, **25**, 39–50.

38. Spencer, D. D., Spencer, S. S., Mattson, R. H. *et al.* (1984) Access to the posterior medial temporal structures in the surgical treatment of temporal lobe epilepsy. *Neurosurgery*, **15**, 667–71.

39. Rausch, R. and Crandall, P. H. (1982) Psychological status related to surgical control of temporal lobe seizures. *Epilepsia*, **23**, 191–202.

40. Polkey, C. E. (1983) Effects of anterior temporal lobectomy apart from the relief of seizures: a study of 40 patients. *J. R. Soc. Med.*, **76**, 354–8.

41. Novelly, R. A., Augustine, E. A., Mattson, R. H. *et al.* (1984) Selective memory improvement and impairment in temporal lobe surgery for epilepsy. *Ann. Neurol.*, **15**, 64–7.

42. Ojemann, G. A. and Dodrill, C. B. (1985) Verbal memory deficits after temporal lobectomy for epilepsy. *J. Neurosurg.*, **62**, 101–7.

43. Mempel, E., Witkiewicz, B., Stadnicki, R. *et al.* (1980) The effect of medial amygdalotomy and anterior hippocampotomy on behaviour and seizures in epileptic patients. *Acta Neurochirurg.*, **Suppl. 30**, 161–7.

44. Hood, T. W., Siegfried, J. and Wieser, H. G. (1983) The role of stereotactic amygdalotomy in the treatment of temporal lobe epilepsy associated with behavioural disorders. *Appl. Neurophysiol.*, **46**, 19–25.

45. Lindsay, J., Ounstead, C. and Richards, P. (1984) Long term outcome in children with temporal lobe seizures. V. Indications and contraindications for neurosurgery. *Develop. Med. Child Neurol.*, **26**, 25–32.

46. Fedio, P. and Martin, A. (1983) Ideative-emotive behavioural characteristics of patients following left or right temporal lobectomy. *Epilepsia*, **24** (Suppl. 2), S117–30.

47. Augustine, E. A., Novelly, R. A., Mattson, R. H. *et al.* (1984) Occupational adjustment following neurosurgical treatment of epilepsy. *Ann. Neurol.*, **15**, 68–72.

48. Turner, D. A. and Wyler, A. R. (1981) Temporal lobectomy for epilepsy: mesial temporal herniation is an operative and prognostic finding. *Epilepsia*, **22**, 623–30.

49. Duncan, J. S. and Sagar, H. J. (1987) Seizure characteristics, pathology and outcome after temporal lobectomy. *Neurology*, (in press).

50. Dodrill, C. B., Wilkins, R. J., Ojemann, G. A. *et al.* (1986) Multidisciplinary prediction of seizure relief from cortical resection surgery. *Ann. Neurol.*, **20**, 2–12.

51. Engel, J. Jr. (ed.) (1987) *Surgical Treatment of the Epilepsies*, Raven Press, New York.

10.2 NEUROPATHOLOGICAL CHANGES IN THE TEMPORAL LOBE ASSOCIATED WITH COMPLEX PARTIAL SEIZURES

W. Jann Brown and Thomas L. Babb

It is now well known that similar pathological substrates in different loci of the brain may induce different types of seizure patterns largely due to the populations of neurones affected, but study of regions other than temporal lobe presently suffer from a lack of the extensive spatiotemporal electrophysiological recording correlations of the type which have been accorded to studies of temporal lobe seizures. The present data are limited to studies of patients in whom hyperexcitability has been demonstrated from spontaneously recorded SEEG information (p. 289) in which the electrical alterations that occur with complex partial seizures are concordant with origin in the hippocampus or other parts of the mesial temporal lobe, with the excitability subsequently transmitted to other parts of the brain [1–3].

The studies reported in this section reflect a population of patients afflicted with drug refractory complex partial seizures. Clinically, patterns of neuronal discharge between and during seizures were studied by the use of arrays of microelectrodes implanted in the limbic system bilaterally in order to determine if the sensitive focus was unilateral [4]. Eligible temporal lobes were resected *en bloc*, and microanatomical studies of these excised tissues have been done in over 200 patients. Represented in the 200 specimens is a wide spectrum of conditions which embraces neoplasm, heterotopia, hamartoma, trauma, hippocampal sclerosis and patients with no demonstrable structural abnormality. The incidence of no structural abnormality was once considered to be as high as 9%; however such a classification is only an indication that no clear abnormality could be found in the specimen provided by the neurosurgeon. As the *en bloc* resections have become more reliable, we have been less likely to miss structural abnormalities.

The antecedent cause for the hippocampal sclerosis found in the greatest proportion of patients with temporal lobe epilepsy has still not been settled despite a span of 160 years of pertinent reporting [5–11].

In the interest of clarity and convenience the pathological substrate in limbic epilepsy is divided below into categories which we have encountered in (1) neocortex and white matter of temporal lobe and (2) those involving archicortex and limbic system. These data reflect all conditions found in 114 unselected patients (see Table 10.1).

10.2.1 Neocortex and subjacent white matter

(a) Hamartoma
Cavanagh [12] reported the presence of 'certain small tumours' encountered

Table 10.1 Incidence of lesions: *en bloc* resected temporal lobes

No. of patients	Tissue diagnosis	% of whole
73	Hippocampal sclerosis*	64
18	Hamartomata†	15.7
12	Gliomata‡	10.5
8	Heterotopia§	7.0
2	Meningiomata	1.7
1	Cyst in white matter (post-traumatic)	0.8
Total 114		99.7

*Includes mesial sclerosis.
†Includes tuberous sclerosis; vascular anomaly.
‡Oligodendroglioma, ganglioglioma, astrocytoma.
§Also epidermoid inclusion cyst.

in the temporal lobe in 10–12% of cases of drug refractory psychomotor epilepsy at the Guy's–Maudsley Neurosurgical Unit, London. Some of these lesions were found either in the hippocampus, and had an associated sclerosis of Ammon's horn in addition to the tumour, or, as in some instances, appeared to be independent of the archicortex. Others have reported similar masses in these loci [10, 13]. Eighteen examples of such non-neoplastic, almost malformational, tissue development (16%) were uncovered in the 114 cases in the present series. Included under the hamartomatous designation is vascular anomaly (Fig. 10.1) and tuberous sclerosis (Fig. 10.2).

In certain instances the neuroglia may form a distinct mass sharply defined from its surround (Fig. 10.3) and microscopic examination of its substance reveals either astrocytes or oligodendroglia (Fig. 10.4) or mixture of both which are indistinguishable from low grade neoplasm and yet the lesion appears to have remained peculiarly quiescent. Historically no such case in our experience has become an active neoplasm and extended itself, evoking renewed seizure activity. The microscopic depictment of either vascular anomaly or tuberous sclerosis is too common to repeat here.

(b) Heterotopia
This type of malformation constitutes 7% (Table 10.1) of the present series. The term as we use it relates to development of either tissues or groups of cells in situations wherein they are not generally found. The presence of squamous epithelium within the brain is a prime example of an ectopic or heterotopic tissue. Such developmentally sequestered epithelial-lined cysts are well known and are found in complex partial seizure surgery. Figure 10.5 shows such a lesion in the uncus of a resected temporal lobe. These lesions are usually connected in some way, however tenuous, with the arachnoid or dura but such

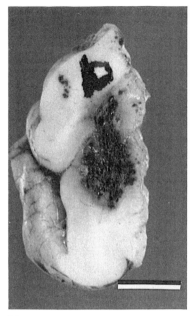

Fig. 10.1

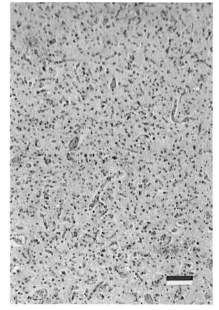

Fig. 10.2

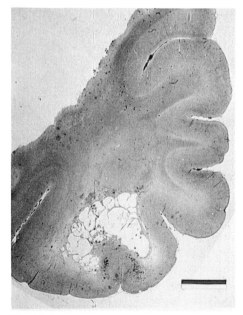

Fig. 10.3

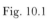

Fig. 10.4

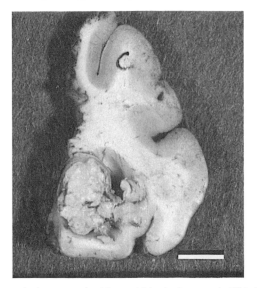

Figure 10.5 Heterotopia in uncus (epidermoid inclusion cyst). This lesion was associated with olfactory auras as components of complex partial seizures. Calibration bar 1.0 cm.

a search is a tedious one, and so it is generally held that the cyst is 'in the parenchyma' as an ectopia.

Other heterotopia that can be found are usually more subtle and may not be visible macroscopically, although the one shown in Fig. 10.6 is visible scattered throughout both mesial and lateral temporal lobe. These small masses are composed of small collections of oligodendroglia, astrocytes and neurones (Fig. 10.6(b)).

Figure 10.1 Cross section through anterior temporal lobe showing hamartoma (vascular anomaly) lateral to resection. Note individual vascular channels at edges. Microscopy showed well developed, even, fibrous, walled channels filled with blood and with some old blood pigment in the interstitial connective tissues. Calibration bar 1.0 cm.

Figure 10.2 Harmartoma (tuberous sclerosis) in white matter of part of middle gyrus lateral to temporal horn of lateral ventricle. The dark stippling consists of focal calcification. Note decreased myelination around the tuber. Calibration bar 1.0 cm.

Figure 10.3 Harmartoma of mixed cysts and astrocytes in inferior temporal gyrus. The pallor in nearby gyrus is due to decrease in oligodendroglia. The lesion superficially resembles a cystic scar but the cyst does not appear in that fashion and more posteriorly the lesion has a solid aspect (see Figure 10.4). Calibration bar 1.0 cm.

Figure 10.4 Shows astrocytic and vascular proliferation of the glial hamartoma of Figure 10.3. Calibration bar 80 μm.

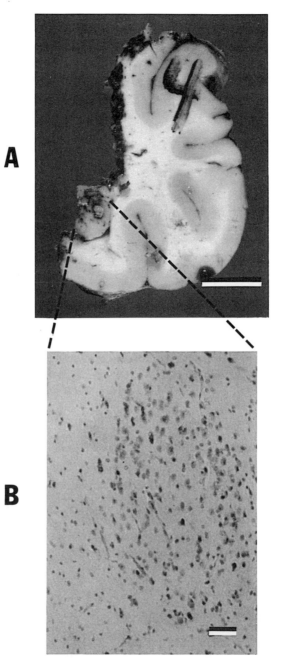

A

B

Table 10.2 Temporal lobe gliomata in complex partial seizures

Case no.	Length of seizure history (years)	Operation	Histology	Post-operative clinical state	Follow-up (years)
1	30	1960	Ganglioglioma	Rare seizure (e.g. 1/yr); Ib*	25
2	7	1968	Astrocytoma Gr II	Slight decrease in seizures; III	17
3	17	1974	Oligodendroglioma	Seizure free; I	11
4	40	1975	Astrocytoma	Seizure free; I	10
5	unknown	1976	Oligodendroglioma	Mild decrease in seizures; III	9
6	4	1976	Astrocytoma Gr I	Seizure free; I	9
7	6	1977	Astrocytoma Gr I	Occasional aura; Ia	8
8	unknown	1977	Astrocytoma Gr II	Seizure free; I	8
9	4	1977	Astrocytoma Gr I	Mild decrease in seizures; III	8
10	10	1978	Oligodendroglioma	Seizure free; I	7
11	23	1980	Ganglioglioma	Seizure free; Ia	5
12	5	1980	Oligodendroglioma (and central Schwannoma)	Seizure free; Ia	5

*Roman numerals adjacent to features of clinical state postoperative indicate a rating of seizure status.

(c) Glioma

Twelve patients or 10% of this case population had frank neuroectodermal neoplasms (Table 10.2). These lesions may be, as suggested by Cavanagh [12], small tumour-like formations with indications in some areas of early neoplastic transformation, or hamartomatous residuals of cerebral development and maturation. However we have elected to use the more narrow definition of hamartoma as employed by Willis [14] in our analysis (see above). Some of the neoplasms shown in Table 10.2 were indeed small and grossly rather sharply delineated (1.5 cm in cross section) (Fig. 10.7); others however occupied much of the lateral neocortex (Fig. 10.8); yet the microscopic appearance of each might not be dissimilar. It is important to appreciate the fact that given either permanent sections or frozen sections

Figure 10.6 Heterotopia sharply-circumscribed and diffusely scattered in mesial and lateral temporal lobe (A). Calibration bar 1.0 cm. (B) Enlargement of heterotopia in subiculum revealing largely masses of ectopic neurones. Other masses in the temporal lobe showed well-differentiated oligodendroglia, as well. Calibration bar 40 μm.

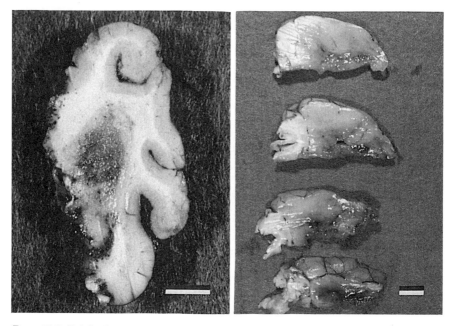

Figure 10.7 Fairly sharp definition of mass in white matter of anterior temporal neocortex. There was no evident neoplasm in the medial resection line by microscopy. This oligodendroglioma is listed as Case no. 10 in Table 10.2. Calibration bar 1.0 cm.

Figure 10.8 Sections of temporal lobe showing diffuse glioma with only inferior gyrus essentially free of astrocytic proliferation. The remainder of the lobe is astrocytoma (see also Figure 10.10). Calibration bar 1.0 cm.

made at surgery, these lesions will be recognized as neoplasms (Figs. 10.9 and 10.10). In the Clinical Neurophysiology Project at UCLA the temporal lobe is delivered after *en bloc* resection; hence the entire neoplasm may be present in the specimen (Fig. 10.7) or, with more extensive neoplastic processes (Fig. 10.8; Case no. 2 in Table 10.2), the neoplasm may be located in the posterior resection surface. While the surgeon does not dare extend his resection posteriorly more than the customary 5.5–6.0 cm from the anterior temporal pole, it is of critical concern to both prognosis and treatment to recognise the extent of the disease.

While most of these neoplasms were neuroglial in origin, occasional combinations with neurones in the absence of tuberous sclerosis were found (Fig. 10.11; Case no. 1 in Table 10.2). An even more exotic tissue amalgamation was found in Case no. 12. The microscopic preparation shows distinct oligodendroglioma which is sharply limited by a small sulcus contiguous to which there is Schwann sheath neoplasm. Both portions of this highly abnormal cortex have distinct forms of connective tissue. The oligodendroglioma has glial processes from astrocytes whereas the peripheral nerve

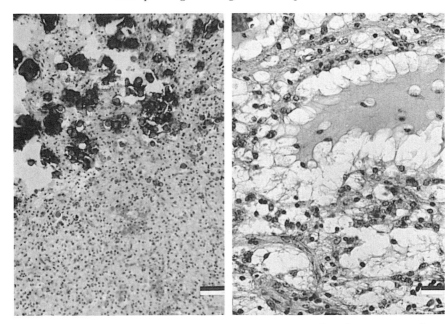

Figure 10.9 Calcification and sheets of oligodendroglioma characteristic of small neoplastic nodules similar to Figure 10.7. Calibration bar 80 μm.

Figure 10.10 Scalloped appearance of proteinaceous fluid in typical neoplastic cyst of astrocytoma. The nearby astrocytes are well-differentiated. Taken from glioma in Figure 10.8. Calibration bar 33 μm.

portion is fibrous. Specific glial acidic protein antibody is reactive with the glial processes but only meagre reaction is present at the edges of the Schwannoma. It has been 25 years since Case no. 1 (ganglioglioma) (Fig. 10.11) had resection of the temporal lobe. She has had only rare seizures (about one per year).

The most advanced astrocytoma in the group was a Grade II with some foci containing marked anaplasia (Fig. 10.12). The patient was irradiated after surgery, and 17 years have elapsed, with only a slight decrease in the incidence and severity of his complex partial seizures. Falconer *et al.* [15] remarked that he found the neoplasms of the temporal lobe clinically indolent and associated with long seizure history 'often even from childhood'. The lesions herein reported are similar, and no patient in the group has died (Table 10.2).

(d) Meningioma

There were two patients with neoplastic proliferations of arachnoidal cap cells; both were remarkable. One is a 23-year-old college student who prior to surgery suffered seizures for ten years. He was struck on the head with a 'stickball' at the age of 11 and rendered unconscious. At the age of 13 he began

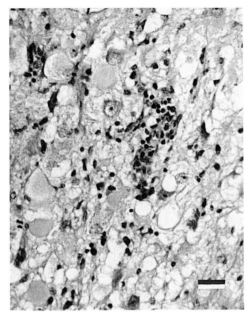

Figure 10.11 Masses of well-differentiated ganglion cells in compact masses mixed with well-differentiated astrocytes. The dark cells in the centre are a small group of lymphocytes. This ganglioglioma occupied the anterior pole of a resected temporal lobe. The patient is alive and seizure free 25 years after surgery. Calibration bar 33 μm.

to have brief episodes of nausea and light headedness at school two to three times each week. The feelings lasted 20–30 s then evolved into confusion. These episodes were drug refractory. A unilateral EEG focus was found in the right temporal lobe. The lobe was resected and small collections of meningiomatous cells were found densely collected along numerous vessels penetrating the cortex of the middle temporal gyrus (Fig. 10.13). He has been seizure free

---

Figure 10.12 Masses of astrocytes, variably-shaped with focal anaplasia from temporal lobe largely composed of neoplasm, and similar to that of Figure 10.8. This section is from Case no. 2 (Table 10.2) who was irradiated after surgery. There has been only slight decrease in seizure incidence (Table 10.2), but of interest is the 17-year survival. Calibration bar 33 μm.

Figure 10.13 The middle gyrus houses a cortex which still contains some neurones, but has infiltration along the penetrating cortical vessels by small masses of proliferated arachnoidal cap cells and rare psamomma bodies. The lesion is sharply-defined and is limited to cortex. There is an underlying pallor of the myelin because many cortical neurones and associated processes are missing. The arrows indicate the extent of the lesion in the cortex. Calibration bar 1.0 cm.

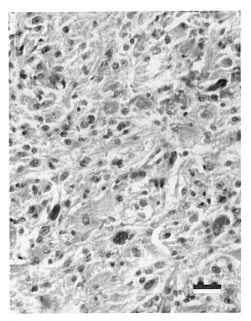

Fig. 10.12

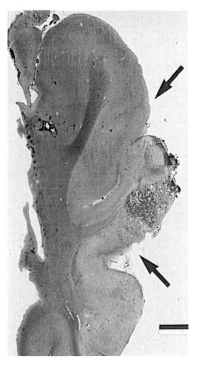

Fig. 10.13

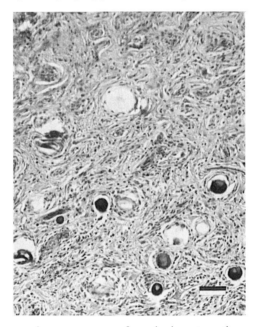

Figure 10.14 Microscopic appearances of meningiomatous tissue within the cortex. Note scattered psamomma bodies. This is typical of both cases of meningioma listed in Table 10.1. Calibration bar 80 μm.

for five years. The second in this group has a more complicated pathological substrate but has some similar features. This 24-year-old man began experiencing auras with the sense of a disgusting taste at the age of eight. Lip smacking accompanied the nausea and an occasional clonic episode. His CT scan was unremarkable, but PET scanning showed a hypometabolic focus in the right temporal lobe. Surgery was carried out, and meningeoangiomatosis similar to the previous case was found in the inferior gyrus and amygdala. Dysplastic changes in the form of tiny collections of glial cells and heterotypic neurones were found adjacent to the anterior hippocampus. Also found was mesial sclerosis with gliosis and neurone loss in regions CA4, CA3, parts of CA2, CA1 and the subiculum.

The neoplastic proliferation of arachnoidal cap cells in both instances penetrated into a short segment of cortex along with abnormal narrow vascular channels, forming a network of sequestered cortex and typical meningioma (Fig. 10.14).

(e) Lesions of injury and vascular occlusion
Cerebral cicatrization occurs as a result of 'healing' of damage due to ischaemic processes, laceration or contusion. Regeneration is not part of this process, and replacement of damaged cortex and white matter by gliosis and

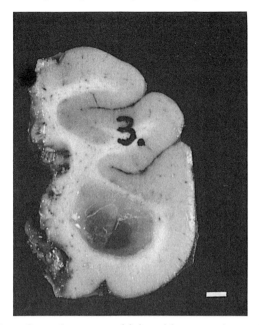

Figure 10.15 Section of anterior temporal lobe with traumatic cyst in inferior gyrus. Note smooth wall, few bridging glial strands. Nearby cortex is preserved even though many axons are obviously cut off by cysts. Calibration bar 1.0 cm.

fibrous scar is largely dependent upon an adequate regional circulation. As the proliferation of astrocytes goes on there is an obvious reorganization going on at the same rate, with residual neurones, dendrites and recurrent collateral axons. Injury induced by complete ischaemia of a part is usually replaced by a fluid-filled cyst as is illustrated by the following brief case history: a 25-year-old man relates that at an early age he suffered an injury to the head of an indeterminant nature. At the age of seven a craniotomy over the right frontal region disclosed a subdural hygroma which was drained. Later, after one and a half years at college, he began to have seizures; initially focal motor with secondary generalized seizures. It was determined that a seizure focus existed in the right temporal lobe. The pole was resected and its cross section is shown in Fig. 10.15. Notice there is preserved cortex surrounding a large glial lined cyst. Sections of the pia and cortex reveal preserved small penetrating cortical vessels stemming from the pia arachnoid. The cortical neuronal laminae in the resected cortex show residual neurones, increased glial cells and capillary profiles. The presumption is that the preserved ganglion cells constitute a hyperactive focus. In the above case seizures ceased after resection. Studies of scarred, contracted gyri of neocortex associated with complex partial or secondarily generalized seizures have been described in some detail by Penfield and Erickson [16].

10.2.2   Archicortex and limbic lobe

(a)   Hippocampal (Mesial) sclerosis

Earlier approaches to surgery of the temporal lobe were tempered by the requirement of either direct visualization of lesions or by dependence upon scalp EEG evidence of abnormality in temporal neocortex. Falconer [17] has pointed out that tissues of the region were largely removed by suction, thus many small subtle lesions such as heterotopia, dysplastic cortex, hamartoma, small scars and cysts were lost and the pathological spectrum not appreciated. Of greater significance, however, was that the mesial components of the limbic lobe and archicortex were left more or less intact in the brain. Penfield and Paine [18] recognized the implications of this when they had to reoperate on patients whose superficial resections of lateral cortex had failed to relieve seizures, but with more radical removal of amygdala, hippocampus and uncus dramatic relief of seizures was achieved. Falconer [19], Talairach and Bancaud [20] and Crandall [21] also reported alleviation of seizures with resections that included the hippocampus. Striking successes of 86%, 77% and 80% respectively are the strongest evidence that most epileptogenic foci responsible for complex partial seizures lie in the mesial structures of the temporal lobe.

As late as 1964 Falconer used criteria for selecting patients for temporal lobe removal that included the following: (1) seizures be frequent, of long history and intractable to drugs, (2) no radiological evidence of expanding lesion, and (3) repeated EEG studies employing on at least one occasion sphenoidal electrodes during intravenous sodium thiopentone narcosis to disclose a focus of spike discharges confined to one temporal lobe or, if bilateral, predominantly in the lobe to be resected. Thus, electrode implantation on a chronic basis was either circumvented or thought unnecessary and surgery was carried out once the criteria in (1), (2) and (3) were attained.

There is however a substantial possibility that complex partial seizures are not limited to limbic lobe origin. So to define more accurately epileptic hyperexcitable foci, Crandall *et al.* [1, 22] directly implanted bilateral chronic electrodes into mesial temporal lobe structures. Subsequent serial sections of such resected lobes have shown us that the electrode tracts, barring inadvertent infection, remained a narrow band of glial scar across the lateral aspect of the lobe to target tissues. Walter [23] has indicated that the unsuspected temporal lobe may be responsible for the seizures as often as 10% of the time when only scalp EEG is used for diagnosis. The determination of where to locate diagnostic electrodes is based primarily on the experience of individuals responsible for defining the pathological substrate in temporal lobe epilepsy.

It is curious that Bouchet and Cazauvieihl [5] are now receiving recognition a century and half after their description of induration of the hippocampus of patients with seizures associated with an aura, although they did not really attribute the peculiar mentation or prodroma in their patients to the hardening of mesial temporal structures. It is understandable therefore why, even though 65 years had passed, when Jackson and Coleman [24] published a detailed report of a physician with similar seizures, they also did not mention changes in the hippocampus. They did report the presence of a focus of infarction in the patient's uncinate gyrus. Stauder [7] once again called attention to the hippocampus by reporting that 91% of postmortem cases of hippocampal sclerosis which he had examined clinically had what we now term complex partial seizures. He further argued that the scarring of the hippocampus was most likely to be found with this type of seizure pattern. He additionally suggested that the *old lesion* might be the *cause* of the ictus instead of the *result of the seizures*. Though sclerosis of the mesial temporal lobe varies widely in its extent and severity [25] some form of it has been found in as high as 90% of lobes resected *en bloc* when the complex seizures have been preceded by an aura. Loss of neurones and focal gliosis have also been reported in the thalamus, amygdala and cerebellum in similar seizure patients [8]. We have not had the opportunity to examine thalamus and cerebellum in our large series of patients.

(b) Quantitative cytology

Though hippocampal sclerosis may be coupled to the recorded hyperexcitability in or near the damaged cortex, the microphysiological and anatomical mechanisms are not understood. We have therefore conducted a series of studies designed to test several hypotheses of the morphological and cytochemical basis of seizure genesis in this altered archicortex.

There have been reports of regional sparing of CA2 neurones in hippocampal sclerosis but there has not been any systematic study of the extent of the damage throughout the hippocampus. We have attempted to define the anterior to posterior distribution of the neurone loss or preservation in this cortex and to relate such findings to both epileptogenesis and favourable or unfavourable outcome following surgical removal of the offending temporal lobe. Depicted in Fig. 10.16 are two examples of hippocampal sclerosis, each of which had different clinical outcomes related to their removal (see below). In one case the damage or loss of neurones and glial scarring is largely confined to the *anterior* segment of the hippocampus (Fig. 10.16(a)). Arranged side by side in the montage is a picture of the posterior hippocampal segment revealing preservation of many neurones in regions of the *posterior* cornu ammonis, especially the prosubiculum (Sommer's sector: arrow) but also including subiculum, fascia dentata, and hippocampus proper (Fig. 10.16(a) Post.). Such patients were shown to have focal interictal spike activity and focal *anterior* seizure onsets in the damaged *anterior* segment [26, 27]. By contrast, in these same patients, the posterior portion appeared cytologically similar to control hippocampi (i.e. no significant cell loss posteriorly). Control hippocampi were from non-neurological cases roughly matched for age [26, 27]. The counting procedures in general were similar to those used by Mouritzen-Dam

Ant   Post

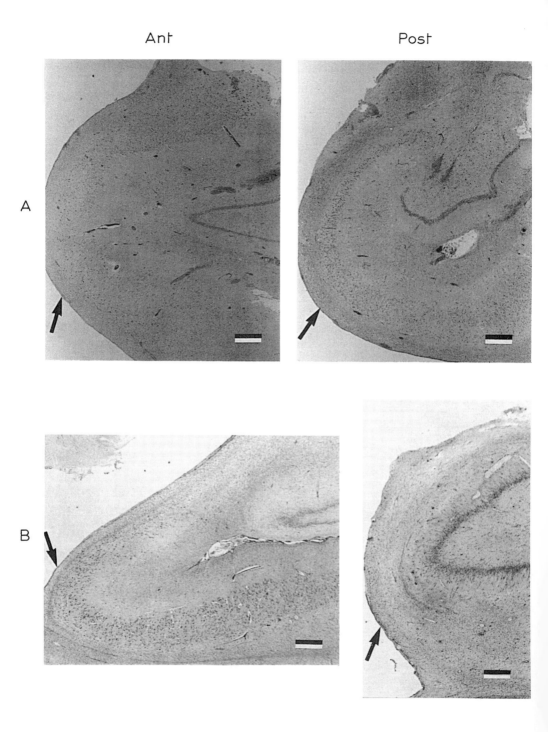

A

B

[28]. Abercrombie's [29] corrections were made for section thicknesses and edge-counting errors.

When damage is largely confined to the anterior segment, resection of the temporal lobe results in either cessation of seizures or a reduction to as few as two or less a year in a four year follow-up period. Such epilepsy we have termed 'primary' temporal lobe epilepsy (i.e. the disease appears clinically cured with resection of this anterior focus). The second set (B) of photographs in Fig. 10.16 shows loss of neurones from the *posterior* segment of hippocampus. Examples of these types of hippocampi may have more neurones in the anterior segment than in posterior hippocampus. For instance, comparison of Sommer's sectors in (B), anterior versus posterior reveals significantly more neurones (arrow) anteriorly and mostly only gliosis (arrow) posteriorly. Further, when widespread spike discharges and regional EEG seizure onsets were found throughout the hippocampus, such cortices were shown to have decreased pyramidal cell densities *both anteriorly* and *posteriorly*. Patients with this type of diffuse injury do not achieve full seizure relief from anterior temporal lobectomy [26, 27].

The question must be asked is there any further information to be gained from examination of regional hippocampal neurone loss, for example, the neurone population of CA3 versus subiculum or CA4? It is well known that Sommer's sector [6], which is largely prosubiculum, is a multilayered pyramidal cortex and is most sensitive to 'the initiating injury'. Edges of this region are really merged into CA1 wherein pyramidal cells appear non-layered. Detailed plots of this and other spatial neurone loss distribution are given in Babb *et al.* [26]. In essence these curves show loss of cells from all regions of cornu ammonis, especially prosubiculum; however in subiculum and presubiculum the loss is not statistically different from control normal brain. Region CA2 was found to have lost slightly fewer cells than other hippocampal regions; however it is none the less *significantly* more damaged than control CA2.

Figure 10.16 (A) Ant: Cross section through anterior hippocampus (Ant) which shows a small segment of fascia dentata (FD), region CA1 and prosubiculum (arrow) which are gliotic (sclerotic). The subiculum and presubiculum have the usual complement of neurones. The most severe involvement is seen in CA1 and prosubiculum (arrow). Resection of this damaged anterior segment cures complex partial seizures. (A) Post: Section through same hippocampus but more posteriorly situated shows CA1, prosubiculum and subiculum to be virtually intact, that is with very little cell loss. (B) Ant: Cross section of anterior (Ant) hippocampus in which neuronal loss is mild in CA1 and prosubiculum (arrow). No cell loss in subiculum and presubiculum. (B) Post: Similar section but more posterior locus reflecting diffuse loss of cells through hippocampus. Fascia dentata is evident as the dense curved line, but other regions are almost devoid of neurones and gliosis is profuse. Such patients do not achieve full seizure relief with resection of anterior temporal lobe. All calibration bars 0.5 mm.

The lateral six-layered temporal cortex, including middle, inferior, fusiform and parahippocampal cortices, in lobes in which hippocampal sclerosis was present, revealed no significant neurone loss [26]. Moreover, neurone densities in hippocampus were not found to be significantly reduced when seizures were initiated by the presence of extrahippocampal lesions such as neoplasms, hamartoma, heterotopia and traumatic cysts, unless the lesion intruded into the hippocampus. There was slight hippocampal neurone loss in such cases, which although not statistically significant, deserves mention and further correlations.

(c) Quantitation of Golgi impregnated neurones

Since it is evident that the neurone population is absolutely decreased in hippocampal sclerosis (Fig. 10.6(a), (b)) there is the implication that connectivity might also be defective. Utilizing the Golgi-Cox reduced silver technique [30] we have routinely examined this aspect of lateral temporal neocortex and neurones of both controls (autopsy and normal subhuman primates) and epileptic hippocampal neurones. Camera lucida drawings were made, for example, of well impregnated pyramidal cells of both conditions in area CA2. In controls, basilar dendrites have numerous spines (Fig. 10.17) with primary apical dendrites and secondary dendrites with spinous branches rising almost directly from the pyramidal cell soma. Measurement of the mean length from the soma to first apical branch in 11 control neurones amounted to 16.5 μm (Fig. 10.17). We have found this same segment of neurone (i.e. the length of apical dendrite from soma to primary branch) from region CA2 in epileptic hippocampus to be two times as long as in controls (Fig. 10.17). The extended apical dendrites denuded of spines were very possibly reinnervated by inhibitory axosomatic synapses commonly found on the nearby pyramidal cell soma. These sprouted inhibitory synapses could cause the increased inhibition that may augment synchronous hippocampal rebound excitement. Both distal dendrite branches and associated spinous sites of excitatory input are *decreased* in epileptic neurones (Fig. 10.17). Does this mean that excitatory inputs to these neurones are less effective? Not necessarily. An alternative view may be that seizures can only be developed by matching coincident firing of neurones over a high threshold [31].

(d) Cytochemical studies of sclerotic cornu ammonis

Ammon's horn pyramidal cells are apparently not seizure-sensitive because of a lack of GABA-mediated recurrent inhibitory input synapses (Fig. 10.18). Rather they appear to have normal or even enhanced recurrent inhibition in the midst of decreased pyramidal output cells. Such recurrent inhibition may paradoxically enhance the synchrony of membrane potentials at a firing theshold and rebound excitation might cause synchronous firing of hippocampal pyramidal cells which are instrumental in recruiting the spared presubicular neurones. The presubicular cortex we have shown above and in

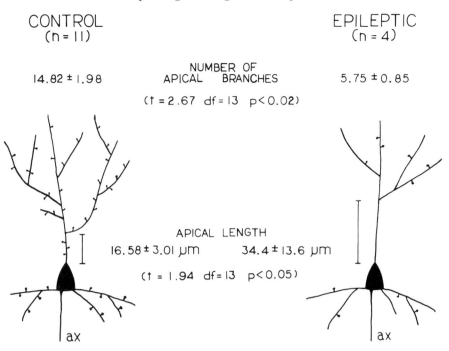

CONTROL
(n = 11)

EPILEPTIC
(n = 4)

NUMBER OF
APICAL BRANCHES

14.82 ± 1.98

5.75 ± 0.85

(t = 2.67 df = 13 p < 0.02)

APICAL LENGTH

16.58 ± 3.01 μm   34.4 ± 13.6 μm

(t = 1.94 df = 13 p < 0.05)

Figure 10.17 This stick drawing is made to scale after examining a series of camera lucida drawings of Golgi impregnations. Compare the lack of spines on receptor dendrites in 'epileptic' neurone with control. Note an apparent elongation as much as two times that of control apical dendrite. This elongated segment is either prone to be enwrapped and insulated by glial slips or serves as sites for plastic reinnervation by somal excitatory or inhibitory boutons. Statistical test outcomes are printed on the illustration after Golgi-Cox preparations measurements.

Babb *et al.* [26] to be either similar to controls or minimally damaged according to quantitative neurone counts of various parts of the hippocampal formation. In Babb and Brown [31] we have further suggested that the presubiculum with its greater population of pyramidal cells which are monosynaptically-driven by hippocampal pyramids would very likely increase seizure spread from presubicular cortex to temporal neocortex or to amygdala. To relate these physiological data to a possible loss of hippocampal inhibition we have quantified GABA interneurones and terminals as revealed by the immunocytochemical localization of the enzyme glutamic acid decarboxylose (GAD), which is the synthesizing enzyme for the inhibitory transmitter GABA. The GAD antibody obtained from Kopin [32] and an avidin–biotin complex conjugated with horeseradish peroxidase [33] were applied to 24 sclerotic human hippocampi and to control monkey hippocampi. In control monkey and rat tissues, counts of GAD positive cells were similar and, even of greater interest, were *not significantly greater* than GAD positive cells in human

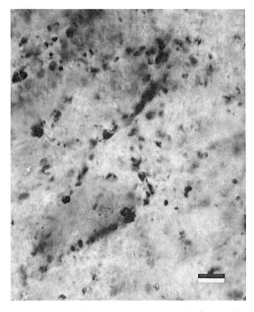

Figure 10.18 Photomicrograph of immunocytochemical reactions of the enzyme glutamic acid decarboxylase (GAD) showing inhibitory boutons (black spots) on pyramidal cell bodies of cornu ammonis. Calibration bar 7.0 μm.

human sclerotic hippocampal subfields, except in region CA3 where there was a 50% GAD positive cell loss [31]. However, in CA3 there was a 70% loss of pyramidal output cells, which indicates that there was not a significant, preferential loss of inhibition in this cortex which might account for hippocampal hyperexcitability and seizure genesis. Normal GAD positive cell densities were present in the presubiculum of the seizure patients as were the pyramidal cell densities. These results, then, suggest very strongly that the concept of 'disinhibition' as a seizure mechanism does not apply to human hippocampal focal seizures.

(e)   Ultrastructural studies
High resolution visualization of inhibitory pyramidal cell soma boutons and excitatory synapses on receptor dendrites of controls and of epileptic cortex was accomplished by electron microscopy. Cross sections of 2 mm of fresh human epileptic and non-sclerotic hippocampus were made with cleaned razor blades directly from *en bloc* temporal lobe resections and then placed in cold Karnovsky aldehyde fixative. After 12 hours, tissues were washed an additional 12 hours with cold 0.125 M phosphate buffer. The entire slice of hippocampus was examined under buffer with a dissecting microscope. Blocks were cut in such a way that a map of the hippocampal cross section could be reconstructed from toluidine blue stained epon-embedded sections.

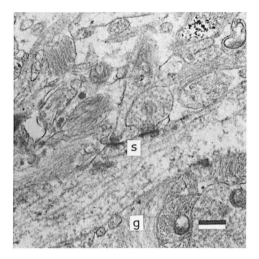

Figure 10.19 Electron micrograph of sclerotic CA2 dendritic region (stratum radiatum) in epileptic hippocampus. Note the dendrite and excitory synapse (s); however glial slips (g) are evident covering much of the dendritic surface. Calibration bar 500 nm.

Photographs were made, and thin sections were doubly-stained with Pb and Ur. Montages were made of serial micrographs using slotted grids so that the entire profile of the neurone could be examined and photographed. Selected segments of cell membranes were also studied with higher magnification to ascertain the extent of glial replacement of recurrent inhibitory synapses on cell somata and possible insulation of asymmetrical excitatory synapses on receptor dendrites (Fig. 10.19).

Ribak *et al.* [34] have reported glial sheathing interspersed between inhibitory symmetrical synapses in neocortex altered by use of alumina gel in monkeys. Ribak *et al.* [34] also suggested that this condition would reduce cortical inhibition and contribute to seizure genesis. Their examination of excitatory synapses further indicated that such glial sheathing on 'epileptic' excitatory synapse receptor sites was also statistically significantly less than that found outside of the epileptic regions. Nevertheless they chose to emphasize decreased inhibitory synaptic function as the cause of alumina-induced focal seizures.

In our preliminary evaluation of synaptic profiles in human epileptic hippocampus, we have found glial sheaths on both pyramidal somata and dendrites. At regions adjacent to these glial fibrils we have found intact, normal-appearing axosomatic and axodendritic synapses. Hence, until we perform more quantitative measures of synapse densities in epileptic versus non-epileptic human hippocampus, we cannot conclude that either inhibition or excitation is significantly altered by glial sheathing. We have such studies underway.

We have not found good evidence of pyramidal neurone loss as a result of complex partial seizures [26]. Uncontrolled tonic-clonic attacks, however, with possible cardiac arrythmia and/or intermittent pulmonary insufficiency are another matter. In complex partial seizures, however, it is known that territorial blood flow in the temporal lobe is actually increased [35, 36]. Despite the increased blood flow and oxygen supply, nutrition can be interfered with in another way. For instance it is possible that the basal lamina of capillaries or the ATP production mechanism of endothelial cells are altered by the presence of attendant gliosis. Accordingly a quantitative and systematic study of the microcirculation in sclerotic and normal hippocampal cortex was carried out. Kasantikul *et al.* [37] found that the basal lamina in sclerotic cortex is three times thicker, and complicated perithelial cells and membranes surround such lamina. In normal hippocampal cortex the basal lamina of capillaries in area CA2 are more delicate than other capillaries. Moreover, with sclerosis the basal lamina of these CA2 capillaries participate to a lesser extent in the sclerosis, which may be in part the basis for a relative 'preservation' of CA2 pyramids compared to other hippocampal pyramids. Furthermore, such capillary endothelia have a reduced mitochondrial population which could seriously compromise this important segment of the blood–brain barrier mechanism thereby altering transport and modifying [K^+] and other ionic levels in and near preserved pyramidal cells. Such perturbations may contribute to either uncontrolled pyramidal cell excitement or interfere with pyramidal cell nutrition despite local increased blood flow and oxygen levels.

10.2.3 Summary and conclusions

One hundred and fourteen unselected patients with drug refractory complex partial seizures were studied by use of chronic indwelling electrodes. Followed by *en bloc* resection of temporal lobes, we analysed lesions of the temporal neocortex and the archicortex. The former included a spectrum of neoplasm, hamartoma, heterotopia, meningioma and traumatic cysts, which are detailed in Tables 10.1 and 10.2. There is an uncommon indolence apparent in the biological activity of the glial neoplasms in these tissues, and all patients are still alive, as long as 25 years after resection of gliomata.

Lesions of the archicortex were largely confined to gliosis or scarring of mesial limbic structures. The majority of patients (64%) fit into this category of central injury. Analysis of the hippocampus in such patients by quantitative microanatomical techniques links anterior hippocampal damage to anterior seizure genesis. In the posterior segment, pyramidal cell densities were often normal or minimally altered. Synaptic reorganizations in the remaining cells are apparently necessary for development of seizure-prone hippocampus to initiate complex partial seizures. Removal of the anterior temporal lobe in this condition gives good seizure relief; whereas should the neurone loss in cornu ammonis be evident over a wide distribution (i.e. to include posterior parts), then seizure relief on resection is variable or ineffective. The cell loss and gliosis in cornu ammonis is probably of early origin because we have not encountered neurone loss from any part of the lateral temporal neocortex unless lesions such as meningioma or hamartoma are immediately adjacent.

When generalized tonic-clonic seizures or episodes of status epilepticus are characteristics of the epilepsy, it is reasonable to point to pulmonary insufficiency and/or cardiac arrhythmias as factors contributing to the neurone loss in hippocampus and in various parts of the cerebral cortex or cerebellum. But with complex partial seizures these severe conditions are not part of the seizure continuum; hence it is reasonable to consider that the damage in the archicortex that signals a seizure-sensitive cortex has been induced earlier and is a continuing process only on a non-specific cell by cell basis. More important is the probability that reorganization or plastic development of new but incomplete or abnormal circuits associated with the subicular complex and thence the hippocampal gyrus generates frequent interictal spikes and focal onsets of seizures.

We have shown an absolute decrease in neurone population in hippocampal sclerosis which implies that the cells' connections are also either absent or defective since some neurones do indeed persist in various patterns in hippocampal cortex and other parts of archicortex. Using Golgi-impregnated neurones from these cortices we have studied their geometric patterns by use of computerized planimetry. In the preceding text we have presented two stylized CA2 region neurones composed from numerous camera lucida drawings of such pyramidal cells. One is from normal cortex and the comparison from epileptic cortex. Some features of reorganization are shown. The epileptic neurones have longer apical dendrites which have no spinous processes and therefore have receptor surfaces available for reinnervation by either local excitatory or inhibitory fibres.

Electron microscopic examination of postsynaptic sites along pyramidal cell soma, apical dendrites and presynaptic axodendritic profiles in stratum radiatum of region CA2, indicates that glial profiles have partially insulated these transmitter sites. Quantitation with electron microscopic preparations is time consuming and results thus far are only suggestive of the concept that there may be loss of both inhibition and excitation in these residual neurones.

The use of GAD immunocytochemistry preparations has thus far supported the idea that ample recurrent inhibitory synaptic input exists in archicortex (hippocampus), the subiculum and presubiculum. The failure to demonstrate a deficiency in such inhibition in this cortex supports conclusions from physiological data that recurrent inhibition may be followed by rebound excitation, which may synchronize neurone firing and generate seizures focally. Quantitation of inhibitory boutons on regions of cornu ammonis and subiculum is presently ongoing. The results will be useful to establish the actual inhibitory bouton population of normal cornu ammonis and subicular neurones and their variance when compared with epileptic cortex.

The possibility of deficiencies in transport dynamics across the blood–brain barrier locally in hippocampus is evident in the thickened basal laminae of microvasculature, increased perithelial cells and their membranes along with decreased endothelial cell mitochondrial area. The latter may be critical in furnishing energy for stabilization of the local ionic milieu of hippocampal neurones.

Acknowledgements

The authors are indebted to the superb neurosurgical techniques of Dr Paul Crandall and Dr Les Cahan who provided *en bloc* temporal lobectomies. Expert tissue processing and photomicrography was provided by Jim Pretorius, Margaret Hall, Marianne Akers, Steve Kaufman and Bill Kupfer. We are especially thankful to all the members of the Clinical Neurophysiology Project (NS02808) for the physiological and clinical data used to interpret our anatomical studies. Special thanks are given to Teresa Osiecki, Gloria Picerno and Katy Kelly, who typed this section.

References

1. Crandall, P. H., Walter, R. D. and Dymond, A. (1971) The ictal electroencephalographic signal identifying limbic system seizure foci. *Proc. Am. Assoc. Neurol. Surg.*, **1**, 1–9.
2. Lieb, J., Walsh, G. O., Babb, T. L. *et al.* (1976) A comparison of EEG seizure patterns recorded with surface and depth electrodes in patients with temporal lobe epilepsy. *Epilepsia*, **17**, 137–50.
3. Lieb, J., Engel, J., Gevins, A. and Crandall, P. H. (1981) Surface and deep EEG correlates of surgical outcome in temporal lobe epilepsy. *Epilepsia*, **22**, 515–38.
4. Babb, T. and Crandall, P. H. (1976) Epileptogenesis of human limbic neurons in psychomotor epileptics. *Electroenceph. Clin. Neurophysiol.*, **40**, 225–43.
5. Bouchet and Cazauvieihl, Y. (1825) De l'epilepsie consideree dans ses rapports avec l'alienation mentale. Recherche sur la nature et le siege de ces deux maladies; memiore qui a remporte le prix au concours establi par M. Esquirol. *Arch. Gen. Med.*, **9**, 510–42.
6. Sommer, W. (1880) Erkrankung des ammonshorns als aetiologisches Moment der Epilepsie. *Arch. Psychiatr. Nervenkr.*, **10**, 631–75.
7. Stauder, K. H. (1936) Epilepsie und Schlafenlappen. *Arch. Psychiatr. Nervenkr.*, **104**, 181–212.
8. Falconer, M. A. and Cavanagh, J. B. (1959) Clinico-pathological considerations of temporal lobe epilepsy due to small focal lesions. *Brain*, **82**, 483–504.
9. Margerison, J. H. and Corsellis, J. (1966) Epilepsy and the temporal lobes. *Brain*, **89**, 499–530.
10. Brown, W. J. 1973) Structural substrates of seizure foci in the human temporal lobe, in *Epilepsy: Its Phenomena in Man* (ed. M. A. B. Brazier), Academic Press, New York, pp. 339–74.
11. Mathieson, G. (1975) Pathology of the temporal lobe, in *Complex Partial Seizures and*

their Treatment (eds J. K. Penry and D. D. Daly), Raven Press, New York, pp. 163–86.

12. Cavanagh, J. B. (1958) 'On certain small tumours encountered in the temporal lobe'. *Brain*, **81**, 389–404.

13. Treip, S. C. (1962) 'Focal lesions in temporal lobe epilepsy', in *Proceedings of the Fourth International Congress for Neuropathology*, George Theime Verlag, Stuttgart, pp. 394–7.

14. Willis, R. A. (1962) *The Borderland of Embryology and Pathology*, 2nd edn, Butterworth and Co. Ltd., London, pp. 351–92.

15. Falconer, M. A., Serafetinides, E. A. and Corsellis, J. A. N. (1964) Etiology and pathogenesis of temporal lobe epilepsy. *Arch. Neurol.*, **10**, 233–48.

16. Penfield, W. and Erickson, T. C. (1941) *Epilepsy and Cerebral Localization*, C. C. Thomas, Springfield, pp. 240–79.

17. Falconer, M. A. (1968) The significance of mesial temporal sclerosis (Ammon's Horn Sclerosis) in epilepsy. *Guy's Hosp. Reports*, **117**, No. 1, 1–12.

18. Penfield, W. and Paine, K. (1955) Results of surgical therapy for focal epileptic seizures. *Canad. Med. Assoc. J.*, **73**, 515–31.

19. Falconer, M. A, Hill, D., Meyer, A. *et al.* (1955) Treatment of temporal-lobe epilepsy by temporal lobectomy. A survey of findings and results. *Lancet*, **i**, 827–35.

20. Talairach, J. and Bancaud, J. (1974) Stereotaxic exploration and therapy in epilepsy, in *The Epilepsies (Handbook of Clinical Neurology*, Vol. 15) (eds P. J. Vinken and C. W. Bruyn), North Holland, Amsterdam, pp. 758–82.

21. Crandall, P. H. (1975) Postoperative management and criteria for evaluations, in *Neurosurgical Management of the Epilepsies* (eds Purpura *et al.*) Raven Press, New York, pp. 265–80.

22. Crandall, P. H., Walter, R. D. and Rand, R. W. (1963) Clinical applications of studies on stereotactically implanted electrodes in temporal lobe epilepsy. *J. Neurosurg.*, **20**, 827–40.

23. Walter, R. D. (1973) Tactical considerations leading to surgical treatment of epilepsy, in *Epilepsy: Its Phenomenon in Man* (ed. M. A. B. Brazier), Academic Press, New York & London, pp. 99–199.

24. Jackson, J. H. and Coleman, W. S. (1898) Case of epilepsy with tasting movements and 'dreamy state' – very small patch of softening in the left uncinate gyrus. *Brain*, **21**, 580.

25. Spielmeyer, W. (1927) Die pathogenese des epileptischen Krampfes. *Zeitschrift Neurol. Psychiatr.*, **109**, 501–20.

26. Babb, T. L., Brown, W. J., Pretorius, J. *et al.* (1984) Temporal lobe volumetric cell densities in temporal lobe epilepsy. *Epilepsia*, **25**(6), 729–40.

27. Babb, T. L., Lieb, J. P., Brown, W. J. *et al.* (1984) Distribution of pyramidal cell density and hyperexcitability in the epileptic human hippocampal formation. *Epilepsia*, **25**(6), 721–8.

28. Mouritzen-Dam, A. (1979) The density of neurons in the human hippocampus. *Neuropathol. Appl. Neurobiol*, **5**, 249–64.

29. Abercrombie, M. (1946) Estimation of nuclear population from micotome sections. *Anat. Rec.*, **94**, 239–47.

30. Lorente de No., R. (1934) Studies on the structure of the cerebral cortex. II. Continuation of the study of the Ammonic system. *J. Psychol. Neurol.*, **46**, 113–77.

31. Babb, T. L. and Brown, W. J. (1986) Neuronal, dendritic and vascular profiles of

human temporal lobe epilepsy correlated with cellular physiology *in vivo*, in *Basic Mechanisms of the Epilepsies* (*Advances in Neurology*, Vol. 44) (eds A. V. Delgado-Escueta *et al.*), Raven Press, New York, pp. 949–66.

32. Oertel, W. H., Schmechel, D. E., Mugnaini, E. *et al.* (1981) Immunocytochemical localization of glutamate decarboxylose in rat cerebellum with antiserum. *Neuroscience*, **6**, 2715–35.

33. Hsu, S. M., Raine, L. and Fanger, H. (1981) The use of avidin biotin-peroxidase complex (ABC) in immunoperoxidase techniques: A comparison betwen ABC and unlabelled antibody (PAP) procedures. *J. Histochem. Cytochem.*, **29**, 577–80.

34. Ribak, C. E., Bradburne, R. M. and Harris, A. B. (1982) A preferential loss of GABA-ergic symmetric synapses in epileptic foci: A quantitative ultrastructural analysis of monkey neocortex. *J. Neurosci.*, **2**, 1725–35.

35. Dymond, A. M. and Crandall, P. H. (1973) Intracerebral temperature changes in patients during spontaneous epileptic seizures. *Brain Res.*, **60**, 249–54.

36. Dymond, A. M. and Crandall, P. H. (1976) Oxygen availability and blood flow in temporal lobes during spontaneous epileptic seizures in man. *Brain Res.*, **102**, 191–6.

37. Kasantikul, V., Brown, W. J., Oldendorf, W. H. and Crandall, P. H. (1983) Ultrastructural parameters and limbic microvasculature in human psychomotor epilepsy. *Clin. Neuropath.*, **2**, 171–8.

10.3   OTHER TYPES OF OPERATION PERFORMED FOR THE RELIEF OF INTRACTABLE EPILEPSY

Anthony Hopkins

10.3.1   Focal cortical excision

By far the greatest number of operations for epilepsy are on the temporal lobe, but the Montreal group have an unrivalled experience of local excision of epileptogenic foci in other areas of the brain [1, 2]. Most of the Montreal experience is on frontal lesions, commonly cicatricial lesions secondary to birth trauma or inflammation. Tumours accounted for 28% of the experience published in 1975 [1], but the surgical procedure was primarily for control of epilepsy rather than the tumour. The results of cortical excision are less good than for temporal lobectomy, but 23% of patients without tumours became free from seizures, and a further 32% showed a marked reduction in seizure frequency. Similar results prevail after surgery for epileptogenic lesions in the central sensori-motor regions [2]. Considerable experience is necessary to decide how much brain can be removed without an unacceptable deficit resulting.

10.3.2   Hemispherectomy

Children with infantile hemiplegia due to birth injury or infarction in early childhood may have intractable seizures arising from the damaged hemisphere. The motor disability may be such that no further physical handicap is caused by removal of the damaged hemisphere. Indeed, in addition to seizure control, there may be striking improvements in behaviour and cognitive development, and in the spasticity of the affected limbs. Unfortunately, recurrent minor bleeding into the large postoperative cavity is associated with a high late postoperative mortality from either the effects of an acute bleed, or obstructive hydrocephalus. Adams [3] has reviewed the surgical procedures whereby these risks can be minimized – by creating a large extradural space at the expense of the subdural space, and by occluding the ipsilateral foramen of Monro by a plug of muscle to isolate the subdural cavity from the ventricular system. An alternative is to remove only part of the hemisphere, but the control of seizures is less good, as some seizure foci remain.

10.3.3   Stereotactic procedures

Stereotactic amygdalotomy (p. 293) is occasionally used in the surgical management of epilepsy, but SEEG recordings show that epileptogenic activity confined to the amygdala is uncommon.

There are reports of a number of stereotactically placed deep white matter lesions, designed to prevent the propagation of seizure discharged far from their site of origin. Targets have included the thalamic nuclei, the internal capsule and the field of Forel. The results have, on the whole, been disappointing.

10.3.4   Division of the corpus callosum

Spread of seizure discharges from one hemisphere to another can take place across the commissures, of which the corpus callosum is of course the largest. Two series [4, 5] reach much the same conclusions about the type of seizure discharge that is likely to be best halted by callosotomy. Rayport and colleagues [4] noted that where preoperative seizure monitoring showed seizures beginning locally, then after callostomy, seizure manifestations could become confined to one hemisphere, an improvement even if seizure frequency remained unchanged. Geoffroy and colleagues [5], operating upon children, noted that those who improved most were those who showed lateralized epileptic discharges with secondary generalization. Children with multifocal or diffuse abnormalities showed little or no improvement.

The results of Geoffroy and colleagues were sufficiently good, in terms of motor and psychological improvement, as well as in some relief of seizures, that they suggest that the operation should be carried out relatively early, even in cases with severe mental deficiency, in order to prevent aggravation of the epilepsy and to facilitate rehabilitation.

There are, however, drawbacks. The Yale group have reported that some patients experience 'more intense' focal seizures after callosal section [6]. In this paper, Spencer and colleagues review the experimental evidence on callosally mediated inhibition in animal models of epilepsy. From this review, Spencer and colleagues suggest that patients with strictly unilateral or strictly homotopic foci would not experience intensification of seizures after callosal section, whereas asymmetric bilateral foci, particularly if one or both were frontal, might well be facilitated by subcortical structures after callosal section.

Other drawbacks to callosal section are the neuropsychological results of hemispheric disconnection [13]. A striking example is quoted by Rayport and colleagues [4]. A woman dressing – 'I open the closet door. I know what I want to wear. As I reach for something with my right hand, my left comes up and takes something different. I can't put it down if it's in my left hand. I have to call my daughter.' Ferrell and colleagues however found that such disconnection syndromes were usually transient [7]. These authors also give useful ethical guidelines to be followed before advising surgery.

10.3.5   Cerebellar stimulation

Stimulation of the cerebellum in some animal models of epilepsy suppresses seizures ([8] for references). In the 1970s several groups, led by Cooper [9] implanted electrodes for chronic stimulation and seizure suppression in a number of patients with intractable epilepsy. Some reports continued to be enthusiastic (e.g. [10]), but most neurologists believe that insufficient attention has been paid by neurosurgeons to the variable course of epilepsy, with partial remissions occurring under intensive investigation and management of whatever type [11]. One small controlled trial with seizure counts during periods of stimulation and no stimulation (although the electrodes remained in place) showed no objectively measurable benefit [12]. Some of the difficulties in assessment are underlined in this trial by the fact that 11 out of the 12 patients subjectively considered that the trial had helped them.

References

1. Rasmussen, T. (1975) Surgery of frontal lobe epilepsy, in *Neurosurgical Management of the Epilepsies* (*Advances in Neurology*, Vol. 8) (eds D. P. Purpura, J. K. Penry and R. D. Walter) Raven Press, New York, pp. 197–205.
2. Rasmussen, T. (1975) Cortical resection for epilepsy arising in regions other than the temporal or frontal lobes, in *Neurosurgical Management of the Epilepsies* (*Advances in Neurology*, Vol. 8) (eds D. P. Purpura, J. K. Penry and R. D. Walter), Raven Press, New York, pp. 207–26.
3. Adams, C. T. B. (1983) Hemispherectomy – a modification. *J. Neurol. Neurosurg. Psychiatr.*, **46**, 617–19.
4. Rayport, M., Ferguson, S. M. and Corrie, W. S. (1983) Outcomes and indications of corpus callosum section for intractable seizure control. *Appl. Neurophysiol.*, **46**, 47–51.
5. Geoffroy, G., Lassonde, M., Delisle, F. and Décarie, M. (1983) Corpus callosotomy for control of intractable epilepsy in children. *Neurology*, **33**, 891–7.

6. Spencer, S. S., Spencer, D. D., Glaser, G. H. *et al.* (1984) More intense focal seizure types after callosal section: the role of inhibition. *Ann. Neurol.*, **16**, 686–93.

7. Ferrell, R. B., Culver, C. M. and Tucker, G. J. (1983) Psychosocial and cognitive function after commissurotomy for intractable seizures. *J. Neurosurg.*, **58**, 374–80.

8. Editorial (1983) Epilepsy, the cerebellum and cerebellar stimulation. *Lancet*, **ii**, 1122–3.

9. Cooper, I. S. (1973) Effect of chronic stimulation of anterior cerebellum on neurological disease. *Lancet*, **i**, 206.

10. Davis, R., Gray, E., Engle, H. and Dusnak, A. (1983) Reduction of intractable seizures using cerebellar stimulation. *Appl. Neurophysiol.*, **46**, 57–61.

11. Sutula, T., Sackellares, J. C., Miller, J. Q. and Dreifuss, F. E. (1981) Efficacy of intensive monitoring and prolonged hospitalisation in refractory epilepsy. *Neurology*, **31**, 243–7.

12. Wright, G. O. S., McLellan, D. L. and Brice, J. G. (1984) A double-blind trial of chronic cerebellar stimulation in twelve patients with severe epilepsy. *J. Neurol. Neurosurg. Psychiatr.*, **47**, 769–74.

13. Reeves, A. G. (1987) Epilepsy and the corpus callosum. Plenum Press, New York.

10.4 AVOIDANCE OF FACTORS THAT INDUCE OR PRECIPITATE SEIZURES

Anthony Hopkins

Many patients themselves identify factors that they believe precipitate seizures. The most clearly defined precipitants are the reflex epilepsies, such as reading epilepsy or musicogenic epilepsy, reviewed on pp. 129–31. Aird [1] distinguishes 'precipitating' or 'triggering' physiological factors such as these from 'inducing factors', in which he includes environmental and endogenous factors that lower seizure threshold. In Aird's study of 500 patients with epilepsy refractory to anticonvulsant treatment, it was found that 'intense emotional reactions' were the most common inducing factors reported by the patients. As Aird points out, the solution or amelioration of personal problems inducing tension depends largely upon the patient, but the neurologist can help by analysing the problem and 'marshalling the forces of constructive support'. It is difficult to know how much any reduction in seizure frequency is due to the effects of increased medical attention improving drug compliance. Furthermore, spontaneous fluctuations in seizure frequency are insufficiently recognized [2], so that increases or decreases in seizure frequency are falsely attributed to changes in life circumstance. Nevertheless, as the next section shows, belief in the unfavourable effects of tension and anxiety is sufficient to encourage psychological intervention as a form of treatment.

It is often difficult to modify the amount of 'tension' in life experienced by a patient, but there are clearly other avoidable factors that induce or precipitate seizures. Most important of these are avoidance of sleep deprivation (p. 126), of excessive fluid intake, and of drugs known to lower seizure threshold (p. 127).

References

1. Aird, R. B. (1983) The importance of seizure-inducing factors in the control of refractory forms of epilepsy. *Epilepsia*, **24**, 567–83.
2. Hopkins, A., Davies, P. and Dobson, G. (1985) Mathematical modelling of patterns of individuals between seizures. *Arch. Neurol.*, **42**, 463–67.

10.5 PSYCHOLOGICAL TREATMENTS

Stephen W. Brown

Opinions about the genesis of individual seizures have consequences for predictions about the outcome of behavioural or psychological intervention. One view stresses the influence of incidental traffic through pools of partially deafferented neurones; another view contends that seizure genesis reflects an unspecified process which builds up until a seizure discharge occurs. In the first view behavioural or psychological interventions may alter incidental traffic and abort seizure onset; in the second, it would be contended that such actions may possibly postpone onset but in all likelihood would have no effect on eventual seizure frequency.

10.5.1 Theoretical background

Current models of epilepsy describe the relationship between abnormal pools of neurones from which the seizure arises and normal brain. Various workers [1–4] have studied cellular changes which occur in an alumina gel epileptic focus produced in the cortex of monkeys. This model of seizure genesis relates directly to the relationship between pools of abnormal neurones within the focus, and the way that physiological events through their influence on such pools can provoke seizure activity. Two types of abnormal neurones are described which may take part in seizure activity. *Group one neurones* are found at the centre of the focus, and are damaged. They do not have an afferent input, and fire continually in a paroxysmal manner showing a high invariant Burst Index. They act as a 'pacemaker' for the epileptic discharge. *Group two neurones* provide a critical mass for the spread of seizure activity. They surround the focus of group one neurones, and are only partially deafferented. They may fire in either a normal or in an epileptic paroxysmal manner. Their activity is highly influenced by the animal's behavioural state. They have the ability to recruit normal neurones into an epileptic discharge, but they can also be synaptically suppressed. A *localized* seizure discharge occurs when group two neurones are recruited by group one neurones, and a *generalized* seizure discharge occurs when group two neurones recruit normal neurones surrounding the focus. Even if seizures may appear clinically to be generalized from the start, it is known that many arise from specific foci, often in the temporal lobe (pp. 10–11). This model shows that the level of activation in group two neurones and in the normal brain surrounding the focus can either inhibit or enhance seizure activity.

If the activity in pools of epileptogenic neurones can be modified by the animal's behaviour, then these same pools should be influenced by learning and conditioning procedures. Forster and colleagues [5] studied the conditioning of focal seizures induced through implanted stimulation electrodes in cats that had previous tetanus toxin lesions of the cortex. When a current was passed through these electrodes, the cat would have a focal seizure. This was the unconditioned stimulus. A conditioned stimulus, a light, was then paired with the unconditioned stimulus, brain stimulation, during the production of a focal fit. It was not possible to condition cats without tetanus lesions such that a light produced a fit. The conclusion was drawn that it is not possible to condition seizures in the undamaged brain, although EEG and behavioural changes in the cats suggested that there was some degree of conditioning, but insufficient to cause an actual seizure. However, it was possible to condition the light to produce a focal fit in those cats which had the tetanus toxin lesion. Forster therefore concluded that fits could only be conditioned in a damaged brain, although they could be conditioned within or across different sensory modalities, so that it was, for example, possible to condition a flickering light to produce focal motor seizures. An unconditioned stimulus in the form of brain stimulation was essential. Conditioning was difficult to establish and exceptionally easy to remove, for one major generalized seizure could abolish weeks of previous conditioning.

Although conditioning in Forster's experiments could be easily removed, he was able to demonstrate the principle that seizures in damaged brains could be conditioned to other external stimuli and across sensory modalities. There is very little work, for obvious ethical reasons, regarding conditioning of seizures in man but one study by Gastaut and colleagues [6] demonstrates the principle. In this study, a patient with photogenic epilepsy had sound stimuli conditioned with the light flashes which produced abnormal epileptogenic photic responses over the occipital cortex. When light was omitted the sound triggered the abnormal epileptic cortical potentials.

Current models of epilepsy therefore specifically allow a relationship between ongoing brain activity (the physiological, behavioural and psychological state of the animal) and the likelihood of seizure occurrence.

10.5.2 Techniques of psychological intervention used in humans

These fall into two areas:

(a) Those specifically intended to affect seizure frequency, e.g.
   overt (positive reinforcement and punishment)

covert (relaxation and covert desensitization)
cue controlled procedures
hypnosis
biofeedback
(b) Fortuitous effects, e.g.
psychodynamic psychotherapy
cognitive therapy

It is unfortunately discouraging that some of the published literature, especially the older case reports, suffers from a lack of rigour. Spunt and colleagues [7] describe it as 'less than overwhelming in quality'. There has been a regrettable tendency to fail to distinguish true epilepsy from pseudoseizures, and a failure to mention important variables such as drug treatment. Some of the better studies are usefully reviewed by Mostofsky & Balaschak [8].

(a) Overt methods

(i)   Positive reinforcement
Periods of seizure-free activity are reinforced by means of praise or tokens. There are several case reports [9–13] with variable follow-up periods rarely exceeding 1 year. Occasional relapse after discontinuation of the regime has been noted.

(ii) Punishment
This may involve punishment of seizure-inducing behaviour, or punishment of seizure occurrence. 'Punishment' may refer to a variety of aversive events ranging from withdrawal of privileges to electric shock. The patient of Ounsted and colleagues [14] deserves mention. A girl with frequent absences was subjected to a burst of photic stimulation whenever a spike-wave paroxysm appeared on the EEG during the experimental situation, and seizure frequency improved. There are some studies using electric shock or different forms of verbal discouragement [15]. The last word on this should go to Spunt and colleagues [7] who write 'despite this success, punishment of seizure activity is less desirable than the use of reinforcement procedures. Epilepsy and its consequences are aversive enough without adding the effects of punishment, which should only be used as a last resort.'

(b) Covert methods
A behavioural technique called 'covert extinction' was described by Caetula in 1971 [16]. Subjects produce the problem behaviour in fantasy and then imagine not receiving any positive reinforcement. This particular method has not been used for the treatment of epilepsy despite the success of other techniques based on manipulating events following a seizure, as described above. However there has been some interest in covert manipulation of events

preceding a seizure. Several workers have described relaxation with covert desensitization to seizure-provoking stimuli [17, 18]. These approaches have in common the association of anxiety with seizure occurrence, and depend on techniques of management of anxiety to prevent the occurrence of seizures.

(c) Cue-controlled methods

These are extensions of covert desensitization, in which the state used to oppose the seizure-provoking stimulus is linked in fantasy to a cue word or strategy. The subject is taught to use the cue to try to abort seizure provoking stimuli when they occur outside the therapeutic session. For example, where anxiety plays a part in seizure precipitation, the patient may be exposed to an anxious situation in fantasy while in a relaxed state and taught to link this with saying or thinking the word 'relax'. The word is then used as a way of evoking a relaxed state when confronted with anxious situations in everyday life [19, 20].

While in some cases where anxiety or increased arousal is a component of the onset of the seizure, cue-controlled relaxation might be suitable; in other cases, teaching the patient to use an arousing strategy might be appropriate. Progressive relaxation has been used in one study [21] to obtain conditions for adequate covert exposure in fantasy, but the subject was instructed to arouse herself by clenching a fist, saying the word 'stop' out loud and trying to feel as aroused as possible when the aura occurred. This was referred to as 'cue-controlled arousal'. The technique is still under evaluation [22, 23].

An interesting recent study by Dahl and colleagues [24] evaluated the results of a behaviour modification program lasting 6 weeks on children with refractory epilepsy. The program included a control for face-to-face contact with the therapist as well as an untreated control group. The authors concluded that 'children, if taught to discover early signs of their seizures, can learn to abort and eventually prevent these . . . behaviour modification . . . may be of substantial help to children with epilepsy who are resistant to conventional drug treatment.'

(d) Hypnosis

The literature on hypnosis, such as it is, is notable for its lack of distinction between true and pseudoseizures, and failure to mention details of drug treatment. One method is to use a cue-controlled technique with exposure and practice while in an hypnotic trance, the trance being perhaps equivalent to the relaxed state used in the cases described previously. Gravitz [25] suggests that hypnotic suggestions directly addressed to the frequency and intensity of seizures may be employed. He reports a case of probably organically determined epilepsy in which, during a course of hypnosis, the seizure frequency dropped from one a day to zero. Here the patient was not only eminently hypnotizable, but also had a high expectation of positive outcome from the treatment, the latter perhaps contributing to the success.

(e) Biofeedback

Sterman [26] reported an 'anticonvulsant' EEG rhythm in cats, the sensorimotor rhythm (SMR). This is a 12–14 Hz sinusoidal waveform recorded from over the sensorimotor cortex. It was thought that operant conditioning of the SMR aimed at increasing its overall occurrence would result in reduced seizure frequency. Early results were encouraging, several groups of workers reported improved control of seizures in their patients, usually after fairly lengthy courses of biofeedback training running into months [27–30]. However, since this promising start, the existence of the SMR in man has been challenged [31]. Some workers have found that seizure reduction occurs in the absence of any increase in the SMR [32], while others [33] found SMR conditioning to be neither sufficient nor necessary for seizure reduction. Lubar and colleagues [34] showed that both biofeedback enhancement of fast (12–15 Hz) rhythms and reduction of slow (3–8 Hz) rhythms seemed to play a part in reduction of seizure frequency, reminiscent of the observation of Ounsted and colleagues [14] that the background EEG of their subject showed a decrease in slow wave components as seizure control improved. Fenwick [35] concluded that teaching the increase of cerebral fast rhythms is effective in reducing seizures. The main disadvantages seem to be the long duration of treatment and the difficulty in identifying factors which might predict a good response. Wyler and colleagues [36] found a slight tendency for more abnormal scores on the Minnesota Multiphasic Personality Inventory to predict good outcome to biofeedback. Good results are said to be obtained in between 43% and 60% of subjects [34], with a tendency for better results to be obtained the longer the treatment is carried out. The technical complexity of the method, coupled with the time-consuming and therefore expensive nature of the treatment, support the search for effective, behaviourally based methods which might have similar effects on the shift in EEG frequency towards faster rhythms. Earlier enthusiasm for biofeedback seems to have waned recently [37]. Some of the success claimed in the early studies could be explained in terms of a general boosting of fast EEG background frequencies, thereby altering the level of arousal in pools of epileptogenic neurones.

(f) Psychodynamic psychotherapy

Early authors tended to see epilepsy as a way of releasing libidinous energy or as a means of escape from an unbearable situation, perhaps a substitute for forbidden sexual or aggressive behaviour. Lehrmann [38] stated 'The partial success of the sedative drug therapy in epilepsy can be accounted for when we bear in mind that these drugs partially accomplish what the symptoms attempt to do – they partially withdraw the patient from reality.' Most epileptologists today would find such a statement naive, and suspect that Lehrmann might have been referring to pseudoseizures rather than true epilepsy. Heilbrunn [39] described submissive traits leading to inherent ego weakness and narcissistic dependency. Interference with the drive for dependent security in the presence of abnormal cerebral electrical activity and lowered seizure threshold is postulated to lead to the motor discharge of a seizure. Typical of more recent reports is the paper by Williams and colleagues [40] regarding the effects of psychotherapy, in part at least psychodynamic in type, on 37 patients with poorly controlled seizures. A good outcome was described in clients with partial seizures, hysterical seizures, normal IQ, normal or only mildly abnormal interictal EEG and who were hypnotizable i.e. suggestible; a poor outcome occurred in cases of generalized true seizures, with mental retardation, an abnormal EEG, and who were not hypnotizable. Not the least of the problems in interpreting the results is the short length of reported follow-up (2–36 months).

(g) Cognitive therapy

This technique of psychotherapy mainly used for affective disorders was developed by Beck [41] and is currently popular with both research workers and clinicians in various fields [42]. Some early reports of cognitive therapy in epilepsy were encouraging [43], but a recent paper [44] describes disappointing results with group cognitive therapy in terms of seizure frequency, although there was a non-significant trend towards improvement compared to a control group. Here a group-based method was used rather than the more common individual approach as this still requires evaluation. It is possible that, as with other approaches, some cases may show idiosyncratic and unexpected improvement:

> A 34 year old woman had suffered tonic-clonic seizures since infancy. She had also experienced absence seizures in childhood but had had none since early adulthood. She continued to experience nocturnal tonic-clonic seizures with no apparent precipitants occurring 3 or 4 times per year, but had no daytime seizures since the age of 12. She took primidone 250 mgs daily, and was reluctant to have her medication changed. She was referred for treatment of recurrent depressive episodes which had begun 10 years previously, consisting of a gradual onset of psychomotor retardation and depressed mood lasting for between 1 and 3 weeks, followed by gradual spontaneous remission; these were becoming more frequent with time. During a course of CT lasting 3 months she experienced one more depressed episode. The content of her negative automatic thoughts elicited as part of therapy revolved largely around the resentment at having the diagnosis of epilepsy, and the stigma she considered it to entail. After the course of cognitive therapy her recurrent depressions ceased, and at 2 year follow-up has had no relapses. It was fortuitously noted that during these 2 years she had no seizures either, this being her longest seizure-free interval for some 30 years [23].

(h) Other factors

Expressed emotion (EE) is a standardized technique for rating the way one family member talks about another in response to a structured interview [45]. The dimensions of EE are criticism, hostility, emotional overinvolvement, warmth and positive remarks, the first three of these contributing to the designation of a family as 'High EE' or 'Low EE'. In one study of families of young adults with epilepsy living with their parents, there was a significant positive correlation between High EE and poor seizure control [46]. It remains uncertain whether serious epilepsy in the family causes high EE to occur or whether high EE makes epilepsy worse. However, the received view in schizophrenia research at the moment [47] is that EE modulates the prognosis of the illness by its effect on the arousal system. It has been shown that it is possible to lower EE by specific interventions, and that this reduces relapse rate in schizophrenia [48], and it is at least possible that similar interventions might have a beneficial effect upon seizure frequency.

10.5.3 Conclusions

Many patients realize that psychological factors play a part in the precipitation of seizures. It is reasonable to look for ways of harnessing these factors in a structured therapeutic manner. There is evidence that in at least some cases of true epilepsy it is possible to alter the frequency of seizures by psychological interventions. The techniques used often include identifying a prodrome or ictally-related mood change, and trying to oppose this in various ways. More formal controlled studies are required in order to identify the individual components that are necessary to bring about a reduction in seizure frequency.

References

1. Lockard, J. S. and Ward, A. A. (1980) *Epilepsy: A Window to the brain mechanisms.* Raven Press, New York.
2. Schwartzkroin, P. A. and Wyler, A. R. (1980) Mechanisms underlying epileptiform burst discharge. *Ann. Neurol.*, **7**, 95–107.
3. Wyler, A. R., Fetz, E. E. and Ward, A. A. (1975) Firing patterns of epileptic and normal neurones in the chronic alumina focus in undrugged monkeys during different behavioural states. *Brain Res.*, **98**, 1–10.
4. Wyler, A. R. and Finch, C. A. (1978) Operant conditioning of tonic firing patterns from precentral neurones in monkey neocortex. *Brain Res.*, **146**, 51–68.
5. Forster, F. M. (1977) *Reflex epilepsy, Behavioural Therapy and Conditional Reflexes.* Charles C. Thomas, Springfield, Illinois.
6. Gastaut, H., Regis, H., Dongier, S. and Roger, A. (1956) Conditionnement élecroencephalographique des décharges épileptique et notion d'epilepsie réflexo-conditonnée. *Revue Neurologique*, **94**, 829–35.
7. Spunt, A. L., Hermann, B. and Rousseau, A. M. (1986) Epilepsy. In *Pharmacological and Behavioural Treatment: An Integrative Approach* (ed. M. Hersen) John Wiley & Sons, New York, pp. 176–96.

8. Mostofsky, D. I. and Balaschak, B. A. (1977) Psychobiological control of seizures. *Psychol. Bull.*, **84**, 723–50.

9. Balaschak, B. A. (1975) Teacher-implemented behaviour modification in a case of organically based epilepsy. *J. Consult. Clin. Psychol.*, **44**, 218–23.

10. Daniels, L. K. (1975) The treatment of grand mal epilepsy by covert and operant conditioning techniques: a case study. *Psychosomatics*, **16**, 65–7.

11. Flannery, R. B. and Caetula, J. R. (1973) Seizures: Controlling the uncontrollable. *J. Rehab.*, **39**, 34–6.

12. Iwata, B. A. and Lorentzen, A. M. (1976) Operant control of seizure-like behaviour in an institutionalized retarded adult. *Behaviour Therapy*, **7**, 247–51.

13. Zlutnick, S. L., Mayville, W. J. and Moffat, S. (1975) Behavioural control of seizure disorders: The interruption of chained behaviour. In *Behaviour therapy and health care: Principles and applications* (eds R. C. Katz and S. J. Zlutnick) Pergamon, Elmsford, New York.

14. Ounsted, C., Lee, D. and Hutt, S. J. (1966) Electroencephalographic and clinical changes in an epileptic child during repeated photic stimulation. *Electroenceph. Clin. Neurophysiol.*, **21**, 388–91.

15. Zlutnick, S. I. (1972) Control of seizures by the modification of pre-seizure behaviour: The punishment of behavioural chain components. *Dissertation Abstracts*, **33**, 6b.

16. Caetula, J. R. (1971) Covert extinction. *Behaviour Therapy*, **2**, 192–200.

17. Parrino, J. J. (1971) Reduction of seizures by desensitisation. *J. Behav. Ther. Exp. Psychiat.*, **2**, 215–18.

18. Standage, K. F. (1972) Treatment of epilepsy by the reciprocal inhibition of anxiety. *Guys Hospital Reports*, **121**, 217–21.

19. Ince, L. P. (1976) The use of relaxation training and a conditioned stimulus in the elimination of epileptic seizures in a child: A case study. *J. Behav. Ther. Exp. Psychiat.*, **7**, 39–42.

20. Wells, K. C., Turner, S. M., Bellack, A. S. and Hersen, M. (1978) Effects of cue-controlled relaxation on psychomotor seizures: An experimental analysis. *Behav. Res. Ther.*, **16**, 51–3.

21. Brown, S. W. and Fenwick, P. B. C. (1984) Psychological methods of seizure control. *Acta Neurol. Scand.*, **70**, 234.

22. Fenwick, P. B. C. and Brown, S. W. (work in progress) Evoked & psychogenic seizures: I Precipitation.

23. Brown, S. W. and Fenwick, P. B. C. (work in progress) Evoked & psychogenic seizures: II Inhibition.

24. Dahl, J., Melin, L., Brorson, L. O. and Schollin, J. (1985) Effects of a broad spectrum behaviour modification treatment program on children with refractory epileptic seizures. *Epilepsia*, **26**, 303–9.

25. Gravitz, M. A. (1979) Hypnotherapeutic management of epileptic behaviour. *Am. J. Clin. Hypnosis*, **21**, 282–4.

26. Sterman, M. B. (1973) Neurophysiologic and clinical studies of sensorimotor and EEG biofeedback training: some effects of epilepsy. In *Biofeedback: Behavior Medicine* (ed. L. Birk) Grune & Stratton, Boston, pp. 507–26.

27. Seifert, A. R. and Lubar, J. F. (1976) Reduction of epileptic seizures through EEG biofeedback training. *Biol. Psychol.*, **3**, 157–84.

28. Lubar, J. F. and Bahler, W. W. (1976) Behavioural management of epileptic

seizures following EEG biofeedback training of the sensorimotor rhythm. *Biofeedback & Self Regulation*, **1**, 77–104.

29. Lubar, J. F. (1977) Electroencephalographic methodology and the management of epilepsy. *Pavlovian J. Biol. Science*, **12**, 147–85.

30. Finley, W. W., Smith, H. A. and Etherton, M. D. (1975) Reduction of seizures and normalisation of the EEG in a severe epileptic following sensorimotor biofeedback training: preliminary study. *Biol. Psychol.*, **2**, 189–203.

31. Fenwick, P. B. C. (1981) Precipitation and inhibition of seizures. In *Epilepsy and Psychiatry* (eds E. H. Reynolds and M. R. Trimble) Churchill Livingstone, Edinburgh, pp. 306–21.

32. Quy, R., Hutt, S. J. and Forrest, S. (1979) Sensorimotor rhythm feedback training and epilepsy. *Biol. Psychol.*, **9**, 129–49.

33. Cott, A., Pavloski, R. and Black, A. (1977) The role of sensorimotor rhythm feedback in the Biofeedback treatment of epilepsy: a preliminary report. *Proceedings of the International meeting on Biofeedback & Self Control*. Tubingen.

34 Lubar, J. F., Shabsin, H. S., Natleson, S. E. *et al.* (1981) EEG operant conditioning in intractable epileptics. *Arch. Neurol.*, **38**, 700–4.

35. Fenwick, P. B. C. (1981) Review of neurophysiological approaches to the treatment of epilepsy. *Brit. J. Clin. Pract.* **Suppl. 18**, 184–7.

36. Wyler, A. R., Robbins, C. A. and Dodrill, C. B. (1979) EEG operant conditioning for the control of epilepsy. *Epilepsia*, **20**, 279–86.

37. Psatta, D. M. (1983) EEG and clinical survey during biofeedback treatment of epileptics. *Neurologia Psihiatria (BUCUR)*, **21**, 63–75.

38. Lehrmann, P. R. (1925) In discussion to Pierce Clark L. Some psychological data regarding the interpretation of essential epilepsy. *J. Nerv. Ment. Dis.*, **61**, 51–9.

39. Heilbrunn, G. (1950) Psychodynamic aspects of epilepsy. *Psychoanal. Quart.*, **19**, 145–57.

40. Williams, D. T., Gold, A. P., Shrout, P. *et al.* (1979) The impact of psychiatric intervention on patients with uncontrolled seizures. *J. Nerv. Ment. Dis.*, **167**, 626–31.

41. Beck, A. T., Rush, A. J., Shaw, B. F. and Emery, G. (1979) *Cognitive Therapy of Depression*, Guildford Press, New York.

42. Blackburn, I. M., Bishop, S., Glen, R. *et al.* (1981) The efficacy of cognitive therapy in depression: a treatment trial using cognitive therapy and pharmacotherapy, each alone and in combination. *Brit. J. Psychiat.*, **139**, 181–9.

43. Tan, S. Y. (1983) Psychosocial functioning of epileptic patients referred for psychological intervention. In *Advances in Epileptology The XIVth Epilepsy International Symposium* (eds M. Parsonage, R. H. E. Grant, A. G. Craig and A. Ä. Ward) Raven Press, New York, pp. 79–87.

44. Tan, S. Y. and Bruni, J. (1986) Cognitive behaviour therapy with adult patients with epilepsy: a controlled outcome study. *Epilepsia*, **27**, 225–33.

45. Koenigsberg, H. W. and Handley, R. (1986) Expressed emotion: from predictive index to clinical construct. *Am. J. Psychiatr.*, **143**, 1361–73.

46. Brown, S. W. and Jadresic, E. (1984) Familial expressed emotion and seizure control. *Acta Neurol. Scand.*, **70**, 234.

47. Sturgeon, D., Kuipers, L., Berkowitz, R. *et al.* (1981) Psychophysiological responses of schizophrenic patients to high and low expressed emotion relatives. *Brit. J. Psychiatr.*, **138**, 40–5.

48. Leff, J. P., Kuipers, L., Berkowitz, R. *et al.* (1982) A controlled trial of social intervention in the families of schizophrenic patients. *Brit. J. Psychiatr.*, **141**, 121–34.

10.6 THE EFFECT OF DIET

Anthony Hopkins

Ketogenic diets have been occasionally used in the management of intractable epilepsy since Wilder's original report in 1921 [1]. The classical diet is based on an estimated daily requirement of 75 kcal/kg body weight; 80% of calories are given as fat, the remainder as protein and carbohydrates. The fats are mainly long chain fats such as butter and cream, and problems of expense as well as palatability arise. With this in mind, the fat component has been replaced, in some centres, by medium chain triglycerides (MCT), largely octanoic and decanoic acids. This in itself is a rather unpalatable oil, and may cause nausea, diarrhoea and abdominal pain. A diet containing 30% long chain fats (butter and cream) and 30% MCT appears to be the most palatable to English children [2], and although not inducing such prominent ketosis (with elevation of acetoacetate and 3-OH butyrate levels) as the classical diet, a number of children benefit. In a study from Oxford [2] 41% of 57 children with epilepsy showed a greater than 90% reduction in seizure frequency within one month of starting the diet. Eighty one per cent of children had a greater than 50% reduction in seizure frequency, and only 19% showed no benefit. The diet appears to be of greater benefit to children with partial seizures and with atonic seizures. Unfortunately, control of seizures may be lost after some months even if adherence to the diet continues.

Studies are at present under way on the efficacy of oligo-antigenic diets in the management of epilepsy, even though there is no clear theoretical basis for any benefit.

References

1. Wilder, R. M. (1921) The effect of ketonuria on the course of epilepsy. *Mayo Clin. Bull.*, **2**, 307.
2. Schwartz, R. H., Eaton, J., Aynsley-Green, A. and Bower, B. D. (1983) Ketogenic diets in the management of epilepsy. In *Research Progress in Epilepsy* (ed. F. Clifford Rose) Pitman, London, pp. 326–32.

CHAPTER ELEVEN

Factors Which Influence the Prognosis of Epilepsy

Ernst Rodin

The general prognosis of epilepsy is considered on p. 11 in Chapter 1. The study of particular factors which influence the prognosis of individual patients with epilepsy is considered in this chapter. Such an analysis is important not only for clinical practice but also in regard to the information it can provide about the causes of the disorder. The clinician needs guidelines which will allow a reasonably accurate prediction as to whether a given patient's seizures will be controllable, and to what extent social or intellectual functions will be affected. The epileptologist who would like to understand the nature of the disease may profit by putting the good and bad prognostic indicators into perspective, and seeing to what extent they hold true across the wide spectrum of seizure patterns, seizure syndromes, and different aetiologies.

For these reasons, this author reviewed the literature in the middle 1960s and performed several large scale statistical studies [1, 2]. Since epilepsy is the tendency to spontaneously recurring seizures, it was decided at that time to include only those patients who had at least three seizures which were clearly epileptic in nature, separated by several weeks, unrelated to external events like alcohol or drug withdrawal, and not associated with any other active neurological disease. These investigations produced eight key variables which defined seizure prognosis: duration of seizure disorder, number of different seizure types in a given patient, frequency of seizures, frequency of injuries resulting from seizures, seizures occurring in clusters, psychomotor seizures, amount of seizure patterns in the EEGs, and the degree of background slowing in the EEG [1–3]. Each prognostic indicator by itself does not necessarily have significance. What mattered was the combination of some or all of these eight parameters in a given patient. It was of great interest to note that the cause of the epilepsy, the presence or absence of neurological abnormalities, and the intelligence quotient (IQ) did not independently contribute additional prognostic information. This may appear paradoxical in view of frequent descriptions in the literature emphasizing the importance of IQ and neurological abnormalities on clinical examination for prognosis of epileptic seizures, but this paradox can be resolved, as will be shown at the conclusion of this chapter. The investigations had one potential drawback – most of the patients were adolescent or in early adult life. It was therefore not clear to what extent these results would be applicable to children or older adults.

A review of the recent literature on the prognosis of epilepsy shows that a number of papers include patients who had only had a single seizure; others include children with febrile convulsions. Thus the view of outcome differs between different investigators, depending on the initial selection criteria which are, unfortunately, not always clearly spelled out.

The following literature review does not pretend to be exhaustive, but provides an overview of the topic arranged mainly by age at time of the first seizure. Whenever possible the prognosis given includes not only that for cessation of seizures, but also for intellectual and social function, and for life expectancy.

11.1 NEONATAL SEIZURES

The information dealing with the prognosis of neonatal seizures (p. 471) comes from a number of diverse studies. The time span included in the definition of the newborn period varies between two and four weeks, the length of follow-up from six months to more than nine years. The diagnostic criteria also are far from uniform [4]. Follow-up studies usually do not include psychological assessment. Statements about 'normal' function of the patient might have needed revision if IQ had been measured rather than relying on clinical judgement alone. Nevertheless, a degree of consensus emerges when the figures presented from various parts of the world are tabulated (Table 11.1). The percentages for morbidity (defined below) for subsequent persistent seizures (i.e. epilepsy), were in part recalculated from the information provided by the authors, and of course reflect the outcome only for those infants that survive. It is apparent that mortality figures differ considerably, reflecting the population under consideration. All of the patients in a study by Knauss and Marshall [5] came from a neonatal intensive care unit, while the sample by Lombroso [6] contained only full term infants. By concentrating on the survivors only, some degree of homogeneity emerges for overall morbidity. This includes cerebral palsy, mental retardation, and epilepsy in various combinations. Persistent morbidity of this kind can be expected in about one-third to one-half of all surviving patients who have had neonatal seizures; chronic epilepsy is a problem in less than one-quarter. Although mortality was clearly related to birth weight, especially in Knauss and Marshall's study, morbidity proved to be essentially the same for infants weighing less than 1500 g at birth (43%), for those who weighed from 1501–2500 g (46%), and for those who weighed more than 2500 g (40%).

The risk factors for morbidity are mainly intracranial haemorrhage, asphyxia, infection, early hypoglycaemia or hypocalcaemia (within the first 72 hours), abnormal findings on neurological examination, congenital malformations, and inborn errors of metabolism. In addition, Mellits *et al.* [7] found, on

Table 11.1 Prognosis of neonatal seizure studies reported after 1970

Author	n	Follow-up duration (years)	Mortality (%)	Morbidity of survivors (%)	Epilepsy (%)
Waldrep and Jabbour, 1972 [53]	15	1	None by definition	40	—
Baudon et al., 1975 [128]	30	1–9	10	50	20
Combes et al., 1975 [129]	129	0.5–3	26	48	7
Kuromori et al., 1976 [130]	123	'adequate'	33	35	18
Knauss and Marshall, 1977 [5]	94	<1–1	46*	43	—
Lombroso, 1978 [6]	210	4–7.6	20	49	—
Holden et al., 1982 [131]	277	7	35	30	18
Watanabe et al., 1982 [132]	264	3–9	None by definition	—†	25

*Figures recalculated to represent total material.
†No information.

the basis of the prospective perinatal collaborative study carried out in the USA, that a five minute APGAR score of less than seven, the need for resuscitation after 5 minutes of age, an early onset of seizures, and a seizure lasting more than 30 min were factors that carried a poor prognosis for survival as well as for mental and physical development. However, *none* of these predictor variables correlated with the subsequent presence or absence of epilepsy at the age of seven years. The only significant parameter in this respect was the number of days during which seizures had occurred in the neonatal period. This variable alone predicted the outcome correctly in 74% of the infants.

A good neurological outcome can be expected if none of the aforementioned risk factors have occurred, if hypocalcaemia is late (i.e. after 72 hours), if there is no identifiable cause, and if the seizures are brief, isolated, and generalized. A further good indicator is if the EEG is either normal, or shows only a unifocal abnormality, and a well developed sleep–waking cycle.

Dehan *et al.* [8] have recently described a subgroup of infants with neonatal seizures who appear to have an excellent prognosis. He refers to the syndrome as 'fifth day seizures'. Seizures start on about the fourth or fifth day after birth in otherwise healthy full term infants; they tend to recur for about 20 hours, and subsequently cease spontaneously. Intravenous diazepam is sometimes helpful but pyridoxine is ineffective. No cause has been found. The finding was confirmed by Pryor *et al.*, [9] Stahl *et al.*, [10] as well as Goldberg and Sheehy [11]. These authors speculated that the syndrome might be due to zinc deficiency, although the data are not entirely convincing. The syndrome appears to be quite common, as it was seen in 20 of 98 infants with neonatal seizures in the original paper. Dehan *et al.*, [12] also made the subsequent point that anticonvulsant treatment appears to be ineffective, and merely prolongs postictal alterations of muscle tone and consciousness. Chronic anticonvulsant medication does not seem to be required as, of 37 infants followed for more than one year, only one had an isolated febrile convulsion and another an isolated afebrile seizure.

In summary, neonatal seizures are associated with a relatively high risk for survival and later morbidity, but a relatively low risk for epilepsy. 'Fifth-day seizures' appear to have a good all round prognosis.

11.2   INFANTILE SPASMS (HYPSARRHYTHMIA)

A review of the results of treatment of patients with the syndrome of infantile spasms (hypsarrhythmia) shows that the outlook is still extremely poor (Table 11.2). Although seizures cease in about one-half of the patients, only between 8% and 23% of patients at follow-up have normal intelligence. However, this is not a uniform condition, but rather a clinical and EEG expression of an immature nervous system to a variety of insults (pp. 101, 473). To use the term, West syndrome, for all of these patients is unjustified. Dr West's son

Table 11.2 Hypsarrhythmia

Author	n	Follow-up duration	Outcome Seizure free (%)	Outcome Intellect normal (%)	Mortality (%)
Chevrie and Aicardi, 1971 [14]	78	mean 30.2 months (range 12–81)	—	14	—
Friedman and Pampiglione, 1971 [20]	105	17–13 years	—	23	25
Sorel, 1971 [133]	145	—	—	17	—
Jeavons et al., 1973 [17]	150	5 years+	45	16	22
Todt et al., 1975 [21]	84	'considerable duration'	60	8	15
Seki et al., 1976 [16]	25	6 years+	56	16	—
O'Donohoe, 1976 [134]	100	5 years+	—	21	19
Pollack et al., 1979* [15]	18	mean 5 years (15 months–16 years)	44	22†	5
Sukuma et al., 1980 [135]	46	1–8 years	52	22	—
Matsumoto et al., 1981 [22]	200	6 years+	44	22	19
Riikonen, 1982 [25]	214	mean 10 years (range 3–19)	40	12	20

*Selected series initially successfully treated with ACTH.
†Normal intellect and seizure-free at follow-up.

clearly suffered from the 'idiopathic' or 'cryptogenic' variety. West had stated 'he was a remarkable fine healthy child when born and continued to thrive till he was 4 months old' [13]. His intellectual deterioration occurred only with the onset of seizures. A review of the papers listed in Table 11.2 shows that in the vast majority of cases the condition is merely superimposed upon pre-existing brain damage rather than arising *de novo*. Unfortunately, the literature is far from concise in its terminology. It is also difficult to extract the pertinent information on the current prognosis of the true West syndrome as defined above. When authors have separated their patients into symptomatic and idiopathic groups, the proportion of the idiopathic or cryptogenic population ranges from 9–51%. However, the term cryptogenic does not necessarily imply absence of prior handicap – some authors use it merely to imply no discernible aetiology. Delay in development, or the occurrence of other types of seizure could have been present before the onset of infantile spasms. For instance, in the series by Chevrie and Aicardi, of the 40 patients in 'groupe primitif', 17% had had prior seizures [14].

A good initial response to treatment may unfortunately not persist, as Pollack *et al.* [15] have demonstrated. In their series of 18 children whose hypsarrhythmia and seizures had disappeared during a three week treatment period with 40 units of ACTH per day, only four (22%) were free from seizures and without intellectual impairment at the last evaluation. The modal age at follow-up was five years (range 15 months to 16 years). However, only five of the patients in this series had been classified as having cryptogenic spasms; the others had a variety of CNS deficits, and six had had other types of seizures before the onset of infantile spasms.

When seizures persist, the EEG tends to change towards that seen in the Lennox-Gastaut syndrome (pp. 102, 474). At times diffuse or focal paroxysms are seen, especially temporal abnormalities; the background activity tends to remain abnormally slow. The subsequent clinical seizures may be tonic-clonic, atonic, myoclonic, atypical absences or of the partial complex variety. Typical absence attacks with 3 cy/s spike wave patterns do not occur [16–19].

The EEG may also give some guide to future mental development. Regardless of the clinical picture, if hypsarrhythmia is seen in the EEG, there is a poor prognosis for intelligence, as Friedman and Pampiglione [20] have shown. Classic hypsarrhythmia which is bilaterally symmetrical tends to have a better prognosis than if there is a constant asymmetry or focal changes in the EEG [21].

All studies agree that birthweight, whether or not the cause is defined, developmental status at time of onset of the infantile spasms, the presence or absence of neurological abnormality and pneumoencephalographic or CT findings influence the prognosis for mental functions. However none of these factors predict subsequent long-standing epilepsy. The only significant finding in this respect is the presence or absence of seizures prior to the onset of infantile spasms [22].

Table 11.3 Hypsarrhythmia–idiopathic cases only

Author	n	Percentage of total (in series)	Onset of treatment	Seizure free (%)	Intellect normal (%)
Chevrie and Aicardi, 1971 [14]	40	51	<1–>73 months (47% <1 month)	—	27
Seki et al., 1976 [16]	12	48	—	56	8
Pollock et al., 1979* [15]	5	28	mean 5 weeks† (2–15 weeks)	—	—
Matsumoto et al., 1981* [22]	—	9	(<1–7 months) mean 5.6 months	50	56
Riikonen, 1982 [25]	29	13	(1 day–24 months)† mean 2.3 months	—	41

*Seven treated within 2 months.
†Total group not specified for subgroup under consideration.

To assess the effectiveness of steroid medication, Table 11.3 was prepared; this lists 'idiopathic' cases only. There is no appreciable difference in regard to seizure cessation between symptomatic and idiopathic groups, but the latter appear to have a somewhat better prognosis for intellectual function. Even so, the prognosis was far from good in Chevrie and Aicardi's series [14]; however, no information was provided as to whether the outcome was different if steroid treatment was given early. The extremely poor outcome in the series of Seki *et al.* [16], which clearly differs from others in Table 11.3, may have been due in part to the fact that of the 20 patients in the entire series, only 12 had received ACTH. Even in those the dose was quite low – 10 units for patients less than one year of age and 20 units thereafter. The number of patients with idiopathic hypsarrhythmia treated with ACTH was not specified.

Sorel and Dusaucy-Bauloye [23] and Gastaut *et al.* [24] pointed out in the late 1950s that if treatment is to be effective as far as intellectual function is concerned, then it needs to be instituted immediately after diagnosis. More than 20 years later, we still do not have a reasonably large scale study comparing the later intellectual function of those with idiopathic hypsarrhythmia treated early compared to the outcome in those in whom treatment was delayed. Some information on this point is available in the studies of Jeavons *et al.* [17], Matsumoto *et al.* [22] and Riikonen [25]. Jeavons *et al.* observed full recovery in five of six patients whose seizures were of the idiopathic variety and had been treated early. Matsumoto *et al.* reported seven children who had been treated within two months of diagnosis, and seven who had received treatment between three and five months after the onset of the illness. Although the numbers are small, they show a definite trend. Five of the seven children treated early were seizure free, but only two of the seven in the other group. Physical development proceeded normally in both groups; intellectual development was normal in six of the early and in only one of the delayed treatment group. A similar difference in regard to outcome was observed by Riikonen. This author noted that the patients in the idiopathic group who had a good outcome had been treated with a mean delay of 1.1 month after diagnosis (range: a few days to three months). Those with a poor outcome had been treated later (mean 4.8 months; range: a few days to 15 months). Sorel has also recently reviewed the topic again, and states that in 80% of children with the idiopathic form 'one can expect a total cure if the treatment has been begun during the first six weeks of development of the illness' [26].

In summary, infantile spasms (hypsarrhythmia) occur mainly as a result of pre-existing brain damage, and therefore carry a poor prognosis for intellectual function. Seizures may cease or change to other seizure types. The EEG background remains slow; there may also be 1–2 per second spike wave patterns or focal changes. Steroids may control seizures in both symptomatic and idiopathic groups, but preserve prospects for intellectual development only in the idiopathic group, and then only if treatment is started immediately after diagnosis.

11.3 SEIZURES DURING THE FIRST YEAR OF LIFE

The prognosis of children who have had seizures during the first year of life, with onset after the first month, was evaluated by Chevrie and Aicardi [27, 28]. Those with symptomatic seizures are much more likely to have persistent seizures five years later (73% vs. 44% for those with idiopathic seizures). Significant differences in regard to persistence of seizures at follow-up were, apart from aetiology, a history of status epilepticus (79%), the occurrence of partial seizures (69%), or generalized seizures (58%), or infantile spasms (52%). Seventy-three per cent of intellectually normal children were seizure free, while this was the case in only 18% of those who were intellectually impaired. The presence or absence of neurological abnormalities was also important but rather less so, 72% vs. 55%. There was also a sex difference – 68% of girls had persistent seizures, but only 51% of boys. Lesions of the CNS that produced neurological signs as opposed to those which were accompanied only by mental retardation did not show differences in seizure outcome. At the time of follow-up 12.2% of the children were dead – comprising 4% of the idiopathic and 19% of the symptomatic group. Mortality was also higher if seizures had occurred under the age of six months, and in patients with partial seizures. However, sex, family history, and presence or absence of prenatal or perinatal abnormalities were not significant in this respect. Neurological abnormalities were present at time of follow-up in 14% of the cryptogenic and 45% of the symptomatic group. Intellect was regarded as normal in 39% of the cryptogenic but only in 6% of the symptomatic group, conversely many more of the symptomatic group were severely retarded (73% as opposed to 32%). On the basis of these figures, the authors concluded that 'the outcome of first year epilepsies are quite severe even when they are not expressed as infantile spasms'. O'Brien *et al.* [29] however, have pointed out that the prognosis is much better if one looks at general paediatric patients rather than those referred to specialists. They followed 28 patients, who had seizures between one and six months of age, for one to four years. Only two had died, and of the 26 survivors only seven had a 'handicap'. Of the 16 survivors with generalized seizures, 15 were regarded as normal (94%). Four of seven with partial or mixed seizures were also normal, but none of the three survivors of the infantile spasm or myoclonic group. The onset of treatment was, in the majority of cases, within less than one week of onset and delayed to six weeks in only one case. The authors noted that a satisfactory outcome was associated with normal physical examination, a normal EEG at time of initial evaluation and easy early control of convulsions. It is, however, not clear from this study whether or not patients with febrile convulsions were included in the generalized group. This certainly was the case in the large series of Matsumoto *et al.* [30] who followed 304 children to the age of six years at least. The mortality was similar to that of Chevrie and Aicardi, namely, 15%. Cessation of seizures had occurred in 58% and normal intellect and physical development in 44%. Corresponding figures from the French study were 56% for seizure cessation and 20% for normal intellect. The difference in regard to intellect may well be due to the inclusion of patients with febrile convulsions in the Japanese series. Patients who had presented initially with febrile convulsions had normal intellect in 82%, while this was the case in only 37.6% of patients who had had afebrile seizures.

In summary, for seizures beginning in the first year of life (after the first month) the prognosis depends on the presence of pre-existing or coexisting brain damage. Control of seizures is easier to achieve for the child who is physically and intellectually intact, and for whom treatment is started early.

11.4   FEBRILE CONVULSIONS
(see also p. 458 of Chapter 15)

Febrile convulsions are the most common type of seizure in childhood, especially between the age of six months to three years. Nelson and Ellenberg found an occurrence of 3.5% in white and 4.2% in black children among the approximately 54 000 offspring of women enrolled in the collaborative perinatal project [31, 32]. Of 1706 children with at least one febrile convulsion which was not due to discernible concomitant neurological disease, vaccination or severe dehydration, one-third had a further convulsion, and 9% had three or more recurrences. The risk factors for development of subsequent afebrile seizures were family history of afebrile seizures, pre-existing neurological abnormalities, and complicated initial seizures. When none of these risk factors were present (60% of the total group) only 1% of the children developed epilepsy. The percentage rose to 2% when one risk factor was present (34% of the total) and to 10% with two or more risk factors (6% of the total). Prolonged postictal paralysis was observed in 0.4% of the group and there were no deaths.

The figures by Annegers *et al.* [33] for the development of epilepsy after a febrile convulsion, based on the population of Rochester, Minnesota, were somewhat higher than those found by Nelson and Ellenberg [32], namely, 6%. The highest risk of occurrence was before the age of five years, but continued higher than expected through to the age 20 and beyond. Patients with pre-existing neurological deficits or with an IQ of less than 70 were at highest risk, with 40% developing recurrent afebrile seizures. The duration of the initial convulsion and presence of focal features were also significant risk factors.

Fois *et al.* [34] divided their 2661 patients into a low risk (72.4%), medium risk (26%), and high risk group (2.5%). The low risk group consisted of patients whose seizure was accompanied by a temperature above 38.5°C, had lasted less than 15 min and had no neurological findings before or after the seizure. Medium risk was defined as one or more of the following: a temperature below 38.5°C, a seizure lasting more than 15 min or accompanied by focal features, the presence of abnormal neurological findings prior to the seizure, and an abnormal EEG. The high risk group consisted of patients whose convulsion was followed by coma and/or postictal hemiplegia which lasted for more than 30 min. In previously neurologically normal children the incidence of subsequent afebrile convulsions was 3.4% in the low risk, 8.3% in the medium risk, and 22.5% in the high risk group. The authors felt that phenobarbital treatment was useful. In the low risk group, which was regularly treated, the relapse rate for febrile convulsions was 7.3%, but 38% in patients who were insufficiently treated. In the medium risk group the percentages were 8.7% for regularly treated, 46.6% for irregular or inadequately treated, and 64.7% for untreated children. Permanent hemiplegia associated with subsequent epilepsy was observed in six of the 40 patients in the high risk group (15%).

Wallace [35] found a 12% rate of spontaneously recurring afebrile seizures in her group of 112 children who were followed for eight to nine years. On the other hand, the rate in the study by Pearce and Macintosh [36] was only 2%. Sample composition and different length of follow-up might well account for the discrepancies.

As far as prognosis for intelligence is concerned, reliable data are sparse because formal IQ testing has rarely been carried out. There are two studies where measured IQs are available, the siblings of the patients being used as controls. The first was by Ellenberg and Nelson [37], who compared the Wechsler Full Scale IQ scores of 431 children from the National Collaborative Perinatal Project at age seven against the sibling closest to them in age. The mean full scale IQ of the children who had convulsed was 93.0 (*SD* 13.9) and that of their sibling 93.7 (*SD* 12.8). The 0.7 point difference was not statistically significant. Significant IQ differences were found, as might be expected, between those children who had shown neurological abnormalities prior to the febrile convulsion, and their siblings, but focal or prolonged seizures were not associated with demonstrable loss of IQ. Eighteen children were still on prophylactic phenobarbital treatment; their mean IQ was 94.9 (*SD* 13.9) versus 92.9 (*SD* 9.7) for their siblings. Blood phenobarbital levels were not available. Schiottz-Christensen and Bruhn (38) compared 14 monozygotic twin pairs, discordant for febrile convulsions, on a large battery of psychological tests, including the Wechsler Intelligence Scale for Children (WISC) or Wechsler Adult Intelligence Scale (WAIS). The mean age at the time of evaluation was 12.6 years (range 6–20 years). In 12 of the 14 pairs the healthy co-twin obtained better results in the majority of tests ($p<.001$). In one pair the results were equal, and in the other the child with febrile convulsions performed better than his co-twin. The Wechsler mean IQ scores were Verbal 97 vs. 100 (not significant), Performance 103 vs. 110 ($p<.001$), and Full Scale 100 vs. 105 ($p<.05$). The authors found no correlation between birth history and intellectual deficit. They wrote that 'it would seem possible therefore that the febrile convulsions themselves could be the cause of the cerebral dysfunction demonstrated'. Since this conclusion appears to conflict with that of

Ellenberg and Nelson [37], who wrote that 'febrile seizures were not associated with a decrement in IQ', it is important to bear in mind the composition of the samples. The Danish study dealt with a homogeneous population of monozygotic twins, while the US study population was of considerable heterogeneity, siblings being used as controls. Furthermore, the Copenhagen controls had an 11 point higher mean IQ than their American counterparts. It has been demonstrated previously that, when intellectual decline takes place in patients with epilepsy, it tends to occur more commonly in those with initially higher IQ scores [1], so that these results are analogous. Furthermore, only the full scale IQ was reported in the US population. The observation that the performance IQ was more affected than verbal IQ is concordant with the literature on the intellectual function of patients with epilepsy, including our most recent follow-up studies of patients with childhood onset seizures [39]. Another report from the UK found no difference in the results of a picture vocabulary test and copying of designs, between the patients who had febrile convulsions and controls. In this study, the WISC was not used [40]. (See also pp. 459–60)

The question whether or not prophylactic treatment after the first febrile convulsion should be carried out is still highly controversial and is reviewed in Chapter 15, p. 457. For patients at high risk of recurrence, the benefits outweigh the potential risks of long term treatment. Failure to prevent febrile seizures with phenytoin was shown by Melchior *et al.* in 1971 [41], and successful prevention with phenobarbital by Faero *et al.* [42]. The latter study was challenged by Heckmatt *et al.* in 1976 [43], but their paper in turn was criticized by Wolf and Forsythe [44]. Early reviews are those of Lennox-Buchthal in 1975 [45], and of Freeman in 1978 [46].

Diazepam may be administered at the time of febrile illness in a predisposed child. The absorption characteristics of various preparations of diazepam were studied by Milligan *et al.* [47]. The intravenous solution given rectally achieved the fastest results. The efficacy of this method (p. 453) has been demonstrated by Knudsen and Vestermark [48], as well as Brown [49], and Ferngren [50].

In summary, children who have pre-existing CNS damage, and/or have a 'complicated' initial febrile seizure, carry a higher risk for developing epilepsy than those with a 'benign' febrile seizure; even in the latter group, the risk is twice that of the general population. The rectal administration of diazepam at the time of a febrile illness in a predisposed child may prevent the development of further seizures.

11.5 PETIT MAL ABSENCES

Dalby followed 160 patients with petit mal between 1959 and 1965 [51]; 46% also had tonic-clonic seizures. Cessation of petit mal episodes occurred in 58%. The subsequent relapse was 7%, occurring two to six years after initial cessation. Where petit mal was the only seizure type 79% of patients became seizure free, but this was the case in only 33% when petit mal was complicated by tonic-clonic seizures. The prognosis was poorer in girls, who also had tonic-clonic seizures more frequently than boys. Later onset of petit mal increased the liability to tonic-clonic seizures and decreased the chances of remission. Delay in treatment resulted in the occurrence of tonic-clonic seizures, with subsequent worse prognosis. Petit mal absences beginning between the ages of five and nine years had the best prognosis. Gastaut *et al* [51a] have studied the long-term course of a selected group of 26 patients with absences continuing after the age of 35 years. Only five of the 26 stopped having absences in a very long follow-up period; 92% had tonic–clonic seizures at some stage of their illness.

Sato *et al.* [52] followed 83 patients for a mean duration of 9.5 years (range 4.7–14.3 years). Forty-eight per cent of the patients were completely seizure free and 58% were free from absence seizures. Twenty-six individuals (31%) were no longer on anticonvulsant medication. Multivariate statistical analysis indicated a good prognosis for those patients with a normal IQ, normal neurological examination, and pure petit mal rather than petit mal absences complicated by tonic-clonic seizures. Tonic-clonic seizures started in 12 children (14%) while they were already being treated for absences. The measured full scale IQ at follow-up was 86.6 vs. 87.6 on initial evaluation. The one point drop was not statistically significant. Patients with a positive family history had a poorer prognosis. Of patients with a positive family history 38% were seizure free compared to 60% without such a history ($p > .04$). A history of absence status also carried a poorer prognosis. Only 35% of these patients became seizure free. In agreement with Dalby's observation, girls did less well than boys. All the patients in this study were videomonitored at the time of follow-up for the presence of petit mal absences, and this may well have influenced the results, comparing the higher remission rates reported by other authors, namely, 77% [54], 81% [55], 82% [56] and 85% [57].

Other reported variations are in the occurrence of tonic-clonic seizures after onset of petit mal absences, ranging from 18% in the series of Waesser *et al.* [58], to 60% in that of Oller-Daurella and Sanchez [59]. However, all authors are agreed that when tonic-clonic seizures complicate the picture, the results of treatment are less good. A long duration of illness does not necessarily carry a poor prognosis for remission of petit mal absences as Gibberd [54] and Wolf and Inoue have shown [56].

Kawai *et al.* [60] studied 10 patients with uncontrollable absences. Three subsequently developed features of the Lennox-Gastaut syndrome, characterized by 2 Hz spike waves, drop attacks, and atypical absences. The evolution of the Lennox-Gastaut syndrome was studied in greater detail by Oller-Daurella [61] in 184 children. Disappearance of the EEG abnormalities and clinical resolution were extremely rare, occurring in only one case. Cessation of seizures, but persistence of clinical handicap, occurred slightly more frequently but most frequently both EEG abnormalities and seizures continued. However, the type of seizure may change to partial seizures, especially temporal lobe attacks. Evolution into pure petit mal absences did not occur.

In summary, children with typical petit mal absences tend to respond well to sodium valproate or succinimides provided they are treated promptly before the development of tonic-clonic seizures. The prognosis is poorer for girls, and when tonic-clonic seizures complicate the picture as a second seizure type. If treatment is delayed, petit mal absences may still respond well, but tonic-clonic seizures disappear only after complete petit mal absence control. Sodium valproate is probably the drug of first choice because of its additional efficacy against primary generalized tonic-clonic seizures, and may prevent the occurrence of these.

11.6 PARTIAL SEIZURES IN CHILDHOOD AND ADOLESCENCE

In 1960 Gibbs and Gibbs [62] reported on the 'good prognosis of midtemporal epilepsy'. They reported 739 patients with spikes in the midtemporal area, finding that this focus is essentially limited to children, mainly between the ages five and 12 years, the peak occurrence being around the age of eight. Of the 120 children who were followed to the age of 18, 85% were then asymptomatic. The EEGs had become normal in 55%; 30% developed 14 and 6 Hz positive spikes, 10% developed a negative spike focus in the anterior temporal area, and 5% continued to have a negative midtemporal spike. Only the patients who developed an anterior temporal spike focus continued to have tonic-clonic and/or partial seizures.

Smith and Kellaway [63] studied 200 children who had 'central foci' in the EEG. The group was similar to that of Gibbs and Gibbs, and was not homogeneous with regard to neurological evaluation or seizure type. Mental retardation had been present in 31%, spasticity or coordination problems in 22%, and behaviour disorders in 11%. Twenty per cent of the patients had episodic symptomatology, regarded by the authors as seizure equivalents, and 59% had clinical epilepsy. The seizures were either generalized tonic-clonic or partial in type. Follow-up studies showed a tendency for the foci to disappear and persistence for more than four years was regarded as rare.

Lombroso [64] subsequently separated from this overall group of patients a subgroup which he termed 'Sylvian seizures'. These were characterized by partial seizures with elementary symptomatology, frequently of sensory variety, but sometimes including motor components. Since the attacks commonly occurred during sleep, focal features could be submerged in a generalized convulsion. He plotted the field distribution of the interictal spikes, and showed that the gradient extended into the Rolandic area rather than into the anterior temporal or frontal regions. Serial tracings in 58 patients showed subsequent normal EEGs in 33, a persistent midtemporal focus in nine, an anterior temporal focus in two, a posterior temporal focus in four, and other seizure patterns including spike wave discharges in ten. Forty-one of the patients (71%) were seizure free five years after the initial record.

The now commonly used term 'benign rolandic epilepsy' for this condition appears to have been coined by Beaussart [65] who felt in 1972 that enough evidence had accumulated to allow the establishment of a separate clinical entity. He called this 'benign epilepsy with rolandic (centrotemporal) spikes'. He reviewed patients whose EEGs had shown Rolandic spikes and noted that these occurred in two main groups of individuals, namely 264 patients with and 221 without epilepsy. He subsequently excluded 43 patients in the group with epilepsy who had associated neuropsychiatric abnormalities. His final report describing the syndrome dealt with 221 children. The modal age of onset was nine years (range 2–14 years). The patients suffered from either partial motor or generalized seizures. In 51% the seizures occurred exclusively during sleep, in 29% whilst awake only, and in 13% of patients both whilst asleep and awake. In 7% information about time of occurrence was not available. Seizures stopped immediately after the onset of treatment in 65%, disappeared between three months and one year in 21% when the dose of medication was raised, and persisted for more than one year, or recurred later in 14%. Rolandic spikes either disappeared with treatment or persisted despite seizure control. Eighty-five patients were followed after cessation of treatment, and all but one remained seizure free. Beaussart felt that in this group of children the focus is 'functional' rather than structural in character. He also felt that there is a strong genetic component (Table 5.2) and noted that the condition is more common than petit mal epilepsy. By 1978 Beaussart and Faou [66] reported on 324 patients with this syndrome who had been followed for one to 22 years. In those patients who had been treated for more than five years, seizures had disappeared in 51%, they occurred with a frequency of less than one a year in 34%, and more than once a year in 16%. One hundred and twenty patients were regarded as cured because treatment had been stopped without any recurrence. In the total group 21 patients had not been treated at all. Of these, seven had had only one seizure. The authors concluded that, with or without treatment, some patients have only one or a few seizures, while others may suffer from seizures for many years. However, there are no criteria which allow one to distinguish reliably these patients at the time of first seizure.

A further study was reported by Blom and Heijbel in 1982 [67], who described a longer follow-up period of a group of children who had previously been reported in 1972 [68]. Of these children 38 had been seizure free from 4–13 years with a mean of 8.4 years. Thirty-five had normal or borderline EEGs at follow-up, and Rolandic spikes had disappeared in all. Ten years later 37 of these patients could be traced and 36 of them had been seizure free from 14–23 years.

Other focal EEG spikes with a good prognosis are those originating in the occipital area [69] and those in the parietal regions which are elicited by stroking the child's foot [70]. The same cannot be said for those children who have anterior temporal lobe spikes. The most detailed follow-up study of children with temporal lobe seizures is that of Lindsay and colleagues [71–75]. The original 100 children were re-evaluated in adult life in 1980 [74]. All 100 patients were available for follow-up. The authors report four groups: (1) seizure free, not taking anticonvulsant medication, and able to support themselves socially and economically (33%); (2) not necessarily seizure free, on anticonvulsant medications, but supporting themselves socially and economically (32%); (3) unable to support themselves, totally dependent upon parents or living in institutions (30%); (4) died prior to the age of 15 (5%). The following eight factors ascertained at the time of the initial evaluation were related to poor outcome: IQ below 90, onset of seizures before the age of two years four months, five or more tonic-clonic seizures, frequent temporal lobe seizures, a left-sided EEG focus, a hyperkinetic behaviour syndrome, catastrophic rages, and the need for special schooling. A family history of epilepsy or febrile convulsions was associated with a good prognosis, and if present could invalidate all these negative factors. Unless totally dependent, females were generally married. However, only those males whose seizures had ceased before adolescence were married. Of the 66 probands who had survived and were not handicapped to the extent that made reproduction impossible, there were 63 offspring by the time of the report. Only 17 of 41 marriageable men were married, and had 22 children, while the 25 women had 41 children. Fourteen of the 24 were unmarried, though marriageable men had no sexual contacts.

Although 85% of the patients had had psychiatric difficulties in childhood, overt psychiatric problems were infrequent in the surviving adults. Seventy per cent of the patients who were not retarded were psychiatrically normal. Nine of the survivors (10%) had developed a schizophreniform psychosis, and seven of these nine patients (8 men, 1 woman) had a left-sided EEG focus. The focus was bilateral in the other two. There was no right-sided focus in this group. All nine patients continued to have seizures. Antisocial conduct in adult life was present in 12 patients, all men. They continued to have seizures and had an EEG focus contralateral to the preferred hand. Treated neurotic and depressive illnesses were uncommon.

Twenty-nine patients had been considered for temporal lobectomy. Sixteen were rejected for various reasons. All of these had subsequently a poor medical and social outcome. On the other hand, all of the 13 patients who had been operated upon recovered from seizures, and their social situation was markedly improved. The authors emphasize that patients whose seizures are improved but not totally controlled by medication should be considered for surgery, as the social outcome is otherwise poor.

Loiseau *et al.* [76] followed 235 patients who had their first partial seizure between ages 12 and 18 years. All had been seen between 1958 and 1978. One hundred and ninety-one had simple partial seizures, 64 complex partial, and 47 secondary generalized tonic-clonic convulsions. The patients were seen immediately after the first seizure, 44% had an isolated seizure in the first year, 12% a second seizure during that year, 20% had more than two but less than 12 during the follow-up period, and 23% had more than 12 seizures. Partial seizures with elementary symptomatology had a better prognosis than compex partial seizures. The prognosis was also poorer when tonic-clonic seizures were present in addition to the partial seizures. The best prognosis was in patients with simple partial seizures as the only seizure type, without any apparent cause, and with a normal EEG.

In summary, approximately half of all patients with central temporal-rolandic spikes do not have even a single clinical seizure. In those who do, the attacks are usually readily controlled; medication can be discontinued by age 13 in most instances especially if the patients are physically and intellectually intact, but there are exceptions. Simple partial seizures have a better prognosis than complex partial seizures. If the latter persist through adolescence into adult life, social outcome is poor. Temporal lobectomy should be more often considered.

11.7   OVERALL CHILDHOOD PROGNOSIS

Several large series of patients have been reported since 1970 covering the spectrum of seizure types. The results are summarized in Table 11.4. Differences in rates of remission are again due largely to sample composition and varying length of follow-up. Decay of success rates over time is apparent in the data of Suzuki *et al.* [77] and those of Sillanpää [78]. The latter study differs from all the other reports, not only in its comprehensive nature, but also because the diagnosis of epilepsy for inclusion in this study required three seizures, each separated by at least one week without associated neurological disease. Febrile convulsions were also excluded. The other studies shown in Table 11.4 employed less stringent criteria. In Sillanpää's investigations, the entire population served by the Turku University Central Hospital Region of Southwestern Finland was surveyed. The prevalence of childhood epilepsy as just defined above, with onset between birth and 15 years, was 3.2 per 1000. The average annual incidence was 0.25 per 1000. His follow-up study consisted of 245 patients with epilepsy who had at one time been fully investigated in a hospital. The duration of follow-up ranged from 84–264 months. A good prognosis was associated with a good response to treatment in the short term, normal psychomotor development, normal neurological examination, and a normal EEG. A poor prognosis was associated with long duration of illness, high seizure frequency at maximum, both daytime and night-time seizures, seizures occurring in clusters, more than one seizure type, frequent status epilepticus, a low IQ, 'completely disturbed' consciousness

Table 11.4 Remission rates for children with epilepsy

Author	n	Follow-up duration of (years)	Remission (%)	Minimum duration remission (years)	Off medication (%)
Rankin, 1972 [136]	128	4–14	51	—	31
Sillanpää, 1973 [78]	245	—	44.6	3	—
Latinville and Loiseau, 1975 [79]	337	5	66	27	33
Suzuki et al., 1976 [77]	185	3–20	62	7	—
Ohtahara et al., 1977 [80]	431	5	76	3 (major) 6 (minor)	—
Geets and Van Calster, 1980 [81]	100	10	68	9	—
Sofijanov, 1982 [137]	512	4–10	51	2	24

during seizures, organic aetiology, abnormal findings on neurological examination, a family history of mental illness, and small head circumference. A normal IQ, defined as 86 or more, was observed in 47% of the patients; 23% were severely retarded, with lesser degrees of retardation in the remaining 30%. On follow-up examination, a decline in IQ had occurred in 61% of the children, and only 3% of the children showed an increase. Factors related to prognosis for intelligence were essentially the same as for seizures, but early onset of seizures was also associated with lower IQ. Schooling had been impossible in 31% of the children, and significantly fewer patients had completed higher education than an age-matched control population. Nearly 30% had required admission to an institution for one or more short periods, while 20% required long term care, in all but two cases on account of severe intellectual limitation or problems with behaviour. Eighteen (7%) of the patients had died, death being related to seizures in eight. There was only one death due to status epilepticus, but five of the 18 patients had drowned – an incidence 100 fold greater than that found for the community.

Latinville and Loiseau [79] added the presence of Rolandic spikes in the EEG, and the presence of tonic-clonic seizures as indicating a good prognosis. Psychomotor seizures were found to have a poorer prognosis by Ohtahara *et al.* [80], and delay of treatment was noted as having an adverse effect by Geets and Van Calster [81].

Patients who had had status epilepticus were investigated by Hayakawa *et al.* [82]. Twenty-eight children had suffered status two to three times. Permanent disability resulted in 13%. Status epilepticus appeared to be more common when mental retardation was present.

The prognosis for academic achievement of the child with seizures depends largely upon the age of onset of seizures, the extent of previous brain injury, and the ability to control attacks. Rutter *et al.* [83] have shown that leaving aside those patients who have suffered cerebral damage, there is some evidence that children with persistent seizures are more prone to have learning disabilities than those who suffer from other chronic cerebral disorders. Although most authorities agree that the intelligence of children with epilepsy uncomplicated by brain injuries is in the average range, measurements (especially with the WISC) have shown them to cluster towards the lower part of the average range, and the scores are slightly lower than those of their siblings [84]. Verbal and performance areas of intelligence tested by the WISC can be differentially affected in seizure patients; the performance IQ tends to decrease more than the verbal subtests when seizures persist uncontrolled. The performance as well as the verbal IQ can rise considerably if seizures are controlled by ordinary rather than excessive amounts of medications. The influence of chronic anticonvulsant medication on intellectual function is being investigated at a number of centres. The current view is that if sedative drugs have to be used, they should be prescribed in the smallest dose that is effective. Nevertheless, for the IQ to remain stable or rise, complete seizure cessation rather than just improvement appears to be necessary. Decrease in intellectual function as a result of seizures does explain the findings of Sillanpää [78], Ross *et al* [85], and the author's group [86–88] which found that patients with chronic seizures tend to end up in lower socioeconomic groups. Our most recent study indicated that if the IQ does decrease, this is not due to loss of previously acquired functions, but to a flattening of the learning curve during the crucial years of schooling. The patients are then ill-prepared for competitive employment [39]. To assess the prognosis for intellectual function, and to some extent therefore for future life performance, measurements of IQ with the WISC or Wide Range Achievement Test (WRAT) should be obtained routinely at the time of first evaluation of a child with seizures, and then subsequently at intervals. In children whose seizure disorder started prior to the age of five, initial testing can be obtained with other test instruments, but by the beginning of school age one or both of the previously two mentioned tests should be employed. It must be emphasized that the clinical impression of even experienced paediatricians or neurologists are unreliable. If one waits for decreased performance at school to be noticed by teachers or parents, then valuable time may be lost.

In summary, control of seizures is more easily achieved in children who are neurologically and mentally intact, and when treatment is started promptly after onset. Intellectual function is determined mainly by the degree of pre-existing or co-existing brain damage, the age of onset of seizures, and the presence or absence of seizure control.

11.8   DISCONTINUATION OF ANTICONVULSANT MEDICATIONS

After a child has been seizure free for some time, the question arises as to how long anticonvulsant medication needs to be continued. There are now several large series available which can provide guidelines. Relapse rates after anticonvulsants have been stopped have been reported as 11% [89], 20% [90], 27% [91], 30.7% [92], 24% [93], and 36.3% [94]. Factors favouring relapse are similar to those which have a poor prognosis for control of seizures in the first place, namely – long duration of epilepsy before control was achieved, the occurrence of more than one seizure type and of partial seizures, the presence of neurological signs or intellectual impairment, high seizure frequency before control was achieved, past history of remission and relapses, early discontinuation of treatment, slow background rhythms or paroxysmal discharges in the EEG, and deterioration of the EEG during withdrawal from medication. Studies have not shown any relationship to age at time of discontinuation, and puberty does not adversely influence the outcome. Most relapses occur within the first year after discontinuation, but some patients relapse after an interval of several years. Groh reported that if the risk factors of freedom from seizures for less than three years, discontinuation of medication over less than six months, the combination of psychomotor seizures with tonic-clonic seizures, a past history of remissions and recurrences while still under treatment, a long interval between initial diagnosis and appropriate treatment, and a persistently abnormal EEG had been taken into account, then recurrences could have been reduced to only 4%. His most recent report based upon these criteria gave a relapse rate of 8% [95]. In a study by Hollowach *et al.* [93] the risk of recurrence by seizure type was 53% for Jacksonian seizures, 40% for more than one seizure type, 25% for psychomotor seizures, 12% for petit mal absences and 8% for tonic-clonic seizures. In children who have become seizure free, especially in the absence of the risk factors, late recurrences are rare. Holowach *et al.* [96] have examined such a patient group 15–23 years after discontinuation of medication. There were only five additional patients who had developed relapses in the interval, bringing the overall rate of recurrence to 28%.

In summary, children can be safely withdrawn from anticonvulsant medications if they have been completely seizure free for a minimum of three to five years and have had none of the risk factors that have been identified as leading to poor prognosis for seizure cessation. Gradual reduction of medication rather than sudden withdrawal is probably advisable.

11.9 ADULT LIFE – PARTIAL SEIZURES

Partial complex seizures of adult life may be difficult to control, especially if associated with tonic-clonic seizures. The natural history tends to be that tonic-clonic seizures decrease in frequency of occurrence or remit altogether as the patient gets older, but partial seizures remain, and may recur several times a month, sometimes in clusters so that the patient is seizure free for two to three weeks or even a month, but subsequently there occur several seizures in one day or over two or three days. In women, clustering may be coupled with the menstrual cycle (p. 374) but clustering of seizures is also commonly encountered in males. These patients, who may have associated mild intellectual changes and personality problems, are the majority of those who attend epilepsy clinics.

Seizure freedom in patients with partial complex seizures was reported as 38% by Ohtaka *et al.* [18], 37% by Pazzaglia *et al.* [97] and 40% by Currie *et al.* [98]. In a sample of 21 patients reported by Kamiya *et al.* [99] there were only two who had achieved complete seizure freedom. A good prognosis in the sample of Ohtaka *et al.* was encountered in patients who did not experience an aura, whose seizures initially occurred with low frequency, whose age of onset was between six years and puberty, who had no temporal spikes in the EEG, who had partial complex seizures as their only seizure type, and for whose epilepsy there was no identified cause. Pazzaglia *et al.* found that a good prognosis was related to short duration of illness, infrequent initial seizures and one seizure type only. The best results were reported by Schmidt *et al.*

[100]. Sixty-three per cent of the patients without and 62% with tonic-clonic seizures were seizure free for at least two years. The presence or absence of tonic-clonic seizures was therefore unrelated to prognosis, but the frequency of tonic-clonic seizures made a marked difference. With rare tonic-clonic seizures the remission rate was 79%, but only 44% with frequent ones.

A great deal has been written in the past decade on the personality of patients with temporal lobe epilepsy (Chapter 18). Careful statistical studies have so far been unable to verify a specific personality syndrome which characterizes the majority of patients who have only partial complex seizures. There is evidence that the combination of tonic-clonic and partial complex seizures clouds the prognosis for mental and emotional functions [101, 102].

Patients with simple partial seizures, on the other hand, usually respond better to medication and 61% were controlled in the series of Pazzaglia *et al.* [97]. Although these patients frequently have focal neurological findings, they tend to do well from the social and behavioural point of view.

In summary, complex partial seizures in adult life present considerable problems in treatment. Seizures are usually of long standing, having persisted from childhood or adolescence, but may also occur for the first time in adult life. If this is the case and there is no structural lesion identifiable, they may respond to prompt treatment. If uncontrollable, they are usually associated with tonic-clonic seizures, and prognosis for remission and for mental functions is then poorer if these are frequent. Simple partial seizures have a better prognosis for seizure cessation and mental function, although they are frequently associated with a neurological handicap.

11.10 POST-TRAUMATIC SEIZURES

This subject is fully addressed in Chapter 13. Useful references are the studies of Jennett *et al.* [103] on the occurrence of seizures after depressed fractures, and of Black *et al.* [104] and De Santis *et al.* [105] on post-traumatic epilepsy in children. Feeney and Walker [106] and Weiss *et al.* [107] have developed formulae which allow the prediction of the risk of occurrence of post-traumatic seizures.

In summary, the risk for post-traumatic seizures depends upon the intensity of the head injury and is higher when the dura is torn, when early seizures have been present, and there has been prolonged post-traumatic amnesia. Frontal and temporal injuries are also more epileptogenic than occipital. While these risk factors influence the occurrence of late seizures, they do not predict the seriousness of the seizure disorder and to what extent the patient will respond to anticonvulsant medication. Jennett in Chapter 13 also discusses the chances of preventing seizures by prophylactic anticonvulsant medication [108–111], and the risks of epilepsy following surgery. The prognosis of postoperative epilepsy is reviewed by Foy [112].

11.11   THE GENERAL PROGNOSIS OF EPILEPSY

A review of the general prognosis of epilepsy in the community is given on p. 11–13 in Chapter 1. Reviewed here are a few further aspects which influence prognosis.

The final result of a large Japanese multi-institutional study involving 20 centres was presented by Okuma *et al.* in 1981 [113]. The outcome of seizures and social adjustment was studied three, five and ten years after the onset of seizures. Seizures had remitted in 58%, and there was no appreciable difference between rates of remission at three and ten years. Normal social adjustment had occurred in 63%, while moderate and severe social maladjustment had occurred in 12%. The population studied included patients with single seizures, and a considerable proportion of children. Highest remission rates were observed in patients with tonic-clonic seizures or simple absences. The lowest rates were in patients with complex partial seizures which occurred in combination with other seizure types. The prognosis was better under the following circumstances: an 'idiopathic' aetiology, an onset of epilepsy at age less than ten years, infrequent seizures, treatment started within the first year, one seizure type only, normal IQ, normal personality, and no appreciable EEG background slowing. Seizures which occurred during sleep rather than whilst awake or in both states, also had a better prognosis. The social adjustment was mainly determined by the extent of seizure control that could be achieved. Additional statistics on remission of seizures for three years are 34% and 43% [114–115], 40% and 32% [116–117], 49% [118], and 42% [119].

The importance of seizure type and neurological abnormalities in determining prognosis is revealed in community as well as in hospital-based studies. Figure 1.4 in Chapter 1 shows the data of Annegers and colleagues [120]. Figure 1.4 shows that residents of Rochester, Minnesota, who had experienced at least two afebrile seizures had a 70% probability of achieving a remission lasting at least five years by the time that 20 years had elapsed since the diagnosis. At this time, 30% continued to have seizures, about 20% were seizure free but still taking anticonvulsant medication, while 50% were seizure free and also not taking medication. The probability for remission in the idiopathic group was 74%, but only 46% for those with neurological abnormalities since birth. Of patients with tonic-clonic seizures 50% were seizure free and medication free, but this was the case in only 35% of patients with complex partial seizures. Age at time of initial diagnosis was also an important factor, namely, 75% probability of remission if onset had occurred prior to age 10, 68% onset between ages 10 and 19, and 63% between ages 20 and 59. The mean annual relapse rate was 1.6%. The cumulative probability for relapse after achieving a remission was 8% in the first five years, 15% by 10 years, and 24% by 20 years. Patients with partial complex seizures had the highest relapse rate, namely 32%, but only 6% of patients with absence seizures relapsed. Relapses were also more common in late onset than in childhood onset seizures. Patients who had not remitted within five years had only a 33% chance of a five year remission during the next ten years.

   The prognosis for seizures of late onset has been studied by Vercelletto and Delobel [121]. One hundred patients with onset after age 60 were investigated. In 52% there was no apparent cause. Most lived normally and were well controlled. Kuhlo and Schwarz [122] followed 106 patients for 6–7 years whose seizures began after the age of 45. Complete freedom from seizures was achieved in 40 patients (38%) but seven of these had had only one seizure. Seizures were infrequent in 39%. They remained the same during the period of observation in 19% and got worse in 5%. Morikawa *et al.* [123] also investigated seizure control in patients who were older than 40 years, the duration of the illness ranging from five months to 53 years with a mean of 23 years. Of the patients 66% had had epilepsy for more than 20 years, and 97% continued to have seizures during the follow-up, but they were infrequent. Eighty-one percent of the patient population had improved, with a reduction in seizures of 75% or more. In a further recent study Lühdorf *et al.* [123a] underlies the relatively satisfactory prognosis of epilepsy in patients aged over 60.

11.11.1   Sex and heredity

The influence of sex and heredity was studied by Pedersen and Krogh [124]. There were more women in the cryptogenic group of epilepsies, and more males in the symptomatic group. Patients with a family history of epilepsy in the cryptogenic group had a poorer prognosis than those without. The prognosis was worse for women than for men.

11.12   PROGNOSIS FOR SOCIAL FUNCTION

Sillanpää [125] found that two-thirds of his patients were potentially employable, but when employed they more commonly found employment in the lower socioeconomic group of jobs. Problems with employment correlated with low IQ, behaviour problems, and higher seizure frequency during the 12 months preceding the study. In our own studies [86–88], we noted that seizure frequency is only one and not necessarily the most important aspect in regard to employment status. There was no statistically significant difference based on seizure frequency alone unless the patients had remitted completely for at least one year. Of 88 patients who had at least one seizure per year, 41 were employed while 47 were not. Of 26 patients who had been seizure free for at least one year, 21 were employed. Employment and especially level of employment is markedly influenced by intellectual and behavioural factors. When our sample of 369 patients was divided into 86 individuals who had only epileptic seizures, and 283 who had associated behavioural and/or intellectual changes, marked significant differences emerged. In the 'epilepsy only' population, there was not a single individual who had been habitually unemployed, while this was the case in one-third of the other group. Levels of occupational achievement also differed markedly between the two groups in favour of the 'epilepsy only' population. The best predictors of future employment were adequate intellect and motivation for work. These two factors could override even marked seizure frequency and social bias. Janz [126] ascertained the employment status of 432 patients and found that 87% were employed. During the follow-up period, which ranged between four and 12 years, 90% had unchanged employment status, 3% had moved up, while 8% had moved down. Upward mobility was associated with seizure freedom or marked improvement of seizure frequency, while decline had occurred mainly in patients who had a combination of tonic-clonic and partial complex seizures.

In summary, social functions are related mainly to intellectual abilities, presence or absence of behavioural problems, and seizure control. The patient population which has seizures without other associated handicaps can be expected to do well with regard to employment and overall life achievements.

The prognosis after a first seizure is considered in Chapter 6 (pp. 151–57), the prognosis after surgery in Chapter 10 (pp. 293–97 and 324–26), and the mortality of epilepsy on pp. 14–16 in Chapter 1.

11.13 CONCLUSIONS

A review of all the information in this Chapter suggests that serious damage to the central nervous system of whatever cause leads predictably to neurological abnormalities, mental and intellectual changes, but not necessarily to seizures. This holds true for all age groups. Thus, there is no doubt that cerebral damage facilitates the initiation of an epileptic process; but the severity of this process, whether it be EEG changes only, a single seizure, some isolated seizures of a single type, or uncontrollable seizures of several different types, obeys laws which we do not as yet understand. Inasmuch as the electrochemical determinants which decide how much brain tissue is potentially epileptogenic at any given point in time are unknown, we can only assess the prognosis of a given patient by the history of the frequency and intensity of the seizures themselves. Thus the paradox which was alluded to in the introduction, namely, that abnormalities on neurological examination and low IQ which are so common in patients with severe intractable epilepsy, did not enter into the prognostic indicators derived through discriminant function analysis, resolves itself. These factors are redundant because they do not independently contribute to prognosis. All patients with slow background rhythms in the EEG, marked EEG seizure patterns, and frequent clinical seizures of various types which tend to occur in clusters, and whose illness has persisted for some time, are brain damaged and intellectually impaired; but severity of brain damage or intellectual limitations do not contribute further information. The other extreme, a single seizure type which repeats infrequently which does not lead to injuries and is accompanied by a normal EEG, virtually guarantees a good prognosis and is encountered mainly in patients who are physically and intellectually intact. These observations can be useful diagnostically. A patient whose EEG and neurological examination including IQ testing is normal, and who complains of uncontrollable frequent seizures, can often be shown to suffer from pseudoseizures rather than epileptic seizures.

The challenge to epileptologists is this – to define the parameters which lead not only to an induced isolated seizure, but underly the process that gives rise to spontaneously repeating attacks occurring at random or in clusters. These are not deducible from currently available methodology, but are the key to the solution of the problem of epilepsy. The most important practical aspect from these considerations is that the epileptogenic process can be interrupted and prevented from assuming proportions which subsequently defy treatment by early effective intervention, in the vast majority of patients. In the case of children with the true West syndrome, this must be done in a matter of days. In patients with other seizure types, within weeks or months. Thus, the old dictum of Hippocrates about the 'sacred illness' is still valid: 'It is curable no less than others unless when from length of time it has become confirmed and stronger than the remedies applied' [127].

REFERENCES

1. Rodin, E. A. (1968) *The Prognosis of Patients with Epilepsy*, Charles C. Thomas, Springfield.
2. Rodin, E. A. (1972) Medical and social prognosis in epilepsy. *Epilepsia*, **13**, 121–31.
3. Rodin, E. A. (1978) Various prognostic aspects in patients with epilepsy. *Folia Psychiatr. Neurol. Jap.*, **32**, 407–18.
4. Freeman, J. M. (1985) *Long-Term Follow-Up of Neonatal Seizures*, paper presented at 16th Epilepsy International Congress 1985, Hamburg.
5. Knauss, T. A. and Marshall, R. E. (1977) Seizures in a neonatal intensive care unit. *Developl Med. Child Neurol.*, **19**, 719–28.
6. Lombroso, C. T. (1978) Convulsive disorders in newborns, in *Pediatric Neurology and Neurosurgery* (eds R. A. Thompson and J. R. Green), Spectrum Press Inc., New York, pp. 205–39.
7. Mellits, E. D., Holden, K. R. and Freeman, J. M. (1982) Neonatal seizures. II. A multivariate analysis of factors associated with outcome. *Pediatrics*, **70**, 177–85.
8. Dehan, M., Quillerou, D., Navelet, Y. *et al.* (1977) Les convulsions de cinquieme jour de vie: un nouveau syndrome? *Arch. Fr. Pediatr.*, **34**, 730–42.
9. Pryor, D. S., Don, N. and Macourt, D. C. (1981) Fifth day fits: a syndrome of neonatal convulsions. *Arch. Dis. Child.*, **56**, 753–8.
10. Stahl, M., Frankenbach, J. M., Von Toenges, V. *et al.* (1985) Fifth-day-fits in

newborns. A new syndrome. (Ger) *Monatsschr. Kinderheilkd.*, **132**, 786–90. (Abstracted (1985) *Excerpta Medica Epilepsy Abstracts*, **18**, 442.)

11. Goldberg, H. J. and Sheehy, E. M. (1982) Fifth day fits: an acute zinc deficiency syndrome? *Arch. Dis. Child.*, **57**, 633–5.

12. Dehan, M., Gabilan, J. C., Navelet, Y. *et al.* (1982) Fifth day fits. *Arch. Dis. Child.*, **57**, 400–1.

13. West, W. J. (1841) On a peculiar form of infantile convulsions (Letter to the Editor). *Lancet*, 724.

14. Chevrie, J. J. and Aicardi, J. (1971) Le pronostic psychique des spasmes infantiles traites par l'ACTH ou les corticoides. Analyse statistique de 78 cas suivis plus d'un an. *J. Neurol. Sci.*, **12**, 351–7.

15. Pollack, M. A., Zion, T. E. and Kellaway, P. (1979) Long-term prognosis of patients with infantile spasms following ACTH therapy. *Epilepsia*, **20**, 255–60.

16. Seki, T., Kawahara, Y. and Hirose, M. (1976) The long term prognosis of infantile spasms. The present condition of cases of infantile spasms in school age. *Folia Psychiatr. Neurol. Jap.*, **30**, 297–306.

17. Jeavons, P. M., Bower, B. D. and Dimitrakoudi, M. (1973) Long-term prognosis of 150 cases of West Syndrome. *Epilepsia*, **14**, 153–64.

18. Ohtaka, T., Miyasaka, M. and Fukuzawa, H. (1978) A study on long-term prognosis of psychomotor seizures. *Folia Psychiatr. Neurol. Jap.*, **32**, 439–43.

19. Hughes, J. R. (1985) Natural history of hypsarrhythmia. *Clin. Electroenceph.*, **16**, 128–35.

20. Friedman, E. and Pampiglione, G. (1971) Prognostic implications of electro-encephalographic findings of hypsarrhythmia in first year of life. *Br. Med. J.*, **4**, 323–6.

21. Todt, H., Wunsche, W. and Korth, G. (1975) Zur Frage des prognostischen Aussagewertes des Elektroenzephalogramms bei Kindern mit BNS-Kraempfen. *Kinderaerztl. Prax.*, **43**, 457–61.

22. Matsumoto, A., Watanabe, K., Negoro, T. *et al.* (1981) Long-term prognosis after infantile spasms: a statistical study of prognostic factors in 200 cases. *Developl Med. Child Neurol.*, **23**, 51–65.

23. Sorel, L. and Dusaucy-Bauloye, A. (1958) A propos de 21 cas d'hypsarrhythmia de Gibbs, son traitement spectaculaire par l'ACTH. *Acta Neurol. Belg.*, **58**, 130–41.

24. Gastaut, H., Saltiel, J., Raybaud, C. *et al.* (1959) A propos du traitement par l'ACTH des encephalites myocloniques de la premiere enfance avec dysrythmie majeure (hypsarrhythmia). *Pediatrie*, **14**, 35–41.

25. Riikonen, R. (1982) A long-term follow-up study of 214 children with the syndrome of infantile spasms. *Neuropediatrics*, **13**, 14–23.

26. Sorel, L. (1985) West's syndrome and its treatment. *Clin. Electroenceph.*, **16**, 122–7.

27. Chevrie, J. J. and Aicardi, J. (1978) Convulsive disorders in the first year of life: neurological and mental outcome and mortality. *Epilepsia*, **19**, 67–74.

28. Chevrie, J. J. and Aicardi, J. (1979) Convulsive disorders in the first year of life: persistence of epileptic seizures. *Epilepsia*, **20**, 643–9.

29. O'Brien, T., Counahan, R., O'Brien, B. *et al.* (1981) Prognosis of convulsions between 1 and 6 months of age. *Arch. Dis. Child.*, **56**, 643–5.

30. Matsumoto, A., Watanabe, K., Sugiura, M. *et al.* (1983) Long-term prognosis of

convulsive disorders in the first year of life: mental and physical development and seizure persistence. *Epilepsia*, **24**, 321–9.

31. Nelson, K. B. and Ellenberg, J. H. (1976) Predictors of epilepsy in children who have experienced febrile seizures. *N. Engl. J. Med.*, **295**, 1029–33.

32. Nelson, K. B. and Ellenberg, J. (1978) Prognosis in children with febrile seizures. *Pediatrics*, **61**, 720–7.

33. Annegers, J. F., Hauser, W. A., Elveback, L. R. *et al.* (1979) The risk of epilepsy following febrile convulsions. *Neurology*, **29**, 297–303.

34. Fois, A., Malandrini, F., Valentini, S. *et al.* (1982) Febrile convulsions: a follow-up of 2661 cases. *Riv. It. Pediatr.*, **8**, 53–60.

35. Wallace, S. J. (1977) Spontaneous fits after convulsions with fever. *Arch. Dis. Child.*, **52**, 192–6.

36. Pearce, J. L. and Mackintosh, H. T. (1979) Prospective study of convulsions in childhood. *NZ Med. J.*, **89**, 1–3.

37. Ellenberg, J. and Nelson, K. B. (1978) Febrile seizures and later intellectual performance. *Arch. Neurol.*, **35**, 17–21.

38. Schiottz-Christensen, E. and Bruhn, P. (1973) Intelligence, behavior and scholastic achievement subsequent to febrile convulsions: an analysis of discordant twin-pairs. *Developl Med. Child Neurol.*, **15**, 565–75.

39. Rodin, E., Schmaltz, S. and Twitty, G. (1986) Intellectual functions in patients with childhood onset epilepsy. *Developl Med. Child Neurol.*, **28**, 25–33.

40. Verity, C. M., Butler, N. R. and Golding, J. (1985) Febrile convulsions in a national cohort followed up from birth. I. Prevalence and recurrence in the first five years of life. *Br. Med. J.*, **290**, 1307–15.

41. Melchior, J. C., Buchthal, F. and Lennox-Buchthal, M. (1971) The ineffectiveness of diphenylhydantoin in preventing febrile convulsions in the age of greatest risk, under three years. *Epilepsia*, **12**, 55–62.

42. Faero, O., Kastrup, K. W., Nielsen, E. L. *et al.* (1972) Successful prophylaxis of febrile convulsions with phenobarbital. *Epilepsia*, **13**, 279–85.

43. Heckmatt, J. Z., Houston, A. B., Clow, D. J. *et al.* (1976) Failure of phenobarbitone to prevent febrile convulsions. *Br. Med. J.*, **1**, 559–61.

44. Wolf, S. M. and Forsythe, A. B. (1976) Failure of phenobarbitone to prevent febrile convulsions. *Br. Med. J.*, **1**, 1277–8.

45. Lennox-Buchthal, M. A. (1975) Comments on prophylactic treatment for febrile convulsions. *Acta Neurol. Scand.*, **60** (Suppl.,), 77–8.

46. Freeman, J. M. (1978) Febrile seizures: an end to confusion. *Pediatrics*, **61**, 806–8.

47. Milligan, N., Dhillon, S., Oxley, J. *et al.* (1982) Absorption of diazepam from the rectum and its effect on interictal spikes in the EEG. *Epilepsia*, **23**, 323–31.

48. Knudsen, F. U. and Vestermark, S. (1978) Prophylactic diazepam or phenobarbitone in febrile convulsions: a prospective, controlled study. *Arch. Dis. Child.*, **53**, 660–3.

49. Brown, J. K. (1982) Personal communication (1979) in *A Textbook of Epilepsy*, 2nd edn (eds J. Laidlaw and A. Richens), Churchill Livingstone, New York, p. 85.

50. Ferngren, H. G. (1974) Diazepam treatment for acute convulsions in children: A report of 41 patients, three with plasma levels. *Epilepsia*, **15**, 27–37.

51. Dalby, M. A. (1969) Epilepsy and 3 per second spike and wave rhythms. *Acta Neurol. Scand.*, **45**, 9–183.

51a. Gastaut, H., Zifkin, B. G., Mariani, E. and Ping, J. S. (1986) The long-term course of primary generalized epilepsy with persisting absences. *Neurology*, **36**, 1021–28.

52. Sato, S., Dreifuss, F. E., Penry, J.K. *et al.* (1983) Long-term follow-up of absence seizures. *Neurology*, **33**, 1590–5.

53. Waldrep, H. C. and Jabbour, J. T. (1972) Neonatal seizures. *J. Tenn. Med. Assoc.*, **65**, 1001–6.

54. Gibberd, F. B. (1972) The prognosis of petit mal in adults. *Epilepsia*, **13**, 171–5.

55. Santavuori, P. (1983) Absence seizures: valproate or ethosuximide? *Acta Neurol. Scand.*, **97**, (Suppl.), 41–8.

56. Wolf, P. and Inoue, Y. (1984) Therapeutic response of absence seizures in patients of an epilepsy clinic for adolescents and adults. *J. Neurol.*, **231**, 225–9.

57. Seki, T., Kawahara, Y. and Hirose, M. (1978) The prognosis of petit mal absence. A follow-up study of more than 3 years. (Jap) *Brain Develop.*, **10**, 161–8. (Abstracted (1979) *Excerpta Medica Neurol. Neurosurg.*, **46**, 416.)

58. Waesser, S., Scheidemann, I., Bergmann, L. *et al.* (1983) Die Prognose bei primaer reiner Absence-Epilepsie. *Psychiatr. Neurol. Med. Psychol.*, **35**, 202–9.

59. Oller-Daurella, L. and Sanchez, M. E. (1981) Evolucion de las ausencias tipicas. *Rev. Neurol. (Barcelona)*, **40**, 81–102.

60. Kawai, I., Fujii, S., Shingu, K. *et al.* (1980) Uncontrollable cases of absence. *Folia Psychiatr. Neurol. Jap.*, **34**, 97–105.

61. Oller-Daurella, L. (1973) Evolution et pronostic du syndrome de Lennox-Gastaut, in *Evolution and Prognosis of Epilepsies*, Proceedings of International Symposium, Venice 1972, (eds E. Lugaresi *et al.*), Aulo Gaggi Publ., Bologna, pp. 155–64.

62. Gibbs, E. and Gibbs, F. (1959/60) Good prognosis of mid-temporal epilepsy. *Epilepsia*, **1**, 448–53.

63. Smith, J. M. B. and Kellaway, P. (1964) Central (Rolandic) foci in children: an analysis of 200 cases. Paper given at American EEG Soc, 17th Ann Meet, San Francisco 1963. Abstracted *Electroenceph. Clin. Neurophysiol.*, **1**, 460P–1P.

64. Lombroso, C. T. (1967) Sylvian seizures and midtemporal spike foci in children. *Arch. Neurol.*, **17**, 52–9.

65. Beaussart, M. (1972) Benign epilepsy of children with Rolandic (centro-temporal) paroxysmal foci. *Epilepsia*, **13**, 795–811.

66. Beaussart, M. and Faou, R. (1978) Evolution of epilepsy with Rolandic paroxysmal foci: a study of 324 cases. *Epilepsia*, **19**, 337–42.

67. Blom, S. and Heijbel, J. (1982) Benign epilepsy of children with centro-temporal EEG foci: a follow-up study in adulthood of patients initially studied as children. *Epilepsia*, **23**, 629–32.

68. Blom, S., Heijbel, J. and Bergfors, P. G. (1972) Benign epilepsy of children with centro-temporal EEG foci. Prevalence and follow-up study of 40 patients. *Epilepsia*, **13**, 609–19.

69. Beaumanoir, A. (1983) Infantile epilepsy with occipital focus and good prognosis. *Eur. Neurol.*, **22**, 43–52.

70. Negrin, P. and DeMarco, P. (1977) Parietal focal spikes evoked by tactile somatotopic stimulation in sixty non-epileptic children: the nocturnal sleep and clinical and EEG evolution. *Electroenceph. Clin. Neurophysiol.*, **43**, 312–16.

71. Lindsay, J., Ounsted, C. and Richards, P. (1979) Long-term outcome in children

with temporal lobe seizures. I. Social outcome and childhood factors. *Developl Med. Child Neurol.*, **21**, 285–98.

72. Lindsay, J., Ounsted, C. and Richards, P. (1979] Long-term outcome in children with temporal lobe seizures. II. Marriage, parenthood and sexual indifference. *Developl Med. Child. Neurol.*, **21**, 433–40.

73. Lindsay, J., Ounsted, C. and Richards, P. (1979) Long-term outcome in children with temporal lobe seizures. III. Psychiatric aspects in childhood and adult life. *Developl Med. Child Neurol.*, **21**, 630–6.

74. Lindsay, J., Ounsted, C. and Richards, P. (1980) Long-term outcome in children with temporal lobe seizures. IV. Genetic factors, febrile convulsions, and the remission of seizures. *Developl Med. Child Neurol.*, **22**, 429–39.

75. Lindsay, J., Ounsted, C. and Richards, P. (1984) Long-term outcome in children with temporal lobe seizures. V. Indications and contra-indications for neurosurgery. *Developl Med. Child Neurol.*, **26**, 25–32.

76. Loiseau, P., Dartigues, J. F. and Pestre, M. (1983) Prognosis of partial epileptic seizures in the adolescent. *Epilepsia*, **24**, 472–81.

77. Suzuki, M., Suzuki, Y., Mitzuno, Y. *et al.* (1976) Long-term prognosis of epilepsy in children. A follow-up report beyond 18 years of age. *Folia Psychiatr. Neurol. Jap.*, **30**, 307–13.

78. Sillanpää, M. (1973) Medico-social prognosis of children with epilepsy. Epidemiological study and analysis of 245 patients. *Acta Paediatr. Scand.*, **237** (Suppl.), 3–104.

79. Latinville, D. and Loiseau, P. (1975) Evolution et pronostic de l'epilepsie chez l'enfant. *Bordeaux Med.*, **8**, 2237–59.

80. Ohtahara, S., Yamatogi, Y., Ohtsuka, Y. *et al.* (1977) Prognosis in childhood epilepsy: a prospective follow-up study. *Folia Psychiatr. Neurol. Jap.*, **31**, 301–13.

81. Geets, W. and Van Calster, L. (1980) Evolution a long terme des crises epileptiques de l'enfant. Influence d'un traitement precoce. *Acta Neurol. Belg.*, **80**, 217–26.

82. Hayakawa, T., Sato, J., Hara, H. *et al.* (1979) Therapy and prognosis of status convulsivus in childhood. *Folia Psychiatr. Neurol. Jap.*, **33**, 445–56.

83. Rutter, M., Graham, P. and Yule, W. (1970) A neuropsychiatric study in childhood, in *Clinics in Developmental Medicine* Nos 35/36, London, Spastics International Medical Publications, London.

84. Rodin, E. A. (1978) Psychiatric disorders associated with epilepsy. *Psychiatr. Clin. N. Am.*, **1**, 101–15.

85. Ross, E. M., Peckham, C. S., West, P. B. *et al.* (1980) Epilepsy in childhood: Findings from the National Child Development Study. *Br. Med. J.*, **280**, 207–10.

86. Rodin, E., Rennick, P., Dennerll, R. *et al.* (1972) Vocational and educational problems of epileptic patients. *Epilepsia*, **13**, 149–60.

87. Rodin, E. A., Shapiro, H. L. and Lennox, K. (1977) Epilepsy and life performance. *Rehab. Lit.*, **38**, 34–9.

88. Rader, B., Shapiro, H. L. and Rodin, E. A. (1978) On placement of multiply handicapped epileptic clients into the open job market. *Rehab. Lit.*, **39**, 299–302.

89. Sakamoto, Y., Kasahara, M. and Satouchi, H. (1978) Long-term prognosis on recurrence of seizures among children with epilepsy after drug withdrawal-elimination. *Folia Psychiatr. Neurol. Jap.*, **32**, 435–7.

90. Groh, Ch. (1975) Zur Frage der Heilbarkeit kindlicher Epilepsien. *Wien Klin. Wschr.*, **87** (Suppl. 40), 1–23.

91. Tamai, I. (1977) Prognosis in infantile epilepsy. Follow-up study of 117 cases after finishing of prolonged anticonvulsant. *Acta Paediatr. Jap. (Overseas Edition)*, **19**, 59.

92. Forster, Ch. and Schmidberger, G. (1982) Prognose der Epilepsie im Kindesalter nach Absetzen der Medikation. *Monatsschr. Kinderheilk*, **130**, 225–8.

93. Holowach, J., Thurston, D. L. and O'Leary, J. (1972) Prognosis in childhood epilepsy. Follow-up study of 148 cases in which therapy had been suspended after prolonged anticonvulsant control. *N. Engl. J. Med.*, **286**, 169–74.

94. Todt, H. (1984) The late prognosis of epilepsy in childhood: results of a prospective follow-up study. *Epilepsia*, **25**, 137–44.

95. Groh, Ch. (1985) *Is It Possible to Lower the Relapse-Rate After Stopping Antiepileptic Medication by Consideration of So-Called Risk-Factors?* Paper presented at the 16th International Congress 1985, Hamburg.

96. Holowach, J., Thurston, D. L., Hixon, B. B. *et al.* (1982) Prognosis in childhood epilepsy. Additional follow-up of 148 children 15 to 23 years after withdrawal of anticonvulsant therapy. *N. Engl. J. Med.*, **306**, 831–6.

97. Pazzaglia, P., D'Alessandro, R., Lozito, A. *et al.* (1982) Classification of partial epilepsies according to the symptomatology of seizures: practical value and prognostic implications. *Epilepsia*, **23**, 343–50.

98. Currie, S., Heathfield, K. W. G., Henson, R. A. *et al.* (1971) Clinical course and prognosis of temporal lobe epilepsy. A survey of 666 patients. *Brain*, **94**, 173–90.

99. Kamiya, S., Minami, K., Kita, S. *et al.* (1977) A long-term clinical course of psychomotor epilepsy. *Folia Psychiatr. Neurol. Jap.*, **31**, 347–58.

100. Schmidt, D., Tsai, J. J. and Janz, D. (1983) Generalized tonic-clonic seizures in patients with complex-partial seizures: natural history and prognostic relevance. *Epilepsia*, **24**, 43–8.

101. Rodin, E., Katz, M. and Lennox, C. (1976) Differences between patients with temporal lobe seizures and those with other forms of epileptic attacks. *Epilepsia*, **76**, 313–20.

102. Hermann, B. P., Dikmen, S. and Wilensky, A. J. (1982) Increased psychopathology associated with multiple seizure types: fact or artifact? *Epilepsia*, **23**, 587–96.

103. Jennett, B., Miller, D. and Braakman, R. (1974) Epilepsy after nonmissile depressed skull fracture. *J. Neurosurg.*, **41**, 208–16.

104. Black, P., Shepard, R. H. and Walker, A. E. (1975) Outcome of head trauma: age and posttraumatic seizures, in *Outcome of Severe Damage to the Central Nervous System*, (*Ciba Foundation Symposium* 34 (New Series)) Elsevier, Amsterdam, pp. 215–26.

105. De Santis, A., Marossero, F., Pagni, C. A. *et al.* (1979) Long-term prognosis of early epilepsy in juvenile head-injured patients. *J. Neurosurg. Sci.*, **23**, 105–8.

106. Feeney, D. M. and Walker, A. E. (1979) The prediction of posttraumatic epilepsy. A mathematical approach. *Arch. Neurol.*, **36**, 8–12.

107. Weiss, G. H., Feeney, D. M., Caveness, W. F. *et al.* (1983) Prognostic factors for the occurrence of posttraumatic epilepsy. *Arch. Neurol.*, **40**, 7–10.

108. Servit, Z. (1960) Prophylactic treatment of posttraumatic epilepsy. *Nature*, **188**, 669–70.

109. Young, B., Rapp, R., Brooks, W. H. *et al.* (1979) Posttraumatic epilepsy prophylaxis. *Epilepsia*, **20**, 671–81.

110. Young, B., Rapp, R. P., Norton, J. A. *et al.* (1983) Failure of prophylactially administered phenytoin to prevent posttraumatic seizures in children. *Child's Brain*, **10**, 185–92.

111. Servit, Z. and Musil, F. (1981) Prophylactic treatment of posttraumatic epilepsy: results of a long-term follow-up in Czechoslovakia. *Epilepsia*, **23**, 315–20.

112. Foy, P. M., Copeland, G. P. and Shaw, M. D. M. (1981) The natural history of post-operative seizures. *Acta Neurochir.*, **57**, 15–22.

113. Okuma, T. and Kumashiro, H. (Chairmen) (1981) Natural history and prognosis of epilepsy: report of a multi-institutional study in Japan. *Epilepsia*, **22**, 35–53.

114. Yamada, H., Yoshida, H. and Ninomiya, H. (1977) A five-year follow-up study of 66 epileptics. *Folia Psychiatr. Neurol. Jap.*, **31**, 339–45.

115. Yamada, H., Yoshida, H. and Ninomiya, H. (1979) A 10-year follow-up study of 97 epileptics. *Folia Psychiatr. Neurol. Jap.*, **33**, 172–82.

116. Hosokawa, K. and Kugoh, T. (1977) Multidimensional clinical study of epileptics under long-term follow-up. *Folia Psychiatr. Neurol. Jap.*, **31**, 359–67.

117. Hosokawa, K. and Kugoh, T. (1978) Prognosis in patients with epilepsy – special reference to change in types of seizure and ingestion of prescribed drugs. *Folia Psychiatr. Neurol. Jap.*, **32**, 447–8.

118. Fukushima, Y. and Kobayashi, H. (1980) Recurrence of seizure in patients with epilepsy whose attacks had been controlled by medication for 10 years or more. *Folia Psychiatr. Neurol. Jap.*, **34**, 302–3.

119. Kitagawa, T. (1981) A clinical and electroencephalographical follow-up study for more than 10 years in patients with epilepsy. *Folia Psychiatr. Neurol. Jap.*, **35**, 333–42.

120. Annegers, J. F., Hauser, W. A. and Elveback, L. R. (1979) Remission of seizures and relapse in patients with epilepsy. *Epilepsia*, **2**, 729–37.

121. Vercelletto, P. and Delobel, R. (1970) Etude des facteurs etiologiques et pronostiques dans les epilepsies debutant apres 60 ans. *Sem. Hop. Paris*, **46**, 3133–7.

122. Kuhlo, W. and Schwarz, J. (1971) Katamnestische Untersuchungen bei sogenannter Spaetepilepsie. (Beginn nach dem 45. Lebensjahr) *Arch. Psychiatr. Nervenkr.*, **215**, 8–21.

123. Morikawa, T., Ishihara, O., Kakegawa, N. *et al.* (1977) A retrospective study on the prognosis of aged patients with epilepsy. *Folia Psychiatr. Neurol. Jap.*, **31**, 375–81.

123a. Lühdorf, K., Jensen, L. K., Plesner, A. M. (1986) Epilepsy in the elderly: prognosis. *Acta Neurol. Scand.*, **74**, 409–15.

124. Pedersen, H. E. and Krogh, E. (1971) The prognostic consequences of familial predisposition and sex in epilepsy. *Acta Neurol. Scand.*, **47**, 106–16.

125. Sillanpää, M. (1977) The influence of childhood epilepsy on potential adult employability. *Int. J. Rehab. Res.*, **1**, 27–33.

126. Janz, D. (1972) Social prognosis in epilepsy especially in regard to social status and the necessity for institutionalization. *Epilepsia*, **13**, 141–7.

127. Hippocrates: Hippocratic writings, translated by Francis Adams (1952). In *Great Books of the Western World, Vol. 10*, Encyclopedia Britannica, Chicago.

128. Baudon, J. J., Bouillie, J. and Gleizes, H. (1975) Aspects cliniques, etiologiques et

pronostiques des convulsions neonatales (a propos de 54 cas). *Rev. Pediat.*, **11**, 457–62.

129. Combes, J. C., Rufo, M., Vallade, M. J. *et al.* (1975) Les convulsions neo-natales circonstances d'apparition et criteres de pronostic. A propos de 129 observations. *Pediatrie*, **30**, 477–92.
130. Kuromori, N., Arai, H. and Ohkubo, O. (1976) A prospective study of epilepsy following neonatal convulsions. *Folia Psychiat. Neurol. Jap.*, **30**, 379–88.
131. Holden, K. R., Mellits, E. D. and Freeman, J. M. (1982) Neonatal seizures. I. Correlation of prenatal and perinatal events with outcomes. *Pediatrics*, **70**, 165–76.
132. Watanabe, K., Kuroyanagi, M., Hara, K. *et al.* (1982) Neonatal seizures and subsequent epilepsy. *Brain Develop.*, **4**, 341–6.
133. Sorel, L. (1971) A propos de 196 observations d'encephalopathie myoclonique infantile avec hypsarythmie (E.M.I.H.). Traitement par A.C.T.H. purifiee. Danger de l'A.C.T.H. synthetique. *Rev. Electroencephal. Neurophysiol.*, **1**, 112–13.
134. O'Donohoe, N. V. (1976) A 15-year follow-up of 100 children with infantile spasms. *Ir. J. Med.*, **145**, 138.
135. Sukuma, N., Murayama, T., Uzuki, K. *et al.* (1980) The prognosis of infantile spasms. Survey of 46 cases. *Folia Psychiatr. Neurol. Jap.*, **34**, 345.
136. Rankin, R. M. (1972) Prognosis of epilepsy in children. *Northwest Med.*, **71**, 455–9.
137. Sofijanov, N. G. (1982) Clinical evolution and prognosis of childhood epilepsies. *Epilepsia*, **23**, 61–9.

CHAPTER TWELVE

Women and Epilepsy

This chapter discusses certain features of epilepsy of particular interest to women – epilepsy and menstruation, epilepsy and pregnancy, and the teratogenic effects of epilepsy and anticonvulsant drugs. Relevant references follow each section.

12.1 EPILEPSY AND MENSTRUATION

Danuta Rosciszewska

12.1.1 Menarche

Gowers in 1893 reported a tendency for epilepsy to begin during puberty [1] and this was reported also by Turner in 1907 [2]. Other authors have also described this phenomenon in single cases [3, 4]. Lennox [5] found an association between the first seizure and menarche in 25% of 387 women with onset of seizures between the ages of 18 and 20. In a smaller group of 47 women whose first seizure occurred during puberty (aged 11–15 years), was found that menarche and the first seizure together occurred within six months in 60%, within one year in 23%, and within two years in 17% of patients.

There is little information on the effect of puberty in girls with already established epilepsy. However, in a study of 115 girls, whose epilepsy had begun at a mean age of 5.1 years, the course of the illness remained unchanged in only one-third of patients [6]. In two-thirds of the remaining girls, seizure frequency increased, or a new type of seizure occurred; in one-third the seizure frequency decreased, or seizures stopped altogether. Generalized tonic-clonic seizures tended to increase, or join other seizure types, as did partial complex seizures. In contrast, absences rarely increased, and sometimes stopped. Exacerbation of epilepsy was more likely in girls whose epilepsy had begun at an earlier age, was of known aetiology, who had had numerous tonic-clonic seizures, and who had neurological or psychological abnormalities on examination, or abnormalities in the EEG. If menarche was later than that of a control population, then the frequency of seizures was likely to be greater during puberty. It is clear, therefore, that clinical features reflecting organic damage to the nervous system predict the likely cause of epilepsy during puberty [6]. No prospective studies have been undertaken on the course of epilepsy during puberty, in which both measurements of ovarian hormones and serum anticonvulsant levels have been made. One retrospective study [6a] showed no important changes in anticonvulsant levels.

12.1.2   Catamenial seizures

Cyclical exacerbation of epilepsy has been observed since antiquity, and used to be attributed to the influence of the moon. Gowers first examined, in 1885, the relationship between seizures and menstruation [7]. Seizures occurring at or near the time of menstrual bleeding have been called catamenial seizures, though different authors use different criteria when defining such seizures. For example, different authors include different numbers of days preceding the first day of bleeding as part of the menstrual period. This may account for some differences between the data presented by different authors. Almquist [8] found almost no evidence of any such relationship, whilst others [5, 9–12] found menstrual exacerbation in between 10% and 63% of women with epilepsy. The highest percentage of all (72%) was reported by Laidlaw [13]. The present author has studied 69 women for four years, and found an increase of seizures before and during menstruation in two-thirds of patients. The distribution of 6900 seizures during 1237 menstrual cycles is shown in Fig. 12.1 [14].

In a few women, seizures may occur *only* during the days immediately preceding menstruation, or during menstruation itself. In our own study [15], only four of 226 women with epilepsy had seizures occurring regularly with every menstruation, and a further six women had occasional seizures during some menstruations only. The term 'catamenial epilepsy' should best be limited to such cases.

Catamenial exacerbation of seizures is more pronounced in women with symptomatic epilepsy, and is often associated with those who are already having frequent seizures. It also appears that those who suffer premenstrual tension are more likely to have seizures on premenstrual days, or at the time of menstrual bleeding [14].

The association between menstruation and seizures has been found in patients with simple partial, complex partial, and generalized tonic-clonic seizures [14, 16, 17]. However, different seizure types are associated with different phases of the menstrual cycle. Patients with absence seizures have most seizures during the late luteal phase, and the least during the menstrual and follicular stages. Conversely, it has been reported that the frequency of partial seizures is least during the luteal phase, the numbers increasing both during menstruation and just before ovulation [17]. In patients with more than one type of seizure, tonic-clonic seizures seem to be more cyclical than other types.

Few EEG studies have been performed, but this author has EEG observations on 41 women with different types of epileptic seizure at different phases of the menstrual cycle [18]. Most have tonic-clonic seizures. A significant increase of paroxysmal discharges was found on the premenstrual days of 24 patients who had catamenial exacerbation of seizures, whereas in 17 women with seizures not related to premenstrual days, the highest frequency of

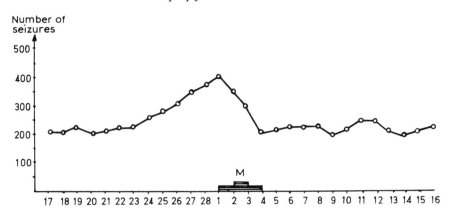

Figure 12.1 Plot of seizure dispersion during the menstrual cycles of 69 women with epilepsy. M – menstrual bleeding. (After [14]).

paroxysmal discharges was seen on days close to ovulation. In both groups, the lowest number of paroxysmal discharges was noted on days six and 22 of the menstrual cycle.

(a) Mechanism of catamenial seizures

One obvious explanation for the variation in seizure incidence during the menstrual cycle is that the seizure frequency is in some way linked to variations in hormonal levels. A number of investigations on models of epilepsy [19–21] have shown a convulsive effect of oestrogens, and an inhibitory effect of progesterone (for further references, see [22]). However, estimations of ovarian hormone levels during the menstrual cycle of those with epilepsy [23] have not confirmed the suggestion [21] that high levels of oestrogens are responsible for the catamenial exacerbation of seizures. Indeed, in 37 women with catamenial seizures, a significant decrease of oestrogens (except for days five and six of the cycle) was found, as compared to a control population. Furthermore, there was no correlation between the circulating levels of oestrogen and the numbers of seizures on different days of the cycle (Fig. 12.2).

The alternative hypothesis is based upon the anticonvulsant properties of progesterone. Figure 12.2 shows that the level of progesterone metabolites was decreased in epileptic women in comparison with the values found in control patients but, when it reached its highest value, the numbers of seizures were least. The difference between the values found in the control and epileptic population was greatest on premenstrual days with the highest incidence of seizures. Measurements of luteinizing hormone confirm decreased progesterone activity during the luteal phase, but not during the follicular phase [24].

These observations are only partly supported by observations on experimental animals. Nicolletti and colleagues [25] found that estradiol and high doses of clomiphene potentiated kainate-induced seizures in the rat the effect being more pronounced in male animals. Low doses of clomiphene were mildly anticonvulsant in both sexes. Medroxyprogesterone partially protected female rats against kainate-induced seizures, but increased the severity of seizures in male rats.

In addition to an altered ratio of oestrogen to progesterone, water retention and disturbances of electrolyte balance may also contribute to the increased propensity of some women to have seizures before or during menstruation. The addition of oral diuretics to anticonvulsant therapy at this time may, therefore, be helpful [3].

Feely and Gibson [26] have described one effective way of treating catamenial epilepsy, by using clobazam for ten days around the time of menstruation. Such intermittent therapy was effective, and seemed to avoid the tolerance often associated with this drug.

A further explanation for the catamenial exacerbation of some patients with epilepsy may be found in the changes in serum phenytoin levels on premenstrual days, demonstrated in Fig. 12.2 [23]. The mechanism of this fall in serum phenytoin on premenstrual days is not clear. It is possible that circulating ovarian steroids may induce the activity of hepatic enzymes which hydroxylate phenytoin [27].

12.1.3   The effect of oral contraceptives

An improvement in seizure frequency has been observed when progesterone was used as an oral contraceptive [3, 4, 28] or as specific medication [28a]. Conversely, an increase in seizure frequency has been observed after the use of oestrogens [29]. Bäckström and his colleagues [30] observed that in four of seven women with complex partial seizures related to menstruation, the spike frequency in the EEG was reduced during the intravenous infusion of progesterone. Mattson and his colleagues [31] showed a worthwhile reduction of previously uncontrolled seizures in six women with epilepsy who were given medroxyprogesterone. However, Dana-Haeri and Richens [16] could not show any effect of norethisterone on seizures associated with menstruation.

There is room for further studies on the interaction of oestrogens, progesterones and free and total circulating levels of anticonvulsants in patients whose epilepsy is worst at the time of menstruation or pill-induced bleeding.

Figure 12.2 Total oestrogen and progesterone metabolite excretion in the group of 37 women with seizures related to the menstrual cycle (E) and in healthy women (C). Phenytoin (DPH) levels in 29 females from the same group, and seizures during the menstrual cycle. M – menstrual bleeding.

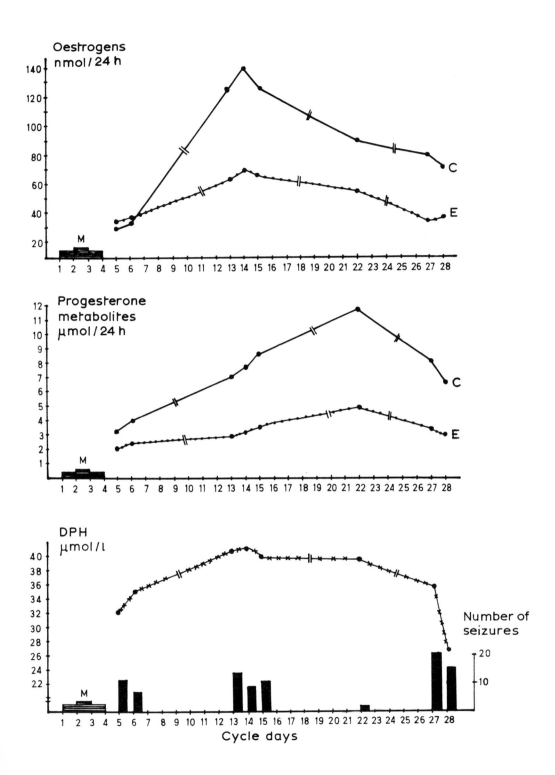

12.1.4   The effect of the menopause on epilepsy

Different authors report different effects of the menopause on seizure frequency – no effect [2, 32], an increase in seizures [33], a recurrence of seizures at the time of the menopause [34], and, finally, a remission of seizures during the menopause [35]. In our own study [15] we found that seizures were more likely to improve during the menopause if the seizures had previously been related to menstruation. Furthermore, epilepsy was more likely to improve during the menopause if epilepsy had begun later in life, and if seizures had always been infrequent. On the other hand, those who had always suffered frequent generalized tonic-clonic or complex partial seizures were more likely to have an exacerbation during the menopause. It appeared that those whose seizures declined in frequency during the menopause had an age of menopause similar to that of the general population, whilst in those with an earlier menopause the seizure frequency remained either unchanged or, in a few cases, increased.

12.1.5   Menstrual dysfunction and complex partial seizures

In addition to the effects of cyclical changes in progesterone and oestrogen upon seizure frequency, the reverse aspect has to be considered. Herzog *et al.* have described amenorrhoea, oligomenorrhoea and cycles of irregular length in many women with complex partial seizures [36]. Women with such menstrual abnormalities are likely to have anovulatory cycles and inadequate luteal phases, characterized by elevated ratios of serum oestrogen to progesterone. This increased ratio may predispose to further seizures. The surges of prolactin released during complex partial seizures (p. 541) may well be the mechanism involved in inducing such menstrual irregularities. In addition, Molaie *et al.* [37] have shown significant elevations in serum prolactin during the non-rapid eye movement sleep of women with complex partial seizures, even though seizures were not occurring. In Herzog's series [36] a polycystic ovary syndrome was much more likely to occur if seizure discharges arose from the left temporal lobe.

12.1.6   Fertility and epilepsy

The preceding section may go some way towards explaining the reduction in fertility of women with epilepsy; a reduction that seems unlikely to be explained solely by limited opportunities of marriage, as women with complex partial seizures are selectively disadvantaged [38]. Fertility rates are however also reduced for epileptic men [38].

References

1. Gowers, W. R. (1893) *A Manual of Diseases of Nervous System*, Blakinson, Philadelphia, pp. 732–53.
2. Turner, W. A. (1907) *Epilepsy, A Study of the Idiopathic Disease*, MacMillan, London, pp. 43–5.
3. Longo, S. and Saldana, G. (1966) Hormones and their influence in epilepsy. *Acta Neurol. Latinoamerica*, **12**, 29–47.
4. Zimmermann, A. W., Holden, K. R., Reiter, E. O. and Dekaban, A. S. (1973) Medroxyprogesterone acetate in the treatment of seizures associated with menstruation. *J. Pediatr.*, **83**, 961–3.
5. Lennox, W. G. and Lennox, M. A. (1960) *Epilepsy and Related Disorders*, Vol. 2, Little, Brown and Co., Boston, pp. 645–50.
6. Rosciszewska, D. and Horwat-Kaczmarek, M. (1985) *Change of Epilepsy Course in Girls During Puberty*, in Abstracts of 16th Epilepsy International Congress, 1985, Hamburg.
6a. Diamantopoulos, N. and Crumrine, P. K. (1986) The effect of puberty on the course of epilepsy. *Arch. Neurol.*, **43**, 873–76.
7. Gowers, W. G. (1885) *Epilepsy and Other Chronic Convulsive Diseases: Their Causes, Symptoms, and Treatment*, William Wood, New York, 255.
8. Almquist, R. (1955) The rhythm of epileptic attacks and its relationship to the menstrual cycle. *Acta Psychiatr. Scand.*, **30** (Suppl. 107), 1–16.
9. Dickerson, W. (1941) The effect of menstruation on seizure incidence. *J. Nerv. Ment. Dis.*, **94**, 160–9.
10. Morrin, S. (1983) *Effect of Certain Hormonal Incidents Upon Seizures in 100 Out-Patient Epileptic Women*, in Abstracts of 15th Epilepsy International Symposium, 1983, Washington, p. 107.
11. Ansell, B. and Clarke, E. (1956) Epilepsy and menstruation: The role of water retention. *Lancet*, **ii**, 1232–5.
12. Schelp, A. O. and Speciali, J. G. (1983) Estudio clinico da epilepsia catamenial. *Arq. Neuro-Psiquiatr. (Sao Paulo)*, **41**, 152–62.
13. Laidlaw, J. (1956) Catamenial epilepsy. *Lancet*, **ii**, 1235–7.
14. Rosciszewska, D. (1980) Analysis of seizure dispersion during menstrual cycle in women with epilepsy, in *Epilepsy. A Clinical and Experimental Research* (ed. J. Majkowski), Karger, Basel, pp. 280–4.
15. Rosciszewska, D. (1974) *Clinical Course of Epilepsy During Puberty Maturity and Climacterium*. Dissertation, Katowice, pp. 25–104.
16. Dana-Haeri, J. and Richens, A. (1983) Effect of norethisterone on seizures associated with menstruation. *Epilepsia*, **24**, 377–81.
17. Bäckström, T., Landgren, S., Zetterlund, B. *et al.* (1984) Effect of ovarian steroid hormones on brain excitability and their relation to epilepsy seizure variation during the menstrual cycle, in *Advances in Epileptology* (15th Epilepsy International Symposium) (ed. R. Porter), Raven Press, New York, pp. 269–77.
18. Grudzinska, B. and Rosciszewska, D. (1980) *Dynamics of EEG Changes During the Menstrual Cycle in Epileptic Women*, in Abstracts of XI Meeting of the Polish Neurological Association, Bydgoszcz, pp. 61–2.
19. Bäckström, T., Blom, S., Landgren, S. *et al.* (1983) *Effect of Female Steroid Hormones*

on the Brain, in Abstracts of 15th Epilepsy International Symposium, Washington, p. 54.

20. Hardy, R. W. (1970) Unit activity in Premarin-induced cortical epileptogenic foci. *Epilepsia*, **11**, 179–86.

21. Logothetis, J., Harner, R., Morrell, F. and Torres, F. (1959) The role of estrogens in catamenial exacerbation of epilepsy. *Neurology* (Minneap.), **9**, 352–60.

22. Magos, A. and Studd, J. (1985) Effects of the menstrual cycle on medical disorders. *Br. J. Hosp. Med.*, **33**, 68–77.

23. Rosciszewska, D., Buntner, B., Guz, I. and Zawisza, L. (1986) Ovarian hormones, anticonvulsant drugs, and seizures during the menstrual cycle in women with epilepsy. *J. Neurol., Neurosurg. Psychiatr.*, **49**, 47–51.

24. Rosciszewska, D., Dutkiewicz, J. and Blecharz, A. (1985) Luteinizing hormone (LH) serum level during the menstrual cycle in female epileptic patients. *Neurol. Neurochirurg. Pol.*, **29**, 205–10.

25. Nicolletti, F., Speciale, C., Sortino, M. A. *et al.* (1985) Comparative effects of estradiol benzoate, the antioestrogen clomiphene citrate, and the progestin medroxyprogesterone acetate on kainic acid-induced seizures in male and female rats. *Epilepsia*, **26**, 252–7.

26. Feely, M. and Gibson, J. (1984) Intermittent clobazam for catamenial epilepsy. *J. Neurol. Neurosurg. Psychiatr.*, **47**, 1279–82.

27. Kutt, H. (1972) Diphenylhydantoin. Interactions with other drugs in man, in *Antiepileptic Drugs* (eds D. M. Woodbury *et al.*), Raven Press, New York, pp. 169–80.

28. Hall, S. M. (1977) Treatment of menstrual epilepsy with a progesterone-only oral contraceptive. *Epilepsia*, **18**, 235–6.

28a. Herzog, A. G. (1986) Intermittent progesterone therapy and frequency of complex partial seizures in women with menstrual disorders. *Neurology*, **36**, 1607–10.

29. Rosciszewska, D. (1973) On the use of oral contraceptive Femigen-Polfa by women with epilepsy. *Neurol. Neurochirurg. Pol.*, **7**, 715–17.

30. Bäckström, T., Zetterlund, B., Blom, S. and Romano, M. (1984) Effect of intravenous progesterone infusions on the epileptic discharge frequency in women with partial epilepsy. *Acta Neurol. Scand.*, **69**, 240–8.

31. Mattson, R. H., Klein, P. E., Caldwell, B. V. and Cramer, J. A. (1982) Medroxyprogesterone treatment of women with uncontrolled seizures. *Epilepsia*, **23**, 436–7.

32. Spratling, W. (1904) *Epilepsy and Its Treatment*, Sundres and Company, Philadelphia, p. 116.

33. Müller, C. (1953) Ovarienfunktion und epilepsie. *Dtsch. Med. Wochenschr.*, **18**, 359–61.

34. Gastaut, H. and Tassinari, C. (1966) Triggering mechanism in epilepsy. *Epilepsia*, **7**, 86–137.

35. Zara, E., Scala, A. and Lavitola, G. (1966) Epilepsia e monopausa. *Osp. Psichiatr. Prov. Napoli*, **34**, 95–104.

36. Herzog, A. G., Seibel, M. M., Schomer, D. L. *et al.* (1986) Reproductive endocrine disorders in women with partial seizures of temporal lobe origin. *Arch. Neurol.*, **43**, 341–46.

37. Molaie, M., Culebras, A. and Miller, M. (1986) Effect of interictal epileptiform discharges on nocturnal plasma prolactin concentrations in epileptic patients with complex partial seizures. *Epilepsia*, **27**, 724–28.

38. Webber, M. P., Hauser, W. A., Ottman, R. and Annegers, J. F. (1986) Fertility in persons with epilepsy: 1935–1974. *Epilepsia*, **27**, 746–52.

12.2 EPILEPSY AND PREGNANCY

Anthony Hopkins

This section discusses the effects of pregnancy upon seizure frequency, the effect of epilepsy upon the fetus, and the effect of pregnancy upon the metabolism of anticonvulsant drugs.

12.2.1 Seizures occurring for the first time in pregnancy

(a) Eclampsia

Seizures occurring late in the third trimester of pregnancy, or rarely within 48 hours of delivery, may be due to eclampsia, but the association of hypertension (diastolic >90 mm Hg), oedema and proteinuria should immediately make this association obvious. The management of eclampsia is outside the scope of this book, beyond remarking that early delivery of the child is the foundation of treatment. From the point of view of seizure control, a neurologist will not go far wrong if he follows the principles of the management of status epilepticus, outlined on p. 432. The use of magnesium sulphate, recommended by many American obstetricians for the control of seizures [1], has not found favour in neurological practice. It probably only controls the overt manifestations of tonic-clonic seizures by neuromuscular paralysis, rather than influencing cerebral paroxysmal activity. Occasionally, the hypertensive ischaemic changes associated with an eclamptic encephalopathy may provide a focus of neural damage based upon which subsequent epilepsy occurs.

(b) First seizures in pregnancy, or epilepsy beginning in pregnancy

As the age-specific annual incidence rate for epilepsy is approximately constant at about 40–50 per 100 000 throughout the childbearing period (p. 7), pregnancy and the onset of non-eclamptic seizures will therefore coincide by chance alone in a number of women. There are of course some women whose first (of many) seizures occurs in pregnancy, but there is no study which provides statistical evidence that pregnancy is likely to start epilepsy.

A rather different problem is that of non-eclamptic seizures which occur for the first time in pregnancy, remit after delivery, and then return only in subsequent pregnancies. Knight and Rhind [1a] found only two such patients amongst their 59 epileptic mothers studied through 153 pregnancies. Furthermore, it is unusual, in the case of pre-existing epilepsy, for seizures to recur during pregnancy after a prolonged seizure-free period. The apparent rarity of these phenomena suggests that pregnancy *per se* is not a particularly potent epileptogenic agent.

Patients who develop seizures during pregnancy may require investigation in the same way as those who develop epilepsy unassociated with pregnancy. CT scanning is reasonably safe for the fetus, which can be largely protected from scattered radiation by appropriate lead curtains and abdominal shielding. MRI scanning is an alternative. Benign tumours such as meningiomas and neurofibromas certainly expand during pregnancy, and the rate of progression of astrocytomas also probably increases. Arteriovenous malformations may also expand or infarct during pregnancy. Finally, in the immediate puerperium, a seizure may be a manifestation of a cerebral venous thrombosis.

(c) Seizure frequency during pregnancy

The effect of pregnancy on the course of epilepsy has been extensively reviewed in recent years. Schmidt [2] lists 27 studies between 1884 and 1980 which show an enormous variation in the frequency of seizures during pregnancy. As examples, in one study, 75% of patients had more seizures and 8% fewer; in another study 33% had more seizures and 52% fewer! The average experience from all studies on a total of 2165 reported patients was an increase in frequency in 24% of women, a decrease in 22% of women, the frequency remaining unchanged in 53% [2]. These figures are close to those found in the British study by Knight and Rhind [1]. They found that whether the epilepsy was idiopathic or symptomatic did not make much difference to these figures, but it should be noted that this early study contained an unusually large number of mothers with so-called 'idiopathic' epilepsy, suggesting that classification of seizures was not accurate by modern standards. Those who had frequent seizures (monthly or more frequently) were four times more likely to have an increased frequency of seizures during pregnancy than those with occasional seizures (less than one in three months). Knight and Rhind also found that mothers carrying a male fetus were twice as likely to deteriorate during pregnancy as those carrying a female fetus. This interesting tendency has been found in two other studies quoted by these authors, but so far remains unexplained.

Remillard and colleagues [3] analysed prospectively the effects of pregnancy upon different types of epileptic seizure. The numbers were not large (52 pregnancies), but patients with secondarily generalized and complex partial seizures were most likely to have an increase in seizures during pregnancy (83% and 67% of mothers respectively), while only 29% of those with primary generalized epilepsy showed such an increase.

Schmidt and his colleagues [4] followed seizure frequency prospectively in 136 pregnancies in 122 epileptic women. Seizure frequency increased during one-third of these pregnancies, but in two-thirds of these, the increase was associated either with poor compliance with suggested anticonvulsant treatment, or deprivation of sleep, though the definition of deprivation of sleep was only 'a delay of more than two hours from the usual working day onset of sleep'. If an increase in seizure frequency did occur, it did so most often in the first two trimesters.

Schmidt and colleagues [4] had the opportunity of studying the course of 23 pregnancies during which the mother was not taking anticonvulsant therapy. In only eight of these did the numbers of seizures increase, and the authors felt that deprivation of sleep was again important in six of these. In pregnant epileptic women as a group, whether on anticonvulsant treatment or not, those who had not had a tonic-clonic seizure in the year before pregnancy, who only had one type of seizure, and who had primarily generalized epilepsy, had the least chance of worsening seizure frequency during pregnancy [4]. These factors are similar to those which also favour good prognosis for seizures in men and non-pregnant women (see Chapter 11).

The studies reviewed by Schmidt [2] are now rather out of date, as there is increased knowledge of the changes during pregnancy of the metabolism of anticonvulsant drugs, a subject reviewed on pp. 385–86. There are therefore opportunities for more skilled control of serum levels of anticonvulsant drugs. Good compliance and adequate serum levels of anticonvulsant drugs are not easily attained. Pregnant women in developed countries are increasingly aware of the teratogenic effects of anticonvulsant drugs (discussed on pp. 391–95). She, or another physician, may therefore reduce or stop the prescribed regimen in an attempt to reduce the chances of having an abnormal baby.

(d)   The effect of epilepsy upon the fetus

Epilepsy could be associated with fetal abnormalities in any one of five ways: (1) There could be a genetic association between the risk of seizures and the risk of fetal abnormality. (2) Seizures could themselves induce metabolic changes, such as hypoxia, which harm the fetus. (3) Trauma associated with seizures could harm the fetus. (4) The presence of epilepsy could provoke an obstetrician into more risky interventions. (5) Medication could harm the fetus. The last aspect is considered by Meadows on pp. 391–95, the others in the following paragraphs.

(1) The genetic association between epilepsy and fetal abnormality can be tested by comparing the fetal abnormality rate of untreated epileptic mothers with the rate for the population as a whole. Nakane and colleagues [5] reviewed the outcome of pregnancies of both treated and untreated epileptic mothers. Of the 14 studies reviewed by them, 4.5% of 825 infants of untreated epileptic mothers were malformed, contrasting with 7.1% of treated epileptic mothers; the rate for the population as a whole is probably about 3%, if follow-up after the neonatal period is carried out for a similar period as in these studies.

Another approach to studying the genetic association between epilepsy and fetal malformation is to compare the children of men with epilepsy, the children of women with epilepsy and the children of a control population without epilepsy. Annegers and Hauser [6] found that children of men with epilepsy did not have an increased rate of congenital malformations of specific types compared to the control population. A recent study from Denmark showed that epileptic men did not have more children with facial clefts than men in the general population [7].

Another approach has been to study the incidence of epilepsy among patients with children with facial clefts – the most frequent abnormality found in the children of epileptic mothers [8]. Friis found that the point prevalence of epilepsy amongst the parents of facial cleft probands was 2.3%, about three times the expected value ($p<0.05$). Any teratogenic effect of anticonvulsant medication would be reflected in a higher number of epileptic mothers than epileptic fathers. However, there was no significant difference between the sex of the parents in the study. Friis and his colleagues [9] have furthermore shown that the incidence of facial clefts among those with epilepsy is twice that expected from the general population.

The studies reviewed above suggest that epilepsy *per se* may be in some way a factor in the genesis of facial clefts. There may be a specific genetic linkage between epilepsy and fetal abnormality but the studies quoted above [6, 7] do not support it. It could be argued that women with epilepsy are limited in their choice of husband, who may be less 'biologically fit'.

(2) Although prolonged maternal hypoxia in status epilepticus could theoretically damage the fetus, the event must be extremely rare. It is, however, of interest that in Nakane's study [4] the highest malformation rate of all was for pregnancies in which seizures had occurred in spite of medication, though the numbers are insufficient to make this association significant. Suggested regimes for managing status epilepticus in pregnancy have been published [10] but, with the exception of the need for fetal monitoring they do not differ significantly from the regimens suggested in Chapter 14.

(3) The author has never encountered fetal damage caused by abdominal trauma during a fit, and knows of no published work to suggest that it has happened. Philbert and Down [11] found no evidence to suggest that obstetric complications such as toxaemia of pregnancy, accidental haemorrhage or hyperemesis are commoner in epileptic mothers. However, a larger study has been undertaken in Washington State [12]. Yerby and colleagues identified all birth certificates in Washington State for the years 1980–1981. There were over 138 000 births in all, but only 204 births to epileptic mothers, identified by coding on the birth certificates. Epileptic pregnancies tended to be complicated more often than randomly matched controls by pre-eclampsia (odds ratio 2.45), the need for amniocentesis (odds ratio 4.59 in second trimester), birth weight of less than 2.5 kg (odds ratio 2.79), and low Apgar scores (odds ratio 3.74 for a score of less than 7 at 5 min). The relative risk of previous fetal loss before 20 weeks gestation was 2.66 for epileptic mothers. Although these are impressive figures, only about one-quarter of the expected number of epileptic mothers were identified by birth certificate coding,

suggesting that these results may not be typical for epileptic women as a whole.

(4) There is however evidence that the presence of maternal epilepsy precipitates more potentially harmful obstetric intervention, such as induction of labour and instrumental delivery [13], although there are often no good grounds for such intervention.

12.2.2 The effect of pregnancy upon the metabolism of anticonvulsant drugs

The first point is that fluid retention and the volume of fetal tissues and placenta increase the volume of distribution of anticonvulsant drugs. This dilution in itself will tend to lower the serum level, if the oral dose is left unchanged.

The plasma protein binding of some drugs may be reduced. Ruprah and colleagues [14] have reported upon the binding of phenytoin to serum proteins in the last trimester. They have shown that the level of binding is considerably reduced, largely due to a fall in serum albumen. In the presence of such reduced binding, any previous relation between the serum phenytoin concentration and therapeutic effect will no longer hold, since a greater proportion of the total drug concentration will be free and pharmacologically active. These authors point out that in such circumstances the clinical value of measuring phenytoin levels in whole serum is greatly reduced unless serum binding capacity is measured. An alternative is to measure salivary phenytoin [14a], which probably reflects the unbound fraction.

The maternal liver may develop an increased capacity for hydroxylation of some anticonvulsant drugs, such as phenytoin [15]. Lander and his colleagues [16] studied the clearance of phenytoin after intravenous injection of phenytoin, and found approximately twice the rate of clearance that is found in non-pregnant patients. Bardy and colleagues [17] report similar findings for phenobarbitone, but, although there were marked variations within and between individuals for clearance of primidone, no overall significant changes were observed, nor did the clearance of carbamazepine change significantly.

The absorption of anticonvulsants from the bowel may be reduced. Ramsey *et al.* [18] report a pregnant woman with seizures who had low serum levels of phenytoin, complicated by the occurrence of status epilepticus, until the oral dose of phenytoin was increased to 1200 mg/day. Metabolic studies showed that, whereas the proportion of unmetabolized phenytoin in the urine remained unchanged, a large proportion (56%, normal range 5–15%) was excreted in the stool, this proportion falling to 23% in the postpartum period. The malabsorption was not specific for phenytoin, affecting also D-xylose and dietary fat.

Interaction with other drugs occurs. For example, benzodiazepines, which may be given to pregnant women, also lower the serum concentration of phenytoin.

If the oral dose of an anticonvulsant drug has been increased during pregnancy, as is sometimes indicated, then it is essential that appropriate adjustments are made after delivery, in order that intoxication is avoided.

The relationship between folic acid and anticonvulsants deserves special mention. Folic acid, often given during pregnancy, is known to cause a reduction in the level of at least one anticonvulsant drug, phenytoin, and may itself have an epileptogenic effect [19]. However, patients taking anticonvulsants may become folate deficient in pregnancy. Hiilesmaa *et al.* [20] showed that, although there was an inverse correlation between serum folate and phenytoin or phenobarbitone levels, the number of epileptic seizures during pregnancy showed no relation to serum folate levels. They suggest that a low dose of 100 μg or 1000 μg of folate is sufficient supplement for pregnant women on these drugs.

12.2.3 The puerperium and the neonate

Even if a baby is born without significant malformation to an epileptic mother, its problems are not necessarily over. Immediately after delivery, the level of anticonvulsants, which have freely crossed the placenta, begin to decline in the baby. The rate of clearance of anticonvulsant drugs from the newborn has been reviewed by Bossi [21]. The half-life for sodium valproate is 14–88 hours, for primidone 7–60 hours, for phenobarbitone 40–500 hours, for phenytoin 15–105 hours, and for carbamazepine 8–28 hours. There is less information for ethosuximide, but a figure of 41 hours has been reported [22].

Desmond *et al.* [23] described the effects of barbiturate withdrawal in the neonate. The clinical signs are hyperexcitability, occasional seizures, tremulousness and impaired suckling. Kaneko and his colleagues studied 42 infants and 32 epileptic mothers for harmful side effects of anticonvulsant therapy [24]. They compared these infants with 50 infants of normal mothers and found less efficient suckling and slower gains in weight in the infants of epileptic mothers. Expectant supervision of such children is usually adequate, but if tremulousness or, in particular, if seizures occur, small doses of phenobarbitone (3–5 mg/kg/day) may be given.

Most mothers on anticonvulsant medication may safely breast feed their children as only moderate quantities of these drugs pass into the milk. The ratio between breast milk level and serum level was reported by Kaneko's group to be 0.19 for phenytoin and 0.41 for carbamazepine, 0.36 for phenobarbitone and 0.70 for primidone [24]. Shorvon (p. 265) gives a ratio of <0.1 for valproate.

Some infants have bled as a result of drug-induced depression of vitamin K-dependent clotting factors, such as prothrombin and Factors V and VII [25, 26]. Davies *et al.* [27] have shown that the concentration of the protein induced by vitamin K absence ('PIVKA') is raised in patients treated by several anticonvulsants. Vitamin K 20 mg/day should be routinely administered for the last two weeks of pregnancy to the mother treated with anticonvulsants, and also given intramuscularly to her newborn infant.

In conclusion, the obstetrician and neurologist have to balance two conflicting interests in managing a pregnant woman with epilepsy. On the one hand, she may be advised to continue to take anticonvulsant drugs during pregnancy, probably in increased oral dosage so that adequate serum levels can be maintained; this is in order to avoid the risks of seizures and in particular the risk of status epilepticus occurring during pregnancy. On the other hand, reducing or stopping anticonvulsant drugs may be suggested in order to reduce the chances of a congenital malformation. A careful review of all the factors relevant to the individual patient and her pregnancy is necessary before a decision can be reached [28].

References

1. Sibai, B. M. and Anderson, G. D. (1986) *Eclampsia in Neurological Disorders of Pregnancy* (ed. P. J. Goldstein) Futura Publishing, New York, pp. 1–18.
1a. Knight, A. H. and Rhind, E. G. (1975) Epilepsy and pregnancy: a study of 153 pregnancies in 59 patients. *Epilepsia*, **16**, 99–110.
2. Schmidt, D. (1982) The effect of pregnancy on the natural history of epilepsy: review of the literature, in *Epilepsy, Pregnancy and the Child* (eds D. Janz *et al.*), Raven Press, New York, pp. 3–14.
3. Remillard, G., Dansky, L., Andermann, E. and Andermann, F. (1982) Seizure frequency during pregnancy and the puerperium, in *Epilepsy, Pregnancy and the Child* (eds D. Janz *et al.*), Raven Press, New York, pp. 15–26.
4. Schmidt, D., Canger, R., Avanzini, G. *et al.* (1983) Change of seizure frequency in pregnant epileptic women. *J. Neurol. Neurosurg. Psychiatr.*, **46**, 751–5.
5. Nakane, Y., Okuma, T., Takahishi, R. *et al.* (1980) Multi-institutional study on the teratogenecity and foetal toxicity of anti-epileptic drugs: a report of a collaborative study group in Japan. *Epilepsia*, **21**, 663–80.
6. Annegers, J. F. and Hauser, W. A. (1982) The frequency of congenital malformations in relatives of patients with epilepsy, in *Epilepsy, Pregnancy and the Child* (eds D. Janz *et al.*), Raven Press, New York, pp. 267–73.
7. Friis, M., Holm, N. V., Sindrup, E. H. *et al.* (1986) Facial clefts in sibs and children of epileptic patients. *Neurology*, **36**, 346–50.
8. Friis, M. L. (1979) Epilepsy among parents of children with facial clefts. *Epilepsia*, **20**, 69–76.
9. Friis, M. L., Boreng-Nielsen, B., Sindrup, E. J. *et al.* (1981) Facial clefts among epileptic patients. *Arch. Neurol.*, **38**, 227–9.
10. Dalessio, D. J. (1985) Seizure disorders and pregnancy. *N. Engl. J. Med.*, **312**, 559–63.
11. Philbert, A. and Dam, M. (1982) The epileptic mother and her child. *Epilepsia*, **23**, 85–99.
12. Yerby, M., Koepsell, T. and Daling, D. (1985) Pregnancy complications and outcomes in a cohort of women with epilepsy. *Epilepsia*, **26**, 631–5.
13. Egenaes, J. (1982) Outcome of pregnancy in women with epilepsy, Norway 1967–

1978: description of material, in *Epilepsy, Pregnancy and the Child* (eds D. Janz *et al.*), Raven Press, New York, pp. 81–5.

14. Ruprah, M., Perucca, E. and Richens, A. (1980) Decreased serum protein binding of phenytoin in late pregnancy. *Lancet*, **ii**, 316–7.

14a. Knott, C., Williams, C. P. and Reynolds, F. (1986) Phenytoin kinetics during pregnancy and the puerperium. *Br. J. Obstet. Gynaecol.*, **93**, 1030–37.

15. Mygind, K. I., Dam, M. and Christiansen, J. (1976) Phenytoin and phenobarbitone plasma clearance during pregnancy. *Acta Neurol. Scandi.*, **54**, 160–6.

16. Lander, C. M., Smith, M. T., Chalk, J. B. *et al.* (1984) Bioavailability and pharmacokinetics of phenytoin during pregnancy. *Eur. J. Clin. Pharmacol.*, **27**, 105–10.

17. Bardy, A. H., Teramo, K. and Hiilesmaa, V. K. (1982) Apparent plasma clearances of phenytoin, phenobarbitone, primidone and carbamazepine during pregnancy: results of the prospect Helsinki study, in *Epilepsy, Pregnancy and the Child* (eds D. Janz *et al.*), Raven Press, New York, pp. 141–5.

18. Ramsey, R. E., Strauss, R. G. and Willmore, L. J. (1978) Status epilepticus in pregnancy: effect of phenytoin malabsorption on seizure control. *Neurology*, **28**, 85–9.

19. Strauss, R. G. and Bernstein, R. (1974) Folic acid and Dilantin antagonism in pregnancy. *Obstetr. Gynecol.*, **44**, 345–8.

20. Hiilesmaa, V. E., Teramo, K., Granstrom, M.-L. and Bardy, A. H. (1983) Serum folate concentrations in women with epilepsy. *Br. Med. J.*, **187**, 577–9.

21. Bossi, L. (1982) Neonatal period including drug disposition in newborns: review of the literature, in *Epilepsy, Pregnancy and the Child* (eds D. Janz *et al.*), Raven Press, New York, pp. 327–34.

22. Koup, J. R., Rose, J. Q. and Cohen, M. E. (1978) Ethosuximide pharmacokinetics in a pregnant patient and her new-born. *Epilepsia*, **19**, 535–9.

23. Desmond, M. M., Schwanecke, R. P., Wilson, G. S. *et al.* (1972) Maternal barbiturate utilisation and neonatal withdrawal symptomatology. *J. Paediatr.*, **80**, 190–7.

24. Kaneko, S., Suzuki, K., Sato, T. *et al.* (1982) The problems of antiepileptic medication in the neonatal period: is breast feeding advisable? in *Epilepsy, Pregnancy and the Child* (eds D. Janz *et al.*), Raven Press, New York, pp. 343–8.

25. Solomon, G. E., Hillgartner, M. W. and Kutt, H. (1973) Coagulation defects caused by phenobarbital and primidone. *Neurology*, **23**, 445–51.

26. Bleyer, W. A. and Skinner, A. L. (1976) Fatal neonatal haemorrhage after maternal anticonvulsant therapy. *JAMA*, **235**, 626–7.

27. Davies, V. A., Argent, A. C., Staub, H. *et al.* (1985) Precursor prothrombin status in patients receiving anticonvulsant drugs. *Lancet*, **i**, 126–28.

28. Hopkins, A. (1987) Epilepsy and anticonvulsant drugs. *Br. Med. J.*, **294**, 497–501.

12.3 THE TERATOGENIC ASSOCIATIONS OF EPILEPSY AND ANTICONVULSANT DRUGS

Roy Meadow

'Teratogenic' is derived from the Greek 'teras' which means malformation or monstrosity. Thus teratogenic means the capacity to induce malformation.

Characteristically most people think of structural or anatomical malformations many of which are detectable immediately at birth, but there can also be functional, physiological and behavioural abnormalities which may not be apparent until much later.

The concept of environmental factors harming the fetus in the womb became firmly established nearly 50 years ago with the discovery of the teratogenic properties of the rubella virus [1]. Even at that time it was clear that the teratogenic effect was not uniform and that it depended upon a susceptible individual being exposed to the harmful environmental factor at a particular moment of pregnancy. Moreover, it was also clear that an agent (the rubella virus) which was relatively innocuous to the mother and sometimes did not even cause her to have appreciable symptoms could cause disastrous consequences such as blindness, congenital heart disease and deafness for her baby. These principles were also shown to apply during the study of the thalidomide disaster [2, 3]. Thalidomide had the pharmacological effect of central nervous system depression and was believed to be a very safe sedative and hypnotic. It rarely caused side effects for women, but by 1961 it was clear that it sometimes caused disastrous damage to the fetus, particularly by way of absent arms and shortened limbs. Once again the studies revealed that only a minority of mothers who took thalidomide during pregnancy had abnormal babies. It also seemed that the drug dosage was not crucial but that the timing in pregnancy when the thalidomide was taken was of great importance. One of the reasons why the teratogenic effects of thalidomide were detected fairly quickly was because of the unusual nature of the defects they induced. If thalidomide had merely induced more common abnormalities such as spina bifida, cleft lip or congenital heart disease it is likely that incrimination of the drug would have taken much longer. The identification of the problem was also made easier as the drug had only recently been introduced. It is clear that if the drug had been in use for a very long time, or alternatively caused more common abnormalities, recognition of this effect might not have occurred.

Since the 1960s most countries have established registers of congenital abnormalities. Any increase of a particular abnormality generates a search for a possible environmental cause. Despite intensive searching, very few drugs have been incriminated. None have been found to be as convincingly teratogenic as thalidomide, except perhaps for the cytotoxic folate antagonists such as aminopterin [4, 5]. However, a number of drugs and a number of environmental factors have been alleged to have a teratogenic action, in that if given to a woman carrying a genetically susceptible fetus, when the fetus is at a susceptible stage in development, congenital abnormality becomes more likely. Anticonvulsants have been incriminated in that way.

In 1968 six infants with cleft lip and palate born to mothers with epilepsy who had taken anticonvulsants in pregnancy were reported [6]. The first of these is shown in Fig. 12.3. Four of the infants had congenital heart lesions and minor skeletal abnormalities also. All had an unusual facial appearance, including a short neck with a low posterior hairline, broadly rooted nose, wide spaced prominent eyes, and deformities of the pinna. The skulls were often of

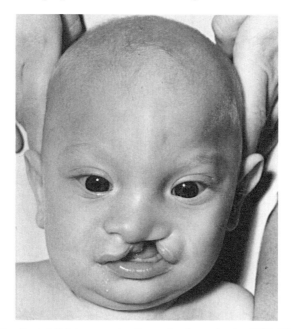

Figure 12.3 The first child to come to the author's notice in 1962. The mother had generalized seizures for which she took phenytoin 300 mg and phenobarbitone 180 mg/day. Her baby had cleft lip and palate, trigonocephaly (the skull looking like a triangle when viewed from above because of the pointed frontal area), marked epicanthic folds and minor bone abnormalities of the hands.

unusual shape, pointed in the frontal area with a prominent ridged suture line; minor bone defects of the hands were common. That report resulted in the author being notified of 40 similar cases that had occurred in England about the same time [7]. It also led to a vast number of studies in different countries into the association between epilepsy, anticonvulsants and congenital malformations. The studies have addressed themselves firstly to establishing an association and then secondly to trying to identify if it is the epilepsy or the anticonvulsants which are primarily responsible for that association.

12.3.1   The nature of the association

More than 20 large scale well-conducted epidemiological surveys of mothers with epilepsy have established that there is a significant increase in congenital malformations in their children [8, 9]. Most of these surveys have been retrospective, but nevertheless have been conducted with care and have used reliable controls. Obviously they are likely to be biased to inclusion of women with more severe epilepsy and are likely to under report minor malformations. They will also fail to record those functional and behavioural abnormalities that only become apparent later in development. However, overall, as shown in Table 12.1, children of epileptic mothers have approximately twice as many malformations as children of mothers without epilepsy. The same finding has

Table 12.1 Incidence of malformations in liveborn children of mothers with epilepsy according to (1) retrospective, and (2) four prospective studies in comparison to control groups

	Children of mothers with epilepsy			Children of mothers without epilepsy (controls)		
	Total	With malformations		Total	With malformations	
	n	*n*	%	*n*	*n*	%
(1)	2737	140	5.1	561 587	14 942	2.7
(2)	404	45	11.1	64 809	3 673	5.7

Reproduced with kind permission from *Epilepsy*, *Pregnancy and the Child* (1982) (eds D. Janz *et al.*), Raven Press, New York [8].

been made from the few reliable prospective studies that have been completed [10, 11, 12]. To put this in perspective, it should be remembered that about 3% of all newborn babies have a major congenital abnormality; therefore if the mother has epilepsy, the chance of her child having a major congenital abnormality is about 6%. Most of the surveys have found that congenital heart disease and clefts of the lip and palate are particularly likely. Congenital heart disease seems to be about 4 times more likely than in the general population and cleft lip and palate ten times more likely [13]. Minor abnormalities of the hands involving hypoplasia of the terminal phalanges, and minor facial anomalies are also common.

12.3.2   Is it epilepsy, anticonvulsant drugs or both which are responsible?

Nearly all the mothers with epilepsy studied in the many surveys were believed to be taking anticonvulsant drugs during their pregnancy. Therefore it is difficult to find reliable surveys comparing the incidence of malformation in the offspring of mothers with epilepsy who were receiving anticonvulsants compared with that for mothers with epilepsy who were not receiving anticonvulsants. Moreover, even when a group of mothers with epilepsy not receiving anticonvulsants can be identified, it is fairly certain that the nature of their epilepsy will be different from those who did receive drugs. It is likely to be less severe and likely to include more simple partial seizures. However, in more than ten controlled studies, the finding is that mothers with epilepsy who are taking anticonvulsant drugs are two to three times more likely to have a baby with a congenital abnormality than mothers with epilepsy who are not taking anticonvulsant drugs [8] (Table 12.2). Studies comparing mothers with epilepsy who do not take anticonvulsant drugs compared with the general population have not shown clearly whether there is a difference in the incidence of congenital malformation. Thus there are prima facie grounds for incriminating anticonvulsant drugs as teratogenic though the possibility is that epilepsy itself (of a severity to require anticonvulsants) is also important.

Table 12.2 Incidence of malformations in children of mothers treated with anti-epileptic drugs and of untreated mothers with epilepsy according to 15 retrospective comparative studies

Children of treated mothers with epilepsy			Children of untreated mothers with epilepsy		
Total	With malformations		Total	With malformations	
n	n	%	n	n	%
2948	229	7.8	943	32	3.4

Reproduced with kind permission from *Epilepsy , Pregnancy and the Child* (1982) (eds D. Janz *et al.*), Raven Press, New York [8].

If anticonvulsants caused a most unusual abnormality (as did Thalidomide), incrimination would probably be easier. However, they do not; in general they cause an increased incidence of the common congenital abnormalities. The one anticonvulsant that may have a more specific teratogenic effect, sodium valproate, is considered later.

12.3.3   The type and severity of epilepsy

Several surveys have studied the type of epilepsy, its severity and the seizure frequency during pregnancy in relation to the occurrence of congenital abnormalities in the baby. No consistent finding emerges; it does not seem that any of these factors is specifically teratogenic [10, 14, 15].

Nevertheless, it is likely that people with epilepsy are genetically more likely to have certain congenital abnormalities than those without epilepsy. Cleft lip and palate has been found to be particularly common in persons with epilepsy (p. 384). Additionally there is an increased incidence of congenital heart disease, which itself is preferentially associated with cleft lip and palate. However, these associations are not strong and in themselves cannot account for the twofold increase of congenital abnormalities in the babies born to mothers with epilepsy receiving anticonvulsants.

The relationship of paternal epilepsy to congenital abnormality in the child is reviewed on p. 384. There have been fewer studies and the studies themselves have been smaller [12, 16–19].

12.3.4 Which anticonvulsants are teratogenic?

The early studies appeared to incriminate mainly phenobarbitone and phenytoin. This probably reflects the fact that these were the drugs principally used at the time of the studies. Some investigators believe that certain anticonvulsants sometimes produce a specific recognizable pattern of abnormalities. American authors particularly have been keen to identify 'the fetal hydantoin syndrome' [20] and the 'trimethadione syndrome' [21]. There is no doubt that the children described as having the hydantoin syndrome have many dysmorphic features – in particular a number of minor abnormalities of the face and the skull including epicanthic folds, strabismus, hypertelorism, abnormal ears, wide mouth with prominent lips, short nose with low nasal bridge, and short or webbed neck. Some regard these features as characteristic of hydantoin ingestion, but it is noteworthy that the first report of abnormalities in 1968 [6] drew attention to these features in children whose mothers had received several different anticonvulsants. The author and others have encountered many children with these features since whose mothers have had anticonvulsants other than phenytoin. In 1970 it was suggested that trimethadione produced a specific characteristic picture [21], but once again since those early reports other babies have been identified with the same features, who have been born to mothers who have had drugs other than trimethadione. Much more recently sodium valproate has been associated with similar dysmorphic features [22]. However, the main concern with sodium valproate is its association with spina bifida. This is unusual because previous reports of congenital abnormalities associated with epilepsy and anticonvulsants have not shown an increased incidence of spina bifida. However, in 1982 a large study from France [23, 24] showed that over 60% of the mothers with epilepsy who had given birth to children with spina bifida had taken sodium valproate during the first three months of pregnancy in a dose of 400–2000 mg/day. Five of these mothers took sodium valproate only, the others took additional anticonvulsants. Confirmation of the link came from the International Clearing House for Birth Defects Monitoring System which suggested that the risk for a mother with epilepsy taking sodium valproate during pregnancy of having a child with spina bifida is approximately 1.2%, which compares with a risk of approximately 0.06% for a woman with neither epilepsy nor anticonvulsant treatment [25].

Several studies have drawn attention to small skull size and slowness at acquiring developmental skills in babies born to mothers with epilepsy who received anticonvulsants [9]. There seems little doubt that as a group they are disadvantaged in that way. It is, however, extremely difficult to separate out the different genetic, social and environmental factors which influence a child's development. It is the old problem of distinguishing between nature and nurture, considering that a significant proportion of children whose parents have severe epilepsy will be living in a disadvantaged environment.

12.3.5   Which anticonvulsants are most teratogenic?

The weight of evidence suggests that anticonvulsant drugs are teratogenic; in addition there are suggestions that some drugs are more teratogenic than others. From that point of view it is worth bearing in mind that the disability resulting from the usual congenital abnormalities varies greatly. Cleft lip and palate may be very distressing for the parents, but nevertheless can usually be corrected well by surgery. Similarly many of the congenital heart lesions are totally correctable. The same is not true for spina bifida, where the majority of children will have permanent disability in the form of paraplegia and neuropathic bladder. Whether or not by the bad luck of being a widely used drug at the time of the first reports of probable anticonvulsant teratogenesis, there is no doubt that phenytoin has been blamed more often for congenital abnormality than most of the other anticonvulsants. The evidence that it is worse is weak, but nevertheless there is a trend throughout all the reports that does suggest that the hydantoin group of drugs may be more damaging than other anticonvulsants. The exceptions to that are the oxazolidinedione drugs such as trimethadione and paramethadione, but their limited use in women of child bearing age diminishes their potential harm to the fetus.

The suggestion also emerges from many studies that phenytoin plus phenobarbitone is more harmful than phenytoin alone.

There have been worrying reports about neuroblastoma occurring in children who are exposed to phenytoin in the womb [26, 27]. These are isolated reports, but taken together do suggest that this unusual tumour is occurring more than one might expect in the children of mothers who took phenytoin during pregnancy [28].

If one is looking for the safest drug, one needs to be cautious because of the lack of detailed studies on the more recently introduced drugs. It is worth remembering that until 1980 sodium valproate was thought to be extremely safe: then came the reports of an increase incidence of spina bifida [29]. The relatively few reports of abnormal babies born to epileptic mothers taking carbamazepine need to be taken cautiously, though at the moment one must concede that it has been linked less often with abnormality than most other drugs [9]. Some drugs that are more often considered as anti-anxiety or tranquillizer rather than anticonvulsant are used nevertheless for people with epilepsy; of these diazepam seems to have been more often incriminated than others, with a suggestive association with cleft lip and palate [30].

12.3.6　The timing of fetal damage

The teratogenic effect of a drug is most likely to occur from 18–56 days after fertilization. A drug can be harmful during the first 17 days but it tends to be an all or none effect – it either prevents implantation and therefore leads to abortion, or has no effect at all. From day 56 onwards, external factors can cause a reduction in the size and number of developing cells but structural abnormality is unlikely. Thus late exposure to a noxious substance may lead to microcephaly and mental retardation, but is unlikely at that time to cause congenital heart disease or a cleft lip. Bearing these dates in mind it is relevant that the teratogenic effect occurs at just about the time of the first missed period, i.e. at the time that the mother is beginning to wonder for the first time whether she might be pregnant, and certainly well before she has consulted her doctor or neurologist about it. This is why the emphasis must be on care before conception, with efforts made to ensure that mothers who are hoping to conceive are in as healthy and favourable state as possible.

In general the fetus shares the same conditions of nutrition and health as the mother. Although most drugs and substances that the mother ingests pass in the placental blood to the fetus, some are handled by the fetus in a different way, which can cause them to have higher or lower concentrations of the drug in their bloodstream than the mother. At present there is limited information about such differences with anticonvulsants but a report on the fetal handling of valproic acid shows that the fetus is exposed to much higher total valproic acid concentrations than the mother [31]. This seems to be the result of decreased maternal serum protein binding as a result of elevated maternal free fatty acid concentrations. Diazepam, which can also be displaced from binding sites by increased free fatty acid levels, is also elevated preferentially [31a]. Elevated free fatty acid levels are present in maternal blood during the perinatal period and also at earlier stages in pregnancy. So it is possible that the fetus is exposed to unusually high levels of valproate (and possibly diazepam) during the vital early days of pregnancy.

12.3.7　Mode of teratogenic effect

The most popular theory concerning the probable teratogenic action of the anticonvulsant drugs is in relation to their influence on folate metabolism [32]. The action of most anticonvulsants in lowering maternal blood serum folate is well known, as is the association in some cases with a frank megaloblastic anaemia. Pregnancy itself tends to lower serum folate levels, and there has been much indirect evidence suggesting that low serum folate is associated with an increased incidence of congenital abnormalities [33]. There is no doubt that folic acid antagonists do induce congenital defects in animals and that they can be teratogenetic for some humans [4, 5]. Others have suggested that breakdown products of particular anticonvulsants, such as phenytoin, are themselves toxic [34].

There have been extensive trials to test the teratogenicity of anticonvulsant drugs in pregnant mice, rats and other animals. However animal studies have limitations, because some species are far more prone to congenital abnormalities than others. Nearly all the anticonvulsants have been shown to be teratogenic in animals, but some anticonvulsants have been more teratogenic in one species, and others more teratogenic in different species. The size of dose used to achieve congenital abnormalities in animals ranges from 3 to 50 times the equivalent therapeutic dose used for humans [9].

There has been great interest in recent years in the role of nutrition, or rather poor nutrition, as an aetiological factor in the genesis of congenital abnormalities, especially spina bifida. The work on this subject is not conclusive, but is highly suggestive that poor nutrition is one of the factors that makes a susceptible person more likely to produce an abnormal child. Although much of the early work was on folate it has become apparent that people who are short of folate are often short of other vitamins and essential nutrients [35]. Therefore in many countries it has become the practice to provide a compound vitamin for pregnant women. As pointed out earlier, for this to be effective during the important stage of organ formation, the woman's nutrition must be in a good state at the time she conceives, and therefore the vitamin supplement needs to be given to women who are *hoping* to become pregnant, rather than at the time of their first visit to the antenatal clinic.

12.3.8 Conclusion

Congenital abnormalities arise from a combination of circumstances in which a genetically susceptible individual [36] is exposed at a critical moment to different environmental factors which cause abnormality to occur. There is some evidence that people with epilepsy may have a genetic susceptibility to certain congenital abnormalities. There is certainty that children born to mothers who have epilepsy and who have received anticonvulsant drugs during the pregnancy have at least twice as many congenital abnormalities as children whose mothers do not have epilepsy. Since mothers with epilepsy not receiving anticonvulsants do not have as many congenital abnormalities it is most probable that anticonvulsant drugs are teratogenic, causing particularly cleft lip and palate and congenital heart disease or, in the case of sodium valproate, spina bifida. An increased incidence of minor physical stigmata also occurs. Most of the commonly used anticonvulsants have been implicated, though trends emerge from the reported studies that do suggest that some drugs may be more teratogenic than others.

12.3.9 Practical implications

For the developing fetus the ideal is to have a healthy, happy mother in a good state of nutrition who is neither too young nor too old. These conditions need to apply before the moment of conception, as well as during the pregnancy. Any drug, whether it be alcohol, aspirin, anticonvulsant or nicotine is best avoided by the mother who is intending to conceive. However, a drug that is important for her health and happiness may be required, and few will doubt that most women of child-bearing age with epilepsy previously receiving anticonvulsants are likely to need anticonvulsants throughout their pregnancy to avoid needless seizures.

Ideally one would like the mother shortly before conception, and particularly for the first four months of pregnancy, not to receive anticonvulsants, but that is unlikely to be sensible for most mothers who have epilepsy. However, it is reasonable to use the current information to work out whether, from the baby's point of view, some anticonvulsants might be preferable to others. The evidence suggests that the fetus should not be exposed to any of the oxazolidinediones. There is also considerable prejudice against the hydantoins, though as mentioned earlier this may merely be because of the frequency with which phenytoin has been used in the past. At present there is least worry about carbamazepine.

Since many congenital abnormalities tend to repeat themselves within families, the doctor should enquire about the presence of a congenital abnormality in other family members including the previous generations. If, for instance, there were a positive family history of spina bifida, it would certainly influence one against giving sodium valproate to a woman of child-bearing age, because of the association between sodium valproate and babies with spina bifida.

From the point of view of the fetus it is likely that exposure to one anticonvulsant is preferable to exposure to two or more, and that lower doses are preferable to high. Any temporary reduction that might be safely considered during pregnancy should be from days 18–40 after conception – that is for three weeks after the first missed period, and ideally for a further two weeks.

Since the occurrence of congenital abnormalities depends on many factors including nutrition, one does not have to believe in the theory that anticonvulsants are harmful because of interference with folate metabolism in order to advise epileptic young women who wish to conceive to ensure good nutrition, and to take a standard compound vitamin supplement containing folate.

REFERENCES

1. Gregg, N. M. (1941) Congenital cataract following German measles in the mother. *Trans. Ophthal. Soc. Aust.*, **3**, 35–46.
2. McBride, W. G. (1961) Thalidomide and congenital abnormalities. *Lancet*, **ii**, 1358.
3. Lenz, W. (1961) Kindliche Missbildungen nach Medikamente-Einnahme wahrend der Gravididat. *Dtsch. Med. Wochenschr.*, **86**, 2555–6.
4. Thiersch, J. B. (1952) Therapeutic abortions with folic acid antagonist 4-aminopteroylglutamic acid (4-amino PGA) administered by oral route. *Am. J. Obstetr. Gynecol.*, **63**, 1298–304.
5. Thiersch, J. B. (1954) Effect of certain 2,4-diaminopyrimidine antagonists of folic acid on pregnancy and rat fetus. *Proc. Soc. Expl Biol. Med.*, **87**, 571–7.
6. Meadow, S. R. (1968) Anticonvulsant drugs and congenital abnormalities. *Lancet*, **ii**, 1296.
7. Meadow, S. R. (1970) Congenital abnormalities and anticonvulsant drugs. *Proc. Ry. Soc. Med.*, **63**, 48–9.
8. Janz, D. (1982) On major malformations and minor anomalies in the offspring of parents with epilepsy: review of the literature, in *Epilepsy, Pregnancy and the Child* (eds D. Janz *et al.*), Raven Press, New York, pp. 211–22.
9. Schardein, J. L. (1985) Drugs affecting the central nervous system: Anticonvulsants, in *Chemically Induced Birth Defects*, Marcel Dekker, New York, pp. 142–90.
10. Hill, R. M., Verniaud, W. M., Horning, M. D. *et al.* (1974) Infants exposed in utero to antiepileptic drugs. *Am. J. Dis. Child*, **127**, 645–53.
11. Kuenssberg, E. V. and Knox, J. D. E. (1973) Teratogenic effect of anticonvulsants. *Lancet*, **i**, 198.
12. Shapiro, S., Harz, S. C., Siskind, B. *et al.* (1976) Anticonvulsants and parental epilepsy in the development of birth defects. *Lancet*, **i**, 272–5.
13. Speidel, B. D. and Meadow, S. R. (1972) maternal epilepsy and abnormalities of the fetus and the newborn. *Lancet*, **ii**, 839–43.
14. Fedrick, J. (1973) Epilepsy and pregnancy. A report from the Oxford record linkage study. *Br. Med. J.*, **2**, 442–8.
15. Nakane, Y. (1979) Congenital malformation among infants of epileptic mothers treated during pregnancy – the report of a collaborative study group in Japan. *Folia Psychiatr. Neurol. Jap.*, **33**, 363–9.
16. Meyer, J. G. (1973) The teratological effects of anticonvulsants and the effects on pregnancy and birth. *Eur. Neurol.*, **10**, 179–90.
17. Annengers, J. F., Hauser, W. A., Elveback, L. R. *et al.* (1978) Congenital malformations and seizure disorders in the offspring of parents with epilepsy. *Int. J. Epidemiol.*, **7**, 241–7.
18. Friis, M. I. (1979) epilepsy among parents of children with facial clefts. *Epilepsia*, **20**, 69–76.
19. Dieterich, E., Steveling, A., Lukas, A. *et al.* (1980) Congenital anomalies in children of epileptic mothers and fathers. *Neuropediatrics*, **11**, 274–83.
20. Hanson, J. W. and Smith, D. W. (1975) Are hydantoins (phenytoins) human teratogens? *J. Pediatr.*, **87**, 285–90.
21. German, J., Kowal, A. and Ehlers, K. H. (1970) Trimethadione and human teratogenesis. *Teratology*, **3**, 349–61.

22. Tein, I. and MacGregor, D. L. (1985) Possible valproate teratogenicity. *Arch. Neurol.*, **42**, 291–3.
23. Robert, E. (1982) Valproic acid and spina bifida: A preliminary report – France. *Morbid. Mortal. Wkly Rep.*, **31**, 565–6.
24. Robert, E. and Guibaud, P. (1983) Maternal valproic acid and congenital neural tube defects. *Lancet*, **ii**, 937.
25. Bjerkedal, T., Czeizel, A., Goujard, J. *et al.* (1982) Valproic acid and spina bifida. *Lancet*, **ii**, 1096.
26. Pendergrass, T. W. and Hanson, J. W. (1976) Fetal hydantoin syndrome and neuroblastoma. *Lancet*, **ii**, 150.
27. Sherman, S. and Roizen, N. (1976) Fetal hydantoin syndrome and neuroblastoma. *Lancet*, **ii**, 517.
28. Ehrenbard, L. T. and Chaganti, R. S. (1981) Cancer in the fetal hydantoin syndrome. *Lancet*, **ii**, 1981.
29. Dalens, B., Ranaud, E. J. and Gaulne, J. (1980) Teratogenicity of valproic acid. *J. Pediatr.*, **97**, 332–3.
30. Schardein, J. L. (1985) Drugs affecting the central nervous system: psychotropic agents, in *Chemically Induced Birth Defects*, Marcel Dekker, New York, pp. 191–6.
31. Nau, H., Helge, H. and Luck, W. (1984) Valproic acid in the perinatal period: Decreased maternal serum protein binding results in fetal accumulation and neonatal displacement of the drug and some metabolites. *J. Pediatr.*, **104**, 627–34.
31a. Krauer, B., Nau, H., Dayer, P. *et al.* (1986) Serum protein binding of diazepam and propanolol in the feto-maternal unit from early to late pregnancy. *Br. J. Obstet. Gynaecol.*, **93**, 322–28.
32. Speidel, B. D. and Meadow, S. R. (1974) Epilepsy, anticonvulsants and congenital malformations. *Drugs*, **8**, 354–65.
33. Smithells, R. W. (1976) Environmental Teratogens of Man. *Br. Med. Bull.*, **32**, 27–33.
34. Blake, D. A. and Fallinger, C. (1976) Embryopathic interaction of phenytoin and trichloropropene oxide in mice. *Teratology*, **13**, 17A.
35. Smithells, R. W. (1982) Neural tube defects: prevention by vitamin supplements. *Paediatrics*, **69**, 498–9.
36. Phelan, M. C., Pellock, J. M., Nance, W. E. (1982) Discordant expression of fetal hydantoin syndrome in heteropaternal dizygotic twins. *N. Engl. J. Med.*, **307**, 99–102.

CHAPTER THIRTEEN

Epilepsy After Head Injury and Intracranial Surgery

13.1 EPILEPSY AFTER HEAD INJURY AND INTRACRANIAL SURGERY

Bryan Jennett

Everyone knows that epilepsy sometimes occurs after head injury and intracranial surgery. Because epilepsy restricts a person's eligibility to drive a motor vehicle it is a serious social handicap in developed countries. It is natural that patients and their doctors usually try to understate the risk of a fit occurring. Much of the controversy about epilepsy after accidental or surgical trauma to the head derives from the implications of this diagnosis for driving [1]. For this reason the legal situation in the UK is summarized first. Fuller details, and the situation in other jurisdictions, are available in Chapter 20.

Epilepsy is one of only four conditions specifically identified in Britain as a bar to holding a licence to drive (others are poor eye sight, disabling giddiness or fainting and severe mental handicap). Once a person has had fits he may not drive until he has been free from any attack for two years – and then a licence is granted for only three years. A person who has had any epileptic attack since the age of five may not hold a vocational licence (to drive a heavy goods or public service vehicle, which includes buses and taxis). The logic behind these regulations is that persons who have had a fit are more likely to have another than are people who have not (so far) ever suffered an epileptic attack. The withdrawal of a licence for only a limited period from a private driver who has had a fit reflects the fact that the chances of a further attack becomes steadily less as time passes (p. 155). The more stringent requirements for vocational drivers reflect evidence that when a large vehicle goes out of control there is greater potential for damage to other road users and pedestrians.

These regulations focus on the risk of further fits once the diagnosis of epilepsy has been made. Until recently neurologists usually regarded a single fit as insufficient to justify the diagnosis of 'epilepsy' – with its implication of a liability to recurrence of fits (p. 2). However, there is increasing evidence that most patients who suffer one fit go on to have more (p. 155) and a period off driving is therefore now usually recommended. It is sometimes asserted that this should not be enforced if it is considered that the first fit had been provoked by an acute disorder that is unlikely to happen again. Recent head injury or intracranial surgery have often been regarded as such provocation – with the implication that one or more fits soon after such events do not justify a period off driving. That view has had to be changed in the light of evidence that such fits indicate a considerably greater risk of future fits than in patients without a history of early seizures.

A greater difficulty is that some patients can be identified after injury or operation as having a substantial risk of developing epilepsy although they have not yet had a fit. By the rule book there might seem to be no good reason to restrict their eligibility to drive. However, the Honorary Medical Advisory Panel to the Department of Transport in the UK, has now recommended that patients at high risk should not drive for a period. This is often resented by patients and also by their neurosurgeons who often disagree both about the level of risk and about its importance for driving. The risk of epilepsy results from the net effect of both surgical manipulation and of pre-existing trauma or disease. However, it is not surprising that surgeons encouraging patients to have elective intracranial surgery, itself a frightening enough prospect, should be as optimistic as possible about the likelihood of good long term recovery, and should resist the notion that their surgical manipulations contribute materially to the risk of epilepsy. In the light of recent legal opinions there is, however, now increasing pressure on surgeons to explain the possibility of significant complications after operation. The irony is that epilepsy is of most consequence for the patient who has made a good recovery and whose activities might otherwise be unrestricted. There is therefore a premium on the ability to predict which patients are at risk – so that they can be advised accordingly whilst other patients are reassured. This section is mainly devoted to the data on which such predictions are based.

13.1.1 Traumatic epilepsy

Most reports on traumatic epilepsy apply either to missile or to non-missile injuries. The former are mostly made up of wounds due to shell fragments, so the often-used word 'gunshot' is a misnomer. Non-missile includes compound depressed fractures resulting from low velocity impact with sharp objects, so that it is misleading to label them blunt or closed injuries. The dura may be intact or penetrated in either missile or non-missile injuries. About one-third of patients with missile injuries develop late epilepsy compared with only 5% of patients with non-missile injuries who have been injured severely enough to be admitted to hospital. However, head injuries in civilian life are so common that trauma is an important cause of acquired epilepsy, both in children and adults.

(a) Early traumatic epilepsy

It has long been recognized that fits that occur soon after injury are less likely to lead to persisting epilepsy than when epilepsy begins later. This led to the belief that early fits were of little significance, but that was before the risks of recurrence had been quantified. In fact the difference is between 25% for further epilepsy after an early fit and 75% after a late fit. But the 25% risk of recurrence after early epilepsy is much greater than in head injured patients who did not have an early fit (see Table 13.3). There was, however, no consensus about how to define 'early' until Jennett's proposal in 1960 to limit this to the first week after injury [2]. Fits much more often begin in the first week than in any one of the next seven weeks; seizures during this week are often limited to focal twitching in the face or hand; and recurrence in the future is much less common (Fig. 13.1).

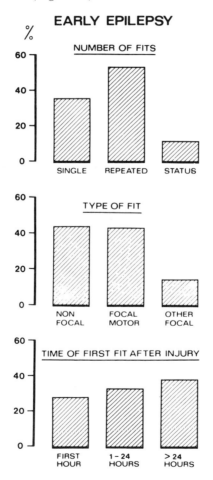

Figure 13.1 Features of early epilepsy. (Reproduced with permission from [5]).

Table 13.1   Incidence of early epilepsy

Age	n	Epilepsy rate (%)	
Adults	2354	2	Stowsand and Bues [3]
<15 years	814	7	
<15 years	4195	5	
< 5 years	—	7	Hendrick and Harris [4]
< 1 year	—	11	
Adults	784	5	
<15 years	202	5	
> 5 years	911	4	Jennett [5]
< 5 years	75	9	
All ages	1000	5	
All ages	1000	4	Courjon [6]

Early epilepsy is now widely accepted as referring to the first week after injury or operation. Early epilepsy occurs in about 5% of head injured patients admitted to hospital in Britain, France and Germany (Table 13.1). It is commoner after more serious injuries (depressed fracture, post-traumatic amnesia (PTA) of more than 24 hours or acute intracranial haematoma); it is therefore more frequent in patients admitted to a neurosurgical unit (13%) than in primary surgical wards where many of the patients are mildly injured. Overall early epilepsy occurs more frequently in children under the age of five, in whom it may occur after mild or even trivial injuries. In about one-third of cases the first fit occurs within an hour of injury, in another third it occurs later during the first day, and in the remainder during the rest of the first week.

In the first few hours or days after injury the occurrence of fits may occasionally indicate that an acute intracranial haematoma is developing – but there are always other signs of such a complication. More often the temporary lowering of conscious level as a result of a seizure, perhaps associated with transient hemiparesis, leads to a mistaken suspicion of serious developments and this can result in unnecessary emergency transfer to a neurosurgical unit. But sometimes generalized fits, especially when status epilepticus occurs in children, lead to secondary hypoxic brain damage. The main significance of early epilepsy is, however, that it indicates a markedly increased likelihood that epilepsy will develop in the future (see below).

(b) Late traumatic epilepsy

Once a fit does occur after the first week the tendency is for fits to continue over many years, although in two-thirds of patients seizures are relatively infrequent if adequate anticonvulsant therapy is maintained. Because of this it is of considerable importance to be able to predict soon after recovery from injury the probability that late epilepsy will develop. The much more frequent occurrence of epilepsy after military injuries reflects the different mechanism of brain damage, over 90% being due to missiles. Civilian injuries associated with depressed fracture or intracranial haematoma most clearly resemble missile injuries in that there is focal brain damage. Only 17% of head injuries in the UK are of this kind and the frequency of epilepsy in this minority of injuries is similar to that after military injuries. Weiss *et al.* [6a] have shown that those who survive penetrating injuries without epilepsy for three years can be 95% certain that they will remain seizure free. Of those with non-missile injuries who were followed for a long period, 25% of those who develop epilepsy have their first *late* fit within one year, but approximately 25% have their first fit after four years have passed. Table 13.2 shows the similar pattern of onset in missile and non-missile injuries.

There is a wide variation in the incidence of late epilepsy after different types of injury, but each of the factors that predispose to this complication are evident within two weeks after injury (Table 13.3). Within the subset of patients who have a compound depressed fracture of the skull there are a small

Table 13.2 Time of onset of seizures in those who develop late epilepsy within 5 years of injury

	Military (Caveness) [7] 1030 Vietnam cases	Civilian (Jennett) [5] 1005 depressed fracture 420 intracranial haematomas
Incidence of epilepsy	28%	29%
Cumulative incidence of epilepsy		
<1 year	67%	66%
1–3 years	95%	91%
3–4 years	98%	96%

Table 13.3

(a) Incidence of late epilepsy after different injuries [5]

	n	% With late epilepsy
Complicated by acute intracranial haematoma*	128	35
No haematoma	854	5
Depressed skull fracture	447	17
No depressed fracture	832	4
After early epilepsy	238	25
No early epilepsy	868	3

(b) In patients with neither haematoma nor depressed fracture [5]

After early epilepsy	124	19
No early epilepsy	168	1
PTA>24 hours	112	5
PTA<24 hours	661	1

Differences in epilepsy incidence in each pair are all significant at $P<0.001$.
*Surgical evacuation within 14 days of injury.
Note: There is as yet no data available for haematomas shown on CT scan but not operated on.

number whose risk of epilepsy is over 60%. However, for some 40% of patients with this kind of injury there is a probability of less than 5% that they will suffer from this complication (Fig. 13.2). Given the predictive power of these simple clinical features the EEG makes little or no useful additional contribution. This is because persisting abnormality in EEG reflects significant brain damage and this is already evident from various clinical criteria. Moreover the correlation between EEG abnormality and late epilepsy becomes significant only one year after injury [5]; by this time more than half the cases of late epilepsy have already declared themselves.

13.1.2   Epilepsy after supratentorial surgery

The most comprehensive study of epilepsy after intracranial surgery for non-traumatic conditions was a review of 1000 patients reported in 1981 [8]. One in five patients who had not previously had a fit developed epilepsy within five years of craniotomy, whether this had been done for a vascular lesion, a benign

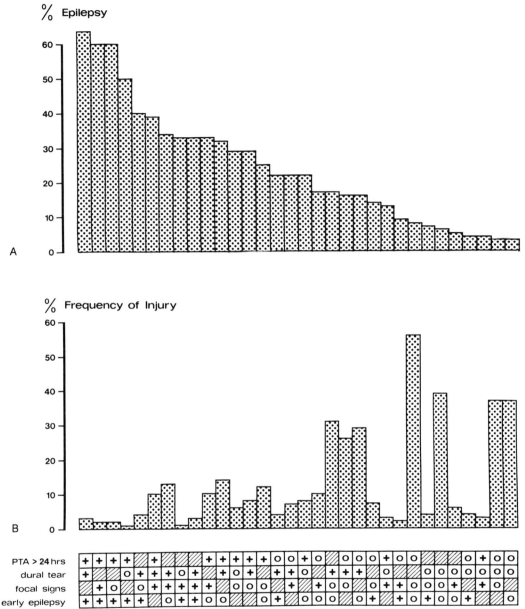

Figure 13.2 (A) Effects of different factors upon the incidence of late epilepsy after compound depressed fracture. (B) The frequency with which different combinations of factors occurred (three factors of four available). Reproduced with permission from [5].

Table 13.4   Epilepsy after supratentorial surgery (for reasons other than trauma)

	n	No seizures before operation (%)	Some seizures before operation (%)
		Frequency of postoperative epilepsy	
Burr hole	392	13	67
Craniotomy	545	19	55
for glioma	115	19	40
for IC haemorrhage	291	21	33
for meningioma	61	22	56

Derived from Foy *et al.* [8].

or a malignant tumour (Table 13.4). Even after a burr hole, most often done for biopsy or placing of a ventricular catheter, the epilepsy rate was 13% in those without previous fits in this study. In another [9] the incidence was 9% overall after placing a catheter, being higher when the catheter was inserted frontally (55%) rather than parietally (7%). When one or more fits had already occurred before operation the postoperative rate was much higher. This study confirmed a number of earlier reports of separate series. That surgery does itself contribute to the risk of epilepsy is evidenced by comparing the frequency of this complication in patients with the same pathological condition only some of whom have had craniotomy. For example no cases of acoustic neuroma whose operation had been confined to the posterior fossa developed epilepsy whilst 22% of 45 patients dealt with by craniotomy had postoperative fits [10]. For posterior communicating artery aneurysms treated by carotid ligation the epilepsy rate was 4% but for those who had a craniotomy it was 20% [11].

As after head injury it has proved possible in Glasgow [12] to identify risk factors and to discover that these occur in only a minority of patients (Table 13.5). In another study, Keranen *et al.* [11a] have underlined that the most important factor is the preoperative state of the patient. Only 2.5% of the 81 Grade I patients developed epilepsy, compared to 33% of the 42 Grade III and IV patients. Other risk factors included the presence of a large intra-cerebral haematoma, the presence of postoperative spasm and an aneurysm on the middle cerebral artery. The important factors contributing to post-operative epilepsy are the brain damage already incurred at the time of spontaneous aneurysmal rupture and the epileptogenic threshold of that particular patient. This may account for the lack of evidence that introduction of the operating microscope has significantly reduced the risk of epilepsy, as surgeons hoped that it would. Obviously the microscope can do nothing to influence the brain damage already sustained at the time of rupture and any subsequent preoperative ischaemic damage. Moreover the use of the operat-

Table 13.5 Influence on postoperative epilepsy of various features associated with aneurysms (n=150) (Reproduced with permission from [12])

Feature	Frequency of occurrence (%)	Epilepsy rate	
		Without feature (%)	With feature (%)
Preoperative epilepsy	7	18	45
Preoperative deficit	29	17	26
Intracranial haematoma	24	17	28
Coma at ictus	26	18	23
Microscope used	78	17	19
Brain resected	22	21	11
Rupture at operation	22	16	26
Early postoperative epilepsy	3	19	20
Focal deficit after operation			
Temporary	33	14	29
Persisting	14	15	43
Either	47	6	33

ing microscope entails considerable retraction of the brain and it is wishful thinking to believe that this does not cause some additional damage. There may be a parallel here in the similar epilepsy rate after missile injuries in World War II as in World War I in spite of improved surgery and a lower infection rate [5].

As with head injuries various risk factors can be combined to identify a number of subsets of patients with widely varying probabilities of developing epilepsy (Table 13.6). In half the patients the risk of epilepsy is only 5% whilst in a small minority the risk is as high as 67%. Even 5% risk is more than 100 times greater than that for normal adults aged 20–59 years, which is about 0.03% per year (Fig. 1.2).

In assessing fitness to drive it has to be recognized that there is also a small risk of recurrent subarachnoid haemorrhage, either from incomplete occlusion of the aneurysm operated on or from another hitherto undetected aneurysm (which are multiple in at least 15% of cases). It is for these reasons that the advice in the UK is that patients who have had a craniotomy for aneurysm are not permitted to drive heavy goods or public service vehicles.

13.1.3 Prophylaxis of epilepsy after head injury or surgery

The attitude of American neurosurgeons towards prophylactic drugs after head injury was surveyed in 1973 [13]. Finding that 40% of neurosurgeons did

Table 13.6 Epilepsy rate according to number of risk factors–preoperative epilepsy, haematoma, rupture at operation and postoperative deficit

(a) Number of risk factors:	Frequency of occurrence (%)	Late epilepsy rate (%)
None	34	6
Any one	39	21
Any two	20	27
Any three	7	64

(b) Predictions based only on preoperative epilepsy and postoperative deficit			
Preoperative epilepsy	Postoperative deficit	Frequency of occurrence (%)	Late epilepsy rate (%)
—	—	49	5
+	—	3	20
—	+	44	32
+	+	4	67

not prescribe anticonvulsants the authors estimated that 100 000 Americans might be suffering unnecessarily from post-traumatic epilepsy each year. The reason given by most surgeons for not giving drugs was uncertainty about the actual risk in individual patients – a reason no longer valid since the data reviewed in this chapter became available. The practice of British

Table 13.7 Prescribing of anticonvulsant drugs after craniotomy for various conditions: proportion of neurosurgeons who always recommended the drugs operatively (%)

75	Brain abscess
60	{ Meningioma Arteriovenous malformation (meningioma)
55	{ Subarachnoid haemorrhage Middle cerebral artery aneurysm Compound depressed skull fracture
45	{ Intracerebral haematoma Anterior or posterior communicating artery aneurysm Glioma Repair for anterior fossa fracture
35	Pituitary tumour
15	Chronic subdural haematoma
15	For patients operated on for any of these conditions
18	For all except subdural haematoma
2	For none of these conditions

neurosurgeons in respect of postoperative anticonvulsants in non-traumatic cases was surveyed in 1982 [14]. The ranking of the proportion of neurosurgeons who *always* gave drugs after surgery for various conditions corresponded well with the order of risks associated with these conditions (Table 13.7). Surgeons said they were influenced in their decision to give drugs by the diagnosis as well as by the occurrence of a fit before or after operation and by other evidence of brain damage (an intracranial haematoma or infection, focal signs or visible evidence of cortical involvement or prolonged coma). A third of surgeons began medication before or during surgery and a half did so immediately after surgery. A third gave drugs for only six months but 40% did so for more than a year.

Evidence for the effectiveness of prophylactic therapy is hard to come by. It requires not only long term follow-up but data about compliance from blood levels [15]. More than one report on phenytoin has been disappointing [16, 17] several patients developing seizures during the second year once drugs have been discontinued [16]. It remains to be established whether maintaining therapeutic levels of drugs during the early months after surgery will confer any lasting protection. There have been some encouraging reports of the use of sodium valproate.

13.1.4 Conclusion

There is a significant risk of epilepsy during the years following certain types of head injury and certain types of intracranial surgery. Although the means to prevent such seizures have still to be developed it is now possible to identify which patients are at high risk and which at low risk. This makes it possible to advise the former about their future activities and to reassure the latter.

References

1. Anonymous (1980) Epilepsy after head trauma and fitness to drive. *Lancet*, **i**, 401–2.
2. Jennett, W. B. and Lewin, W. S. (1960) Traumatic epilepsy after closed head injuries. *J. Neurol. Neurosurg. Psychiatr.*, **23**, 295–301.
3. Stowsand, D. and Bues, E. (1970) Frühanfälle und ihre Verläufe nach Hirntraumeln im Kindesalter. *Z. Neurol.*, **198**, 201–11.
4. Hendrick, E. B. and Harris, L. (1968) Post-traumatic epilepsy in children. *J. Trauma*, **8**, 547–56.
5. Jennett, B. (1975) *Epilepsy After Non-Missile Head Injuries*, 2nd Ed., William Heinemann, London.
6. Courjon, J. A. (1969) in *The Late Effects of Head Injury* (eds A. E. Walker *et al.*), Charles C. Thomas, Springfield, Ill.
6a. Weiss, G. H., Salazar, A. M., Vance, S. C. *et al.* (1986) Predicting post-traumatic epilepsy in penetrating head injury. *Arch. Neurol.*, **43**, 771–73.
7. Caveness, W. F., Meirowsky, A. M., Risk, B. L., *et al.* (1979) The nature of post-traumatic epilepsy. *J. Neurosurg.*, **50**, 545–53.

8. Foy, P. M., Copeland, G. P. and Shaw, M. D. M. (1981) The incidence of post-operative seizures. *Acta Neurochirurg.*, **55**, 253–64.

9. Dan, N. Q. and Wade, M. J. (1986) The incidence of epilepsy after ventricular shunting procedures. *J. Neurosurg.*, **65**, 19–21.

10. Cabral, R., King, T. T. and Scott, D. F. (1976) Incidence of post-operative epilepsy after a transtentorial approach to acoustic nerve tumours. *J. Neurol. Neurosurg. Psychiatr.*, **39**, 663–5.

11. Cabral, R., King, T. T. and Scott, D. F. (1976) Epilepsy after two different neurosurgical approaches to the treatment of ruptured intracranial aneurysms. *J. Neurol. Neurosurg. Psychiatr.*, **39**, 1052–6.

11a. Keranen, T., Tapaninaho, A., Hernesniemi, J. and Vapalahti, M. (1986) Late epilepsy after aneurysm operations. *Neurosurgery*, **17**, 897–900.

12. Jennett, B., Ward, P. and Murray, L. (1984) Risk of epilepsy after head injury and intracranial surgery. *J. Neurol. Neurosurg. Psychiatr.*, **47**, 104.

13. Rapport, R. L. and Penry, J. K. (1973) A survey of attitudes towards the pharmacological prophylaxis of post-traumatic epilepsy. *J. Neurosurg.*, **38**, 159–66.

14. Jennett, B. (1983) Anticonvulsant drugs and advice about driving after head injury and intracranial surgery. *Br. Med. J.*, **286**, 627–8.

15. Serist, Z. and Musil, F. (1981) Prophylactic treatment of post-traumatic epilepsy: results of long term follow-up in Czechoslovakia. *Epilepsia*, **23**, 315–20.

16. North, J. B., Penhall, R. K., Haneich, A. *et al.* (1983) Phenytoin and post-operative epilepsy. *J. Neurosurg.*, **58**, 672–77.

17. Young, B., Kapp, R. P., Norton, J. A. *et al.* (1983) Failure of prophylactically administered phenytoin to prevent post-traumatic seizures. *J. Neurosurg.*, **58**, 236–41.

13.2   THE NEUROPATHOLOGY OF EPILEPSY FOLLOWING CRANIAL TRAUMA

Thomas L. Babb and W. Jann Brown

13.2.1   Penetrating injuries

The neuropathology of penetrating and non-penetrating cerebral injuries is quite distinct. Figure 13.3 illustrates one example of a low velocity penetrating

Figure 13.3 Histopathology of lateral temporal cortex in a case of surgically-treated focal post-traumatic epilepsy resulting from a 12-year-old stab wound through the temporal bone. (A) Low power photomicrograph to show sharply-defined defect in superior temporal gyrus extending from pia-arachnoid to the subjacent myelin (arrow). Nearby cortical lamina is intact. Hematoxylin and eosin stain. Calibration bar 200 μm. (B) Higher power view of same defect as A. Note the neuropil shows a shearing, splitting injury rather than the large volumetric loss of brain as typically found in vascular occlusion. Note also adjacent normal neuron lamination on each side of the penetrating injury. Many of the nuclei in the injured region are fibrous astrocytes mixed with oligodendroglia but no obvious loss of brain substance. Calibration bar 80 μm.

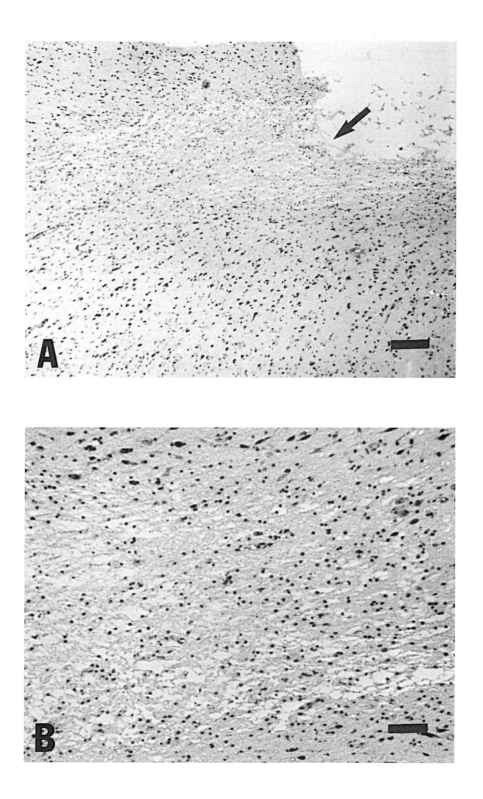

injury caused by a shot wound to the left temporal lobe of a 30-year-old woman. Nine months after the injury she developed complex partial seizures that were sufficiently troublesome to require *en bloc* temporal lobectomy. The lobe had a sharply-defined cut across the superior temporal gyrus directed toward the mesial parts of the lobe (Fig. 13.3A). In Fig. 13.3B the same region is revealed under higher power. The long term effect of the shearing defect of the neuropil is shown. There is no actual extensive volumetric loss of brain aside from secondary changes due to disruption of the microvasculature, dendrites, neurones and their axons and sheaths. The stromal astrocytes have proliferated but sparingly, and there is no large cyst as is commonly found with vascular occlusion.

This case has clearly shown penetration of bone, piercing of the dura mater and some loss of neuropil. This mode of intracerebral trauma invariably develops into a dense scar mixture of gliosis and fibrous tissue. This type of lesion injures blood vessels and may cause even more extensive secondary brain loss associated with long term development of the meningocerebral cicatrix. This dense scar may cause compression or traction atrophy of underlying neuropil. We do not yet know why similar intracerebral trauma may *not* lead to epilepsy, why some of these post-traumatic epileptic scars may not continue to cause seizures, and why it is the region surrounding the scar that is epileptogenic (see Chapter 2).

13.2.2   Closed head injuries

Because blunt head injuries cause differential acceleration–deceleration of brain compared to cranium, the locus of brain damage may be very diffuse. In fact, such trauma has been shown to be *remote or opposite* to the impact (*contre-coup*) in a variety of cases of post-traumatic epilepsy [1]. Courville has emphasized that the 'localization' of brain contusions seems to be related to irregularities in the anterior and middle cranial fossae. However, *contre-coup* contusions do not seem prevalent in the parietal and occipital lobes following frontal impacts. Blunt head impacts may produce a variety of brain contusions, the most likely being (1) the basal frontal lobe, which abuts the orbital plate of the frontal bone and medially the ethmoid bone (crista galli) and (2) the anterior temporal lobe which is surrounded by the wings of the sphenoid bone, and laterally by the temporal bone.

A recent report to the US National Institute of Neurological Disorders and Stroke [2] has described *focal* brain damage and four categories of *diffuse* brain damage resulting from non-penetrating impacts to the heads of humans or baboons. This report did not describe post-traumatic epilepsy as such as the studies were designed to describe the pathology following blunt head trauma in general. This study confirmed Courville's earlier conclusion that angular acceleration of the head results in *focal* brain damage '. . . characteristically at the frontal and temporal poles and on the inferior surfaces of the frontal and temporal lobes where brain tissue comes in contact with bone protuberances in the base of the skull [2].' However, these authors also reported that *focal contusions* were not always opposite (*contre-coup*) to the impact because such contusions were always more severe in frontal and temporal lobes even following frontal impact.

Focal haematomas following blunt impact were described as subdural in this report, as true epidural haemorrhage occurs only with skull fracture and rupture of meningeal arteries. The pathogenesis of these focal subdural bleeds was localized to rupture of bridging veins when there was rapid head acceleration [2]. Other types of *focal* brain damage were pituitary stalk rupture, avulsion of cranial nerves, pontomedullary rents, and the changes associated with raised intracranial pressure [2].

Diffuse brain damage was categorized into four types: (1) axonal injury, (2) hypoxia, (3) brain swelling, and (4) multiple petechial haemorrhages [2]. With severe impacts or accelerations, axonal injuries may be seen microscopically as large numbers of axon retraction balls, which presumably represent extrusion of axoplasm, seen if the brain is carefully fixed and examined within days of the impact. After a week of survival from the impact, the major myelinated tracts have clusters of monocytes and macrophages, which are responding to the injury of oligodendroglia [2]. Gurdjian and Webster [3] have described neuronal destruction in post-traumatic epilepsy and emphasized the disappearance of oligodendroglia in direct proportion to the neuronal loss and astrocytic proliferation. With survival periods of months or longer, Adams *et al.* [2] have demonstrated long tract degeneration of the Wallerian type throughout the brain. When we consider that much of the volume of the brain consists of axons, such injuries should be and often are visible as morphological changes in gyri and fissures of the brain visualized by computerized tomography. Salazar and colleagues [4] reported a very high incidence of post-traumatic epilepsy when the loss of brain volume, as judged by CT scanning, exceeded 75 ml.

Diffuse hypoxic brain damage is reported as a second major diffuse result of blunt impact. Hypoxia may be regional or diffuse. It is probably caused by a variety of conditions including high intracranial pressure, arterial vasospasm and hypotension. Gradations of hypoxic damage in different brain regions rather than whole brain hypoxia are found with non-penetrating trauma.

Diffuse brain swelling may occur in either one or both cerebral hemispheres. The mechanism appears to be a 'secondary' vasogenic oedema in which water and electrolytes permeate the brain substance. The primary cause may be rapid vasodilatation, increased cerebral blood volume and a defective blood–brain barrier [2]. If there were early post-traumatic seizures or status epilepticus, abnormal pH and pCO_2 levels may impair the vascular uptake of water and aggravate the brain swelling.

Diffuse petechial haemorrhages may be limited to regions such as the brainstem [5] following blunt trauma. However similar punctate haemorrhages are found in the white matter of the temporal and frontal lobes [2]. Such numerous small clots probably result from ruptures of small arteries sheared by the rapid acceleration of the brain. Although this shearing mechanism may seem analogous to the traction of axons, the vessels are more elastic than axons and the acceleration forces must be greater to produce such multiple haemorrhages [2].

It should be clear from the foregoing review of the various types of brain damage caused by blunt head trauma that there will be a variety of neurological deficits other than epilepsy, which is found in only 5–10% of such head injuries. As we have repeated, post-traumatic epilepsy has a high incidence only when there is severe, usually focal, brain damage. In blunt or closed head injuries epilepsy may be less likely than many other deficits such as hemiparesis, ataxia or scotoma. Future studies of focal or diffuse brain damage following blunt trauma must be related to the onset and frequency of post-traumatic seizures before we can accurately identify anatomical mechanisms underlying epilepsy following closed head injuries.

References

1. Courville, C. B. (1985) Traumatic lesions of the temporal lobe as the essential cause of psychomotor epilepsy, in *Temporal Lobe Epilepsy* (eds M. Baldwin and P. Bailey), C. C. Thomas, Springfield, pp. 220–39.
2. Adams, J. H., Graham, D. E. and Gennarelli, T. A. (1985) Contemporary neuropathological considerations regarding brain damage in head injury, in *Central Nervous System Trauma* (eds D. P. Becker and J. T. Povlishock), National Institutes of Health, Bethesda, Md.
3. Gurdjian, E. S. and Webster, J. E. (1958) *Head Injuries*, Little, Brown and Co., Boston.
4. Salazar, A. M., Jabbari, B., Vance, S. C., *et al.* (1985) Epilepsy after penetrating head injury. I. Clinical correlates. *Neurology*, **35**, 1406–14.
5. Tomlinson, B. E. (1970) Brain-stem lesions after head injury, in *The Pathology of Trauma* (eds S. Sevitt and H. B. Stoner), *J. Clin. Pathol.* **23** (Suppl. 4), 178–86.

CHAPTER FOURTEEN

The Management of Status Epilepticus

Barbara E. Swartz and Antonio V. Delgado-Escueta

The management of status epilepticus can be viewed as a problem with three dimensions. The first dimension is of necessity the initiation of steps which will protect the patient from the known general metabolic deficits induced by the seizures themselves. The second is the identification and correction of precipitating factors where this is possible in the acute stage. The third is the initiation of pharmacological treatment which is specifically and selectively indicated for the particular type of status epilepticus.

We are in an exciting era of rapid advances in epilepsy. The technological advantages of neuroradiological investigations, i.e. computerized axial tomography (CT), positron emission tomography (PET) and magnetic resonance imaging (MRI) scanning, will undoubtedly affect our classification of the epilepsies or status itself into primary or secondary types, Thus, in the pre-CT era Oxbury and Whitty [1] categorized nine patients with status as suffering 'idiopathic' epilepsy, but two to seven years later identified brain tumours in seven of these. The increasing use of continuous monitoring of brain electrical activity while viewing clinical behaviour during intermittent seizures by closed circuit television and electroencephalography has dramatically improved our classification of the epilepsies (Chapter 3). These techniques are being applied in some centres to status epilepticus as well [2, 3, 4]. This can allow easier differentiation of status subtypes such as tonic-clonic status epilepticus, which is a secondarily generalized seizure type 70–80% of the time [2, 5, 6] from that of clonic-tonic-clonic status epilepticus which is more likely to appear in a patient with a primary generalized epilepsy of a genetic basis [7]. Recently a report of temporal lobe status epilepticus studied by depth electrodes has appeared which correlated a prolonged aura phenomenon with status epilepticus involving only the left hippocampus [8]. While this is not presently of significance in the management of status epilepticus, it is of import for the future studies of pathogenesis and prognosis in status epilepticus.

Through systematic prospective clinical trials, we are gaining skill in treating status epilepticus pharmacologically [9, 10]. It is still true that most articles on treatment of status epilepticus acknowledge that all of the main-line anticonvulsant drugs work reasonably well while none are ideal [11]. However, the authors feel that over the course of the next five to ten years increased use of selective drugs for particular types of status will be implemented. Therefore, while we still advocate a fairly standard regimen for the treatment of status epilepticus, we urge practising clinical neurologists to keep abreast of new developments in this area.

14.1 CAUSAL AND PRECIPITATING FACTORS

Status epilepticus is generally divided into idiopathic or symptomatic groups. It is also useful to distinguish between those symptomatic cases of status epilepticus due to acute neurological or systemic disease, and those which appear in the setting of a chronic neurological state. With this classification, Hauser [12] noted that while some studies showed a preponderance of status epilepticus in a setting of chronic neurological disease [1, 6], other studies showed an equal distribution among the three classes both in children [13] and in adults [14]. If one combines the studies as comprehensively listed by Hauser in 1983 (a total of 755 patients), 42% of status epilepticus occurs in the chronic symptomatic setting, 23% occurs in the acute symptomatic setting and 35% occurs in the idiopathic group. The ratio of symptomatic to idiopathic cases is therefore 2:1. This is in contrast to status in neonates where a much higher ratio is reported [15], but consistent with a recent series showing that 24% of cases of status occurred in patients with a previous seizure history. The specific symptomatic causes include cranial trauma, cerebrovascular diseases, metabolic derangements [16], brain tumours (more often frontal than at other sites) [5], encephalitic, perinatal and miscellaneous causes [17, 18]. Miscellaneous causes include intoxication by and withdrawal from drugs, including both prescription and 'recreational' drugs such as cocaine, particularly when it is combined with strychnine. In addition, brain and spinal operations, brain oedema of diverse aetiologies, degenerative and demyelinating diseases, inflammatory and infectious diseases (meningitis, encephalitis, or septic emboli) can all cause status epilepticus. Metabolic derangements include renal failure, overhydration [19], hypoglycaemia, hypocalcaemia and hypokalaemia [16].

Precipitating factors may be those which reduce seizure threshold on a substrate of pre-existing organic pathology, thereby contributing to the development of status. In known epileptics the most common causes of status epilepticus are the intentional or inadvertent withdrawal of anticonvulsant drugs or activation by fever [5, 20]. Infections, primarily of the respiratory tract, may account for 25% of cases of precipitated status epilepticus [19]. Other precipitating factors include withdrawal from alcohol or other sedatives [21], metabolic disturbances (hypocalcaemia, hypo- or hyperglycaemia, hyponatraemia, hepatic or renal failure), drug intoxication (isoniazid, tricyclic antidepressants, neuroleptics, strychnine) [4], physical exertion, radiation therapy, pregnancy and delivery [22].

The effective management of status epilepticus requires prompt recognition and correction of the above factors.

14.2 SUBVARIETIES OF STATUS EPILEPTICUS

It may not be possible to establish a cause for the status until after the seizures have been controlled. The clinician may, however, be able to make some assumptions regarding aetiology and plan proper management through careful clinical assessment. We use the framework of Table 14.1 as a means of quick seizure classification.

Table 14.1 Classification of status epilepticus

Primary generalized convulsive status
   Tonic-clonic status
   Myoclonic status
   Clonic-tonic-clonic status
Secondarily generalized convulsive status
   Tonic-clonic status with partial onset
   Tonic status
   Subtle generalized convulsive status
Simple partial status
   Partial motor status
   Unilateral status
   Epilepsia partialis continua
   Partial sensory status
   Partial status with vegetative, autonomic or affective symptoms
Non-convulsive status
   Absence status – typical or atypical
   Complex partial status

14.2.1 Generalized tonic-clonic status (grand mal)

Tonic-clonic status epilepticus is the most common and most serious form of status epilepticus. A number of independent studies have demonstrated that 70–80% of patients with tonic-clonic status epilepticus will have a partial onset to their seizures. Thus, one should attempt to observe or elicit in the history signs of partial motor onset or adversive head and eye movements. Tonic-clonic status epilepticus most frequently results from acute cerebral insults such as cerebral infarcts, meningitis, encephalitis, head trauma, and cerebral anoxia secondary to cardiorespiratory disease. It may also be caused by withdrawal from anticonvulsant drugs in those with chronic epilepsy or those with metabolic derangements or uncontrolled seizures on the basis of an old cerebral infarct [2, 4]. If tonic-clonic status epilepticus is the initial manifestation of an epilepsy, a space occupying lesion must be considered. One should be suspicious of this diagnosis when previously healthy adults present in tonic-clonic status epilepticus. Some authors [1, 4, 5] report that 20–25% of tonic-clonic status epilepticus results from brain tumours.

14.2.2 Myoclonic and clonic-tonic-clonic status epilepticus

Myoclonic status epilepticus consists of generalized, brief muscular contractions repeating frequently but without loss of consciousness. These may evolve to clonic-tonic-clonic seizures or generalized clonic seizures with more frequent jerks and with impairment of consciousness. These patterns are generally seen in primarily generalized epilepsies such as the juvenile myoclonic epilepsy of Janz, myoclonic astatic epilepsy of Doose, and various heredofamilial progressive myoclonic encephalopathies [7]. However either pattern may also be seen under the same conditions in which random myoclonic jerks occur, such as renal encephalopathy, dialysis dementia, severe cerebral anoxia [4] and Creutzfeldt-Jacob disease (personal observation).

14.2.3 Tonic status epilepticus

Generalized tonic status epilepticus is a much rarer entity than tonic-clonic status epilepticus. As first described by Gastaut *et al.* [23], tonic seizures occur most commonly in the Lennox–Gastaut syndrome. However, a well documented case of tonic status epilepticus has appeared in which the patient was a boy aged 17 of normal intelligence with a history of tonic-clonic seizures who evidently took his phenytoin irregularly [24]. The case is important in that the boy presented as a confusional state. While this is a generalized epilepsy, these authors and others [25] note that ictal motor activity may be so attenuated that the correct diagnosis may not be made without EEG and polygraphic recording.

14.2.4 Subtle generalized convulsive status epilepticus

Patients reported recently by Treiman *et al.* [26] had marked impairment of consciousness, subtle motor manifestations, sometimes limited to one side of the body, with frequent eyeblinks and nystagmus. This type of status may be due to a structural brain lesion or a severe encephalopathy. It is important to recognise this syndrome as the EEG may reveal only periodic lateralized or generalized epileptiform discharges (PLEDS), and yet this condition can evolve in a setting of incompletely treated tonic-clonic status and carries a poor prognosis. Simon and Aminoff described a type of status, in the setting of severe anoxic-ischaemic brain damage, in which the only motor manifestation of electrographic status was vertical eye movements [26a].

14.2.5 Unilateral status epilepticus

Although 'unilateral epilepsy' is not included in the International Classification of the Epilepsies, this form of status was discussed by Roger *et al.* [25]. It is most frequent in young children presenting as hemiclonic status, often associated with hemiplegia [27]. However, it has also been reported as a benign type of epilepsy with status in an adolescent [28].

14.2.6 Simple partial status epilepticus

The patient with simple partial status epilepticus retains consciousness in the face of continuous partial seizures which may be motor, somatosensory, special sensory, autonomic, psychic or a combination of these.

Two types of simple partial status have been recognized [2, 29]. One can be considered as 'Jacksonian' status which may or may not become generalized. Status begins with a twitching of the foot or hand. It may then spread along the limb and to other ipsilateral muscles in a march reflecting the somatotopic organization of the motor cortex. If generalization occurs the patient loses consciousness. When the tonic-clonic phase ends, this pattern may repeat itself. This type of seizure without generalization has been called 'epilepsia partialis continua' by some authors [30]. Others reserve this term for that entity which was described originally by Kozhewnikow in 1895 [31] in which brief focal contractions may remain in one site or progress without a somatotopic pattern. Simple partial motor status may be seen with metabolic derangements such as non-ketotic hyperglycaemia [30] or drug toxicity [32] as well as with focal lesions such as a neoplasm or infarct.

14.2.7 Non-convulsive status epilepticus

Absence status with prolonged periods of variable degrees of psychic clouding has been recognized since Lennox's description of the petit mal epilepsies [33]. The Marseille school [34] further identified immobility, mutism and reactive automatisms as important signs. The term 'petit mal' status or typical absence status may be used in a restrictive sense when a continuous twilight state is accompanied by diffuse, synchronous, 3 Hz spike and wave rhythms [35]. The terminology is confusing, however, because 'petit mal status' may be thought to include also propulsive petit mal status (infantile spasms in status), impulsive petit mal status (myoclonic status of Janz) [17], and even myoclonic astatic status (akinetic seizures). We have listed the last two syndromes under myoclonic status (p. 420).

We feel that Gastaut's recommendation to simplify the terminology is appropriate [36]. Thus, 'typical' absence status would refer to the restricted definition above. 'Atypical' absence status would include children presenting with secondarily generalized epilepsy (mainly Lennox syndrome), and features a more marked mental confusion with recurrent spike waves at less than 3 Hz, arrhythmic spike-wave complexes, or even diffuse high amplitude background slowing with superimposed bursts of spike-wave and occasional bursts of fast activity. In this group, the atypical absence status may last days to months and carries a poor prognosis [37]. A similar picture may appear in adults, particularly postmenopausal women with or without a past history of absences, although often with a history of generalized seizures. In this group the prognosis is good [35]. Guberman *et al.* [38] have drawn attention to how non-convulsive status may be mistaken initially for a psychiatric disorder. Language, albeit with reduced fluency, may be retained despite other cognitive impairment.

14.2.8 Complex partial status epilepticus

This used to be considered a rare form of status making up only 2–3% of reported series of status [4, 39]. However, increasing recognition of this entity is probably due to improved recording techniques such as stereoencephalography (p. 289), and recognition of the various forms that the syndrome can take (four case reports noted between 1973 and 1979, and 31 patients reported from 1980–1985). Fluctuations in the level of responsiveness of the patient and occasional oral-buccal automatisms may occur [40]. In the largest series to date, Treiman and Delgado-Escueta [41] collected 11 cases of complex partial status epilepticus. They found that the critical distinction from prolonged absence (spike-wave stupor) is the cyclical nature of the behavioural phases. These phases consist of: (1) a continuous twilight state with partial and amnestic responsiveness, partial speech and quasi-purposeful automatisms alternating with (2) staring, total unresponsiveness, speech arrest and stereotyped automatisms. The cyclic behaviour noted above appears to recapitulate the manifestations of Type I partial complex seizures [42] which are of hippocampal-amygdalar origin. It is possible that complex potential status epilepticus from other loci (Type II) may present differently, but no well documented cases have appeared, possibly due to the tendency of these seizures to spread rapidly to temporal lobes or to generalize. The characteristics of coma, somnolence, hallucinations and psychotic behaviour are more typical of absence status [7, 43] as is a duration lasting days or even weeks [36]. However, as some manifestations of complex partial status could be misinterpreted as psychosis, for example catatonic episodes [44] and visual hallucinations [45], careful observation of all behaviours is important.

A more restrictive type of complex partial seizure status has been reported. One patient with a chronic sense of anxiety and 'maximal fear' showed associated spiking on sphenoidal leads, and general EEG desynchronization [46]. Wieser and associates [47] have reported two patients studied by depth electrodes in whom prolonged experiential phenomenon (hearing music) or olfactory and/or gustatory sensations [8] were associated with continuous seizure activity in one site – Heschl's gyrus and hippocampus, respectively. These status states lasted for three hours in the patient who experienced music and for three days in the other patient. Some aura-like phenomena are therefore simple partial seizure status epilepticus but this only becomes clear on depth electrode EEG recording.

14.3 RISKS AND COMPLICATIONS OF TONIC-CLONIC STATUS EPILEPTICUS

Tonic-clonic status epilepticus is a serious neurological emergency due to the protean dysfunctions produced in thermoregulatory, cardiovascular and metabolic systems. It cannot be allowed to persist beyond one hour if severe permanent brain damage is to be avoided [48–51]. The mean duration of status in patients without neurological sequelae is one and one-half hours, while patients who die have been in status for an average of 13 hours [4, 20].

One of the earliest changes is a profound fall in blood pH due to lactic acidosis from maximally exercized muscles. This has been shown to occur within 1–4 min in baboons [50]. Aminoff and Simon [52] reported that 84% of their 70 patients developed acidosis. In approximately 40% the pH fell below 7.0. Following cessation of seizures, the pH returns to a mean of 7.3 within 30 min [53]. In the absence of cardiac failure the degree of neuropathological damage does not correlate with the severity of acidosis in either human or, animal studies [49, 52]. There is also little evidence for acute potassium shifts due to acidosis [54] although hyperkalaemia associated with myonecrosis is well documented and may occur in seizures. Consequently, myoglobulinuria and lower nephron necrosis may be later sequelae.

Elevation of temperature occurs in more than 75% of patients with status epilepticus [52] and is the only factor other than duration of status that correlates with the extent of neuropathological damage in controlled animal experiments [49]. The magnitude of the change in temperature is not necessarily a function of the presence of infection or the duration of status [55].

Following a generalized seizure, norepinephrine and epinephrine levels increase dramatically up to forty-fold, and remain elevated for 30–60 mins [55a]. These large increases in epinephrine may contribute to the cause of sudden unexplained death in epileptic patients due to the precipitation of cardiac arrhythmias. Large increases in cerebral blood flow during status have been noted to appear within 1 min after the onset of status [52]. This initial nine-fold increase drops to a two-fold increment after 1–2 hours of seizures. On the other hand, the rate of cerebral oxygen consumption ($CMRO_2$) rises over this time to two to three times control values, thus giving rise to a relative mismatch between oxygen supply and demand [56]. Brown and Brierley [57] demonstrated that permanent cell damage in the hippocampus, thalamus and middle cerebral cortical layers develops after 60 min of convulsive status even in artificially ventilated animals, the metabolic dysfunctions of which are corrected. These changes are concordant with those noted in autopsies of infants and adults dying in acute status [58] and to those described by Sommer [59] among those with chronic epilepsy. In addition, Chapman *et al.* [60] demonstrated that histopathological damage is already present by 60 min at a time prior to the development of such a mismatch between oxygen supply and demand. Similarly, Kreisman *et al.* [48] identified a 'transitional period' occurring approximately 30 min after the onset of status, after which regional oxygen insufficiency adds to further damage. At the molecular level, changes which can lead to cellular destruction appear to be already present within the first two to three convulsions. These changes include elevations of neuronal calcium and accumulation of toxic levels of arachidonic acid, prostaglandins, and leucotrienes that can lead to brain oedema and cell death [52, 56, 60, 61].

Large elevations in pulmonary vascular pressures may lead to the development of pulmonary oedema [55], which may contribute to sudden death in status [62]. Other consequences of status, such as fluxes in cyclic nucleotides, prolactin, growth hormone, ACTH, cortisol, insulin, and glucagon, are still being investigated for their possible relevance to neuronal damage.

14.4   PROGNOSIS IN STATUS EPILEPTICUS

While the mechanisms of brain damage discussed above may be expected to operate in any type of status, the substrate, such as the age of the brain involved, and the underlying pathology, as well as the degree of generalization of the convulsions will undoubtedly vary prognosis across different groups. We cannot, therefore, be comprehensive in this Chapter but present a summary.

14.4.1   Adult tonic-clonic status epilepticus

In adults, mortality due to the seizures themselves ranges from 0–2% [14, 52]. Acute mortality due to non-seizure causes may range from 0–16% and late mortality from 0–6% in these series. Among patients without a history of epilepsy but with symptomatic status mortality may reach 28%, although only 9% die in the acute stage. These data refer to adults who fall within the aetiological groups discussed earlier. The low number of deaths due to the seizures appears to reflect improved management over the past 10–20 years.

The ability to ascribe morbidity to status is confounded by pre-existing epilepsy and other illnesses, more so in adults than in children. Oxbury and Whitty [1] reported that five of 47 patients reviewed after status showed neurological deterioration. Only two of these had 'idiopathic' seizures. In seven of 84 survivors of status, Aminoff and Simon [52] noted deterioration in intellect and neurological functioning which could not be attributed to other causes. A prospective study of patients pre- and post-status would be useful, possibly using the Wechsler Adult Intelligence Scale (WAIS) on which some patients with epilepsy perform poorly in some sub-tests [63].

14.4.2 Childhood tonic-clonic status epilepticus

The prognosis of status epilepticus in older children is difficult to assess accurately because most studies include children of different ages. However, judging by the large series of Aircardi and Chevrie [13], the incidence of neurological and mental abnormalities (almost always occurring together) was 57%, of which 34% seemed to be acquired at the time of status. These abnormalities included diplegia, extrapyramidal syndromes such as choreoathetosis and other movement disorders, cerebellar signs, bilateral pyramidal tract signs and even decerebrate or decorticate posturing. In the childhood years, seizures seem to beget seizures; the same series reports that 23% of those with status had a previous history of seizures while 57% had seizures afterwards when followed for more than one year. The hemiconvulsive hemiplegia syndrome occurring in children under three years of age is often followed by psychomotor or partial motor seizures several years later [64]. Seizures after an episode of status may be of a different type than those occurring before, [65, 66] suggesting that the status causes further pathological changes, themselves epileptogenic.

14.4.3 Neonatal status epilepticus

The situation is different in neonates, for in this group little or no decrease in mortality accompanying status epilepticus has occurred in recent years [67]. Morbidity has also not changed, with 35% of those neonates showing later sequelae. Three factors appear to determine prognosis in this age group: (1) the earlier the age at which status occurs, the worse the prognosis (2) the less obvious the ictal behaviour, the worse the prognosis; (3) the more disorganized the EEG, the worse the prognosis. An accurate neurological and developmental assessment of the newborn and possibly more recent investigations such as evoked potentials may help predict outcome. These issues are fully discussed by Lombroso [67, 68].

14.4.4 Complex partial status epilepticus

There are few good models for complex partial seizures in animals. In an acute model, Brown *et al.* [69] injected cobalt into one ventral hippocampus of cats and observed bilateral, but not independent, temporal lobe discharges. However, microscopical examination, even using electron microscopy, failed to reveal any changes in the non-injected side. With special staining for glutamic acid decarboxylase (GAD – the synthetic enzyme for GABA), Ribak and colleagues showed selective loss of GAD containing synapses [70], using an alumin-cream injection model of chronic epilepsy in primates. Collins *et al.* [71] have developed a useful model of temporal lobe epilepsy in rodents. Following injections of kainic acid, and the subsequent development of temporal lobe seizures, dendritic swelling of hippocampal CA1, CA3 and CA4 neurones and their associated glia was observed after only one hour of partial seizures.

We feel strongly that partial complex status epilepticus is also a neurological emergency. The studies cited above on tonic-clonic status epilepticus in man and animals reveal the hippocampus to be a site of selective vulnerability to seizures. An autopsy-proven case of severe hemispheric brain damage following unilateral status epilepticus has recently been reported. The hemisphere not involved in the seizure discharge was virtually spared [72]. In addition, at least three cases have been reported in which prolonged or permanent memory deficits followed complex partial seizure status [44, 73].

14.4.5 Absence status

It is difficult to prognosticate about this type of status, given the wide variety of subtypes and aetiologies which may lead to it as discussed above. Brett [37] reported on 22 children whom we would classify as atypical absence status, with status lasting days to months, accompanied by myoclonus and by slow spike and wave abnormalities on EEG. In 68% of these there was a previous history of epilepsy. At long term follow-up of the total, 27% of the children were normal, 18% had died of various causes (one in tonic-clonic status epilepticus) and 14% had degenerative neurological diseases subsequently identified. Forty-one per cent deteriorated for unexplained reasons. Doose and colleagues have reported a statistical correlation between both myoclonic astatic and petit mal status and later dementia [74, 75].

A review of 50 cases of absence status in adults and children reported in the Japanese literature concluded that cases of typical absence in childhood were associated with a fair prognosis, while atypical absence of childhood had a poor prognosis. The adult group all fell into the atypical classification and had 'fair' prognoses. The 'poor' group were related to the persistence of psychiatric symptoms or diagnoses. It appeared that these were present in nine patients, with only four having a history of such. The definitions of 'poor' and 'fair' were not given [43]. Psychiatric symptoms which antedated or appeared simultaneously with absence status were also noted in ten of 12 patients reported by Berkovic and Bladin [76]. In five of these, the symptoms remitted with control of seizures. In the other five it is not clear whether symptoms antedated absence status or not.

At the present state of our knowledge then, we assume that the prognosis of absence status is a function of the underlying pathophysiology. It can range from excellent, as has been reported following post-metrizimide myelography [77] to poor (Lennox–Gastaut syndrome). Therapy should be rapidly instituted. Given the alterations in responsiveness [78] and impairment of other cognitive processes [79, 80] which occur in absence seizures or status, the need for controlled studies testing for subtle deficits in cognition following absence status is apparent.

14.5   THE MANAGEMENT OF STATUS EPILEPTICUS

The rational approach to status epilepticus begins with the *identification of the type of status*. The discussion above should aid in clinical recognition of the varieties of status listed in Table 14.1. Whenever there is a doubt of the diagnosis, an emergency EEG should be performed immediately. This can clearly be of great assistance in distinguishing complex partial status epilepticus from absence status (although not necessarily typical from atypical forms) [81]. The distinction of subvarieties of absence status is not critical, since all respond to a varying degree to benzodiazepines, although atypical absence status has only a 15–60% response rate [82]. Other possible areas of confusion arise in the patient with tonic status epilepticus [24, 25] and with subtle generalized convulsive status (p. 420), which is a life threatening form of status. In patients who present with poriomania, the prolonged ambulatory behaviour of epileptic patients for which they are amnesic [83], which can occur interictally in complex partial status, or with an acute confusional state, the EEG may demonstrate cycles of temporal lobe paroxysms or atypical absence patterns, respectively. Acute conversion states and suspected pseudoseizures need careful clinical assessment and EEG verification to avoid the physical and emotional morbidity that can befall these patients when they are treated too aggressively. Videorecording of behaviour with EEG telemetry is a useful adjunct to differentiate these seizure types [3]. EEG is particularly important in the evaluation of neonatal seizures [81]. Table 14.4 on p. 434 lists the EEG findings and appropriate therapies for the principal varieties of status epilepticus. Of course, when generalized tonic-clonic or clonic-tonic-clonic status is apparent, one cannot delay treatment to wait for an EEG.

Previous publications from this centre have stressed that the second principle of management is the *treatment and correction of the causes and precipitating factors of status epilepticus* [2, 7, 84]. A brief neurological examination may determine the presence of a focal cerebral lesion, such as an acute cerebral infarct, a rapidly expanding intracerebral lesion or cranial trauma. Blood tests to search for hyper- and hypoglycaemia, hypoxia, hyponatraemia, hypocalaemia, and uraemia should be done immediately, and blood and urine obtained for screening for toxic substances at the same time. However, when clonic-tonic-clonic status is the problem the third principle of management should be instigated before more lengthy procedures such as computerized cranial tomography, skull films or lumbar puncture are performed. Some tests and therapy can be carried out simultaneously, for example anticonvulsant infusion during performance of a lumbar puncture, if meningitis is suspected.

The third principle of rational management is the most obvious: to *stop the seizures.* The goal is to halt status within 20 min (the 'transitional period') [48]. If the patient continues to convulse beyond 60 min in spite of adequate drug therapy, general anaesthesia should be initiated. If not already performed at this point, the patient should be placed on artificial ventilation with cardio-respiratory monitoring in an intensive care unit, and any metabolic disturbances should be controlled.

14.6 AVAILABLE REGIMENS

Just as there are many drugs now approved for epilepsy and others in clinical trials (see Chapter 9), many drugs have been tried in status epilepticus, although few with controlled, double-blind prospective studies. Table 14.2 lists the properties of an ideal drug for status epilepticus. Many authors have noted in the past that no such ideal drug exists [11, 40]. It seems a number of authors consider that diphenylhydantoin fits these criteria closest [85, 86], although the pharmacokinetics of zero order elimination in a drug with a long half-life (22+ hours) dictates a delay before a steady state concentration is reached. It has been estimated that 15–30 min are required before phenytoin reaches peak concentrations in brain, and it takes this long on the average to stop generalized status [2]. Therefore, as diazepam is rapidly distributed, entering the brain within 10 s, and as it is a very effective drug, a protocol which employs the simultaneous infusion or bolus injection of diazepam to a total of 20 mg with diphenylhydantoin injection beginning simultaneously has been proposed and widely utilized [2, 7, 84]. These authors point out that intravenous diazepam stops seizures within 5 min in 80% of patients, but seizures may recur in 10–20 min due to redistribution in lipid pools. The combination of diazepam and phenytoin will cause arrest of seizures in nearly all cases of primary generalized tonic-clonic, clonic-tonic-clonic and myoclonic status, and status due to drug or alcohol withdrawal, and in 65% of patients with secondary generalized tonic-clonic status, anticonvulsant drug withdrawal and progressive encephalopathies.

Other authors, however, consider the 5-hydroxy, 1,4-benzodiazepine,

Table 14.2 Properties of an ideal drug for treatment of status epilepticus

---

(1) Rapidly effective against all types of status
(2) Available for intravenous administration
(3) Potent, so that small volumes can be given rapidly
(4) Safe: no cardiorespiratory depression, no depression of consciousness, no systemic side effects
(5) Rapidly enters the brain
(6) Long distribution half-life
(7) Short elimination half-life
(8) Useful in oral form as a chronic antiepileptic drug

---

lorazepam, to be an ideal first line anticonvulsant. Its biological half-life is shorter, about 15 hours, and it has no active metabolites, so toxic accumulation is less likely than with diazepam. However, it has a less extensive tissue distribution than diazepam, being less lipophilic, and therefore the half-life is effectively longer [87, 88]. Lorazepam reaches peak brain concentrations somewhat less rapidly (15–30 min) for the same reason [89] but the onset of useful action in clinical studies has been less than 3 min [90]. Combining six studies between 1979 and 1981, lorazepam was effective in stopping status in 88% of 113 adults and 75 children [91–96]. In one study, the group most refractory appeared to be myoclonic status, in which lorazepam controlled only 55% of cases [90]. One double-blind comparison of lorazepam and diazepam for control of partial seizures showed diazepam to be effective in 70% of cases, compared to 86% for lorazepam group, but these differences were not significant [85]. A preliminary report from an ongoing prospective, double-blind cross-over study comparing lorazepam with diphenylhydantoin in generalized convulsive status shows a success rate of 20/26 for lorazepam as a first drug and 6/10 as a second drug, while phenytoin was successful in controlling 12/22 as the first drug and 5/6 as the second. Patients with subtle generalized convulsive status did not respond to either drug [97]. In general, lorazepam appears to be as safe as diazepam in clinical studies. Leppik and colleagues [85] found that lorazepam produced respiratory depression in the same number of patients as did diazepam. Other side effects such as drowsiness, ataxia, confusion, agitation, hallucinations have been reported, but these are reversible complications. Three cases of paradoxical tonic status were precipitated when the drug was used in atypical absence [92, 96]. Transitory respiratory arrest or depression has also been reported in a patient without previous lung disease [91]. Lorazepam appears not to cause cardiac side effects, and long term complications have not been reported.

Lorazepam may in the future be recommended as a first line drug for status epilepticus, but it is presently not approved by the Federal Drug Administration for this use. To fulfill FDA requirements, a nationwide, co-operative study involving ten medical centres is evaluating treatments in a blinded, randomized fashion to determine which method is best: phenobarbitone alone, a diazepam–phenytoin combination, phenytoin alone or lorazepam. This will better define the first and second line drugs of choice. In centres where it is presently being used, lorazepam is administered at 0.1 mg/kg as an intravenous bolus [96]. If seizures continue, the same dose can be repeated in 15 min. A mean serum level of 52 ng/ml at 120 min after bolus was correlated with efficacy in the study of Walker and colleagues [91]. These authors used a fixed dose of 4 mg given intravenously over 2 min. Seizure control lasted between 2 and 72 hours, which is longer than the control usually achieved with diazepam. It is always necessary to be prepared for depression of respiration.

There is no data on what efficacy, if any, may be expected from constant diazepam infusion in the event that lorazepam fails. However our experience with this regimen has shown that diazepam infusions stopped convulsive status in seven of 13 patients with progressive neurological lesions who had previously received combinations of diazepam bolus, phenytoin, and phenobarbitone. The combination of phenytoin and diazepam bolus and drip achieved control in 88% of patients including those with progressive lesions in a prospective study [10]. A recent review concludes that solutions of 0.125 mg/ml are stable for 6–8 hours [98]. This is within the range that Delgado-Escueta and Bajorek recommended [7], but we additionally recommend now that the intravenous solution be changed every 6 hours. Diazepam can be given in 0.9% NaCl, dextrose solutions, Ringer's or Ringer's lactate solutions. Care should be taken to use polyolefin sets with short lengths of tubing [98]. Levels should be kept in the range of 0.2–0.8 μg/ml to assure control. This regimen reduced the number of refractory patients from 35% to 12% [10].

In previous protocols, Delgado-Escueta and colleagues have recommended phenobarbitone as a second line drug. In spite of its effectiveness and ease of rapid administration, it was not recommended as a first line drug because of its depressant effects on respiration and mental awareness and because no controlled trial of its efficacy in status epilepticus has been reported. In the present protocol, patients who fail to be controlled on the first two lines of drug therapy will have already received 20 mg diazepam, 18 mg/kg diphenylhydantoin and 0.1 mg/kg lorazepam. If convulsions persist it is reasonable to proceed to therapy with the administration of anaesthetizing doses of barbiturates or inhalation anaesthesia.

There are no controlled trials comparing one barbiturate with another or with other anaesthetics in the management of status epilepticus, although in the UK short-acting barbiturates such as thiopentone are preferred. Goldberg and McIntyre [99] reported some success with the use of barbiturate anaesthesia in a pilot study. Patients who had failed to respond to diazepam and diphenylhydantoin with or without phenobarbitone were admitted to an intensive care unit and placed on artificial ventilation. They received an initial bolus of 5 mg/kg pentobarbitone. The EEG was monitored and additional pentobarbitone was given if necessary to produce a 'suppression burst' pattern. Infusion was continued at a rate of 1–3 mg/kg/hour for four hours. After this time, the infusion rate was decreased and the EEG checked for generalized discharges. If these were present the procedure was repeated for another four hours; if not, the pentobarbital was withdrawn over 12–24 hours.

Other barbiturate anaesthetics may be equally useful [100, 101]. In a retrospective study Burton and Holland [102] reviewed their experience with non-anaesthetizing doses of thiopentone given either intravenously or per rectum. Eight patients in status received this as a first drug and another 31 had had various anticonvulsants prior to this, without control of status. 1 gm thiopentone was diluted in 500 ml of normal saline, and administered using a 'micro-drip' set at 1 ml/min or 2 mg/min for 30 min, then reduced to 0.5 ml/min if seizures were controlled. If seizures were not controlled the dose was increased until clinical seizures ceased. Both intravenous and rectal routes brought about immediate control in nine patients, which meant seizures were controlled within one hour and did not recur while thiopentone was being administered. Also, status did not recur during the admission. Six of the intravenous group and 13 treated rectally had breakthrough seizures, but not status, occurring usually when the dosage was decreased. One in each group failed to be controlled. Three patients developed respiratory depression during infusion but two had received large boluses of thiopentone previously and one had been on diazepam infusion. All three recovered without sequelae and 12 had no complications. Of 23 treatment episodes using the rectal route, no complications occurred in 20. Three became obtunded but responded to a decreased rate of infusion. Proctoscopy performed on several patients after rectal infusions after treatment revealed no abnormality. This is an encouraging report and we would hope a prospective clinical trial could assess this drug further.

A case report of treatment of status epilepticus in a four month old infant treated with thiopentone anaesthesia has also appeared [103]. The child, who suffered from pneumococcal meningitis, had received maximal doses of phenytoin, phenobarbitone, and diazepam by bolus injection and intravenous infusion. Thiopentone 10 mg/kg brought the EEG to 'brain silence', and in addition decreased the intracranial pressure from above 30 mm Hg to below 20 mm Hg. In severely refractory cases of status, the thiopentone dose can simply be increased to anaesthetic levels. Thiopentone is metabolized to pentobarbitone, the levels of which in the CSF can reach between 15%–40% of the serum level when infused. Serum levels show a prompt response to changes in the rate of infusion [104]. The potential for decreasing intracranial pressure and decreasing cerebral hypoxic damage [105] also make barbiturates rational drugs for further studies.

If seizures are not controlled after steps 1 to 4 of Table 14.3, and an anaesthetist is not immediately available, one is left to select a variety of agents which have even less controlled data to help determine their efficacy. Paraldehyde may be effective in some cases of tonic-clonic status resistant to first and second line drugs [106]. The drug must have been properly stored in glass, light-resistant containers, and freshly opened. Any open containers must be discarded after 24 hours, owing to the formation of acetic acid. The serum concentration should be monitored. Anaesthetic levels are 12–30 mg/100 ml while the minimum lethal level is 50 mg/100 ml. Safe control should be achieved with 200 mg/kg infused over five minutes followed by a drip of 20 mg/kg/h [107]. Some consider it a second line drug in neonates. Curless and colleagues [108] report that in 16 trials of childhood status in which diazepam and phenytoin had failed, paraldehyde gave a good therapeutic response in 37% of children and side effects did not occur in those cases not given an initial bolus.

The sedative and hypnotic chlormethiazole is sometimes of use in refractory

Table 14.3 Management of tonic-clonic status epilepticus

Steps	Time from initial observation and treatment (mins)	Procedure
1	0	Assess cardiorespiratory function as the presence of tonic-clonic status is verified. If unsure of diagnosis, observe one tonic-clonic attack and verify the presence of unconsciousness after the end of the tonic-clonic attack. Insert oral airway and administer O_2 if necessary. Insert an indwelling intravenous catheter. Draw venous blood for levels of anticonvulsants, glucose, electrolytes, urea and for blood count and for blood culture if appropriate. Draw arterial blood for pH, pO_2, HCO_3^-. Monitor respiration, blood pressure, and ECG. If possible, monitor EEG.
2	5	Start intravenous infusion through indwelling venous catheter with normal saline containing vitamin B complex. Give a bolus injection of 50 ml 50% glucose.
3	10	Infuse diazepam intravenously no faster than 2 mg/min until seizures stop, or to total of 20 mg. Also start infusion of phenytoin no faster than 50 mg/min to a total of 18 mg/kg. If hypotension develops, slow infusion rate. (Phenytoin, 50 mg/ml in propylene glycol, may be placed in a 100 ml volume control set and diluted with normal saline. The rate of infusion should then be watched carefully. Alternatively, phenytoin may be injected *slowly* by intravenous bolus injection.)

If diazepam and phenytoin do not achieve control of seizures, EEG monitoring at intervals, or the use of a cerebral function monitor [110a] and endotracheal intubation is recommended during the remaining steps.

Steps	Time from initial observation and treatment (mins)	Procedure
4	30–50	If seizures re-occur or persist, four options exist: (i) 0.1 mg/kg lorazepam as intravenous bolus. Repeat the same dose in 15 min if control is not achieved. (ii) Diazepam intravenous drip: 50–100 mg of diazepam is diluted in 500 cc of dextrose-saline or other solute (see text) and run in at 40 ml/h. Levels should be monitored to assure therapeutic range of 0.2–0.8 μg/ml; solution should be changed every six hours. (iii) Intravenous phenobarbitone: start bolus infusion of phenobarbitone no faster than 100 mg/min until seizures stop, or a loading dose of 20 mg/kg has been given.

Table 14.3 – cont.

Steps	Time from initial observation and treatment (mins)	Procedure
		(iv) Thiopentone may be given at non-anaesthetizing doses, i.e. 2 mg/min in normal saline by a micro-drip set for 30–60 min. Reduce dose to 0.5 mg/min when controlled. Dose can be increased to anaesthetic levels if necessary to achieve control. EEG monitoring to ascertain a 'burst-suppression' pattern and seizure control is required. Alternatively, other anaesthetizing barbiturates can be used.
5	60–80	If seizures continue, general anaesthesia with halothane and neuromuscular junction blockade is instituted.

Once control is achieved, EEG monitoring is recommended continuously or as frequently as is technically possible in the obtunded patient, to ensure that status has not recurred.

status [109, 110]. After mixing 8 g/l in 4% dextrose, 5–10 mg/kg/h can be used [110]. Problems with this drug include hyperpyrexia, thombophlebitis if infused for 12 hours or more, and the softening of plastic intravenous sets within 4–6 hours.

The recommended protocol shown in Table 14.3 is designed for tonic-clonic status epilepticus but should be applied to any form of convulsive or non-convulsive status epilepticus with some exceptions. The protocols shown in Tables 14.3 and 14.4 are intended for patients from the juvenile to adult age groups. The problems of management of status epilepticus in the neonate are unique, due to differences in pharmacokinetics and seizure presentation [15]. There may also be difficulties in establishing rapid venous access. In particular, many paediatricians favour phenobarbitone over diphenylhydantoin [111, 112]. Others have had good results with rectal diazepam in infants [113, 114]. We have limited experience with this preparation and would refer the reader to those references for further information.

Other exceptions to the protocol appear in Table 14.4. One particular difficulty arises in some patients who have tonic status or atypical absence status, for these patients may be made worse by sedative drugs. Valproic acid is generally useful for these conditions, but it is unavailable as a parenteral preparation. A preparation of valproic acid to be given per rectum has been described [115, 116]. Vajda reports that a mean dose of 2100 mg/day per rectum was useful in controlling tonic-clonic, complex partial, tonic, partial

Table 14.4 Type of status, EEG characteristic, and recommended management

Type of status	EEG characteristic	Recommended management
Primary generalized:		
Clonic	8–10 Hz sharp waves or diffuse periodic discharges at 0.3–1 Hz	Protocol as Table 14.3
Clonic-tonic-clonic	1.5–5 Hz spike-wave complexes	Protocol as Table 14.3
Tonic-clonic	1.5–5 Hz spike-wave complexes or diffuse 16 Hz spikes	Protocol as Table 14.3
Secondarily generalized:		
Tonic-clonic with partial onset	Focal 12–18 Hz spikes spreading diffusely or focal 1 Hz spikes and spike-waves spreading diffusely	Protocol as Table 14.3
Subtle generalized convulsive status	Periodic lateralized discharges often bilateral with or without synchrony. Background slowing	Protocol as Table 14.3
Tonic status	Generalized paroxysmal fast activity at 16–35 Hz	Intravenous diphenylhydantoin infusion as protocol on Table 14.3. Sedatives, especially benzodiazepines, should be avoided. Seizures may stop spontaneously, or rectal sodium valproate may be effective [2]
Non-convulsive status:		
Complex partial	Rhythmic spikes, sharp waves or low voltage fast activity, unilateral or with a temporal predominance alternating with a postictal slow record with voltage attenuation and progressive normalization	Protocol as Table 14.3
Absence status Typical	3 Hz spike and wave complexes, diffuse and synchronous. May vary between 2.5–3.5 Hz continuous or intermittent paroxysms	Diazepam or lorazepam bolus as Table 14.3. Or 1–2 mg clonazepam, intravenous bolus, repeat in 5 min if no result*

Table 14.4 – cont.

Type of status	EEG characteristic	Recommended management
Atypical	4–6 Hz spike and waves; 3–5 Hz slow waves with occasional spikes; irregular slow spike and wave; high voltage triphasic sharp waves at 2–3 Hz, 1 Hz bursts of sharp waves and spikes. Any pattern may be continuous or intermittent	If 2 intravenous doses of any benzodiazepine are without effect, rectal sodium valproate may be an option†
Simple partial status:		
Partial motor status	Focal spikes, sharp waves, or spike and waves occurring rhythmically at variable frequencies. Or rhythmic slow waves with circumscribed spread. There may or may not be background slowing	Protocol as Table 14.3, steps 1–3. In a conscious patient the simultaneous initiation of oral carbamazepine at a therapeutic dosage is recommended (800–1200 mg a day). Other non-anaesthetizing second or third line drugs may be tried.
Partial sensory status		
Partial status with other symptoms		
Unilateral status	Generalized slow waves of high amplitude possibly in conjunction with myoclonic jerks; intermittent superimposed recruiting rhythms progressing to diffuse unilateral spike and wave complexes	Protocol as Table 14.3. Although this is a partial status the generally poor outcome of this group of patients warrants aggressive management
Epilepsia partialis continua	8–30 Hz rhythms in sensory-motor area	Protocol as Table 14.3, steps 1–4. Unless seizures generalize, anaesthesia should be avoided

* In typical absence, some authorities recommend trying intravenous acetazolamide first, due to its low toxicity. The dose is 250 mg for persons less than 250 kg and 500 mg for persons more than 35 kg [111].
† References [115] and [116].

motor and myoclonic status [116]. Viani and colleagues [115] have also reported the use of rectal sodium valproate in infantile and neonatal status. Controlled trials will be necessary to judge the comparative value of this regimen over others.

14.7 CONCLUSION

The destructive effect of uncontrolled seizures necessitates an aggressive approach to the control of all types of status epilepticus. As our understanding of the pathophysiology of the epileptic process grows, we will be able to identify better the various types of status, and thus design selective, specific and effective treatments. In the meantime, the use of EEG monitoring with or without video observations can help us to identify the subtler forms of status, and intervene to reduce further the morbidity of this condition.

REFERENCES

1. Oxbury, J. M. and Whitty, C. W. M. (1971) Causes and consequences of status epilepticus in adults: A study of 86 cases. *Brain*, **94**, 733–44.
2. Treiman, D. M. and Delgado-Escueta, A. V. (1980) Status epilepticus, in *Critical Care of Neurological and Neurosurgical Emergencies*, (eds R. A. Thompson and J. R. Green), Raven Press, New York, pp. 53–99.
3. Mattson, R. H. (1983) Closed-circuit televised videotape recording and electro-encephalography (CCTV-EEG) in convulsive status epilepticus, in *Status Epilepticus: Mechanisms of Brain Damage and Treatment Advances in Neurology*, Vol. 34) (eds A. V. Delgado-Escueta *et al.*), Raven Press, New York, pp. 37–49.
4. Celesia, G. G. (1976) Modern concepts of status epilepticus. *JAMA*, **235**, 1571–4.
5. Janz, D. (1961) Conditions and causes of status epilepticus. *Epilepsia*, **2**, 170–97.
6. Janz, D. and Kautz, G. (1964) The aetiology and treatment of status epilepticus. *Dtsch. Med. Waochenschr.*, **88**, 2189.
7. Delgado-Escueta, A. V. and Bajorek, J. G. (1982) Status epilepticus: Mechanisms of brain damage and rational management. *Epilepsia*, **23** (Suppl. 1), S29–41.
8. Wieser, H. G., Hailemariam, S., Regard, M. and Landis, T. (1985) Unilateral limbic epileptic status activity: StereoEEG, behavioural and cognitive data. *Epilepsia*, **26(1)**, 19–29.
9. Mattson, R. H. (1983) The design of clinical studies to assess the efficacy to toxicity of antiepileptic drugs. *Neurology*, **33** (Suppl. 1), 1–37.
10. Delgado-Escueta, A. V. and Enrile-Bacsal, F. (1983) Combination therapy for status epilepticus: Intravenous diazepam and phenytoin, in *Status Epilepticus: Mechanisms of Brain Damage and Treatment (Advances in Neurology*, Vol. 34) (eds A. V. Delgado-Escueta *et al.*) Raven Press, New York, pp. 395–8.
11. Duffy, F. H. and Lambroso, C. T. (1978) Treatment of status epilepticus, in *Clinical Neuropharmacology*, Vol. 3 (ed. H. L. Klavans), Raven Press, New York, pp. 41–56.
12. Hauser, W. A. (1983) Status epilepticus: Frequency, etiology, and neurological sequelae, in *Status Epilepticus: Mechanisms of Brain Damage and Treatment. (Advances in Neurology*, Vol. 34) (eds A. V. Delgado-Escueta *et al.*), Raven Press, New York, pp. 3–13.
13. Aicardi, J. and Chevrie, J. J. (1970) Convulsive status epilepticus in infants and children: A study of 239 cases. *Epilepsia*, **11**, 187–97.

14. Hauser, W. A. (1980) *Epidemiology, Morbidity, and Mortality of Status Epilepticus*, presented at the International Symposium of Status Epilepticus, Santa Monica, California.

15. Mora, E. U., Olmes-Garcia de Alba, G., Garcia, D. V. and Valdez, J. M. (1984) Neonatal status epilepticus I: Clinical aspects. *Clin. Electroenceph.*, **15(4)**, 193–201.

16. Celesia, G. G. (1983) Prognosis in convulsive status epilepticus, in *Status Epilepticus: Mechanisms of Brain Damage and Treatment (Advances in Neurology*, Vol. 34) (eds A. V. Delgado-Escueta *et al.*), Raven Press, New York, pp. 55–60.

17. Janz, D. (1963) *Die Epilepsien, Spigjielle Pathologie und Therapie*, Georg Thieme Verlag, Stuttgart.

18. Janz, D. (1983) Etiology of convulsant status epilepticus, in *Status Epilepticus: Mechanisms of Brain Damage and Treatment (Advances in Neurology*, Vol. 34) (eds A. V. Delgado-Escueta *et al.*), Raven Press, New York, pp. 47–59.

19. Hunter, R. H. (1959–60) Status epilepticus: History, incidents and problems. *Epilepsia*, **4**, 162–88.

20. Rowan, II. J. and Scott, D. F. (1970) Major status epilepticus: A series of 42 patients. *Acta Neurol. Scand.*, **46**, 573–84.

21. Victor, M. and Brausch, J. (1967) The role of abstinence in the genesis of alcoholic epilepsy. *Epilepsia*, **8**, 1–20.

22. Schmidt, D. (1982) The effect of pregnancy on the natural course of epilepsy, in *Epilepsy, Pregnancy and the Child* (eds D. Janz *et al.*), Raven Press, New York.

23. Gastaut, H., Roger, J., Ouahchi, S. *et al.* (1963) An electroclinical study of generalized epileptic seizures of tonic expression. *Epilepsia*, **4**, 15–44.

24. Sommerville, E. R. and Bruni, J. (1983) Tonic status epilepticus, presenting as confusional state. *Ann. Neurol.*, **5**, 549–52.

25. Roger, J., Lob, H. and Tassinari, C. A. (1974) Status epilepticus, in *The Epilepsies (Neurology*, Vol. 15) (eds O. Magnus, A. M. Lorentz de Haas), North Holland Publishing Co., Amsterdam, pp.145–88.

26. Treiman, D. M., DeGiorgio, C. M., Salisbury, S. M. and Wickboldt, C. L. (1984) Subtle generalized convulsive status epilepticus. *Proc. Am. Epilepsy Soc.*, Abstracts, p. 20.

26a. Simon, R. P. and Aminoff, M. J. (1986) Electrographic status epilepticus in fatal anoxic coma. *Ann. Neurol.*, **20**, 351–55.

27. Mises, J., Plouin, P., Bour, F. and Lerique-Koechlin, A. (1981) A propos d'une forme d'epilepsie hemiconvulsive avec hemiplegie chez l'enfant. *Rev. EEG Neurophysiol.*, **11**, 445–9.

28. Aguglia, U. and Gastaut, H. (1983) Benign unilateral seizures or epilepsy? *J. Neurol. Neurosurg. Psychiatr.*, **46**, 871–7.

29. Delgado-Escueta, A. V., Wasterlain, C. G., Treiman, D. M. and Porter, R. J. (1983) Summary, in *Status Epilepticus: Mechanisms of Brain Damage and Treatment (Advances in Neurology*, Vol. 34) (eds A. V. Delgado-Escueta *et al.*), Raven Press, New York, pp. 537–42.

30. Singh, B. M. and Strobos, R. J. (1980) Epilepsia partialis continua associated with nonketotic hyperglycemia: Clinical and biochemical profile of 21 patients. *Ann. Neurol.*, **8**, 155–60.

31. Koshewnikow, A. Y. (1895) Eine besondere form von cortical en epilepsie. *Neurol. Zentralbl.*, **14**, 47–8.

32. Yarnell, P. R. and Chu, N. (1975) Focal seizures and aminophylline. *Neurology*, **25**, 819–22.
33. Lennox, W (1945) The petit mal epilepsies: Their treatment with tridione. *JAMA*, **129**, 1069–73.
34. Gastaut, H., Roger, J. and Lob, H. (1967) *Les Etats de Mal Epileptiques*, Masson, Paris.
35. Andermann, F. and Robb, J. P. (1972) Absence status. A reappraisal following review of 38 patients. *Epilepsia*, **13**, 177–87.
36. Gastaut, H. (1983) Classification of status epilepticus, in *Status Epilepticus: Mechanisms of Brain Damage and Treatment (Advances in Neurology*, Vol. 34) (eds A. V. Delgado-Escueta *et al.*), Raven Press, New York, pp. 15–35.
37. Brett, E. M. (1966) Minor status epilepticus. *J. Neurol. Sci.*, **3**, 52–75.
38. Guberman, A., Cantu-Reyna, G., Stuss, D. and Broughton, R. (1986) Nonconvulsive generalized status epilepticus: clinical features, neurophysiological testing, and long-term follow-up. *Neurology*, **36**, 1284–91.
39. Forster, C., Ross, A. and Kugler, J. (1969) Psychomotor status epilepticus. *EEG Clin. Neurophysiol.*, **27**, 211.
40. Nakada, T., Lee, H., Kwee, I. L. and Lerner, A. M. (1984) Epileptic Kluver-Bucy syndrome: Case report. *J. Clin. Psychiatr.*, **45**, 87–8.
41. Treiman, D. M. and Delgado-Escueta, A. V. (1983) Complex partial status epilepticus, in *Status Epilepticus: Mechanisms of Brain Damage and Treatment (Advances in Neurology*, Vol. 34) (eds A. V. Delgado-Escueta *et al.*), Raven Press, New York, pp. 69–81.
42. Delgado-Escueta, A. V. and Walsh, G. O. (1985) Type I complex partial seizures of hippocampal origin: Excellent results of anterior temporal lobectomy. *Neurology*, **35(2)**, 143–54.
43. Nakane, Y. (1983) Absence status: with special reference to the psychiatric symptoms directly related to the occurence of seizure activity. *Folia Psychiatr. Neurol. Jap.*, **37(3)**, 227–38.
44. Engel, J., Jr, Ludwig, B. L. and Fetell, M. (1978) Prolonged partial complex status epilepticus: EEG and behavioural observations. *Neurology*, **28**, 863–9.
45. Lugaresi, E., Pazzaglia, P. and Tassinari, C. A. (1971) Differentiation of absence status and temporal lobe status. *Epilepsia*, **12**, 77–87.
46. Henriksen, G. F. (1973) Status epilepticus partialis with fear as clinical expression. Report of a case and ictal EEG findings. *Epilepsia*, **14**, 39–46.
47. Wieser, H. G. (1980) Temporal lobe or psychomotor status epilepticus, A case report. *Electroenceph. Clin. Neurophysiol.*, **48**, 558–72.
48. Kreisman, N. R., Rosenthal, M., LaManna, J. C. and Sick, T. J. (1983) Cerebral oxygenation during recurrent seizures, in *Status Epilepticus: Mechanisms of Brain Damage and Treatment (Advances in Neurology*, Vol. 34) (eds A. V. Delgado-Escueta *et al.*), Raven Press, New York, pp. 231–9.
49. Meldrum, B. S. and Brierly, J. B. (1973) Prolonged epileptic seizures in primates: Ischemic cell change and its relation to ictal physiological events. *Arch. Neurol.*, **28**, 10–17.
50. Meldrum, B. S. and Horton, R. W. (1973) Physiology of status epilepticus in primates. *Arch. Neurol.*, **29**, 1–9.
51. Meldrum, B. S., Vigoraux, R. A. and Brierley J. B. (1973) Systemic factors and

epileptic brain damage: Prolonged seizures in paralyzed artificially ventilated baboons. *Arch. Neurol.*, **29**, 82–7.

52. Aminoff, M. J. and Simon, R. P. (1980) Status epilepticus: Causes, clinical features and consequences in 98 patients. *A. J. Med.*, **69**, 657–66.

53. Orringer, C. E., Eustace, J. C., Wunsch, C. D. and Garder, L. B. (1977) Natural history of lactic acidosis after grand-mal seizures. *N. Engl. J. Med.*, **297**, 796–9.

54. Fulop, M. (1978) Serum potassium in lacticacidosis and ketoacidosis. *N. Engl. J. Med.*, **300**, 1087.

55. Simon, R. P. (1985) Physiologic consequences of status epilepticus. *Epilepsia*, **26** (Suppl. 1), S58–66.

55a. Benowitz, N. L., Simon, R. P. and Copeland, J. R. (1986) Status epilepticus divergence of sympathetic activity and cardiovascular response. *Ann. Neurol.*, **19**, 197–99.

56. Meldrum, B. S. (1983) Metabolic factors during prolonged seizures and their relation to nerve cell death, in *Status Epilepticus: Mechanisms of Brain Damage and Treatment (Advances in Neurology*, Vol. 34) (eds A. V. Delgado-Escueta *et al.*), Raven Press, New York, pp. 261–75.

57. Brown, A. W. and Brierley, J. B. (1973) The earliest alterations in rat neurones after anoxia and ischaemia. *Acta Neuropathol. (Berl.)*, **23**, 9–22.

58. Corsellis, J. A. N. and Bruton, C. J. (1983) Neuropathology of status epilepticus in humans, in *Status Epilepticus: Mechanisms of Brain Damage and Treatment (Advances in Neurology*, Vol. 34) (eds A. V. Delgado-Escueta *et al.*), Raven Press, New York, pp. 129–40.

59. Sommer, W. (1980) Erkrankung des ammonshornes al aetiologisches moment der epilepsie. *Arch. Psychiatr. Nervenkr.*, **10**, 631–75.

60. Chapman, A., Meldrum, B. S. and Siesjo, B. K. (1977) Cerebral metabolic changes during prolonged epileptic seizures in rats. *J. Neurochem.*, **28**, 1025–35.

61. Chapman, A., Inguai, M. and Siesjo, B. K. (1980) Free fatty acids in the brain in bicuculline-induced epilepticus. *Acta Physiol. Scand.*, **110**, 335–6.

62. Terrence, C. F., Rae, G. R. and Pepper, J. A. (1981) Neurogenic pulmonary edema in unexpected, unexplained death of epileptic patients. *Ann. Neurol.*, **9**, 448.

63. Giordani, B., Berent, S., Sackellares, J. *et al.* (1985) Intelligence test performance of patients with partial and generalized seizures. *Epilepsia*, **26(1)**, 37–42.

64. Gastaut, H., Poiser, F., Payan, G. *et al.* (1960) H.H.E. Syndrome: Hemiconvulsions, hemiplegia, epilepsy. *Epilepsia*, **1**, 418–47.

65. Ounsted, C., Lindsay, J. and Norman, R. (1966) *Biological Factors in Temporal Lobe Epilepsy*, William Heinemann, London.

66. Falconer, M. A., Serafetinides, E. A. and Corsellis, J. A. N. (1964) Etiology and pathogenesis of temporal lobe epilepsy. *Arch. Neurol.*, **10**, 233–48.

67. Lombroso, C. T. (1983) Prognosis in neonatal seizures, in *Status Epilepticus: Mechanisms of Brain Damage and Treatment (Advances in Neurology*, Vol. 34) (eds A. V. Delgado-Escueta *et al.*), Raven Press, New York, pp. 101–14.

68. Lombroso, C. T. (1978) Convulsive disorders in newborns, in *Pediatric Neurology and Neurosurgery* (eds R. A. Thompson and J. R. Green), Spectrum, New York, pp. 205–39.

69. Brown, W. J., Mitchell, A. G., Babb, T. L. and Crandall, P. H. (1980) Structural and physiologic studies in experimentally induced epilepsy. *Expl Neurol.*, **69**, 543–62.

70. Ribak, C. E., Harris, A. B., Vaughn, J. E. and Roberts, E. (1979) Inhibitory GABAergic nerve terminals decrease at sites of focal epilepsy. *Science*, **205(4402)**, 211–14.

71. Collins, R. C., Lothman, E. W. and Olney, J. W. (1983) Status epilepticus in the limbic system: Biochemical and pathological changes, in *Status Epilepticus: Mechanisms of Brain Damage and Treatment* (*Advances in Neurology*, Vol. 34) (eds A. V. Delgado-Escueta *et al.*), Raven Press, New York, pp. 277–88.

72. Soffer, D., Melamed, E., Assaf, Y. and Cotev, S. (1986) Hemispheric brain damage in unilateral status epilepticus. *Ann Neurol.*, **20**, 737–39.

73. Treiman, D. M., Delgado-Escueta, A. V. and Clark, M. A. (1981) Impairment of memory following prolonged complex partial status epilepticus. *Neurology (Minneap.)*, **31**, 109.

74. Doose, H., Gerken, H., Leonhardt, R. *et al.* (1970) Centrencephalic myoclonic-astatic petit mal. *Neuropaediatrie*, **2**, 59–78.

75. Doose, H. and Volzke, E. (1979) Petit mal status and dementia. *Neuropaediatrie*, **10**, 10–14.

76. Berkovic, S. F. and Bladin, P. F. (1983) Absence status in adults. *Clin. Expl Neurol.*, **19**, 198–207.

77. Pritchard, P. B. and O'Neal, D. B. (1984) Nonconvulsive status epilepticus following metrizamide myelography. *Ann. Neurol.*, **16(2)**, 252–4.

78. Porter, R. J. and Penry, J. K. (1983) Petit mal status, in *Status Epilepticus: Mechanisms of Brain Damage and Treatment* (*Advances in Neurology*, Vol. 34) (eds A. V. Delgado-Escueta *et al.*), Raven Press, New York, pp. 61–8.

79. Goode, D. J., Penry, K. and Dreifuss, F. E. (1970) Effects of paroxysmal spike-wave on continuous visual motor performance. *Epilepsia*, **11**, 241–54.

80. Binnie, C. D. (1980) Detection of transitory cognitive impairment during epileptiform EEG discharges: Problems in clinical practice, in *Epilepsy and Behavior* (eds B. M. Kulig, M. Meinardi and G. Stores), Swets & Zeitlinger, Lisse, pp. 91–7.

81. Doose, H. (1983) Nonconvulsive status epilepticus in childhood: clinical aspects and classification, in *Status Epilepticus: Mechanisms of Brain Damage and Treatment* (*Advances in Neurology*, Vol. 34) (eds A. V. Delgado-Escueta *et al.*), Raven Press, New York, pp. 83–92.

82. Tassinari, C. A., Daniele, O., Michelucci, R. *et al.* (1983) Benzodiazepines: Efficacy in status epilepticus, in *Status Epilepticus: Mechanisms of Brain Damage and Treatment* (*Advances in Neurology*, Vol. 34) (eds A. V. Delgado-Escueta *et al.*), Raven Press, New York, pp. 465–75.

83. Mayeaux, R., Alexander, M. P., Benson, F. *et al.* (1979) Poriomania. *Neurology*, **29**, 1616–19.

84. Delgado-Escueta, A. V., Wasterlain, C., Treiman, D. M. and Porter, R. J. (1982) Management of status epilepticus. *N. Engl. J. Med.*, **306**, 1337–40.

85. Leppik, I. E., Patrick, B. K. and Cranford, R. E. (1983) Treatment of acute seizures and status epilepticus with intravenous phenytoin, in *Status Epilepticus: Mechanisms of Brain Damage and Treatment* (*Advances in Neurology*, Vol. 34) (eds A. V. Delgado-Escueta *et al.*), Raven Press, New York, pp. 447–52.

87. Van der Kleijn, E., Baars, A. M., Vree, T. B. and Van der Dries, A. (1983) Pharmacokinetics of drugs used in treatment of status, in *Status Epilepticus: Mechanisms of Brain Damage and Treatment* (*Advances in Neurology*, Vol. 34) (eds A. V. Delgado-Escueta *et al.*), Raven Press, New York, pp. 421–40.

88. Greenblatt, D. J. and Divoll, M. (1983) Diazepam vs lorazepam: Relationship of drug distribution to duration of clinical action, in *Status Epilepticus: Mechanisms of Brain Damage and Treatment* (*Advances in Neurology*, Vol. 34) (eds A. V. Delgado-Escueta *et al.*), Raven Press, New York, pp. 487–92.

89. Ruelius, H. W. (1978) Comparative metabolism of lorazepam in man and four animal species. *J. Clin. Psychiatr.*, **(Section 2)**, 11–15.

90. Homan, R. W. and Walker, J. E. (1983) Clinical studies of lorazepam in status epilepticus, in *Status Epilepticus: Mechanisms of Brain Damage and Treatment* (*Advances in Neurology*, Vol. 34) (eds A. V. Delgado-Escueta *et al.*), Raven Press, New York, pp. 493–99.

91. Walker, J., Homan, R., Vaskec, M. *et al.* (1979) Lorazepam in status epilepticus. *Ann. Neurol.*, **6**, 207–13.

92. Amand, G. and Evrand, P. (1976) Injectable lorazepam in epilepsy. *Rev. EEG Neurophysiol. Clin.*, **6**, 532–3.

93. DeOliveira, R. S. P. (1978) Treatment of convulsive seizures with a new benzodiazepine, lorazepam. *Rev. Bras. Clin. Therap.*, **7**, 295–8.

94. Griffith, P. A. and Karp, H. R. (1980) Lorazepam in therapy for status epilepticus. *Ann. Neurol.*, **7**, 493.

95. Sorrel, L., Mechler, L. and Harmont, J. (1981) Comparative trial of intravenous lorazepam and clonazepam in status epilepticus. *Clin. Therap.*, **4**, 326–36.

96. Waltregny, A. and Dargent, J. (1976) Preliminary report: Parenteral lorazepam in induced epileptic states in man. *Acta Neurol. (Belg.)*, **76**, 173–9.

97. Treiman, D. M., DeGiorgio, C. M., Ben-Menachem, E. *et al.* (1985) Lorazepam versus phenytoin in the treatment of generalized convulsive status epilepticus: Report of an ongoing study. *Neurology*, **35(4)**, (Suppl. 1), S284.

98. Bell, H. E. and Bertino, J. S. (1974) Constant diazepam infusion in the treatment of continuous seizure activity, in *Critical Care Therapeutics* (ed. J. S. Dasta), *Drug Intell. Clin. Pharmacol.*, **18**, 965–70.

99. Goldberg, M. A. and McIntyre, H. B. (1983) Barbiturates in the treatment of status epilepticus, in *Status Epilepticus: Mechanisms of Brain Damage and Treatment* (*Advances in Neurology*, Vol. 34) (eds A. V. Delgado-Escueta *et al.*), Raven Press, New York, pp. 499–504.

100. Logie, A. W and Christian, P. S. (1981) Status epilepticus treated by barbiturate anaesthesia (letter). *Br. Med. J. (Clin. Res.)*, **282(6268)**, 991.

101. Jones, E. S. and Luksza, A. (1981) Status epilepticus treated by barbiturate anaesthesia (letter). *Br. Med. J. (Clin. Res.)*, **282(6265)**, 7111.

102. Burton, K. and Holland, J. T. (1984) Convulsive status epilepsy: Is there a role for thiopentone-induced narcosis? *Clin. Expl Neurol.*, **20**, 47–56.

103. Goiten, R. J., Mussaffi, H. and Melamed, E. (1983) Treatment of status epilepticus with thiopentone sodium anaesthesia in a child. *Eur. J. Pediatr.*, **140**, 133–5.

104. Airey, I. L., Smith, P. A. and Stoddart, J. C. (1982) Plasma and cerebrospinal fluid barbiturate levels during prolonged continuous thiopentone infusion. *Anaesthesia*, **37(3)**, 328–31.

105. Smith, A. (1975) Barbiturate protection in cerebral hypoxia. *Anesthesiology*, **47**, 285.

106. Brown, T. R. (1983) Paraldehyde, chloromethiazole and lidocaine for treatment of status, in *Status Epilepticus: Mechanisms of Brain Damage and Treatment (Advances in Neurology*, Vol. 34) (eds A. V. Delgado-Escueta *et al.*), Raven Press, New York, pp. 509–18.

107. Bostrom, E. (1982) Paraldehyde toxicity during treatment of status epilepticus. *Am. J. Dis. Child.*, **136(5)**, 414–15.

108. Curless, R. G., Helzman, B. H. and Ramsay, R. E. (1983) Paraldehyde therapy in childhood status epilepticus. *Arch. Neurol.*, **40(8)**, 477–80.

109. Harvey, P. K., Higenbottom, T. M. and Lob, L. (1976) Clormethiazole in the treatment of status epilepticus. *Br. Med. J.*, **1**, 603.

110. Lingam, S., Bertwhistle, H., Elliston, H. M. and Wilson, J. (1980) Problems with intravenous chlormethiazole (heminevrin) in status epilepticus. *Br. Med. J.*, **1**, 155.

110a. Prior P. F. and Maynard, D. E. (1986) *Monitoring cerebral function*. Long-term monitoring of EEG and evoked potentials. Elsevier, Amsterdam.

111. Menkes, J. H. (1985) *Textbook of Child Neurology*, Lea & Febiger, Philadelphia, Chap. 12, pp. 608–76.

112. Dodsan, W. E. (1982) Nonlinear kinetics of phenytoin in children. *Neurology*, **32**, 42.

113. Agurell, S., Berlin, A., Ferngran, H. and Hellstrom, B. (1975) Plasma levels of diazepam after parenteral and rectal administration in children. *Epilepsia*, **16**, 277–83.

114. Frunzani, E., Carbini, C. and Lambertini, A. (1983) Rectal diazepam: a clinical and EEG study after a single dose in children. *Epilepsia*, **24**, 35–41.

115. Viani, F., Jussi, M. I., Germani, M. *et al.* (1984) Rectal administration of sodium valproate for neonatal and infantile status epilepticus. *Devl Med. Child. Neurol.*, **26(5)**, 678–9.

116. Vajda, F. J. (1983) Valproic acid in the treatment of status epilepticus, in Status Epilepticus: Mechanisms of Brain Damage and Treatment (Advances in Neurology, Vol. 34) (eds A. V. Delgado-Escueta *et al.*) Raven Press, New York, pp. 519–29.

CHAPTER FIFTEEN

Febrile Convulsions

Sheila J. Wallace

15.1 DEFINITION

The broadest definition of a febrile convulsion is any seizure occurring in association with any pyrexial illness. Unless all seizures associated with fever are included in this definition it is difficult to choose suitable limits by which it can be decided whether or not a seizure can be classed as febrile. Most confusion has arisen in relation to infection of the central nervous system or its coverings, and chronic neurological disorder. In the first instance, in keeping with the present usually satisfactory recovery from bacterial meningitis in developed countries, it has been shown that children with seizures and with cerebrospinal fluid pleocytosis have as good an outcome as those without cells in the cerebrospinal fluid [1]. The demonstration that viral infection is by far the most usual precipitating event of a febrile convulsion [2] and that this is related to EEG changes comparable with those in encephalitis [3], makes attempts to divide children with febrile convulsion into those with and without encephalitic illnesses nonsensical. Similarly, there is no doubt that children with cerebral palsy and other chronic neurological disorders can have seizures when febrile and not at other times. Minor deviations from normal neurodevelopmental progress are common in children who convulse when febrile, so that, if the definition of febrile convulsion excludes children with neurological deficits, it is difficult to know how severe such deficits should be for the definition to be no longer applicable.

The most useful approach is to recognize that the seizure is an indication of an acute central nervous system disorder, and that it may be, in some cases, symptomatic of an acute intracranial infection and/or an important long-term neurological disorder.

15.1.1 Other causes of acute loss of consciousness in young children

The differential diagnosis of febrile convulsion includes reflex anoxic seizures, vasovagal attacks, benign paroxysmal vertigo, rigors, tetany and cardiac arrhythmias. The distinction rests upon a detailed history of the event (p. 483).

15.2 DISTINCTION OF FEBRILE CONVULSIONS FROM EPILEPSY PRECIPITATED BY FEVER

A number of authors, notably Livingston [4], have suggested that seizures which occur during rises in body temperature can be divided into two groups: simple febrile convulsions, and, epileptic seizures precipitated by fever. Using this classification simple febrile convulsions are defined as brief generalized seizures, seldom lasting longer than a few minutes, occurring soon after an elevation of temperature, in children in whom there is no clinical or laboratory evidence of cerebral infection or intoxication and in whom the EEG is normal after the patient has been afebrile for at least a week. The presence of a positive family history of simple febrile convulsions is considered supportive evidence. On the other hand, epilepsy precipitated by fever is deemed to have occurred if seizures are prolonged, have partial features, if the child is over the age of five years and if EEG abnormalities comparable with those seen in overt epilepsy are recorded. Livingston [4] recommends that children in the latter group be treated with prophylactic anticonvulsants in a manner comparable to the treatment of established epilepsy. In practice, the prognosis cannot be defined as simply as would be suggested by this classification. Indeed, Livingston concludes his remarks by suggesting that follow-up is necessary as some patients in the group with simple febrile convulsions later have epilepsy.

15.3 INCIDENCE

The incidence of febrile convulsions in the general population has been estimated at between 19 and 36 per 1000 [5–12]. Despite more enlightened practices of rearing children, and better social conditions, implying a reduction in respiratory illness in children, the incidence has remained remarkably unaltered over the past 30 years.

15.3.1 Incidence related to sex

In almost all studies the proportion of boys has been greater than that of girls, the ratio of boys to girls being about 1.2:1 [11]. In one study, in the combined sibships of 134 children with febrile convulsions, information on convulsive disorders was available for 396 children. Of 206 boys and 190 girls 48% and 39% respectively had had convulsions when febrile, a ratio of 1.2:1 within these sibships [13].

15.4 BIOLOGICAL SIGNIFICANCE OF AGE AND SEX

Febrile convulsions are strongly age related. Millichap [14] examined the age of the first febrile convulsion in 7000 patients reported in the literature. He found that approximately 4% had their first seizure before the age of six months, and 75% between six months and three years, with a peak age of onset between nine and 18 months. In all, 95% of children who had febrile convulsions had their first episode before the age of five years. More recently Verity *et al.* [12] reported that half of 303 children with febrile convulsion ascertained in the British Births Survey (1970) had their first febrile convulsion during the second year of life. Taylor [15] has drawn attention to a tendency in his series for girls to have their first seizures with fever at younger ages than boys, a tendency also noted by Wallace [13]. However, a similar sex difference was not noted by Bamberger and Matthes [6] or Herlitz [16]. Taylor and Ounsted [17] have further elaborated on the risks of convulsions at different ages. They found that children with positive family histories are at maximal risk at a later period than those with negative family histories for convulsive disorders. In addition, they suggested that, as girls tend to have convulsions earlier than boys, then girls are brought disproportionately into the age range during which it is postulated that associated cerebral damage is more likely to occur.

15.4.1   Age as a factor in convulsions in young animals

The investigation of other young animals, for example DBA mice, has shown that they also pass through a critical period in their cerebral development, during which convulsions in response to fever are particularly likely to occur [18]. The electrical stability usually found in the neonatal brain compared with slightly older children may explain the relative infrequency of febrile convulsions in the first six months of life [19].

15.5   IMPORTANCE OF DEVELOPMENT BEFORE THE FIRST CONVULSION

In considering the neurodevelopmental status of the child prior to the first convulsion, it is relevant to start before the child's conception, and proceed to examine events during the pregnancy, perinatal and postnatal periods up to the time of the convulsion.

15.5.1   Events prior to conception

The mothers of children who convulse with fever have a greater than expected incidence of chronic ill-health. Epilepsy, thyroid disease, atopic conditions, gall bladder disease, rheumatism and peptic ulcers in particular have been noted [8, 20]. Examination of parental fertility suggests that this is suboptimal where the children have febrile convulsions, and that subfertility is particularly common where a male infant has febrile convulsions [20]. An increased loss of fetuses before 20 weeks gestation has been reported in the previous pregnancies of mothers of children with febrile convulsions when these are compared with a control population [21].

Thus there are reasons for suspecting that, for some affected children, the potential for suboptimal neurological development may be present even before conception.

15.5.2 Events during gestation

Adverse events which have occurred during intrauterine life and which might predispose to convulsions have been widely recognized [6, 22–26]. In particular, either threatened abortion or antepartum haemorrhage have been noted [22, 25, 26]. Medication of some kind has been necessary during the pregnancies in an unexpectedly high number of cases [25, 26]. Diuretics, anticonvulsants, antibiotics, antiemetics and antidepressives were taken much more commonly during the pregnancies resulting in the birth of a child with later febrile convulsions than in pregnancies preceding the birth of seizure-free siblings [26]. Thus two factors which might be relevant to suboptimal neurological development have been observed. Mothers are generally less well when pregnant with children who subsequently have febrile convulsions, and drugs which might have adverse effects on the developing nervous system are ingested more often.

15.5.3 The perinatal period

Some authors have suggested that prematurity may be a predisposing factor for febrile convulsions [27, 28] but others have found, on comparison with control populations, that children with febrile convulsions are not more likely to have been born before term [26, 29]. Comments on abnormalities of labour and delivery have been made [22–25, 30–32], but in none of these studies was control data available. In an interesting report on twins discordant for febrile convulsions, Schiottz-Christensen [33] found no significant difference between the incidences in convulsing or non-convulsing twins of being born first or second, type of presentation, assisted delivery or other unspecified abnormality in the perinatal period. However, Verity *et al.* [34] report a significant excess of breech deliveries in children with febrile convulsions compared with the general population. In a study which compared children with febrile convulsions with their siblings, there was an excess of deliveries by Caesarean section amongst the convulsing children as a whole, and the males with febrile convulsions were more likely to have had fetal distress during labour [26]. In some studies children with febrile convulsions are reported to have birth weights comparable to controls [34] or twin pairs [33]. However, when the birth weights have been corrected for gestational age, sex, birth order, and maternal height, a significant excess of children with febrile convulsions have been found to be small for gestational age [26]. This further suggests suboptimal prenatal development.

Referring to the immediate postnatal period as normal or abnormal, Schiottz-Christensen [33] was unable to demonstrate that the twin with subsequent febrile convulsions was disadvantaged. On the other hand, poor feeding during the neonatal period has been found to be significantly commoner in males with febrile convulsions than non-convulsing male siblings [26].

There is enough information in these studies to conclude that abnormalities in the perinatal period may predispose some children to convulse when febrile.

15.5.4 Development after birth, and before the first convulsion

There is surprising ambivalence among different authors as to whether children with recognizable neurological deficits can be properly considered to have febrile convulsions rather than precipitation of epilepsy by fever. This distinction is artificial. Even those who profess to exclude children with ongoing neurological abnormalities give figures for the incidence of such disorders [8, 35, 36]. In addition, virtually all large cohorts of children with febrile convulsions have been studied retrospectively. This has led to considerable variability in the reporting of prior neurodevelopmental abnormality [6, 16, 24, 35, 37, 38]. Where a very detailed neurodevelopmental history was taken at the time of the first seizure, 28% of children admitted to hospital with febrile convulsions were considered to have had prior neurological problems in comparison with 16% of seizure-free siblings [39]. In the population study of Nelson and Ellenberg [40], 22% of those who convulsed with fever had been classed as 'not normal' on tests administered before the first seizure. These authors were unable to give a truly comparable figure for children without convulsions but report that 12% were considered neurologically suspect or abnormal at four months of age [41]. Rather surprisingly, only just over 4% of 303 patients with febrile convulsions identified from the British Birth Survey (1970) were considered to be neurologically abnormal prior to their first convulsion [12]. Since approximately 3 per 1000 of the general childhood population have cerebral palsy, it is clear that frank neurological abnormality is commoner than anticipated amongst children with febrile convulsions.

Slowness in development prior to the initial seizure has also been noted [16, 24, 27, 38, 42, 43]. In particular Ellenberg and Nelson [42] showed that almost 20% of a cohort of children with febrile convulsions taken from their population study had been developmentally abnormal or suspect prior to their first seizures.

It is clear that neurological abnormality, whether expressed as abnormal clinical signs, or slowness in development must be considered as predisposing to febrile convulsions.

15.6 FAMILY HISTORY OF SEIZURE DISORDERS

In all series of children in whom inheritance has been explored, there is a higher than expected incidence of convulsive disorders amongst relatives.

Bamberger and Matthes [6] reported that 27.5% of 523 index cases had relatives in whom some form of convulsive disease had occurred. Doose *et al.* [38] found a positive family history in 29% of 576 children, and Horstmann and Schinnerling [44] in 29.9% of 108 cases. Where only close relations of the patient have been examined, rather lower percentages tend to be found. A positive history for convulsions has been reported in the parents in 9.5% of one cohort of 776 children [16] and in 21.2% of another group of 151 [27]. When they have been compared with control populations, children with febrile convulsions have been found to have significantly higher incidences of positive family histories of convulsions [7, 13]. In a retrospective study of 64 same sex twins of whom at least one had convulsed when febrile, Schiottz-Christensen [45] suggested that, in particular, genetic factors were important for girls, but that such factors were only some of a number of reasons why a child might have a febrile convulsion. On the other hand, in another study where boys and girls were compared for a history of convulsions in their parents, there was a significantly greater likelihood that the parents of the boys would have had convulsions [13]. In this series, the girls with febrile convulsions had an incidence of convulsive disorders in relatives comparable to that of girls who were admitted to hospital febrile, but not convulsing, whereas boys with febrile convulsions had a significantly greater likelihood of a positive family history than boy controls [13].

A number of studies of the genetics of febrile convulsions have been performed [45–48]. Frantzen *et al.* [46] enquired about childhood convulsions and adult epilepsy at the time of the first seizure and between five and seven years later. They found that of 228 children, 40% had a relative with febrile convulsions and 20% a relative with epilepsy. In 10% of cases both conditions existed. The incidence of febrile convulsions, at three times that in the general population, was comparable in parents and siblings. On further analysis of their material Frantzen *et al.* believed that there was no evidence that there were cases of non-genetic origin amongst their patients and suggested that their findings were compatible with inheritance by a single dominant gene. Nevertheless, their study does not confirm that all children who convulse when febrile are genetically predisposed to do so. That the genetic message may be strictly related to age was, however, suggested by the finding that recurrence rates of febrile convulsions were significantly higher in children where the age at onset was 14–35 months and the family history was positive for febrile convulsions, compared with those with a history of no seizures or adult epilepsy in the family, or an older age at onset. Ounsted [47] showed that febrile convulsions and the epilepsies as a whole do not segregate from the genetic point of view. However, the demonstration that the patient and sibling patterns of risk for febrile convulsions alone, or for febrile convulsions followed by continuing epilepsy are quite different, led Ounsted to suggest that children whose febrile convulsions were followed by continued epilepsy had acquired acute cerebral damage at the time of the first convulsion. A further analysis of the data led to the conclusion that the genetic message to convulse when febrile is inherited in an autosomal dominant manner [49]. Conversely, Tsuboi [48], after an analysis of 450 children with febrile convulsions, felt that autosomal dominant inheritance was unlikely, but could not be ruled out because incomplete expression is possible. Tsuboi concluded that multifactorial inheritance was probable but the arguments given in this paper in favour of this statement are far from convincing.

Thus there is general agreement that inherited factors predispose to febrile convulsions but that other factors and events highlight this inherent predisposition.

15.7 THE PRECIPITATING EVENT

In the preceding parts of this chapter the factors which may predispose a child to convulse when febrile are considered. However, it will be appreciated that a precipitating event during the critical age period is necessary if this type of seizure disorder is to be manifest.

15.7.1 The infecting agent

For many centuries physicians have been aware that children may convulse when suffering from otherwise banal ailments [50]. Seasonal incidences in febrile convulsions have been noted [6, 24, 51]. A suggestion that such seizures are most likely to occur when particular infecting agents are present in epidemic concentrations in the community has been substantiated by a study of the role of respiratory viruses as the cause of the febrile illnesses [51], and by a very detailed analysis of the evidence for viral infection in children with febrile convulsions [2]. Although upper respiratory tract infections are the commonest precipitating illnesses on clinical grounds [6, 16, 24, 27, 30, 31, 35, 52, 53], enteroviruses, mycoplasma pneumoniae and Q-fever have also been implicated [3, 51].

When a viral infection is conscientiously sought, it can be found in up to 86% of patients [2]. However, other causes of fever should not be totally ignored. Gastrointestinal infection, in particular with shigella or salmonella organisms, has been recorded in from 4–13% of cases [6, 16, 24, 27, 30, 52]. Within populations of children with febrile convulsions, between 0.9–4% are reported to have convulsed following vaccination when smallpox was still being actively prevented [6, 16, 24, 27, 30]. However, when the incidence of febrile convulsions in association with current vaccination schedules was examined, it was found that diphtheria, tetanus and pertussis antigens given together were associated with convulsions in 0.09 per 1000 doses. Seizures also occurred after polio vaccination in 0.6 per 1000 doses and after measles vaccination in 0.93 per 1000 doses [7]. It was concluded that only for measles was there a significant, though very small, risk of febrile convulsions being precipitated by vaccination.

Many authors exclude children with intracranial infections from the definition of febrile convulsions, but where the long term outcome of such children has been examined, it is no different from those in whom there are no cells in the cerebrospinal fluid [1]. Between 2–8% of children who present febrile and with convulsions are found to have bacterial or viral meningitis [13, 54].

Various estimates have been made of the frequency of febrile convulsions in the course of the illnesses which they commonly accompany. Thirty years ago, approximately 11% of febrile Danish children who were admitted to hospital had had convulsions [52]. Seizures have been estimated to complicate upper respiratory tract infections, including influenza and otitis media, in almost 8% of children, and to complicate measles in 2.5% [6], but these incidences are certainly exaggerated, being based on hospital admissions. Measles was accompanied by convulsions in only 0.7% in a non-hospital population closely observed for the first five years of life [55].

With the definite exception of bacterial meningitis and the possible exception of shigellosis, convulsions seem rarely to complicate illnesses attributable to bacteria. Up to 17% of young children with bacterial meningitis may present with convulsions [56, 57]. Several authors have been interested in the possibility that shigella organisms may produce a neurotoxic agent [58–60]. In one large series of children with gastroenteritis, 4.8% of those with shigella infections convulsed, in comparison with 1.2% in whom the gastroenteritis was due to other causes [60]. If the shigella organisms do produce a neurotoxin, this remains to be identified.

The wide variety of childhood ailments with which febrile convulsions may be associated emphasizes the concept of predisposition of the host to convulse when challenged by fever, particularly if this is secondary to viral infection.

15.7.2   General effects of the infecting agent

The most obvious indication of systemic infection is a fever. In viral or bacterial infections, exogenous pyrogens precipitate the release of endogenous pyrogens which lead to an upward setting of the thermoregulatory centres in the hypothalamic and preoptic areas. Early experimental evidence [61] suggested that the ensuing pyrexia was caused by the release of acetylcholine in the caudal hypothalamus, which in turn activated nicotinic receptors concerned in thermogenesis. It was felt then that these chemical changes might be directly related to the genesis of febrile convulsions. However later studies have concluded that there is no simple relationship between experimental febrile convulsions and the cholinergic system [62, 63].

It may be necessary for the cortex to be damaged for a seizure to occur in association with fever. The seizure threshold in cats and rat pups that have been subjected to cerebral ischaemia has been found to be lower than in controls [64, 65]. Thus the presence of even minor neurological lesions may be relevant in predisposing a child to convulse when feverish.

In the clinical field, much interest has been shown in the height of the temperature at which the seizure occurs, and in the rate of rise of temperature. There are practical difficulties in the exploration of these factors since both are difficult to monitor. However, between 50% and 80% of children in hospital samples are recorded as having temperatures of 39°C or higher at the time of the seizure [6, 16, 22, 27, 30, 31, 52, 66]. Fischler [60] noted that, in shigellosis, children who convulsed tended to have higher temperatures than those who did not convulse. In children in whom simultaneous continuous EEGs and temperatures were recorded for 24 hours immediately after an initial febrile convulsion, seizure discharges appeared almost exclusively during periods of sustained high fever [67].

Secondary effects of fever have been considered, but neither electrolyte imbalance [58, 68], nor temporary pyridoxine deficiency [69] appear important precipitants of the convulsion with fever.

In summary, fever is a necessary accompaniment of a febrile convulsion. The fever is usually a symptom of a viral infection, and factors other than the fever itself are probably important in the precipitation of the seizure. These other factors remain incompletely defined, but the pre-seizure neurological status of the host is probably crucial.

15.8   THE INITIAL SEIZURE

In the past, a somewhat cavalier attitude to a febrile convulsion was usual. Nevertheless Buchan [50] noted as early as 1802 that 'if the fit continues for only a short space and returns seldom there is reason for hope; but if it continues long, and returns frequently, the prospect is bad'. In recognition of the more serious consequences of prolonged attacks, most authors now report the outcome for short and long seizures separately. Under-reporting of partial onsets in convulsions which later become generalized is probably commonplace. The panic associated with a child's first febrile seizure makes the witness, usually the mother, a relatively poor source of information.

15.8.1   Incidences of prolonged, repeated or partial seizures

Most authors define a prolonged convulsion as one which lasts for at least 30 min. However others regard 15 min as the critical duration. Convulsions lasting longer than 30 min are reported in at least 20% of patients in hospital series [6, 7, 24, 68, 70]. Before diazepam was readily available, febrile convulsions of more than one hour's duration were recorded in 13–14% of hospital series [30, 31]. It is of some interest that none of 36 children in whom a seizure was the alerting sign for meningitis convulsed for more than 30 min [57]. An initial partial febrile convulsion with or without secondary generalization has been noted in up to 19% of patients, and repeated seizures within the same illness in up to 30% [68]. In population studies where febrile convulsions are categorized as either complicated (defined as partial, prolonged for 15 min or more, or repeated within 24 hours) or simple, between one-fifth and one-third of children have initial seizures which are other than simple [34, 40]. On the other hand, in a study where very detailed histories of the convulsions were obtained at the time of presentation 62% of a hospital series had attacks which were of at least 30 min duration, repeated within the same illness or had partial features [68]. It has been noted that children with a complex initial convulsion are rather more likely to be admitted to hospital [12], but the apparently higher incidence of complex seizures cannot be entirely explained on this basis, and it must be concluded that partial features are often ignored in the panic which frequently surrounds an initial febrile convulsion.

15.8.2   Factors predisposing to an initial complex febrile convulsion

In some studies, girls have appeared more susceptible to a prolonged or partial initial febrile convulsion [16, 17, 71], but in others the incidence of complex seizures has been reported to be equal in boys and girls [68, 72]. Children with a history both of seizures in first degree relatives and perinatal abnormalities have been found to be significantly at risk of a complex initial febrile convulsion, as were those girls with a history suggestive of previous clinical neurological abnormality [68]. Although there is general agreement that younger children have a higher risk of complex initial seizures, the critical age below which such attacks are considered likely has varied between 12 and 18 months [22, 38, 68, 71]. No study has convincingly shown that the duration of the seizure is related to the rate of rise of temperature or to the duration of fever.

15.8.3   Evidence for cerebral damage in association with febrile convulsions

The evidence that cerebral damage might occur during febrile convulsions is often circumstantial. In one series where the children had a high incidence of complex seizures, 20% acquired new neurological deficits and 15% became mentally retarded [71]. Conversely, where the patients have been hospitalized but not otherwise selected, about 5% are considered to have acquired neurological signs [14, 39]. In large population studies where standardized neurological techniques have not been applied, acquisition of new neurological deficits appears to be unusual [34, 73]. The much higher incidence of later epilepsy in children who have had prolonged initial seizures has frequently been emphasized [6, 8, 22, 24, 27, 30, 38, 40, 74], but it is often not clear whether the prolonged seizures are secondary to factors which might predispose to both complex febrile convulsions and epilepsy.

In a postmortem study of children dying during illnesses in which prolonged convulsions had occurred, the major pathological changes were found in the frontal, occipital and temporal lobes, basal ganglia and in the Purkinje cells of the cerebellum [75]. The changes were comparable with those seen after hypoxia or ischaemia [76].

In an attempt to estimate the degree of cerebral hypoxia which might occur in association with febrile convulsions, cerebrospinal fluid lactate and pyruvate levels have been measured [77, 78]. In 50% of the children who had multiple short seizures, or a single seizure lasting more than 30 min, increased cerebrospinal fluid lactate and an increased lactate:pyruvate ratio indicated biochemical signs of cerebral hypoxia. The lactate levels were normal in all those with simple febrile convulsions whose CSF (cerebrospinal fluid) was examined.

On the basis of subsequent clinical features, and pathological and biochemical findings, there is good evidence that prolonged febrile convulsions have the potential for causing abnormalities in both cerebral structure and function.

15.9 MANAGEMENT OF THE FEBRILE SEIZURE

At the time of the febrile seizure, it is important to minimize anoxia and other general effects of the attack, to terminate the convulsion if it is still in progress, to identify and if necessary treat the underlying infection and to acknowledge the parents' anxieties and allay them if possible.

15.9.1 Attention to general effects

As for any other seizure, the airway should be cleared and oxygen given if necessary. Reduction in body temperature to as near normal as possible should be attempted using a fan, and/or tepid sponging, and rectal paracetamol given as suppositories. It may be useful to set up an intravenous line.

15.9.2 Anticonvulsants for the acute attack

If the convulsion does not terminate spontaneously within 10 min, diazepam should be given as the anticonvulsant of first choice. If possible, diazepam 0.1 mg/kg body weight should be administered intravenously. However, intravenous injection may be technically difficult in children under the age of 3 years and rectal diazepam (in solution, not as a suppository) 0.5 mg/kg body weight is almost as rapidly effective as diazepam by the intravenous route. If, after a further 15 min, the seizure is still in progress, a second comparable dose of diazepam may be given. It is unusual for the seizure to continue after this but should it do so, care in a unit equipped for tracheal intubation and ventilation is mandatory. Only in such a unit can either a continuous diazepam infusion *or* intravenous phenobarbitone (10–15 mg/kg body weight) *or* rectal or intramuscular paraldehyde be given under close observation for possible respiratory depression.

15.9.3 Treatment of the infection

Since almost 90% of children with febrile convulsions will have their convulsions precipitated by viral infections [2], specific treatment of the cause of the fever is usually impossible. Clearly, for the 10% who have fevers secondary to bacterial infections, and particularly for those with bacterial meningitis, appropriate antibiotic therapy is indicated. It is useful in all cases to minimize the pyrexia by giving regular antipyretics until the fever settles.

15.9.4 Parental anxieties

At least 70% of parents who witness their child's first febrile convulsion believe at the time that the child has died [79, 80]. Understandably, acute parental anxiety usually accompanies a convulsion. There is also a fear of meningitis [79], which can almost always be allayed by examination of the cerebrospinal fluid. Later the parents are concerned by the possibilities of recurrence of convulsions, epilepsy and mental retardation. The risk factors for these sequelae are considered on pp. 458–59. It is important that these risk factors are taken fully into account when the outlook for an individual child with an initial convulsion is discussed with the parents.

15.10 INVESTIGATION AT THE TIME OF THE SEIZURE

Laboratory and radiological investigations performed at the time of a seizure may be relevant to the accompanying infection, to secondary metabolic changes or to the seizure itself.

15.10.1 Blood count, serum electrolytes, calcium, phosphate

Neutropenia has commonly been identified and is thought to be indicative of viral infection [72], but on the whole the blood count is unhelpful in the management of the illness [54, 81]. Hyponatraemia is a frequent finding [82], but appears to be a non-specific response to fever [68]. Calcium and phosphate levels are almost invariably normal [54, 83].

15.10.2 Serum and cerebrospinal fluid immunoglobulin levels

Since febrile convulsions are a response to infection, the paucity of reports on investigations of the immune system is rather surprising. In some children low serum levels of IgA may be of relevance [84, 85]. On the basis of immunoglobulin estimations in CSF, active immune responses have been identified in children with febrile convulsions. It is concluded that these responses are secondary to the presence of viral antigens within the central nervous system [86, 87].

15.10.3 Lumbar puncture

Considerable attention has been given to the necessity for or the desirability of examination of the CSF in children with febrile convulsions. Although only approximately 6% of children who present feverish and convulsing have meningitis, 41% of those with bacterial meningitis have seizures [88]. In about one-third the convulsion is the presenting sign. On purely clinical grounds it is almost impossible to exclude meningitis in the postictal state [54, 81, 89]. It is especially difficult to be certain of neck stiffness and minor alterations in alertness in younger children and babies. Those paediatricians who have addressed themselves particularly to these difficulties conclude that lumbar punctures should always be performed when febrile convulsions present before the age of 18 months [54] or, more cautiously, at less than three years [81]. Clearly, if there is any suspicion of meningitis on clinical grounds, or if recovery from the convulsion appears unduly delayed, examination of the CSF is mandatory, whatever the child's age.

In summary, lumbar puncture is recommended in all who are aged less than 18 months and in older children with clouding of awareness or other signs suggesting intracranial infection.

15.10.4 Radiological examination

Skull radiology is almost invariably normal in children with febrile convulsions and should not be requested as a routine [81, 83, 89, 90]. More sophisticated neuroradiological investigation is indicated only when there is a suspicion of a serious underlying illness.

15.10.5 Electroencephalography (EEG)

Several authors have studied EEGs following a febrile convulsion. In recognition that abnormalities might be related to the underlying infection [91], there has sometimes been deliberate delay in recording [23]. In the first week after a febrile convulsion, normal EEGs have been found in between 50% and 71% of patients [6, 22, 30, 31, 92]. Slowing of background rhythms has been noted in between one-fifth and one-third of cases [6, 30, 31]. Marked slowing has been associated with complex febrile convulsions in children over two years, with fevers of over 39°C, with an illness of more than 36 hours, and when gastroenteritis has been the underlying infection [31], or with young age and long duration of fever [22]. Paroxysmal abnormalities and spikes are rare in routine EEGs recorded during the week following the febrile convulsion, and are unhelpful in prognosis [93, 94]. Thus, although an EEG may give some information about the underlying cerebral disturbance, they do not provide useful predictive data. They should be recorded only when it is considered that they might provide help in the immediate management.

15.11   RECURRENCE OF FEBRILE CONVULSIONS

The true recurrence rate for febrile convulsions based on a population in which anticonvulsant prophylaxis has not been given is difficult to identify from the literature as a whole. Where the anticonvulsant status has not been noted, and follow-up has been for at least three years, between 20% and 58.5% of children are reported to have had further febrile convulsions [6, 12, 16, 23, 24, 27, 29, 38, 40, 91, 95, 96]. In children with a previous febrile convulsion and on no anticonvulsant therapy at times of later fevers, further seizures have been recorded in 47% and 51% [97, 98]. Of the children who have had febrile convulsions on two occasions, approximately one-third will have three or more episodes [99].

15.11.1   Factors increasing the risk of recurrence

In a study of children who were definitely not receiving anticonvulsant prophylaxis, those whose parents were unskilled or unemployed, whose first degree relatives had had seizures and who were aged less than 20 months at the time of a first febrile convulsion invariably had another seizure; and those with at least two of these three adverse factors were significantly more likely than those with one or no such factor to convulse again [98]. In other studies, abnormalities of pregnancy and low birth weight [25], complex initial seizures [25, 97] and neurological abnormality [25, 73, 97, 99] have been significantly related to recurrence. Thus at the time of the first febrile convulsion children at significant risk of recurrent attacks can be identified.

15.12   PROPHYLAXIS AGAINST RECURRENCE

Since recurrent febrile convulsions can both adversely affect cognitive development (p. 460) and predispose to later epilepsy [99, 100] (p. 458), they should be prevented if possible. Detailed antipyretic instruction will not, alone, reduce the risk of recurrence [101]. Dependent on the anticonvulsant chosen, therapy can be given on an intermittent or continuous basis.

15.12.1 Intermittent anticonvulsant therapy

Diazepam is the only antiepileptic drug which is effective when given at the time of a feverish illness. It must be administered rectally and can be given in solution in a dose of 5–7.5 mg every 12 hours while the temperature is elevated [102], or as a suppository in a dose of 5 mg every 8 hours during periods of fever [103]. Using diazepam in this manner the recurrence rate can be reduced to just over 10% with most of the further febrile convulsions occurring in children whose parents had not appreciated that they were unwell early enough. Where the parents are considered able to appreciate the onset of fever, the use of intermittent diazepam during febrile illnesses is the prophylaxis of choice.

15.12.2 Continuous anticonvulsant therapy

Continuous therapy is indicated in children with factors carrying a significant risk of recurrence, where the parents are thought to be unable to recognize the onset of fever, or who are unwilling to give medication per rectum. Phenobarbitone [25, 104–108] and sodium valproate [107, 108] used singly are the only anticonvulsants which have been demonstrated to reduce significantly the risk of recurrence. Phenobarbitone 4–5 mg/kg/day produces serum levels which are usually high enough to prevent recurrences. Sodium valproate is used in a dose of 20–30 mg/kg/day. Phenytoin is difficult to use in young children and has not been successful in reducing the recurrence rate in children aged less than three years, and who, therefore, are at greatest risk of recurrences [109]. Carbamazepine has not prevented recurrences when used either as a first choice [110] or after phenobarbitone has failed [111].

15.12.3 Side effects from prophylactic medication

Diazepam when given during the feverish illness may cause some drowsiness but in no case has this been sufficient to obscure important clinical signs [102].

Phenobarbitone causes unacceptable overactivity in 20% of children with febrile convulsions [112]. Adverse effects on behaviour which are not severe enough to warrant discontinuance of therapy are noted in about another 20% [112–115]. Studies of the possible effects of barbiturates on cognitive development have shown that, provided unacceptable behaviour changes do not occur, intellectual development proceeds normally when phenobarbitone is given for up to 35 months in the prophylaxis of febrile convulsions [100, 115–117].

Sodium valproate causes significantly fewer behavioural problems than phenobarbitone [113]. Sodium valproate does not adversely effect cognitive development if given over a two year period [100]. No report of serious irreversible side effects has appeared in the literature when sodium valproate has been used as prophylaxis against febrile convulsions [107, 108, 118–121].

15.13 FEBRILE SEIZURES AND LATER EPILEPSY

Although there is general agreement that the incidence of epilepsy is greater in people who have had febrile convulsions than in the general population, the degree of risk varies greatly between studies. When children with febrile convulsions in a population study were followed to age seven years, 2% had epilepsy – that is to say recurrent non-febrile seizures – in comparison to 0.5% in those who had not had a febrile convulsion [40]. However, in a hospital series, only two-thirds of those with epilepsy when aged 9–14 years had their first afebrile seizure before the age of seven years [93], suggesting that seven years of age is too early for a categorical statement to be made about the probability of later epilepsy. A recent study from the Rochester group shows that when children with febrile convulsions were followed up for up to 30 years (mean 18 years), the life-table cumulative risk of subsequent epilepsy was 2% by the age of 5, 4.5% by age 10, 5.5% by age 15, and 7% by age 25 [99].

15.13.1 Seizure types in epilepsy following febrile convulsions

Almost any type of epilepsy may follow febrile convulsions, but generalized tonic-clonic seizures are those most often reported [16, 24, 40, 44, 122]. Typical absences are rare sequelae. On the other hand, when analysing the antecedents in patients with partial epilepsy, almost one-quarter were noted to have had previous febrile convulsions [123], and, in a long term population study, the risk for later partial epilepsy was almost twice that for generalized epilepsy [99]. Two studies [40, 122] reported a high incidence of myoclonic or minor motor seizures. In one of these studies complex partial seizures were not mentioned [40], yet the sequence of events where a hemiconvulsion is followed by a hemiplegia, usually transient, and later by complex partial seizures [124] is now well recognized. It can only be concluded that the classification of the epilepsies which may follow febrile convulsions has been less than ideal.

15.13.2 Risk factors for epilepsy

When risk factors for the later development of epilepsy have been examined, epilepsy has usually been considered in a composite manner. When children with febrile convulsions were followed to the age of seven years, factors significantly related to later epilepsy included suspect or abnormal development prior to the initial seizure, complex (prolonged, repeated or focal) features in the first febrile convulsion, and a history of seizures when afebrile in a parent or prior born sibling [73]. Annegers *et al.* have analysed the contribution of three different risk factors – prolonged convulsion, focal features, and repeated episodes within 24 hours – to the subsequent development of epilepsy [99]. One-third of the children had none of these factors, and their actuarial risk of subsequent epilepsy was 2.4% – not much greater than the population risk illustrated in Fig. 1.2. If all three factors were present the child had a 49% risk of subsequently developing epilepsy. Different combinations of factors had intermediate effects.

When the possibility that partial and generalized epilepsies might follow different precipitating events has been examined, persisting generalized tonic-clonic seizures were most commonly found in those children with unskilled or unemployed parents, those who had had perinatal abnormalities, and those who showed continuing neurological abnormalities, whereas complex partial seizures were significantly related to the occurrence of a prolonged febrile convulsion with unilateral features [93]. Of the children who developed complex partial seizures after a unilateral febrile convulsion of more than 30 min duration, those in the younger age range, and particularly girls in whom the initial convulsion had been right-sided (left hemisphere), were most likely to develop complex partial seizures [125].

15.14 LONG TERM EEG STUDIES

Long term EEG studies following febrile convulsions have been performed for two main reasons. It has been felt that characteristic patterns might give information about genetic tendencies to febrile convulsions, and that the evolution to epilepsy might be usefully monitored by the EEG.

In 89 children from whom 1046 EEGs were recorded up to the ages of 11–13 years, patterns considered to be genetically determined (bilateral synchronous spike and wave, photosensitivity and 4–7 Hz waves) were found in 81% of cases [126]. Spike and wave discharges were very inconsistent and strongly age dependent, being found maximally between five and six years. In this study, although no correlation was found between the EEG findings and the family history, the authors concluded that as the EEG patterns were those generally considered to be genetically determined, then there was support for the belief that febrile convulsions occur as the result of a heterogeneous response to polygenetic inheritance. However it seems doubtful that this conclusion is justified on the basis of EEG findings alone.

Other authors have noted the appearance of spikes in middle childhood in patients whose earlier EEGs have shown no evidence of epileptic activity [127, 128]. In neither study has the appearance of spikes been found to correlate with clinical events.

In brief, so far, long term EEG studies appear to be of more academic than practical importance.

15.15 OUTLOOK FOR INTELLECTUAL DEVELOPMENT

Later mental retardation (IQ of less than 70) is found in between 6% and 18% of children admitted to hospital with their initial febrile convulsion [23, 27, 37,

43, 52]. No comparable figures are available for non-hospital populations, but problems with speech were noted to be significantly more prevalent in children with febrile convulsions identified in the British Birth Survey (1970) [34]. This survey also showed that children with unilateral or prolonged febrile convulsions tended to be disadvantaged in tests of copying designs and of vocabulary at age five years.

Despite the presence of some children of lower ability within groups who have had febrile convulsions, the mean intelligence is well within the normal range in all studies where cognitive development has been assessed [42, 43, 100, 115, 117]. However, the overall intelligence rating may mask specific learning difficulties. In a study of twin pairs discordant for febrile convulsions, the convulsing twin was found to be significantly disadvantaged on measures of logical memory (retention), the Weschler digit symbol test, block design and Part B of the trail making test [129]. Specific reading retardation was noted in 19% of a hospital based, but otherwise unselected, cohort who were tested when aged between 8 and 14 years [130], and in 35% of children whose initial febrile convulsion was right sided (left hemisphere) and prolonged or repeated within the same illness [125].

Factors which predispose to or are associated with below average ability in children with febrile convulsions are low social class and perinatal abnormalities [43], prior or continuing neurological disorders [42, 43], recurrence of febrile convulsions [100], and progression to epilepsy [73, 130].

15.16 SUMMARY

Febrile convulsions occur in approximately 2.5% of all children. They are strongly age-dependent. A positive family history, less than optimal pre- and perinatal development, and/or neurodevelopmental delay, may predispose an individual child to convulse when challenged by a viral infection. It is important to terminate the convulsion within 30 min. Recurrences may be prevented by either diazepam solution given rectally at the time of subsequent fevers or by continuous phenobarbitone or sodium valproate. The overall risk of later epilepsy is about five times that in the general population, but is very significantly increased by the presence of neurodevelopmental disorders. Although usually of average intelligence, children with febrile convulsions have a higher than expected incidence of reading difficulties.

REFERENCES

1. Frantzen, E. (1971) Spinal findings in children with febrile convulsions. *Epilepsia*, **12**, 192.
2. Lewis, H. M., Parry, J. V., Parry, R. P., *et al.* (1979) Role of viruses in febrile convulsions. *Arch. Dis. Child.*, **54**, 869–76.
3. Wallace, S. J. and Zealley, H. (1970) Neurological, electroencephalographic and virological findings in febrile children. *Arch. Dis. Child.*, **45**, 611–23.

4. Livingston, S. (1968) Infantile febrile convulsions. *Devl Med. Child Neurol.*, **10**, 374–6.

5. Annegers, J. F., Hauser, W. A., Elveback, L. R. and Kurland, L. T. (1979) The risk of epilepsy following febrile convulsions. *Neurology*, **29**, 297–303.

6. Bamberger, P. and Matthes, A. (1959) *Anfalle im Kindesalter*, Karger, Basel, pp. 368–432.

7. Harker, P. (1977) Primary immunisation and febrile convulsions in Oxford 1972–5. *Br. Med. J.*, **2**, 490–3.

8. Hrbek, A. (1957) Fieberkrämpfe im Kindesalter. *Ann. Paediatr.*, **188**, 162–82.

9. Schuman, S. H. and Miller, L. J. (1966) Febrile convulsions in families: findings in an epidemiological survey. *Clin. Pediatr.*, **5**, 604–8.

10. Van den Berg, B. J. and Yerushalmy, J. (1969) Studies on convulsive disorders in young children. I. Incidence of febrile and non-febrile convulsions by age and other factors. *Pediatr. Res.*, **3**, 298–304.

11. Ohtahara, S. O., Ishida, S., Yamatogi, Y., *et al.* (1981) Febrile convulsions in Tamano City, Okayama: A neuro-epidemiologic study. *Brain Devl.*, **3**, 103.

12. Verity, C. M., Butler, N. R. and Golding, J. (1985) Febrile convulsions in a national cohort followed up from birth. I. Prevalence and recurrence in the first five years of life. *Br. Med. J.*, **290**, 1307–10.

13. Wallace, S. J. Unpublished data.

14. Millichap, J. G. (1968) *Febrile Convulsions*, Macmillan, New York.

15. Taylor, D. C. (1969) Differential rates of cerebral maturation between the sexes and between hemispheres. Evidence from epilepsy. *Lancet*, **ii**, 140–2.

16. Herlitz, G. (1941) Studien uber die sogenannten initialen Fieberkrämpfe bei Kindern. *Acta Paediatr.*, **29** (Suppl. 1), 1–142.

17. Taylor, D. C. and Ounsted, C. (1971) Biological mechanisms influencing the outcome of seizures in response to fever. *Epilepsia*, **12**, 33–45.

18. Hertz, L., Schousboe, A., Formby, B. and Lennox-Buchthal, M. (1974) Some age-dependent biochemical changes in mice susceptible to seizures. *Epilepsia*, **15**, 619–32.

19. Purpura, D. P. (1969) Stability and seizure susceptibility of immature brain, in *Basic Mechanisms of the Epilepsies* (eds H. H. Jasper, A. A. Ward and A. Pope) Little, Brown, and Co., Boston, pp. 481–505.

20. Wallace, S. J. (1974) The reproductive efficiency of parents whose children convulse when febrile. *Devl Med. Child Neurol.*, **16**, 465–74.

21. Van den Berg, B. J. and Yerushalmy, J. (1974) Studies on convulsive disorders in young children. V. Excess of early fetal deaths among pregnancies preceding the birth of children with febrile or non-febrile convulsions. *J. Pediatr.*, **84**, 837–40.

22. Lennox, M. A. (1949) Febrile convulsions in childhood: a clinical and electro-encephalographic study. *Am. J. Dis. Child.*, **78**, 868–82.

23. Millichap, J. G., Madsen, J. A. and Aledort, L. M. (1960) Studies in febrile seizures. V. Clinical and electroencephalographic study in unselected patients. *Neurology*, **10**, 643–53.

24. Degen, R. and Goller, K. (1967) Die sogenannten Fieberkrämpfe des Kindesalters und ihre Beziehungen zur Epilepsie. *Nervenarzt*, **38**, 55–61.

25. Wolf, S. M., Carr, A., Davis, D. C., *et al.* (1977) The value of phenobarbital in the child who has had a single febrile seizure: a controlled prospective study. *Pediatrics*, **59**, 378–85.

26. Wallace, S. J. (1972) Aetiological aspects of febrile convulsions. Pregnancy and perinatal factors. *Arch. Dis. Child.*, **47**, 171–8.
27. Zellweger, H. (1948) Fieber- oder Infektionskrämpfe. *Helv. Paediatr. Acta*, **3** (Suppl. 5), 58–140.
28. Yanai, N. (1967) Febrile convulsions in children. *Devl Med. Child Neurol.*, **10**, 255.
29. Ekholm, E. and Niemineva, K. (1950) On convulsions in early childhood and their prognosis. *Acta Paediatr. Scand.*, **39**, 481–501.
30. Laplane, R., Humbert, R., Laget, P., *et al.* (1958) Suites immediates et lointaines des convulsions febriles avant quatre ans. *Rev. Neurol.*, **99**, 26–38.
31. Frantzen, E., Lennox-Buchthal, M. and Nygaard, A. (1968) Longitudinal EEG and clinical study of children with febrile convulsions. *Electroenceph. Clin. Neurophysiol.*, **24**, 197–212.
32. Peterman, M. G. (1952) Febrile convulsions. *J. Pediatr.*, **41**, 536–40.
33. Schiottz-Christensen, E. (1973) Role of birth history in the aetiology and course of febrile convulsions. A twin study. *Neuropaediatrie*, **4**, 238–44.
34. Verity, C. M., Butler, N. R. and Golding, J. (1958) Febrile convulsions in a national cohort followed up from birth. II. Medical history and intellectual ability at 5 years of age. *Br. Med. J.*, **290**, 1311–15.
35. Cary, W. (1956) Febrile convulsions in infancy and childhood. *Med. J. Aust.*, **43**, 254–6.
36. Debre, R., Thieffry, S., Neyroud, M. and Lerique, A. (1948) Les convulsions hyperpyretiques. *Arch. Fr. Pediatr.*, **5**, 62–5.
37. Aicardi, J. and Chevrie, J.-J. (1976) Febrile convulsions: neurological sequelae and mental retardation, in *Brain Dysfunction in Infantile Febrile Convulsions* (eds M. A. B. Brazier and F. Coceani), Raven Press, New York, pp. 247–57.
38. Doose, H., Petersen, C. E., Volke, E. and Herberger, E. (1966) Fieberkrämpfe und Epilepsie. I. Atiologie, Klinisches Bild und Verlauf der sogenannten Infekt- oder Fieberkrämpfe. *Arch. Psychiat. Nervenkr.*, **208**, 400–12.
39. Wallace, S. J. (1976) Neurological and intellectual deficits: convulsions with fever viewed as acute indications of life-long developmental defects, in *Brain Dysfunction in Infantile Febrile Convulsions* (eds M. A. B. Brazier and F. Coceani), Raven Press, New York, pp. 259–77.
40. Nelson, K. B. and Ellenberg, J. H. (1976) Predictors of epilepsy in children who have experienced febrile seizures. *N. Engl. J. Med.*, **295**, 1029–33.
41. Nelson, K. B. and Ellenberg, J. H. (1980) They don't do very well. *Pediatrics*, **65**, 679.
42. Ellenberg, J. H. and Nelson, K. B. (1978) Febrile seizures and later intellectual performance. *Arch. Neurol.*, **35**, 17–21.
43. Wallace, S. J. and Cull, A. M. (1979) Long-term psychological outlook for children whose first fit occurs with fever. *Devl Med. Child Neurol.*, **21**, 28–40.
44. Horstmann, W. and Schinnerling, W. (1963) Zur prognose der sogenannten Fieberkrämpfe. *Monatsschr. Kinderheilkd.*, **111**, 52–7.
45. Schiottz-Christensen, E. (1972) Genetic factors in febrile convulsions. *Acta Neurol. Scand.*, **48**, 538–46.
46. Frantzen, E., Lennox-Buchthal, M., Nygaard, A. and Stene, J. (1970) A genetic study of febrile convulsions. *Neurology*, **20**, 909–17.
47. Ounsted, C. (1955) Genetics and social aspects of the epilepsies of childhood. *Eugenics Rev.*, **47**, 33–49.

48. Tsuboi, T. (1977) Genetic aspects of febrile convulsions. *Hum. Genet.*, **38**, 169–73.
49. Ounsted, C. (1971) Some aspects of seizure disorders, in *Recent Advances in Paediatrics* (eds D. Gairdner and D. Hull), Churchill Livingstone, London, pp. 363–400.
50. Buchan, W. (1802) Of the epilepsy, or falling sickness, in *Domestic Medicine; or the Family Physician*, J. Pillans & Sons, Edinburgh, pp. 417–21.
51. Stokes, M. J., Downham, M. A. P. S., Webb, J. K. G., *et al.* (1977) Viruses and febrile convulsions. *Arch. Dis. Child.*, **52**, 129–33.
52. Friderichsen, C. and Melchior, J. (1954) Febrile convulsions in children, their frequency and prognosis. *Acta Paediatr. Scand.*, **43** (Suppl. 100), 307–17.
53. Lerique-Koechlin, A., Mises, J., Teyssoniere de Gramont, M. and Loosky-Nekhorocheff, I. (1958) L'EEG dans les convulsions febriles. *Rev. Neurol.*, **99**, 11–25.
54. Rutter, N. and Smales, O. R. C. (1977) Role of routine investigations in children presenting with their first febrile convulsion. *Arch. Dis. Child.*, **52**, 188–91.
55. Miller, F. J. W., Court, S. D. M., Walton, W. S. and Knox, E. J. (1960) *Growing Up in Newcastle-upon-Tyne*, Oxford University Press, London.
56. Samson, J. H., Apthorp, J. and Finley, A. (1969) Febrile seizures and purulent meningitis. *JAMA*, **210**, 1918–19.
57. Ratcliffe, J. C. and Wolf, S. M. (1977) Febrile convulsions caused by meningitis in young children. *Ann. Neurol.*, **1**, 285–6.
58. Donald, W. D., Winkler, C. H. and Bargeron, L. M. Jr. (1956) The occurrence of convulsions in children with shigella gastroenteritis. *J. Pediatr.*, **48**, 323–7.
59. Kowlessar, M. and Forbes, G. B. (1958) The febrile convulsion in shigellosis. *N. Engl. J. Med.*, **258**, 520–6.
60. Fischler, E. (1962) Convulsions as a complication of shigellosis in children. *Helv. Paediatr. Acta*, **17**, 389–94.
61. Tangri, K. K., Misra, N. and Bhargava, K. P. (1976) Central cholinergic mechanism of pyrexia, in *Brain Dysfunction in Infantile Febrile Convulsions* (eds M. A. B. Brazier and F. Coceani), Raven Press, New York, pp. 307–17.
62. McCaughran, J. A., Edwards, E., Zito, R. S. and Schecter, N. (1982) Experimental febrile convulsions: Short and long-term effects on the cholinergic system in the rat. *Epilepsia*, **23**, 434.
63. McCaughran, J. A., Edwards, E. and Schecter, N. (1984) Experimental febrile convulsions in the developing rat: effects on the cholinergic system. *Epilepsia*, **25**, 250–8.
64. Teschan, P. and Gellhorn, E. (1950) Temperature and convulsive activity. *Arch. Int. Pharmacodyn.*, **84**, 57–67.
65. Olson, J. E., Horne, D. S., Holtzman, D. and Miller, M. (1985) Hyperthermia-induced seizures in rat pups with pre-existing ischaemic brain injury. *Epilepsia*, **26**, 360–4.
66. Melekian, R., Laplane, R. and Debray, P. (1962) Considerations cliniques et statistiques sur les convulsions au cours des deshydrations aigues. *Ann. Pediatr.*, **9**, 290–302.
67. Minchom, P. E. and Wallace, S. J. (1984) Febrile convulsions: elecroencephalographic changes related to rectal temperature. *Arch. Dis. Child.*, **59**, 371–3.
68. Wallace, S. J. (1975) Factors predisposing to a complicated initial febrile convulsion. *Arch. Dis. Child.*, **50**, 943–7.

69. McKiernan, J., Mellor, D., Court, S., *et al.* (1980) Hydroxykinurenine/hydroxy-anthranilic acid ratios and febrile convulsions. *Arch. Dis. Child.*, **55**, 873–5.

70. Chevrie, J.-J. and Aicardi, J. (1975) Duration and lateralisation of febrile convulsions. Etiological factors. *Epilepsia*, **16**, 781–9.

71. Aicardi, J. and Chevrie, J.-J. (1970) Convulsive status epilepticus in infants and children. *Epilepsia*, **11**, 187–97.

72. Lennox-Buchthal, M. A. (1973) Febrile convulsions. A reappraisal. *Electroenceph. Clin. Neurophysiol.*, **32** (Suppl. 32), 1–132.

73. Nelson, K. B. and Ellenberg, J. H. (1978) Prognosis in children with febrile seizures. *Pediatrics*, **61**, 720–7.

74. Lennox, M. A. (1949) Febrile convulsions in childhood: their relationship to adult epilepsy. *J. Pediatr.*, **35**, 427–35.

75. Fowler, M. (1957) Brain damage after febrile convulsions. *Arch. Dis. Child.*, **32**, 67–76.

76. Aicardi, J. and Chevrie, J.-J. (1983) Consequences of status epilepticus in infants and children, in *Status epilepticus: Mechanisms of Brain Damage and Treatment* (eds A. V. Delgado-Escueta *et al.*), Raven Press, New York, pp. 115–25.

77. Simpson, H., Habel, A. H. and George, E. L. (1977) Cerebrospinal fluid acid-base status and lactate and pyruvate concentrations after short (less than 30 minutes) first febrile convulsions in children. *Arch. Dis. Child.*, **52**, 836–43.

78. Simpson, H., Habel, A. H. and George, E. L. (1977) Cerebrospinal fluid acid-base status and lactate and pyruvate concentrations after convulsions of varied duration and aetiology in children. *Arch. Dis. Child.*, **52**, 844–9.

79. Clare, M., Aldridge Smith, J. and Wallace, S. J. (1978) A child's first febrile convulsion. *Practitioner*, **221**, 775–6.

80. Baumer, J. H., David, T. J., Valentine, S. J., *et al.* (1981) Many parents think that their child is dying when having a first febrile convulsion. *Devl Med. Child Neurol.*, **23**, 462–4.

81. Wolf, S. M. (1978) Laboratory evaluation of the child with febrile convulsions. *Arch. Dis. Child.*, **53**, 85–7.

82. Rutter, N. and O'Callaghan, M. J. (1978) Hyponatraemia in children with febrile convulsions. *Arch. Dis. Child.*, **53**, 85–7.

83. Heijbel, J., Blom, S. and Bergfors, P. G. (1980) Simple febrile convulsions. A prospective incidence study and an evaluation of investigations initially needed. *Neuropaediatrie*, **11**, 45–56.

84. Lewis, H., Valman, H. B., Webster, D. and Tyrrell, D. A. J. (1980) Viruses in febrile convulsions. *Lancet*, **ii**, 150.

85. Isaacs, D., Webster, A. D. B. and Valman, H. B. (1984) Serum immunoglobulin concentrations in febrile convulsions. *Arch. Dis. Child.*, **59**, 367–9.

86. Ariizumi, M., Kuromori, N., Utsumi, Y. and Shiihara, H. (1981) Febrile convulsions, childhood epilepsy and csf IgG index. *Brain Devl.*, **3**, 109.

87. Eeg-Olofsson, O. and Wigertz, A. (1982) Immunoglobulin abnormalities in cerebro-spinal fluid and blood in children with febrile seizures. *Neuropaediatrics*, **13**, 39–41.

88. Wallace, S. J. (1985) Convulsions and lumbar puncture. *Devl Med. Child Neurol.*, **27**, 69–71.

89. Jaffe, M., Bar-Joseph, G. and Tirosh, E. (1981) Fever and convulsions – Indications for laboratory investigations. *Pediatrics*, **67**, 729–31.

90. Nealis, J. G. T., McFadden, S. W., Asnes, R. A. and Ouellette, E. M. (1977) Routine skull roentgenograms in the management of simple febrile seizures. *J. Pediatr.*, **90**, 595–6.

91. Lennox, W. G. (1953) Significance of febrile convulsions. *Pediatrics*, **11**, 341–57.

92. Lerique, A. (1955) Electroencephalograph in febrile convulsions. *Electroenceph. Clin. Neurophysiol.*, **7**, 451.

93. Wallace, S. J. (1977) Spontaneous fits after convulsions with fever. *Arch. Dis. Child.*, **52**, 192–6.

94. Matsuo, M., Kurokawa, T., Tomita, S., *et al.* (1981) EEG findings during the period of febrile convulsions and transition to afebrile seizures. *Brain Devl.*, **3**, 104.

95. Pearce, J. L. and Mackintosh, H. T. (1979) Prospective study of convulsions in childhood. *NZ Med. J.*, **89**, 1–3.

96. Van der Berg, B. J. (1974) Studies on convulsive disorders in young children. III. Recurrence of febrile convulsions. *Epilepsia*, **15**, 177–90.

97. Wallace, S. J. (1974) Recurrence of febrile convulsions. *Arch. Dis. Child.*, **49**, 763–5.

98. Wallace, S. J. and Aldridge Smith, J. (1981) Recurrence of convulsions in febrile children on no anticonvulsant, in *Advances in Epileptology: XIIth Epilepsy International Symposium* (eds M. Dam, L. Gram and J. K. Penry), Raven Press, New York, pp. 499–502.

99. Annegers, J. F., Hauser, W. A., Shirts, S. B. and Kurland, L. T. (1987) Factors prognostic of unprovoked seizures after febrile convulsions. *New Eng. J. Med.*, **316**, 493–98.

100. Aldridge Smith, J. and Wallace, S. J. (1982) Febrile convulsions; Intellectual progress in relation to anticonvulsant therapy and to recurrence of fits. *Arch. Dis. Child.*, **57**, 104–7.

101. Camfield, P. R., Camfield, C., Shapiro, S. and Cummings, C. (1980) The first febrile seizure – antipyretic instruction plus either phenobarbital or placebo to prevent a recurrence. *J. Pediatr.*, **97**, 16–21.

102. Knudsen, F. U. (1983) *Intermittent Rectal Diazepam Prophylaxis Versus No Prophylaxis in Febrile Children*, paper delivered at the XVth Epilepsy International Symposium, Washington, 1983.

103. Knudsen, F. U. (1981) Successful intermittent prophylaxis in febrile convulsions: preliminary results of a prospective controlled trial, in *Advances in Epileptology: XIIth Epilepsy International Symposium* (eds M. Dam, L. Gram and J. K. Penry), Raven Press, New York, pp. 165–8.

104. Faer, O., Kastrup, K. W., Lykkegaard Nielsen, E., *et al.* (1972) Successful prophylaxis of febrile convulsions with phenobarbital. *Epilepsia*, **12**, 109–12.

105. Thorn, I. (1975) A controlled study of prophylactic long-term treatment of febrile convulsions with phenobarbital. *Acta Neurol. Scand.*, **60** (Suppl. 75), 67–73.

106. Wallace, S. J. (1975) Continuous prophylactic anticonvulsants in selected children with febrile convulsions. *Acta Neurol. Scand.*, **60** (Suppl. 75), 62–6.

107. Wallace, S. J. and Aldridge Smith, J. (1980) Successful prophylaxis against febrile convulsions with valproic acid or phenobarbitone. *Br. Med. J.*, **280**, 353–4.

108. Ngwane, E. and Bower, B. D. (1980) Continuous sodium valproate or phenobarbitone in the prevention of 'simple' febrile convulsions. *Arch. Dis. Child.*, **55**, 171–4.

109. Melchior, J. C., Buchthal, F. and Lennox-Buchthal, M. (1971) The ineffective-

ness of diphenylhydantoin in preventing febrile convulsions in the age of greatest risk, under three years. *Epilepsia*, **12**, 55–62.

110. Monaco, F., Sechi, G. P., Mutani, R., *et al.* (1980) Lack of efficacy of carbamazepine in preventing the recurrence of febrile convulsions, in *Antiepileptic Therapy: Advances in Drug Monitoring* (eds S. I. Johannessen *et al.*), Raven Press, New York, pp. 75–9.

111. Camfield, P. R., Camfield, C. S. and Tibbles, J. (1982) Carbamazepine does not prevent febrile seizures in phenobarbitone failures. *Neurology*, **32**, 288–9.

112. Wolf, S. M. and Forsythe, A. B. (1978) Behaviour disturbance, phenobarbital and febrile seizures. *Pediatrics*, **61**, 728–31.

113. Wallace, S. J. (1981) Prevention of recurrent febrile seizures using continuous prophylaxis: sodium valproate compared with phenobarbital, in *Febrile Seizures* (eds K. B. Nelson and J. H. Ellenberg), Raven Press, New York, pp. 135–42.

114. Bacon, C. J., Cranage, J. D., Hierons, A. M., *et al.* (1981) Behavioural effects of phenobarbitone and phenytoin in small children. *Arch. Dis. Child.*, **56**, 836–40.

115. Camfield, C. S., Chaplin, S., Doyle, A.-B., *et al.* (1979) Side-effects of phenobarbital in toddlers; behavioural and cognitive aspects. *J. Pediatr.*, **95**, 361–5.

116. Hellström, B. and Barlach-Christoffersen, M. (1980) Influence of phenobarbital on the psychomotor development and behaviour in pre-school children with convulsions. *Neuropaediatrie*, **11**, 151–60.

117. Wolf, S. M., Forsythe, A., Studen, A. A., *et al.* (1981) Long-term effect of phenobarbital on cognitive function in children with febrile convulsions. *Pediatrics*, **68**, 820–3.

118. Cavazzuti, G. B. (1975) Prevention of febrile convulsions with dipropylacetate (Depakine). *Epilepsia*, **16**, 647–8.

119. Herranz, J. L., Armijo, J. A. and Arteaga, R. (1984) Effectiveness and toxicity of phenobarbital, primidone and sodium valproate in the prevention of febrile convulsions, controlled by plasma levels. *Epilepsia*, **25**, 89–95.

120. Mamelle, N., Mamelle, J. C., Plasse, J. C., *et al.* (1984) Prevention of recurrent febrile convulsions – a randomised therapeutic assay: sodium valproate, phenobarbital and placebo. *Neuropaediatrics*, **15**, 37–42.

121. Williams, A. J., Evans-Jones, L. G., Kindley, A. D. and Groom, P. J. (1979) Sodium valproate in the prophylaxis of simple febrile seizures. *Clin. Pediatr.*, **18**, 426–30.

122. Tsuboi, T. and Endo, S. (1977) Febrile convulsions followed by non-febrile convulsions. A clinical, electroencephalographic and follow-up study. *Neuropaediatrie*, **8**, 209–23.

123. Danesi, M. A. (1985) Classification of the epilepsies: An investigation of 945 patients in a developing country. *Epilepsia*, **26**, 131–6.

124. Gastaut, H., Poirier, F., Payan, H., *et al.* (1960) H.H.E. Syndrome. Hemiconvulsions, hemiplegia, epilepsy. *Epilepsia*, **1**, 418–47.

125. Wallace, S. J. (1982) Prognosis after prolonged unilateral febrile convulsions, in *Advances in Epileptology: XIIIth Epilepsy International Symposium* (eds H. Akimoto *et al.*), Raven Press, New York, pp. 97–9.

126. Doose, H., Ritter, K. and Volzke, E. (1983) EEG longitudinal studies in febrile convulsions: Genetic aspects. *Neuropaediatrics*, **14**, 81–7.

127. Des Termes, H., Mises, J., Plouin, P., *et al.* (1977) Les 'foyers de pointes' au cours

de l'evolution des convulsions hyperpyretiques. Etude electro-clinique a propos de 35 cas. *Rev. Electroenceph. Neurophysiol. Clin.*, **7**, 455–8.

128. Thorn, I. (1982) The significance of electroencephalography in febrile convulsions, in *Advances in Epileptology: XIIIth Epilepsy International Symposium* (eds H. Akimoto *et al.*), Raven Press, New York, pp. 93–5.

129. Schiottz-Christensen, E. and Bruhn, P. (1973) Intelligence, behaviour and scholastic achievement subsequent to febrile convulsions: an analysis of discordant twin-pairs. *Devl Med. Child Neurol.*, **15**, 565–75.

130. Cull, A. M. (1975) *Some Psychological Aspects of the Prognosis of Febrile Convulsions*, MPh Thesis, University of Edinburgh.

CHAPTER SIXTEEN

Epilepsy in Childhood

Niall V. O'Donohoe

Epilepsy is an important paediatric problem. Seizures are the commonest symptom encountered by the paediatric neurologist. The high incidence of seizures in early childhood means that most of those developing epilepsy do so before the age of 20 years [1], an indication of the vulnerability of the developing nervous system to seizure discharge. The age of onset of epilepsy varies with different varieties of epilepsy. The earliest peak is in infancy and reflects prenatal and perinatal causes such as malformation of and injury to the brain. A high but declining incidence continues through childhood and adolescence, a consequence of the frequent occurrence of primary generalized epilepsies during these periods of development. The epidemiology of epilepsy in childhood is beset with difficulties since the condition is often misdiagnosed or concealed and because there are variations in different geographic locations and socioeconomic environments. A prevalence of 4.1 per 1000 among children followed to their eleventh birthday was observed in the British National Child Development Study in which epilepsy was defined as the occurrence of two or more spontaneous afebrile seizures [2].

In childhood, as in adult life, epilepsy presents clinically as a paroxysmal disorder with recurring seizures as symptoms. Correct diagnosis and differentiation from other non-epileptic paroxysmal disorders are essential and often difficult. The seizure type should be identified, if this is possible, and an attempt should be made to establish an aetiological diagnosis. Seizures may broadly be divided into generalized seizures, bilaterally symmetrical and without local onset, and partial seizures which have a local onset. Partial seizures may become secondarily generalized with accompanying loss of consciousness. Lennox [3] proposed that 'as a brain disorder epilepsy is a disease but as a seizure it is a symptom'. Epilepsy cannot really be called a disease entity because virtually all the serious diseases of humankind may result in seizures. However, despite the multiplicity of exogenous factors which may result in epilepsy, most human epilepsies, whether generalized or partial, share a common genetic basis which contributes significantly to epileptogenesis. The current concept of the aetiology of childhood epilepsies is that they are multifactorial in causation with genetic and acquired factors operating to varying degrees in each case [4]. The genetically determined potentially epileptic brain dysfunction reveals itself in the EEG as generalized spike-wave discharges. These are the neurophysiological expression of a diffuse corticoreticular hyperexcitability [5]. Inherited epileptogenicity interacts with other aetiological factors, some of them probably also genetic, but the majority exogenous and encompassing the long list of pathological states recognized as causing epilepsy. Organic brain lesions represent a 'realization factor' for the clinical expression of the epileptic phenotype. In an apparently primary or idiopathic epilepsy, a trivial brain lesion may seem to be the factor that brings the epilepsy to clinical expression; in children manifesting epilepsy apparently exclusively on a basis of brain damage, additional genetic factors will be found in 70% of the subjects [6]. We do not know precisely how the interaction works or why the genetic predisposition becomes clinically apparent in one child while a sibling with the same predisposition remains healthy. Part of the explanation may reside in the kindling process by which a repeated stimulus in the brain may lead to a permanent augmentation of response [7] (p. 56).

The childhood epilepsies are chronic disorders, a group of syndromes rather than a disease entity [8]. They may broadly be divided as follows [9]:

(1) Primary or essential or functional or genetic epilepsies, i.e. independent of an identifiable brain lesion, and
(2) Secondary or symptomatic or lesional epilepsies, i.e. dependent on the presence of a brain lesion.

Clearly, this is an oversimplification of the classification problem, which is considered fully in Chapter 3. The main difference between the two categories resides in the special weight of the genetic and exogenous factors in each individual epilepsy. The difference between the two groups is more relative than absolute. However, the division remains a useful one in practice and is especially relevant to the question of prognosis. Both groups include epilepsies which are generalized or partial, characterized by generalized seizures or by partial seizures, either simple or complex. The primary epilepsies are characterized by the onset of a specific type of epilepsy at a particular age. They are usually associated with normal neurodevelopmental status, relatively mild and infrequent seizures, and a good prognosis with or without treatment [10].

Most epileptic syndromes in childhood are age-dependent, however, reflecting the influence of brain maturation on the epileptic process (Table 16.1). Lennox [3] wrote 'the type of epilepsy which occurs in a child represents a confluence of age, heredity, and structural brain abnormality'. A chronological approach to the various epilepsies is logical, therefore, with division into epochs extending from the neonatal period through infancy and childhood to adolescence. At all stages of childhood the role of biological changes as triggering factors for the occurrence of seizures should be considered, for example, infection, fever, emotional upset, excessive fatigue or lack of sleep,

Table 16.1 Some epileptic syndromes at different ages in infancy, childhood, and adolescence

---

Neonatal seizure states

Infantile spasms (West's syndrome): 3–8 months

The myoclonic epilepsies of early childhood (including the Lennox-Gastaut syndrome): 1–6 years

Febrile convulsions: 6 months to 5 years

The primary generalized epilepsies
  (1) petit mal: 5–10 years
  (2) grand mal: 3–10+ years

Photosensitive epilepsy: 6–15 years

Primary partial epilepsies including benign focal or Rolandic epilepsy of childhood: 7–10 years

Secondary partial epilepsies with complex symptomatology including temporal lobe epilepsy: any age from early childhood onwards

The epilepsies of adolescence including juvenile absence epilepsy, myoclonic epilepsy of adolescence (Janz syndrome), and epilepsy with grand mal on awakening

---

overhydration, biochemical changes such as hypoglycaemia, and the effects of the precipitate withdrawal of drugs.

16.1 NEONATAL SEIZURES

At no time of life is the brain more likely to be subjected to insults leading to seizures than in the neonatal period, and this explains the high incidence then [11]. In the neonatal period and up to three months of age, inhibitory influences predominate, there is incomplete development of synapses and of commissural connections and, in addition, developmental abnormalities of the brain may be present. Seizures in the neonate are usually partial, fragmented, disorganized and subtle in their presentation. When present, they are usually indicative of serious underlying disease or abnormality. More intensive care and observation of the newborn have been accompanied by an appreciable increase in the recorded incidence of seizures in the early weeks of life. The most common cause is hypoxic-ischaemic encephalopathy; modern imaging techniques such as ultrasonography have demonstrated that intracranial haemorrhage is now the second commonest cause [12]. Other causes include intracranial infection, developmental defects, metabolic disorders such as hypoglycaemia and hypocalcaemia, and withdrawal of narcotics. Hypocalcaemia may occur in the early hours or days in association with hypoxic-ischaemic encephalopathy and prematurity, or after 7–10 days of life in infants artificially fed with high phosphate containing milks. Modifications in milk formulae have led to a virtual disappearance of this type of neonatal tetany. Various types of seizures occur in the neonate. These include so-called subtle seizures, manifested by clonic eye deviation, repetitive blinking, various oral-buccal-lingual movements, repetitive arm and leg movements and periods of apnoea [13]. Generalized tonic seizures and multifocal or localized clonic seizures may also occur. Seizures need to be distinguished from the phenomenon known as 'jitteriness' which is not accompanied by abnormalities of ocular movement but is characterized by tremulousness. Jitteriness may be a consequence of anoxia-ischaemia, of metabolic disturbance or of drug withdrawal and is not considered epileptic in nature [14].

The neonate with seizures requires urgent assessment and treatment. CSF examination, blood and urine culture, ultrasonography and EEG may be required. The EEG is useful in identifying subtle seizures and also has prognostic value. A normal EEG is associated with a prospect of normal development at four years in over 80% of cases; conversely an EEG which is flat, shows burst suppression changes, or has a multifocal discharge pattern is associated with a 12% or lesser chance of normal development later [15]. EEG patterns must, however, be related to the developmental maturity of the infant since, for example, records showing burst suppression may be found in normal premature babies.

The overall prognosis for neonates with seizures is closely related to the underlying cause. In general, the prognosis has improved considerably in recent years. Mortality has declined from 40% to 15%, though the incidence of neurological sequelae in survivors has remained unchanged at 35% [11, 13]. Treatment of affected newborn children should be directed at the cause if possible as, for example, where infection or metabolic abnormality is responsible. Support for respiration, control of blood pressure [16], the administration of intravenous dextrose and the use of anticonvulsant drugs are employed. Phenobarbitone is presently the drug of choice, given intravenously. A loading dose of 10 mg/kg is administered followed 20 min later by 5 mg/kg which may be repeated. The maintenance dose is 5–6 mg/kg/day [17]. Phenobarbitone may have some protective effect on neurones by decreasing the metabolism of damaged cells. An elevation of previously depleted high energy phosphate compounds has been demonstrated by ^{31}P NMR spectroscopy following the use of this drug in neonatal seizures [18].

It should be remembered that there is a small group of neonates whose seizures have no attributable cause. This includes a rare familial disorder characterized by frequent and often refractory convulsions and followed by remission and normal intellectual development [19]. There are also 'fifth-day fits' which resolve spontaneously and may be caused by transient metabolic disorder [20].

16.2   SEIZURES OF EARLY CHILDHOOD

In the early months of life, seizures are uncommon and, as in the neonate, often partial, fragmented and clinically unremarkable. Yet, when they are present, they are often indicative of serious brain abnormality and dysfunction. In fact, at any time during the first year of life, seizures, whether generalized or partial, may be symptomatic of serious disease of the brain and may imply a poor prognosis for normal physical and mental development later [21, 22]. The inhibitory influences gradually decline in the nervous system and conduction of discharges improves so that, by the age of six months, generalized seizures are possible. These may be manifested as febrile convulsions which occur frequently from this age until after four years (Chapter 15) or by the very serious generalized myoclonic epilepsies, of which the most important are infantile spasms and the generalized myoclonic epilepsies of early childhood.

Infantile spasms are characterized by the occurrence of generalized seizures in which brief and repeated flexor spasms of the trunk and limbs are observed; rarely the spasms are extensor. The peak age of onset is between three and eight months, usually at 5–6 months [23]. There is a cessation of normal psychosocial development; a deterioration in adaptive behaviour and a withdrawal phenomenon are usual. The condition is often called West's syndrome after the man who first described it [24]. The EEG pattern is severely disorganized; this is called hypsarrhythmia. Males predominate, familial incidence is rare and a family history of epilepsy is unusual, except when tuberous sclerosis is the cause. Infantile spasms are a non-specific response to a variety of insults. The condition is age-related and depends on a degree of brain maturation having been attained. Diagnosis may be difficult. The condition is sometimes mistaken for colic, or for a startle response.

Consideration of any large series of cases of infantile spasms reveals that there are three identifiable groups: a cryptogenic or primary group, consisting of children who develop normally prior to the onset of spasms; a symptomatic or secondary group often with clearcut aetiological factors and abnormal development prior to spasms; and a small group of doubtful origin. The symptomatic group accounts for 60% of the cases, and the cryptogenic group for about 30%. The onset of the spasms may appear to follow pertussis immunization but the relationship is either coincidental or the immunization acts as a 'trigger' for the development of spasms in an individual predisposed to the condition for some reason [25]. Computed tomography shows cerebral abnormalities in 80% of some series [26], consisting of malformations, calcifications and/or atrophy. Evidence of tuberous sclerosis has been found in up to 20% of some series [27]. The characteristic depigmented 'ash-leaf' patches on the skin should be sought, using Wood's light if necessary.

ACTH has been the preferred form of therapy since 1958 and daily dosage varies from 10 to 180 units [28]. The duration of treatment has varied from 3 weeks to 6 months or longer but there is no convincing evidence that larger doses for longer periods of time are more effective in producing a better long-term outlook for mental development and control of epilepsy. It is important to arrange CT examination prior to ACTH therapy because the hormone itself causes reversible ventricular dilatation [29]. However, at least in animals, ACTH has no influence on the neuronal development of the growing brain [29a]. ACTH is not without risk in these young children [29b], so it is of interest that nitrazepam has recently been shown to be of equal effect in reducing seizure frequency [29b]. The long-term effect of nitrazepam on development however is not yet known.

The prognosis for children with infantile spasms is grave (Table 11.2). Less than a fifth of those affected will be physically and mentally normal later [30]. Indeed, the more careful and detailed the follow-up, the fewer will be the number of fully-recovered children. The prognosis is best in those who demonstrate normal development prior to spasms; where other seizures do not precede the spasms; where the onset is at 6 months or later; where the perinatal history has been uneventful; where diagnosis and treatment were prompt; and where remission of spasms occurred rapidly and was not followed by relapse [31]. As with other primary and secondary epilepsies in childhood, the former (or cryptogenic) do best, including those apparently provoked by immunization, and recovery may be expected in nearly half of these [32].

Another group of serious epilepsies in which age, the degree of brain maturation, structural brain abnormality either congenital or acquired, and also heredity play important roles are those called the *myoclonic epilepsies of early childhood* [33]. This is a heterogeneous group of disorders and not a single entity [34a]. They range from the severe and intractable 'Lennox-Gastaut syndrome' to forms of primary myoclonic epilepsy developing in previously normal children over the age of three years, who often respond well to anticonvulsant therapy. The value of using the term 'Lennox-Gastaut syndrome' to describe severe cases of myoclonic epilepsy of early onset which, like West's syndrome, are age-related and non-specific in aetiology, and which often demonstrate progressive intellectual dilapidation and continuing severe epilepsy even into adult life, is disputed but has some practical merits. A proportion of children with infantile spasms continue to have severe epilepsy, and are indistinguishable from so-called 'Lennox-Gastaut' cases. Myoclonic epilepsies of the severe type are the most malignant form of epilepsy in childhood and constitute more than 70% of the really intractable cases [35]. A variety of generalized seizures occurs including severe drop attacks, head nodding and salaam seizures, prolonged absences, generalized and partial myoclonic jerks, tonic seizures in sleep, tonic-clonic grand mal seizures and episodes of minor epileptic status [36]. The conditions causing the predominant secondary or symptomatic group of myoclonic epilepsies are as diverse as with infantile spasms and include developmental brain abnormalities, perinatal brain injury, acquired postnatal brain damage and, once again, tuberous sclerosis.

Mental handicap is very frequently associated with these epilepsies but the degree of handicap is variable. In one follow-up study of these epilepsies, 84.5% had some degree of mental handicap and 61.2% continued to have seizures [37]. The resemblance to the fate of those with infantile spasms is clear. In the case of the myoclonic epilepsies, the large secondary group has an earlier onset, reflecting the severity of the cerebral insult, and prognosis is poor, whereas the uncommon primary cases begin later and do better. In the latter groups, hereditary factors play an important aetiological role [38].

Diagnosis is based on the clinical history and the nature of the seizures, and on the presence of characteristic slow spike-wave discharges in the EEG. However, these are not always present and may be replaced by diffuse polyspikes and slow waves or even a hypsarrhythmic pattern. Continuous slow spike-wave complexes may accompany the obtundation of minor epileptic status [36]. The atypical absences of this variety of epilepsy should be carefully distinguished from true petit mal with its later onset, typical EEG pattern, and satisfactory response to treatment. There is often a temporal relationship between a worsening myoclonic epileptic disorder and the occurrence of ataxia, and a progressive degenerative brain disorder may be suspected. However, the ataxia usually disappears when the 'epileptic encephalopathy' is treated. Myoclonic phenomena occur with degenerative disease, notably in neuronal ceroid lipofuscinosis and in subacute sclerosing panencephalitis (more often seen in later childhood) and also in association with ataxia in the 'dancing eye syndrome' [39]. In those neuronal storage diseases termed gangliosidoses, the neurones contain abnormal amounts of complex lipids known as gangliosides and are ultimately destroyed. Clinical presentation is usually in infancy with rapid developmental regression and seizures which are generalized and often myoclonic in type [34a, 40].

The treatment of these epilepsies is difficult; no other seizure disorder in childhood is as unyielding to medication as these. All the established anticonvulsants are used, either alone or in combination, but the most successful are the benzodiazepines [41] and sodium valproate [42]. Ethosuximide is sometimes helpful, and ACTH may be used successfully in situations where seizures are very frequent and 'epileptic encephalopathy' results [43]. The ketogenic diet may be helpful in perhaps a third of the cases [44] (p. 337). The general care of children with this frightening condition, which Lennox [3] called the charter member of the ancient order of the 'Falling Sickness', is of great importance. Parents need regular support and advice from their doctors in attempting to deal with the many management and educational problems which are associated with the protracted illness. It may be necessary to protect the child's head and face from trauma in the attacks. Both infantile spasms and the severe myoclonic epilepsies have an equally poor prognosis, with mental retardation having an almost equally high incidence in both epileptic syndromes [45].

16.3 SEIZURES IN LATER CHILDHOOD

From the age of three to four years up to about ten years of age, convulsions in association with fever, common in early childhood, become rarer although they may continue to occur in a small proportion of children even up to the age of ten years. Primary epilepsies, which are genetically transmitted, and nearly always phenotypically expressed as primary generalized seizures, predominate during this period. Their clinical and EEG changes indicate simultaneous involvement of both hemispheres. The initial motor signs are bilateral and reflect the generalized neuronal discharges. Consciousness is quickly impaired or lost. The clinical features do not include signs or symptons referable to an anatomical or functional system localized to one hemisphere. The outstanding exception to these general rules is the epileptic syndrome variously known as benign focal epilepsy of childhood, or Rolandic or Sylvian epilepsy (p. 478).

Convulsive (grand mal) and non-convulsive (absence) epilepsies are the common primary epilepsies at this age. The *tonic-clonic grand mal seizure* is the archetypal convulsion. Approximately 75% of children with epilepsy have this type of attack at some time, either as the only manifestation of their epilepsy or in combination with other seizure types. Grand mal seizures due to primary generalized epilepsy are most frequently seen after the age of five years, are associated with the genetic marker of regular 3 Hz spike waves discharges in the EEG, and usually respond readily to therapy with sodium valproate, carbamazepine, or phenytoin. The prognosis for permanent remission is good and intellectual and behavioural difficulties are rare. However, at this or any other age, grand mal seizures may also occur with the secondary generalized epilepsies associated with diffuse or multifocal brain disease and these have a more uncertain prognosis and response to therapy. Furthermore, any partial seizure may almost immediately become secondarily generalized, and be indistinguishable clinically from a primary generalized grand mal convulsion.

Typical (petit mal) absences in their pure or simple form are a relatively uncommon form of childhood epilepsy, occurring in about 2–5% of patients. The EEG characteristic is the symmetrical bilaterally synchronous 3 Hz spike-wave complex. Absences are frequent, of abrupt onset and termination, last 5–15 s, are accompanied by staring, drifting of the eyes upwards and flickering of the eyelids, and may be induced by hyperventilation. Stereotyped automatic behaviour may accompany absences in many cases, consisting of lip smacking, chewing and some hand movements [46]. It is considered that bursts of spike-wave activity need to last at least 3 s before some degree of impairment of consciousness is apparent. The appearance of automatisms is related to the duration of the absence. In the classic genetic studies of this variety of epilepsy [47], it was noted that siblings and offspring of the patient had a 35% chance of expressing the same EEG trait during their lifetime, and an 8% chance of having absence attacks (Chapter 5). It has been suggested that these genetic risks are not in keeping with single gene Mendelian inheritance, and that other genetic and environmental factors must interact with whatever produces the spike-wave EEG trait before clinical absences occur [48]. For example, two gene loci may need to interact to produce the classic phenotype with appearance of the epilepsy at about the age of 5–9 years. An unknown proportion of cases of absence epilepsy may be sporadic or due to phenocopies, that is clinically similar disorders but with different genotypes. Absence seizures occurring during late childhood and adolescence may represent such cases, with atypical clinical features, the occurrence of grand mal attacks, relative resistance to therapy and the tendency for the epilepsy to persist into adult life [10]. An important form of juvenile or adolescent absence occurs in juvenile myoclonic epilepsy or impulsive petit mal (p. 481). In the diagnosis of petit mal, it is important to distinguish other types of absence attacks, for example, those occurring in the generalized myoclonic epilepsies, and similar disturbances of awareness due to complex partial seizures of temporal lobe origin, associated with prolonged dreamy states and with unusual or bizarre auras and sensations.

Petit mal epilepsy in its pure form has an excellent prognosis (p. 350), and is very responsive to modern drugs such as ethosuximide and sodium valproate. Complete remission occurs in over 75% of cases [49]. Treatment with clonazepam may be effective in resistant cases, The prognosis is favourable when the onset is between five and nine years, when there is no other associated form of seizure such as grand mal attacks, when the EEG is typical, and when mental and neurological status are normal [50].

Generalized seizures, either tonic-clonic convulsions or, less frequently, absences may be precipitated by external stimuli. The most frequently occurring stimulus is a rapidly flashing light, or the rapid flicker produced by a normally functioning television screen. The photoconvulsive response in the EEG (p. 177) is an indication of a genetically determined susceptibility to epilepsy of the primary generalized type, but the actual occurrence of epileptic seizures is low [51]. Reflex epilepsy of the photosensitive type usually begins in the decade 6–15 years, and then wanes during the years of adolescence and early adult life [52]. In most cases, television-viewing at a distance of not less than 3 m is all that is required for prevention. Treatment with sodium valproate may be necessary for individuals who are very sensitive to light and for those who additionally have spontaneous seizures (occurring without reflex stimulation).

Partial epilepsies are due to disturbances in well-defined areas of the brain which produce a variety of symptons depending on the site of the epileptic focus. Consciousness is by definition retained in simple partial seizures, and impaired or altered in complex partial seizures. Consciousness is usually lost if the seizure becomes secondarily generalized. Partial epilepsies in childhood may be due to a variety of non-progressive brain lesions and may then be termed secondary. Perinatal brain damage, damage due to CNS infections or metabolic disturbances, and the effects of trauma from many causes may be responsible. Partial and generalized seizures are frequent in children with cerebral palsy and may also complicate hydrocephalus treated by shunting procedures [52]. Cerebral tumours are a rare cause of epilepsy in childhood since at this age the majority of neoplasms arise in the cerebellum and brainstem rather than in the cerebral hemispheres. However, any child with a progressive epilepsy and/or evolving neurological signs should be investigated for tumour by CT scan [54].

The role of genetics in most partial epilepsies is an important one. There is evidence that there is an interaction between genetic and environmental factors in their causation [4]. The incidence of seizure disorders among first-degree relatives of patients with partial seizures is higher than average and there is also a higher incidence of EEG abnormalities. Genetic factors are of paramount importance in the aetiology of the primary partial epilepsy which is now considered to be the commonest variety of all the epilepsies occurring in childhood, constituting about 16% of the total [4]. This epileptic syndrome is called by various titles including *benign focal epilepsy of childhood*, benign partial epilepsy, benign centrotemporal epilepsy, benign focal epilepsy with Rolandic spikes (BFERS), Rolandic epilepsy or benign childhood epilepsy with centrotemporal spikes. The characteristic interictal EEG trait is the presence of high-voltage spikes followed by slow waves appearing singly or in groups in one or both Rolandic areas (Fig. 16.1). A history of epilepsy has been found in family studies in 13% of patients with this condition and Rolandic spikes in 34% of siblings [55] (p.141).

The syndrome characteristically affects both sexes with males predominating. The commonest age of onset is between seven and ten years; although it may present earlier it rarely begins after 12 years. The outstanding feature of the attacks is their occurrence during sleep. The EEG discharges (Fig. 16.1) are activated by REM sleep and by deep slow wave sleep. Initially the attack has the characteristics of a partial seizure which may then become secondarily generalized [56, 57]. The first nocturnal attack may be observed by siblings sleeping in the same bedroom, or attacks may be observed by parents while the patient is taking a nap during a car journey. Attacks associated with sleep almost invariably cause great parental alarm and anxiety. Diurnal attacks also occur in some cases and have remarkable and unique features. Clonic jerking of one side of the face (hemifacial seizures), paraesthesiae or jerking in one limb and oropharyngeal signs consisting of salivation, gurgling, contractions of the jaw, numbness of the lips, and tingling or jerking in the tongue may occur. Some children have feelings of suffocation and an inability to swallow or speak, while at the same time retaining normal consciousness and awareness.

The clear definition of this variety of epilepsy has been an important advance. The development of epilepsy in a child at any age leads to considerable family anxiety and parents may react by over protection or rejection of the patient. This epilepsy, due essentially to a self-limiting disturbance of function in the brain, is a benign condition and this is consoling for anxious parents as is also the fact that there are rarely associated cognitive or behavioural problems. Seizures are infrequent in many cases with or without treatment and

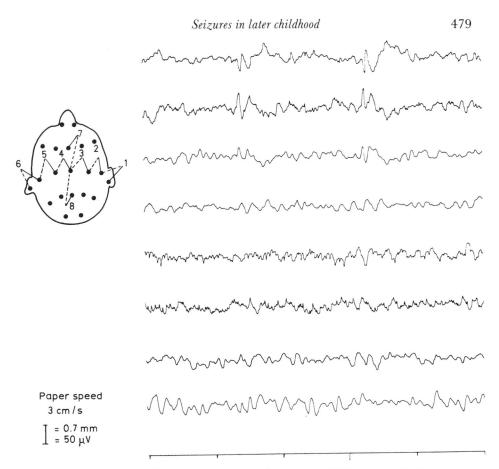

Paper speed
3 cm / s

= 0.7 mm
= 50 μV

Figure 16.1 Boy aged 11½ years and awake with eyes open. EEG shows spike discharges in the right Sylvian area.

remission is invariable, usually by mid-adolescence [58, 59]. The EEG abnormality may persist for a time after the clinical epilepsy has ceased.

In treating partial seizures of simple or elementary symptomatology, carbamazepine is probably the drug of first choice today because of its lack of side-effects and low toxicity. Phenytoin is the other drug which is widely used. Monotherapy with either drug should be the rule. Carbamazepine is particularly valuable in treating benign focal epilepsy of childhood where the drug may be effective in small doses given at bedtime only. Treatment may be withheld altogether if attacks are very infrequent.

Partial seizures of complex symptomatology arising as a result of lesions involving the temporal lobes and limbic system may start at any age in childhood, even before five years. However, they are more frequent after this age and during adolescence. Complex partial seizures are among the most commonly encountered seizure types when all age groups are considered [60] (p. 10).

Among the lesions found in resected material from the temporal lobes have been hamartomas, small angiomas, areas of tuberose sclerosis, and scarring in the hippocampus due to mesial temporal sclerosis (Section 10.2). Mesial temporal sclerosis has been cited as the example *par exellence* of a lesion involving the limbic system. The two most important factors in its causation may be prolonged febrile convulsions in early childhood and a genetic predisposition to epilepsy [61]. However estimates of the role of febrile convulsions in causing mesial temporal sclerosis and temporal lobe epilepsy suggest that this sequence of events is responsible for not more than approximately 10% of cases [62].

Excessive local neuronal discharge in one or other temporal lobe can cause a remarkable variety of minor seizure patterns. Bizarre sensory phenomena, visceral and special sense experiences, auditory and other hallucinations, speech disturbances and strange emotional feelings, including especially those of fear and depersonalization, may occur. 'The epileptic patient may experience his aura as weird, terrifying or ominous in its inexplicable foreignness to his personality' [63] and children may find it very difficult to describe their strange sensations to parents and physicians. Prolonged absences with automatisms occur in this secondary partial epilepsy and these have to be distinguished from absences due to other causes. Secondary generalized tonic-clonic seizures may occur if discharges spread to produce bilateral cortical involvement.

Confirming the diagnosis of temporal lobe epilepsy is difficult at any age and depends on identifying and localizing the EEG abnormalities, if necessary by the use of sleep recordings or other special EEG techniques (pp. 288–91). Characterization of the clinical features of complex partial seizures may be documented by closed circuit television and videotape recording combined with simultaneous EEG recordings [46] (Chapter 2). High resolution CT scanning techniques may be employed to outline the anatomy of the mesial temporal areas preoperatively [64] (p. 218).

The prognosis for children with complex partial seizures is uncertain. In a large group of children followed into adult life, 33% were seizure-free and independent, 32% were socially and economically independent but were still receiving anticonvulsant treatment and were not necessarily seizure-free, 30% were dependent on their parents or on institutional care and 5% had died. The aetiology was more likely to have been undetermined in those who did well than in those who did badly, where a known brain insult was more often identifiable. Adverse factors included lower than average intelligence, early onset of seizures, frequent grand mal seizures, frequent complex partial seizures, a left-sided epileptic focus, severe behavioural disturbance and a need for special schooling [65, 66].

The medical management of temporal lobe epilepsy in childhood presents much the same problems as in adults (Chapter 9). Carbamazepine is the drug of first choice with phenytoin the alternative therapeutic agent [67]. Other drugs such as primidone or sodium valproate may also be used, although the former may produce side-effects and the latter is of limited efficacy in this seizure disorder. In resistant cases, all antiepileptic drugs and combinations of these may have to be tried. Surgical excision of the temporal lobe may be resorted to in intractable cases (Section 10.1). Many believe that this procedure should be done early rather than late, as soon as it becomes clear that the patient's epilepsy is resistant to medication and if the other criteria for surgery are satisfied [68].

16.3.1 Seizures in adolescence

Epilepsy which begins in childhood may improve or deteriorate during adolescence. True petit mal and benign focal epilepsy tend to improve or remit altogether. Complex partial seizures usually continue and may be complicated increasingly by the development of behavioural disorders. Absence-like attacks beginning during adolescence are more likely to be of temporal lobe origin than due to petit mal. Primary brain tumours arising in the cortex are more frequent in this epoch of life and may present with seizures. Photosensitive epilepsy can present for the first time in adolescence; the initial attack may occur in the darkness of a discothèque. Primary generalized epilepsy of the grand mal type may commence during adolescence and attacks can be precipitated by lack of adequate sleep, excessive fatigue, over-indulgence in alcohol and drug abuse or withdrawal. Characteristically, the seizures occur on awakening and may begin with clonic movements followed by a brief tonic-clonic seizure and loss of consciousness. The response to sodium valproate is good as a rule and a permanent remission occurs eventually in the majority of cases [10].

A closely related epileptic syndrome presenting in adolescent patients is that which is variously called *myoclonic epilepsy of adolescence* and not *impulsive* ~~*impulsive*~~ *petit mal of Janz* [69]. Myoclonic jerks occur bilaterally and particularly involve the upper limbs. Repeated jerks may occur shortly after awakening and, in girls, the attacks may coincide with menstruation. The patient may drop what he is holding or objects may be thrown haphazardly ('the flying cornflakes syndrome'). Generalized tonic-clonic seizures may occur but are rare and usually nocturnal. The EEG may be normal or show bilateral irregular spike-waves or polyspike discharges. There may be clinical and EEG evidence of photosensitivity. Typical petit mal absences associated with spike-wave complexes at 3 Hz may occur. Sodium valproate or a benzodiazepine drug are the most effective therapeutic agents, although the condition is often rather resistant to control by drugs [42]. Even when control is achieved, the EEG abnormalities tend to persist and relapse may occur if treatment is withdrawn. During adolescence, the possibility of *subacute sclerosing panencephalitis* should always be remembered as a possible cause of myoclonic seizures. The associated dementia and the classic EEG pattern make the diagnosis clear.

Even today, twenty years after the discovery of a viral aetiology and the association with measles virus, no effective treatment is available for this terrible disease [70].

Behavioural and learning disorders as concomitants of epilepsy in childhood and adolescence are often greater problems than are the seizures themselves. There is no single or characteristic mental state or behaviour pattern consequent on chronic epilepsy. The factors which tend to increase psychiatric morbidity are: early age of onset and chronicity of epilepsy, adverse environmental circumstances e.g. disturbed family background, also certain specific types of epilepsy, especially those which produce complex partial seizures, and the presence of structural or organic brain disease. The majority of children with epilepsy are of average intelligence and behave normally and a proportion, just as in the population at large, are of superior intelligence. Those with primary epilepsies are more likely to be of normal intellect and to behave normally. Parental attitudes to their child's epilepsy may determine whether or not behavioural problems arise. Over protection is common [71]. Public prejudice about epilepsy is still widespread, even among doctors and teachers. Children who develop epilepsy in their early years experience multiple visits to doctors and hospital, years of drug treatment and its possible side-effects, sometimes injuries sustained during seizures, restrictions on normal activities if the epilepsy is severe, and the effects of prejudice about their condition [72]. Hyperactive behaviour may be associated with some of the serious epilepsies of early life as, for example, with the myoclonic epilepsies and with complex partial seizures. The possible role of drugs such as the barbiturates or even occasionally sodium valproate in exacerbating such behaviour should be remembered. Surveys of large groups of children with epilepsy have shown that psychiatric disorders may occur in a third of them, compared with only 6% of their normal peers. The rate of psychiatric disorder is much higher when structural brain disease is present [73].

Learning problems are also common in children with epilepsy and occur in a third or more of those affected [74]. Lethargy, poor concentration, inattentiveness and poor reading skills are frequent complaints [75]. These difficulties and impaired cognitive function may be caused by drug therapy although the newer anticonvulsants (carbamazepine and sodium valproate) are less likely to act in this way, especially when monotherapy is practised and excessive dosage avoided [76]. Boys are more at risk of developing cognitive difficulties than are girls; this difference seems to be independent of drug therapy. Boys are particularly disadvantaged as regards reading and, in this respect, the presence of left hemisphere focal spike discharges in the EEG has been linked with inferior reading skills [77]. The spike-wave paroxysms of petit mal may be associated with inattentiveness and perceptual deficits. The academic achievements of children with epilepsy may also be affected by environmental factors such as over-protection by parents, unsatisfactory attitudes of teachers and by the general prejudice about epilepsy [78] (Chapter 17).

16.4 DIFFERENTIAL DIAGNOSIS OF EPILEPSY IN CHILDREN

A quarter of those referred with a diagnosis of epilepsy do not have the condition. This statistic applies equally to adults and children [79]. Careful history-taking remains the essential cornerstone of accurate diagnosis. A detailed description of the attack should include enquiries about any postictal features such as confusion, headache or sleep. Details about circumstances surrounding the attack should be obtained since single or occasional seizures may be precipitated in susceptible individuals by illness, fever, fatigue, emotional upset, or by reflex factors such as flicker. The single isolated seizure should lead to a careful analysis as in adults (Chapter 6). Clinical examination may reveal clues to the aetiology of epilepsy in the skin, central nervous system, fundi or in other systems. Formal neurological examination should include vital measurements (particularly of the head circumference) and inspection for any asymmetries in skull, face or limbs. Evidence of chronic disorders of movement and posture should be sought since many of the cerebral palsies, even when mild, may be associated with secondary or symptomatic epilepsy.

Breath-holding attacks may be mistaken for epilepsy in the very young. The classic attack in which breath-holding, cyanosis and loss of consciousness follow a short period of crying in expiration, is relatively easy to distinguish from an epileptic seizure [80]. A different form of attack occurs in a minority of children in whom unconsciousness supervenes immediately after a sudden unexpected stimulus such as a blow to the head. Pallor is a striking feature of this latter attack and the pathophysiology is one of vagal-mediated cardiac asystole and respiratory arrest. Either variety may, if the attack is prolonged, be followed by a generalized tonic-clonic seizure due to cerebral anoxia and ischaemia. In the second type of attack, bilateral ocular compression (the oculocardiac or oculovagal reflex) has been used as a diagnostic procedure to induce reflex cardiac asystole in susceptible subjects [81, 82].

Syncopal attacks at any age may be mistaken for epilepsy and occur even in infancy. A typical faint in older children is preceded by feelings of weakness, dizziness, nausea and a sinking sensation in the abdomen. Stiffening and slight jerking may occur in a prolonged attack. Urinary incontinence may also be seen in children. Deathly pallor is the rule and rapid recovery of consciousness is usual. Any episode of loss of consciousness which occurs after exercise should be suspected of having a cardiac cause, and an ECG may reveal an arrhythmia or a congenital conduction defect [83].

There are many other conditions which may be confused with epilepsy in the young child. These include benign paroxysmal vertigo in which sudden brief attacks of unsteadiness occur without loss of consciousness. The prognosis is good with remission occurring by five years of age. Night terrors, in which episodes of screaming are associated with sudden arousal from deep sleep during the early part of the night, may be confused with seizures. Children in the toddler age group may perform ritualistic movements with the hands while also looking vacant and do so especially when tired and bored. Their remote withdrawn behaviour alarms parents and a misdiagnosis of petit mal is often made. The children are immediately distracted from their activities when called and this activity (sometimes associated with masturbation) is completely innocent and disappears with time [33].

Hypoglycaemic attacks occasionally present a problem in differential diagnosis but they usually occur in the morning after a period of fasting. Migraine is common in childhood and sometimes migraine and epilepsy are present in the same patient. However, the clinical phenomena of the two conditions are usually distinct. When the clinical phenomena are closely associated, the migraine attack is either the triggering factor for a seizure or else the severe migraine-type headache follows the seizure as a prominent postictal feature [84]. Non-epileptic seizures or pseudoseizures (p. 539) in which the patient simulates true seizures, are not uncommon in adolescents. The distinction from true epilepsy may be difficult without observation in the hospital and the use of EEG and videotape monitoring techniques [85]. The measurement of prolactin levels after apparent seizures may also be useful [86]. In a condition now usually entitled 'Munchausen syndrome by proxy', mothers give fraudulent histories of seizures and other symptoms in order to gain hospital admission for their children. The psychopathology of the parents is complex and there are associations with non-accidental injury and with other varieties of parental-induced injury [87].

16.4.1 Investigation of epilepsy in childhood

The EEG is the most important investigation in establishing a diagnosis of epilepsy. It is a non-invasive, painless, and relatively inexpensive technique. The EEG can be studied during attention or at rest and also during sleep. The degree of functional abnormality may vary from one state to the other in a child with epilepsy. The EEG has limitations as an investigative tool, however, since it records electrical signals from a limited area of the brain only, namely from the convexity of the hemispheres. Obtaining satisfactory EEG recordings in small children requires special technical skills and the interpretation of the paediatric EEG requires knowledge and experience since there are considerable differences between the EEGs of adults and children [88]. The EEG is sometimes used to decide whether a patient's symptoms are epileptic or psychogenic or due to some other cause such as syncope. However, it must be remembered that the EEG may be normal in epilepsy and epileptic discharges in an EEG do not mean that the patient's symptoms are necessarily due to epilepsy. Improvements in the EEG does not always parallel improvement in the patient's clinical epilepsy. For example, in benign focal epilepsy of childhood, the frequency of epileptic discharges in the centrotemporal areas bears no direct relationship to the severity or otherwise of the clinical epilepsy, and discharges may persist long after the clinical epilepsy has remitted [89]. The approach to a patient's epilepsy should always be primarily clinical and the EEG should not be regarded with greater veneration than any other clinical factor.

Intensive monitoring of children with epilepsy (as described in Chapter 3) provides information on seizure frequency, types of seizures, response to treatment, and also serves as an objective method to distinguish between true and non-epileptic seizures. The three methods currently available are telemetry, videotape recording and ambulatory EEG monitoring. Simultaneous clinical and EEG videotape monitoring provides permanent visual images and simultaneous EEG tracings of the patient and seizures. However, the patient is confined to a chair or bed during the recording whereas ambulatory EEG monitoring examines the patient during normal daily activity [90].

Various other investigations, including CSF examination, biochemical measurements, and radiography, may be required to elucidate the cause of the patient's epilepsy. Imaging of the brain, especially computerized tomographic scanning (CT), is used increasingly in children with epilepsy in a search for structural abnormalities (Chapter 8). It is least likely to show any abnormality in the primary generalized epilepsies and most likely to give positive results in the secondary generalized and partial epilepsies. In one large study of CT findings in children presenting with all varieties of seizures [91], an overall incidence of abnormalities of 33% was found. The presence of an abnormal neurological examination increased the incidence of abnormalities to 64%. In children with complex partial seizures, with partial seizures of simple symptomatology and with generalized seizures of known aetiology, the scans were abnormal in 30%, 52% and 40% respectively. However, in patients with generalized seizures of primary type, CT was abnormal in only 8% of cases. The CT scan is extremely useful in children with chronic epilepsy who develop sudden changes in their seizure pattern, neurological examination or EEG; normal appearances help to exclude treatable conditions or progressive disease such as tumour [92].

16.4.2 Treatment of epilepsy in childhood

The care and management of the patient with epilepsy means more than the prescription of antiepileptic drugs. In addition to their seizures, many patients will have intellectual and cognitive problems, behavioural difficulties and perhaps a neurological deficit. A correct diagnosis of epilepsy and any associated problems is the first essential. A precise seizure diagnosis and, if attainable, an aetiological diagnosis should be made. Any conditioning or precipitating factors for the seizures should be noted as, for example, sleep, fever, illness, emotional upset, acute or chronic fatigue, alcohol or drug abuse.

There are few experiences more frightening for parents than witnessing their child having a convulsion and the basis of management should be sympathetic and knowledgeable advice, bearing in mind that epilepsy is still a word which inspires misunderstanding and fear in many people [33].

Restrictions on children with epilepsy should be limited by the need to allow them to lead as normal a life as possible and by the necessity of avoiding over-protection, especially of the school-going child [93]. Swimming should be prohibited for those with frequent seizures but allowed with supervision if reasonable seizure control has been achieved. Drowning is probably more likely to happen in the bathtub and supervision is essential there for younger children; older children and adolescents should shower. Climbing to dangerous heights should be avoided and body contact sports are not recommended. Sports such as tennis, athletics and golf may be encouraged and should satisfy the child's competitive instincts. Many children with epilepsy have fewer seizures when their attention is engaged than when they are bored or discontented.

The control of seizures is the essential and most important problem for all patients with epilepsy. The use of antiepileptic drugs is the standard form of therapy today although not all children with epilepsy require drug therapy [94]. There are strong arguments for attempting to find out whether a child's epilepsy can be controlled by one drug alone and monotherapy is now the rule in the initial treatment of the patient with seizures. To do this successfully, however, the clinician should preferably have facilities available for accurate estimations of drug levels in the blood. The careful selection of antiepileptic drugs designed to control particular types of epilepsy and the control of therapy by monitoring serum levels have been the really significant advances in management in recent years. It should be remembered, however, that the clinical response of the patient is still of paramount importance in management. The use of the term 'therapeutic blood level' has been unfortunate and 'optimal blood level' would be preferable [95]. It is a common experience for doctors dealing with epilepsy that, in many cases, seizure control is obtained with blood levels that might be termed 'sub-therapeutic' and this is particularly true of many of the primary generalized and primary partial epilepsies of childhood. The child should be regarded as an individual patient and not as a laboratory index.

As with adults, interactions occur between the antiepileptic drugs themselves and with other therapeutic agents and endogenous substances (pp. 231–33). Sodium valproate is an inhibitor of drug metabolism and, if added to the treatment regimen of a child already receiving phenobarbitone or phenytoin, may cause short-lived rises in the concentrations of these drugs into the toxic range. In the case of phenytoin, the situation is further complicated by the fact that both it and sodium valproate are strongly protein-bound. Regular drug monitoring is essential in such situations. Carbamazepine, on the other hand, induces enzyme activity and, if added to phenytoin, may lead to a sharp fall in the level of the latter drug. Enhancement of the metabolism of vitamin D may lead to metabolic bone disease when antiepileptic drug therapy is prolonged [96]. Depletion of the body folate may also be a consequence of enzyme induction by these drugs [97].

Many variables affect how drugs are utilized by infants and children; indeed, the metabolism of antiepileptic drugs during infancy and childhood differs at all stages and at different ages from that in adults [98]. Signs of acute toxicity are difficult to detect in young infants or in mentally handicapped children. The effects of chronic drug toxicity in developing children are largely unknown and possible adverse effects on bone metabolism, endocrine function, cognition and behaviour may have long-lasting effects. Reynolds [99] referred to the large number of patients with epilepsy and to the early age of onset in many and noted that there was no other group of patients who consumed so many drugs for so long. He commented that existing knowledge about these drugs was often not applied to the treatment of patients, resulting in the administration of excessive numbers of drugs in excessive amounts.

The only absolute indication for drug therapy in childhood epilepsy is the repeated occurrence of seizures at frequent or fairly frequent intervals. When antiepileptic medication is prescribed it is only likely to be successful if the patients take their drugs conscientiously, regularly and in adequate doses over prolonged periods of time. Such a degree of patient compliance is essential if a satisfactory response to therapy is to be achieved and careful instructions concerning the importance of regular medication should be given. Changing from one drug to another should be done carefully, gradually withdrawing one drug and simultaneously introducing another in a stepwise fashion.

Reference to the use of individual antiepileptic drugs has already been made in discussing the various epileptic syndromes of infancy, childhood and adolescence. In the last two decades, clinicians have learned to use a smaller range of drugs more precisely and effectively and with less recourse to the type of polypharmacy which was so often deleterious to the patient in the past. Individual drugs are now seen as relatively specific agents for particular epilepsies and used accordingly. The drugs used today include phenobarbitone, primidone, phenytoin, carbamazepine, the benzodiazepines, and sodium valproate for the generalized epilepsies, ethosuximide and sodium valproate for generalized epilepsies characterized by the non-convulsive absence attacks such as occur in petit mal, and carbamazepine, phenytoin, and perhaps phenobarbitone or primidone for the partial epilepsies. The important new drugs of the past 25 years have been carbamazepine, the benzodiazepines and sodium valproate. The benzodiazepine diazepam is the drug of choice for terminating a seizure and for treating status epilepticus in children. Diazepam may be given intravenously or rectally, but is ineffective as an anticonvulsant when given orally and is slowly absorbed after intramuscular injection. Clonazepam and nitrazepam are benzodiazepines given orally as antiepileptic drugs although both may produce undue drowsiness in some patients. Clobazam, a recently introduced benzodiazepine with a molecule similar to diazepam but with altered nitrogen radicals, has anti-convulsant properties but only mild sedative side-effects. It has been used successfully in intractable generalized epilepsies in childhood but tolerance to the drug develops quickly [100].

Carbamazepine is probably the best general antiepileptic drug presently available, especially for partial seizures including those arising from the temporal lobe and limbic system. Approximately two-thirds of children with such seizures will benefit [101] and the drug is particularly effective in benign focal epilepsy of childhood [58]. The drug occasionally causes a rash and temporary leucopenia can occur but serious blood dyscrasias are extremely rare in children [102]. Sodium valproate is another excellent drug, especially for generalized epilepsies including absences. Hair loss, excessive appetite and weight gain occasionally limit its use, especially in adolescence [103]. The development of hepatotoxicity is a serious but rare idiosyncratic reaction which is quite unpredictable. It may happen weeks or months after the start of treatment and is attributed to an aberration in the metabolism of the drug. The accumulation of toxic metabolites may then damage the liver. The influence of concomitant drugs causing enzyme induction, the effect of an associated viral infection, or the presence of some genetically determined enzyme defect in the liver have been proposed to explain the reaction [104]. The onset of anorexia, vomiting, lethargy and loss of seizure control should suggest the possible development of this complication and the drug should be stopped at once.

One of the outstanding advantages of both carbamazepine and sodium valproate is that they are unlikely to impair cognitive function during long term administration [76]. The same cannot be said for many of the older antiepileptic drugs. Although phenobarbitone and primidone are effective drugs in epilepsy and relatively inexpensive, they may cause drowsiness, dulling of attention and perception and impaired vigilance at any age, and therefore they may interfere with learning and school performance. They frequently have a paradoxical stimulatory effect on a proportion of young children causing irritability, aggressiveness, overactivity, and altered sleep patterns [105]. Parents often find such behaviour intolerable.

Among the other long-established drugs, ethosuximide is still widely used for controlling absence attacks, particularly those due to true petit mal, and it is a very safe drug. Phenytoin is highly effective for both generalized and partial epilepsies but is capable of causing both acute and long term adverse effects including ataxia, gum hypertrophy, hirsuties and thickening of sub-cutaneous connective tissue producing coarsening of the facies. This last effect should prohibit its use, unless absolutely necessary, in adolescent girls. Careful monitoring of serum levels will help to prevent serious toxicity, including cerebellar damage and a chronic encephalopathy, but some of the side-effects can occur at so-called 'therapeutic' levels of the drug [106].

Aside from drug therapy, special diets inducing a constant state of ketosis have been used for intractable epilepsy with limited success [44] (p. 337) and surgery for resistant temporal lobe seizures will probably be used increasingly in the paediatric and adolescent age-groups in the future (p. 295).

Many of the ill-effects of antiepileptic drugs derive from protracted therapy and this is a matter of great importance in childhood where developing tissues are exposed to the possible adverse effects of drugs. There are many factors which influence duration of treatment, including the type of epilepsy being treated, the severity and frequency of the seizures, the presence or absence of structural brain abnormality, evidence of a strong family predisposition to epilepsy, and the age of the patient. There are no hard and fast rules for withdrawing drug treatment and each case must be considered on its merits and in the light of EEG and other data [107] (pp. 245–46). In view of the risks of prolonged medication, it is probably better to err on the side of withdrawing treatment sooner rather than later, provided that it is done cautiously and under supervision. It is better to risk an occasional recurrence than to continue treatment unnecessarily [108].

The prognosis for children with epilepsy is difficult to evaluate and is probably best related to individual epileptic syndromes and to different ages (Chapter 11). Epilepsy which begins in the first year of life has an uncertain outcome and onset in the first six months implies a particularly poor prognosis [21]. Status epilepticus in children shows a peak incidence in the first year of life, often with a high risk to life or with serious sequelae [109]. The poor prognosis following infantile spasms and the generalized myoclonic epilepsies has been mentioned although primary or cryptogenic cases may do well if recognized early and treated promptly. Throughout childhood and adolescence, the prognosis tends to be better when the patient's epilepsy is mainly due to constitutional or hereditary factors, i.e. a primary epilepsy, rather than when it is secondary to structural abnormality of the brain or acquired cerebral damage. Patients who are normal in other respects apart from their epilepsy, tend to do better in general [110]. The chances for a child or adolescent to achieve complete freedom from seizures depend particularly on the intensity of the seizure disorder and its duration, and both aspects are usually prominent features when the epilepsy is secondary to or symptomatic of a serious underlying brain disorder. It has been estimated that a child with epilepsy who has been free of seizures for four years while taking antiepileptic drugs has about a 70% chance of remaining in permanent remission when drugs are withdrawn [111]. Early onset, chronicity of epilepsy, associated neurological and/or intellectual deficits, different seizure types occurring in the same individual, are all indicative of a poor prognosis.

The prevention of epilepsy is an important matter for all those concerned with child care. Better understanding of the causes of epilepsy, both genetic and acquired, improved prenatal, perinatal and neonatal care and more effective treatment of potentially brain-damaging illnesses in infancy and childhood, will all contribute to a reduction in the incidence of later epilepsy. Education of the medical profession and of the lay public about this common and world-wide problem is particularly important. The teaching of epileptology should take its proper place in the medical curriculum [112]. Public attitudes and the attitudes of the medical and nursing professions to those with epilepsy are still far from ideal. A change is needed if the consequences of epilepsy, psychological, social and economic, are to be avoided, thereby ensuring better lives for those with the condition.

REFERENCES

1. Porter, R. J. (1984) *Epilepsy: 100 Elementary Principles*, W. B. Saunders Co., London and Philadelphia, p. 6.
2. Ross, E. M. and Peckham, C. S. (1983) Seizure disorder in the National Child Development Study, in *Research Progress in Epilepsy* (ed F. C. Rose), Pitman, London, pp. 46–59.
3. Lennox, W. G. (1960) *Epilepsy and Related Disorders*, Vol. 1, Churchill Livingstone, London.
4. Andermann, E. (1980) Multifactorial inheritance in the epilepsies, in *Advances in Epileptology: The XIth Epilepsy International Symposium* (eds R. Canger, F. Angeleri and J. K. Penry), Raven Press, New York, pp. 297–310.
5. Gloor, P. (1982) Towards a unifying concept of epileptogenesis, in *Advances in Epileptology: The XIIIth Epilepsy International Symposium* (eds H. Akimoto, *et al.*) Raven Press, New York, pp. 425–8.
6. Doose, H. (1980) Genetic factors in childhood epilepsy, in *Advances in Epileptology: The XIth Epilepsy International Symposium* (eds R. Canger, F. Angeleri and J. K. Penry), Raven Press, New York, pp. 289–96).
7. Glaser, G. H. (1983) Kindling. *Devl. Med. Child Neurol.*, **25**, 376–9.
8. Roger, J., Dravet, C., Bureau, M., *et al.* (1985) *Epileptic Syndromes in Infancy, Childhood and Adolescence*, John Libbey Eurotext Ltd, London and Paris.
9. Gastaut, H. (1983) A proposed completion of the current international classification of the epilepsies, in *Research Progress in Epilepsy* (ed. F. C. Rose), Pitman, London, pp. 8–13.
10. Delgado-Escueta, A. V., Treiman, D. M. and Walsh, G. O. (1983) The treatable epilepsies. *N. Eng. J. Med.*, **308**, 1508–14.
11. Goldberg, H. J. (1983) Neonatal convulsions – a 10 year review. *Arch. Dis. Child.*, **58**, 976–8.
12. Levene, M. I. (1985) Aetiology of neonatal seizures, in *Paediatric Perspectives on Epilepsy* (eds E. Ross and E. Reynolds), John Wiley and Sons, Chichester and New York, pp. 11–16.
13. Hill, A. and Volpe, J. J. (1981) Seizures, hypoxic-ischaemic brain injury, and intraventricular haemorrhage in the newborn. *Ann. Neurol.*, **10**, 109–21.
14. Volpe, J. J. (1977) Neonatal seizures. *Clin. Perinatol.*, **4**, 43–63.
15. Rose, A. L. and Lombroso, C. T. (1970) Neonatal seizure states. *Pediatrics*, **45**, 404–25.
16. Perlman, J. M., McMenamin, J. B. and Volpe, J. J. (1983) Fluctuating cerebral blood-flow velocity in respiratory distress syndrome. *N. Eng. J. Med.*, **304**, 204–9.

17. Ouvrier, R. A. and Goldsmith, R. (1982) Phenobarbitone dosage in neonatal convulsions. *Arch. Dis. Child.*, **57**, 653–7.
18. Younkin, D. P., Delivoria-Papadopoulos, M., Maris, J. *et al.* (1986) Cerebral metabolic effects of neonatal seizures measured with in vivo ^{31}P NMR spectroscopy. *Ann. Neurol.*, **20**, 513–19.
19. Carton, D. (1978) Benign familial neonatal convulsions. *Neuropadiatrie*, **9**, 167–71.
20. Pryor, D. S., Don, N. and Macourt, D. C. (1981) Fifth day fits: a syndrome of neonatal convulsions. *Arch. Dis. Child.*, **56**, 753–8.
21. Editorial (1985) First year fits. *Br. Med. J.*, **290**, 1095–6.
22. Cavazzuti, G. B., Ferrari, P. and Lalla, M. (1984) Follow-up study of 482 cases with convulsive disorders in the first year of life. *Devl. Med. Child Neurol.*, **26**, 425–37.
23. Jeavons, P. M. and Bower, B. D. (1964) Infantile Spasms. A review of the literature and a study of 112 cases, in *Clinics in Developmental Medicine*, No. 15, Spastics Society and Heinemann Medical, London. pp. 1–82.
24. West, W. J. (1841) On a peculiar form of infantile convulsions. *Lancet*, **i**, 724–5.
25. Bellman, M. (1983) Infantile spasms, in *Recent Advances in Epilepsy*, No. 1 (eds T. A. Pedley and B. S. Meldrum), Churchill Livingstone, Edinburgh and London, pp. 113–38.
26. Singer, W. D., Haller, J. S. and Sullivan, L. R., *et al.* (1982) The value of neuroradiology in infantile spasms. *J. Pediatr.*, **100**, 47–50.
27. Pampiglione, G. and Moynahan, E. J. (1976) Tuberous sclerosis syndrome: clinical and EEG studies in 100 children. *J. Neurol. Neurosurg. Psychiatr.*, **39**, 666–73.
28. Singer, W. D., Rabe, E. F. and Haller, J. S. (1980) The effect of ACTH therapy upon infantile spasms. *J. Pediatr.*, **96**, 485–9.
29. Deonna, T. and Voumard, C. (1979) Reversible cortical atrophy and corticotrophin (letter). *Lancet*, **ii**, 207.
29a. Holmes, G. L. and Weber, D. A. (1986) Effects of ACTH on seizure susceptibility in the developing brain. *Ann. Neurol.*, **20**, 82–8.
29b. Dreifuss, F., Farwell, J., Holmes, G. *et al.* (1986) Infantile spasms: comparative trial of nitrazepam and corticotrophin. *Arch. Neurol.*, **43**, 1107–10.
30. Matsumoto, A., Watanabe, K. and Negoro, T., *et al.* (1981) Long term prognosis after infantile spasms: a statistical study of prognostic factors in 200 cases. *Devl. Med. Child Neurol.*, **23**, 51–65.
31. Riikonen, R. (1984) Infantile spasms: modern practical aspects. *Acta Paediatr. Scand.*, **73**, 1–12.
32. O'Donohoe, N. V. (1976) A 15-year follow up of 100 children with infantile spasms. *Ir. J. Med. Sci.*, **145**, 138.
33. O'Donohoe, N. V. (1985) *Epilepsies of Childhood*, 2nd ed., Butterworths, London and Boston.
34. Aicardi, J. and Chevrie, J. J. (1971) Myoclonic epilepsies of childhood. *Neuropadiatrie*, **3**, 177–90.
34a. Berkovic, S. F., Andermann, F., Carpenter, S. and Wolfe, L. S. (1986) Progressive myoclonus epilepsies: specific causes and diagnosis. *New Engl. J. Med.*, **315**, 296–305.
35. Brown, J. K. and Livingstone, J. (1985) The malignant epilepsies of childhood: West's syndrome and the Lennox-Gastaut syndrome, in *Paediatric Perspectives on*

Epilepsy (eds E. Ross and E. Reynolds), John Wiley and Sons, Chichester and New York, pp. 29–40.

36. Brett, E. M. (1966) Minor epileptic status. *J. Neurol. Sci.*, **3**, 52–75.

37. Ohtahara, S., Yamatogi, Y. and Ohtsuka, Y. (1977) Prognosis of the Lennox syndrome. A clinical and electroencephalographic study. *Epilepsia*, **18**, 130–1.

38. Doose, H., Gerken, H. and Leonhardt, R., *et al.* (1970) Centrencephalic myoclonic-astatic petit mal. Clinical and genetic considerations. *Neuropadiatrie*, **2**, 59–78.

39. Kinsbourne, M. (1962) Myoclonic encephalopathy of infancy. *J. Neurol. Neurosurg. Psychiatr.*, **25**, 271–6.

40. Brett, E. M. and Lake, B. D. (1983) Progressive neurometabolic brain diseases, in *Paediatric Neurology* (ed. E. M. Brett), Churchill Livingstone, Edinburgh and London, pp. 128–77.

41. Gastaut, H. (1982) The effect of benzodiazepines on chronic epilepsies in man (with particular reference to clobazam), in *Clobazam (Royal Society of Medicine International Congress and Symposium Series*, No. 43), Academic Press and Royal Society of Medicine, London, pp. 141–50.

42. Jeavons, P. M. (1982) Myoclonic epilepsies: therapy and prognosis, in *Advances in Epileptology: The XIIIth Epilepsy International Symposium* (eds H. Akimoto *et al.*), Raven Press, New York, pp. 141–4.

43. Snead, O. C., Benton, J. W. and Myers, G. J. (1983) ACTH and prednisone in childhood seizure disorder. *Neurology*, **33**, 966–70.

44. Bower, B. D. (1980) Epilepsy in childhood and adolescence, in *The Treatment of Epilepsy* (ed. J. H. Tyrer), MTP Press, Lancaster, pp. 251–74.

45. Kurokawa, T., Nagahide, G., Fukuyama, Y., *et al.* (1980) West syndrome and Lennox-Gastaut syndrome: a survey of natural history. *Pediatrics*, **65**, 81–8.

46. Penry, J. K., Porter, R. F. and Dreifuss, F. E. (1975) Simultaneous recordings of absence seizures with videotape and EEG. *Brain*, **98**, 427–40.

47. Metrakos, K. and Metrakos, J. D. (1961) Genetics of convulsive disorders. 11. Genetic and electroencephalographic studies in centrencephalic epilepsy. *Neurology*, **11**, 474–83.

48. Andermann, E. (1982) Multifactorial inheritance of generalized and focal epilepsy, in *Genetic Basis of the Epilepsies* (eds V. E. Anderson *et al.*), Raven Press, New York, pp. 355–74.

49. Sato, S., Dreifuss, F. E. and Penry, J. K. (1976) Prognosis factors in absence seizures. *Neurology*, **26**, 788–96.

50. Roger, J. (1974) Prognostic features of petit mal absence. *Epilepsia*, **15**, 433.

51. Doose, H., Gerken, H., Hein-Volgel, K. J. and Volzke, E. (1969) Genetics of photosensitive epilepsy. *Neuropadiatrie*, **1**, 56–73.

52. Jeavons, P. M. and Harding, G. F. A. (1975) Photosensitive Epilepsy, in *Clinics in Developmental Medicine*, No. 56, Spastics International and Heinemann Medical, London.

53. Graebner, R. W., and Celesia, G. G. (1973) EEG findings in hydrocephalus and their relation to shunting procedures. *Electroenceph. Clin. Neurophysiol.*, **35**, 517–21.

54. Cohen, M. E. and Duffner, P. K. (1984) Brain tumours in children: principles of diagnosis and treatment, in *The International Review of Child Neurology* (eds J. French, I. Rapin and J. S. Pritchard) Raven Press, New York pp. 1–378.

55. Heijbel, J., Blom, S. and Bergfors, P. G. (1975) Benign epilepsy of children with

centrotemporal EEG foci. A study of incidence rate in outpatient care. *Epilepsia*, **16**, 657–64.

56. Beaussart, M. (1972) Benign epilepsy of children with Rolandic (centro-temporal) paroxysmal foci: a clinical entity. Study of 221 cases. *Epilepsia*, **13**, 795–811.

57. Ambrosetto, G. and Gobbi, G. (1975) Benign epilepsy of childhood with Rolandic spikes, or a lesion? EEG during a seizure. *Epilepsia*, **16**, 793–6.

58. O'Donohoe, N. V. (1980) Benign focal epilepsy of childhood. *Ir. Med. J.*, **73** (Suppl.), S62–6.

59. Lerman, P. (1985) Benign partial epilepsy with centro-temporal spikes, in *Epileptic Syndromes in Infancy, Childhood and Adolescence* (eds J. Roger *et al.*), John Libbey Eurotext Ltd, London and Paris, pp. 150–8.

60. Hauser, W. A. and Kurland, L. T. (1975) The epidemiology of epilepsy in Rochester, Minnesota, 1935 through 1967. *Epilepsia*, **16**, 1–66.

61. Falconer, M. A. (1970) Historical review: the pathological substrates of temporal lobe epilepsy. *Guy's Hosp. Rep.*, **119**, 47–60.

62. Leviton, A. and Cowan, L. D. (1981) Do febrile seizures increase the risk of complex partial seizures? An epidemiologic assessment, in *Febrile Seizures* (eds K. B. Nelson and J. H. Ellenberg), Raven Press, New York, pp. 65–74.

63. Flor Henry, P. (1969) Psychosis and temporal lobe epilepsy. *Epilepsia*, **10**, 363–95.

64. Wyler, A. R. and Bolender, N. F. (1983) Preoperative CT diagnosis of mesial temporal sclerosis for surgical treatment of epilepsy. *Ann. Neurol.*, **13**, 59–64.

65. Lindsay, J., Ounsted, C. and Richards, P. (1979) Long term outcome in children with temporal lobe seizures. I. Social outcome and childhood factors. II. Marriage, parenthood, and sexual indifference. III. Psychiatric aspects in childhood and adult life. *Devl. Med. Child Neurol.*, **21**, (1) 285–98; (II) 433–40; (III) 630–6.

66. Lindsay, J., Ounsted, C. and Richards, P. (1980) Long term outcome in children with temporal lobe seizures. IV. Genetic factors, febrile convulsions and remission of seizures. *Devl. Med. Child Neurol.*, **22**, 429–39.

67. Gamstorp, I. (1983) Partial seizures, in *Antiepileptic Drug Therapy in Pediatrics* (eds P. L. Morselli, C. E. Pippenger and J. K. Penry), Raven Press, New York, pp. 163–72.

68. Jensen, I. (1977) Temporal lobe epilepsy: on whom to operate and when, in *Epilepsy: The VIIIth Epilepsy International Symposium* (ed. J. K. Penry), Raven Press, New York, pp. 325–30.

69. Janz, D. and Christian, W. (1957) Impulsiv–petit mal. *Dtsch. Z. Nervenheilk*, **176**, 346–86.

70. Editorial (1985) Subacute sclerosing panencephalitis and lymphocytes. *N. Eng. J. Med.*, **313**, 952–54.

71. Lindsay, J. (1972) The difficult epileptic child. *Br. Med. J.*, **2**, 283–5.

72. Taylor, D. C. (1973) Aspects of seizure disorders. II. On prejudice. *Devl. Med. Child Neurol.*, **15**, 91–4.

73. Rutter, M., Graham, P. and Yule, W. (1970) A neuropsychiatric study in childhood, in *Clinics in Developmental Medicine*, Nos 35/36, Spastics International and Heinemann Medical, London. pp. 1–272.

74. Holdsworth, L. and Whitmore, K. (1974) A study of children with epilepsy

attending normal schools. I. Their seizure patterns, progress and behaviour in school. *Devl. Med. Child Neurol.*, **16**, 746–58.

75. Stores, G. (1973) Studies of attention and seizure disorders. *Devl. Med. Child Neurol.*, **15**, 376–82.

76. Reynolds, E. H. (1983) Mental effects of antiepileptic medication: a review. *Epilepsia*, **24**, (Suppl. 2), S85–95.

77. Stores, G. and Hart, J. (1976) Reading skills of children with generalized or focal epilepsy attending ordinary school. *Devl. Med. Child Neurol.*, **18**, 705–16.

78. Stores, G. (1981) Problems of learning and behaviour in children with epilepsy, in *Epilepsy and Psychiatry* (eds E. H. Reynolds and M. R. Trimble), Churchill Livingstone, Edinburgh and London, pp. 34–8.

79. Jeavons, P. M. (1983) Non-epileptic attacks in childhood, in *Research Progress in Epilepsy* (ed. F. C. Rose), Pitman, London, pp. 224–30.

80. Lombroso, C. T. and Lerman, P. (1967) Breatholding spells (cyanotic and pallid infantile syncope). *Pediatrics*, **39**, 563–81.

81. Gastaut, H. and Gastaut, Y. (1958) Electroencephalographic and clinical study of anoxic convulsions in children: their place in the framework of infantile convulsions. *Rev. Neurol.*, **99**, 100–25.

82. Stephenson, J. B. P. (1978) Reflex anoxic seizures ('white breath-holding): non-epileptic vagal attacks. *Arch. Dis. Child.*, **53**, 193–200.

83. Rennie, J. M. and Arnold, R. (1984) Asystole in the prolonged QT syndrome. *Arch. Dis. Child.*, **59**, 571–3.

84. Deonna, Th. and Ziegler, A. (1984) Paroxysmal visual disturbances of epileptic origin and occipital epilepsy in children. *Neuropediatrics*, **15**, 131–5.

85. Finlayson, R. E. and Lucas, A. R. (1979) Pseudoepileptic seizures in children and adolescents. *Mayo Clin. Proc.*, **54**, 83–7.

86. Trimble, M. R. (1981) Hysteria and other non-epileptic convulsions, in *Epilepsy and Psychiatry* (eds E. H. Reynolds and M. R. Trimble), Churchill Livingstone, Edinburgh and London, pp. 92–112.

87. Meadow, R. (1984) Fictitious epilepsy. *Lancet*, **ii**, 25–8.

88. Peterson, I. and Eeg-Oloffsson (1971) The development of the electro-encephalogram in normal children from the age of 1 through 15 years. Non-paroxysmal activity. *Neuropadiatrie*, **2**, 247–304.

89. Aicardi, J. (1979) Benign epilepsy of childhood with Rolandic spikes. (BECRS). *Brain Dev.*, **1**, 71–3.

90. Stores, G. (1984) Intensive EEG monitoring in paediatrics. *Devl. Med. Child Neurol.*, **26**, 231–4.

91. Yang, P. J., Berger, P. E., Cohen, M. E. and Duffner, P. K. (1979) Computed tomography and childhood seizure disorders. *Neurology*, **29**, 1084–8.

92. Bachman, D. S., Hodges, F. J. and Freeman, J. M. (1976) Computed axial tomography in chronic seizure disorders of childhood. *Pediatrics*, **58**, 828–32.

93. O'Donohoe, N. V. (1983) What should a child with epilepsy be allowed to do? *Arch. Dis. Child.*, **58**, 934–7.

94. Taylor, D. C. and McKinlay, I. (1984) When not to treat epilepsy with drugs. *Devl. Med. Child Neurol.*, **26**, 822–7.

95. Vajda, F. J. E. and Aicardi, J. (1983) Reassessment of the concept of a therapeutic range of anticonvulsant plasma levels. *Devl. Med. Child Neurol.*, **25**, 660–71.

96. Dent, C. E., Richens, A., Rowe, D. J. F. and Stamp, T. (1970) Osteomalacia with long term anticonvulsant therapy in epilepsy. *Br. Med. J.*, **4**, 69–72.

97. Reynolds, E. H. (1975) Chronic antiepileptic toxicity. A review. *Epilepsia*, **16**, 319–52.

98. Morselli, P. L. (1983) Development of physiological variables important for drug kinetics, in *Antiepileptic Drug Therapy in Pediatrics*, (eds P. L. Morselli, C. E. Pippenger and J. K. Penry), Raven Press, New York, pp. 1–12.

99. Reynolds, E. H. (1976) Unsatisfactory aspects of the drug treatment of epilepsy. *Epilepsia*, **17**, 13–15.

100. Shimizu, H., Abe. J., Futagi, Y., *et al.* (1982) Antiepileptic effects of clobazam in children. *Brain Dev.*, **4**, 57–62.

101. Gamstorp, I. (1976) Carbamazepine in the treatment of epileptic disorders in infancy and childhood, in *Epileptic Seizures–Behaviour–Pain* (ed. W. Birkmayer), Hans Huber, Bern, Stuttgart and Vienna, pp. 98–103.

102. Hendriksen, O., Johannessen, S. I. and Munthe-Kaas, A. W. (1983) How to use carbamazepine, in *Antiepileptic Drug Therapy in Pediatrics* (eds P. L. Morselli, C. E. Pippenger and J. K. Penry), Raven Press, New York, pp. 237–40.

103. Egger, J. and Brett, E. M. (1981) Effects of sodium valproate in 100 children with special reference to weight. *Br. Med. J.*, **283**, 577–80.

104. Jeavons, P. M. (1984) Non-dose-related side effects of valproate. *Epilepsia*, **25**, (Suppl. 1), S50–5.

105. Wolf, S. M. and Forsythe, A. (1978) Behaviour disturbance, phenobarbital and febrile seizures. *Pediatrics*, **61**, 728–31.

106. Dam, M. (1983) Phenytoin: an update, in *Recent Advances in Epilepsy*, No. 1 (eds T. A. Pedley and B. S. Meldrum), Churchill Livingstone, Edinburgh and London, pp. 25–34.

107. Gordon, N. S. (1976) The control of anti-epileptic drug treatment. *Devl. Med. Child Neurol.*, **18**, 535–7.

108. Robinson, R. (1984) When to start and stop anticonvulsants, in *Recent Advances in Paediatrics*, No 7 (ed. R. Meadow), Churchill Livingstone, Edinburgh and London, pp. 155–74.

109. Aicardi, J. and Chevrie, J. J. (1970) Convulsive status epilepticus in infants and children. A study of 239 cases. *Epilepsia*, **11**, 187–97.

110. Annegers, J. F., Hauser, W. A., Elveback, L. R. and Kurland, L. T. (1980) Remission and relapses of seizures in epilepsy, in *Advances in Epileptology: The Xth International Epilepsy Symposium.* (eds J. A. Wada and J. K. Penry), Raven Press, New York, pp. 143–7.

111. Emerson, E., D'Sousa, B. J., Vining, E. P., *et al.* (1981) Stopping medication in children with epilepsy: predictors of outcome. *N. Eng. J. Med.*, **304**, 1125–9.

112. Parsonage, M. (1983) Education of medical undergraduates and postgraduates about epilepsy, in *Advances in Epileptology: The XIVth Epilepsy International Symposium*, (eds M. Parsonage, *et al.*), Raven Press, New York, pp. 1–8.

CHAPTER SEVENTEEN

Sociological Aspects of Epilepsy

Graham Scambler

Life with epilepsy generally involves more than adjustment to intermittent loss of control, long term drug therapy and medical surveillance. People with epilepsy also have to learn to cope with a degree of public antipathy towards their condition. Indeed, many of those who have written of the psychosocial problems associated with epilepsy have confidently asserted that these are almost always caused by public discrimination arising out of the perception of epilepsy as stigmatizing. This chapter starts by asking what evidence there is to support this assertion. An account is then given of how people with epilepsy themselves see their condition and of the different ways in which it can affect their lives – during childhood, as spouses and parents, and in employment. Finally, some of the main implications of the growing social scientific literature for the medical 'management' of epilepsy and, more broadly, for the relationship between doctor and patient are discussed.

17.1 EPILEPSY AS STIGMA

17.1.1 Public perceptions

Temkin has shown that the treatment of epilepsy as stigmatizing – often as a form of spirit possession – has been historically pervasive [1]. What remains of this legacy in the final quarter of the twentieth century? It is evident that epileptic phenomena are still interpreted negatively and demonologically in many third world communities. A recent community study in Nigeria, for example, found that, after heredity, 'witchcraft' was the cause most commonly attributed to epilepsy by the lay populace [2]. Danesi has testified that most Nigerians with epilepsy feel heavily stigmatized and regard it as something to be hidden [3]. But what of the modern industrial or postindustrial societies of the West? Is epilepsy still seen and experienced as stigmatizing in the cultures of Europe and the US?

A number of studies have examined lay beliefs and attitudes concerning epilepsy. Perhaps the most influential is the sequence of surveys undertaken at five-yearly intervals since 1949 by the American Institute of Public Opinion [4]. The latest report, of the 1979 survey, indicates that 95% of American adults are familiar with the word epilepsy, and that, of these 63% have known someone with epilepsy and 59% have actually witnessed an epileptic seizure. Taken together, the surveys show a gradual increase in public awareness of what epilepsy is and of how it is caused. For instance, in 1949 only 59% of respondents disputed that epilepsy is a form of 'insanity', compared with 92% in 1979.

These surveys by Caveness and his colleagues also suggest a growing public tolerance of epilepsy. Changing responses to two particular questionnaire items illustrate this trend. Respondents were asked: 'Would you object to having any of your children in school or at play associate with persons who sometimes had seizures (fits)?' Twenty-five per cent replied 'yes' in 1949, 17% in 1954, 18% in 1959, 13% in 1964, 9% in 1969, 5% in 1974, and 6% in 1979. The second question was: 'Do you think epileptics should be employed in jobs like other people?' Thirty-five per cent said 'no' in 1949, 22% in 1954, 11% in 1959, 9% in 1964, 12% in 1969, 8% in 1974, and 9% in 1979. In each of the seven surveys 'liberal' responses were most prevalent in the better educated, professional, younger and urban sectors of the population.

While the balance of the evidence available, in Europe as well as in the US, would seem to support this indication of enhanced lay knowledge and tolerance of epilepsy since the war, there are three qualifications that need to be made. First, many of the relevant studies have relied, like Caveness, on questionnaires, and the questionnaire has several limitations as an instrument of research. For example, not all questions can be reasonably answered within the framework of a finite number of choices. Consider the question: 'Do you think epileptics should be employed in jobs like other people?' Although Caveness has acknowledged a tendency among participants in his studies to want to *qualify* their answers (e.g. 'if treated for the disease', 'if capable', 'if some plan is provided to prevent injury' [5]), his reports allow only for an unqualified 'yes', or 'no' or 'don't know'. It is far from clear how such 'forced' responses are to be interpreted.

Second, a minority of studies have produced findings at variance with those of Caveness. To take a single example, Bagley's British survey, utilizing a social distance scale, suggested there is still considerable public antagonism towards people with epilepsy [6]. One of his findings was that people with epilepsy are more often rejected than those with cerebral palsy or mental illness. Interestingly, an American study carried out a decade later, and also using a social distance scale, reported that people with epilepsy are less often rejected than those with cerebral palsy or mental illness [7]. Axiomatically, caution is required in interpreting apparently inconsistent results like these. Are the opposing findings explicable in terms of the time-gap between the two studies, or in terms of the different cultures in which the studies were conducted, or are they artifactual?

The third qualification is probably the most important. It is well known that the relationship between beliefs and attitudes on the one hand, and behaviour on the other, is a precarious one. Even if it is accepted therefore that the public is generally better informed and less hostile towards epilepsy today than it was a generation ago, it does *not* follow that discrimination based on stigma is necessarily diminished or dying out. There is in fact abundant anecdotal evidence of episodes of stigmatization, but there is no solid European or American evidence concerning either the prevalence of these episodes or of the degree of risk of stigmatization faced by people with epilepsy. There is need for studies of discriminatory practices against people with epilepsy which deploy convincing measures of discrimination that are independent of putative victims' accounts. These would almost certainly incorporate comparison groups of non-epileptics.

17.1.2 Self perceptions

If there are no satisfactory investigations of the extent of public stigmatization, research has been done on the perceptions of stigma of people with epilepsy themselves. Ryan and colleagues have claimed that many people with epilepsy in the United States do not feel stigmatized by their condition [8]. They found, for example, that as many as 81% of those who completed postal questionnaires felt they had been treated fairly by employers. Approximately 70% felt they had been neither unduly restricted nor treated differently because of their seizures. It may be significant, however, that the index of 'perceived stigma' used by Ryan and her colleagues contained several items on whether or not respondents had actually *experienced* discrimination based on stigma. A comment by Blaxter, arising out of her general survey of disability in Britain, is pertinent here: 'Epilepsy came into a special category. In fact, none of the sample's epileptics gave any evidence at all that they had experienced any social stigma, but each one expressed surprise and gratitude at this and told generalized stories about the problems which epileptics "usually" faced' [9]. This suggests that it may be useful to distinguish between actually experiencing stigmatization and expecting or fearing it.

Just such a distinction underlies the work of Scambler and Hopkins [10]. They use the term 'enacted stigma' to refer to actual instances of discrimination against people with epilepsy on the grounds of their perceived unacceptibility or inferiority. This specifically excludes episodes of what might be called 'legitimate' discrimination – for example, banning them from driving. They employ the term 'felt stigma' to refer primarily to the fear of enacted stigma. In their British community study, they found that while only a third of their sample could recall ever having experienced enacted stigma at all, even in the form of casual ridicule, nearly 90% reported suffering intermittently from felt stigma.

Scambler and Hopkins suggest that when the diagnosis of epilepsy is communicated to them, people quickly learn to see their status as 'epileptics' as socially undesirable. Typically, they develop a 'special view of the world' in which felt stigma predominates. When 'activated' by 'situational stimuli' –

witnessed seizures, for example – this 'special view of the world' predisposes them above all else to conceal their condition and its medical label from others, to try to 'pass' as normal [11]. This was the first-choice strategy for the great majority of Scambler and Hopkins' respondents, a finding apparently at odds with Schneider and Conrad's report that in their study in the US concealment was just one of a number of strategies routinely employed by adults with epilepsy [12].

This policy of non-disclosure, Scambler and Hopkins go on to claim, has the effect of reducing the opportunities others have for discriminating against people with epilepsy. To use their own concepts, felt stigma leads to a policy of secrecy and concealment, which in turn leads to a reduced rate of enacted stigma. The authors add that one crucial consequence of this is that felt stigma tends to be more disruptive of the quality of life of people with epilepsy than enacted stigma. The question of the extent to which felt stigma is justified, however, remains for the moment unanswered.

A summary at this juncture might run as follows. Most of the literature supports the view that popular reactions to epilepsy have mellowed in the last generation. People are now better informed and their attitudes to epilepsy less inimical. It would be unwise to assume, however, that discrimination based on the perception of epilepsy as stigma is largely a thing of the past. Stigmatization clearly still occurs, although there are no reliable estimates of its prevalence. There is strong evidence, however, that people with epilepsy themselves regard stigmatization as a very real threat and that this can be a lasting source of anxiety and tension in its own right.

17.2   EPILEPSY IN THE FAMILY CIRCLE

17.2.1   A family secret

Epilepsy often starts in childhood and several authors have intimated that people with epilepsy frequently learn to see their condition as stigmatizing as a result of parental tuition. Schneider and Conrad have labelled many parents of children with epilepsy 'stigma coaches'. They write: 'Our data indicate that the more the parents convey a definition of epilepsy as something "bad", and the less willing they are to talk about it with their children, the more likely the child is to see it as something to be concealed' [13]. In his British study of the families of children with epilepsy, West argues that some parents may actually feel ashamed to have a child with epilepsy, although he acknowledges that this affiliational aspect of felt stigma is difficult to demonstrate since parents' accounts tend to centre on the implications for the child rather than for the family as a whole [14].

Scambler and Hopkins also report stigma coaching among parents [10]. Many parents in their study tried to ensure that the word 'epilepsy' was never used, not only outside the family circle but also within it. Only half of those brothers and sisters who shared the parental home with sufferers knew of the diagnosis. Interestingly even fewer, 21%, of the children of a parent with epilepsy knew of the diagnosis. In fact only half of those children who were aged 16 or more and had actually seen their parent having a seizure had been told of the diagnosis of epilepsy. These figures suggest that parents are even more reluctant to discuss their own epilepsy than they are the epilepsy of a child.

The same study demonstrated an unwillingness on the part of adolescents with epilepsy to disclose to boy or girl friends. They generally faced a choice between what Schneider and Conrad call 'anticipatory preventive telling' [13] – disclosing in the hope of influencing others' reactions should a seizure occur – and a more or less precarious concealment. Of those who had had more than a single boy or girl friend and were themselves aware of the diagnosis of epilepsy, 13% had always disclosed it, 26% had done so at least once, and 61% had never done so. Almost a third of those who had disclosed at least once felt they had endured broken relationships in consequence.

Most of those who adopted a policy of concealment in relation to boy or girl friends stressed that they would disclose, as a matter of principle, if they ever became engaged to be married. However, anticipating behaving appropriately is one thing, doing so quite another. The authors suggest that felt stigma was responsible for the fact that only 33% of the marriages that took place after onset were preceded by a full disclosure incorporating the word 'epilepsy'; and only a further 36% by a partial disclosure involving words like 'attacks' or 'dizzy spells'. There was no disclosure at all in 31% of cases. There was no evidence that such concealment jeopardized marriages at a later date.

17.2.2 The problem of over-protection

Stigma coaching on the part of anxious parents is usually an attempt to protect the child with epilepsy from exposure to stigmatization. This injunction to secrecy, however, is only one aspect of the problem of parental over-protection. The notion that parents tend to be over-protective and that this is potentially harmful is not new. In 1960 Lennox wrote: 'Many parents believe it their duty to keep the child always in sight and forbid all activities which involve any danger' [15]. Writing before Lennox, Ounsted employed the neologism 'hyperpaedophilia' to refer to this same parental attitude [16]. Ounsted found, as have others since, that parental over-protection nourishes behaviour disorders in offspring with epilepsy.

Lerman has similarly argued that over-protection and over-indulgence often lead to behavioural and personality problems which mitigate against normal maturation and, later, successful employment [17]. His account of what 'typically' happens is exaggerated, but it does reflect an established pattern of research findings. Parents generally react to the diagnosis of epilepsy, he claims, with a mixture of apprehension, shame, anxiety, frustration and helplessness. This leads to 'an oppressive atmosphere of secrecy and despair' which has an adverse effect on the child. The child cannot discuss his or her condition openly and soon comes to see it as something bad. Stigmatization may be experienced at the hands of schoolmates, friends and neighbours who are in the know. The child often becomes confined to the home and socially isolated. The intricate skills of social relationships are never learned and he or she remains 'insecure, overdependent, emotionally immature', and is 'inept' when adulthood is reached. Such dire long term consequences are rarer than Lerman implies, although they certainly occur. Nevertheless, Scambler and Hopkins found that family, and especially parental, overprotection was the most common cause of any anger or resentment expressed by those with epilepsy against members of their families [18].

17.2.3 Achieving family equilibrium

A diagnosis of epilepsy frequently throws families into confusion or disequilibrium. Somehow a state of equilibrium has to be restored. The homeostatic mechanisms at work in contexts like this can be extremely complex [19]. If the person with epilepsy is a child, then the parents may well seek to restore family equilibrium through a policy of containment: the world outside of the family is defined as potentially hazardous and the child exhorted neither to trust in others nor to venture too far alone. Parents may feel a need to make some kind of systematic sense of the intrusion of epilepsy into family life. They are particularly likely to construct their own lay theories about the cause of their child's epilepsy. Tavriger writes: 'It would appear that the anxiety engendered by epilepsy demands from some parents alleviation in the form of a theory as to its cause, no matter how illogical' [20].

Adults with epilepsy are equally motivated to theorize about the causes of their conditions. Indeed this seems to be a common response amongst adults to the onset of most chronic illnesses: Blaxter refers to it as the 'strain towards rationality' [9]. When Scambler and Hopkins asked their respondents if they had any questions they would like to put to a physician, 56% of the resultant queries concerned aetiology [18]. It is revealing that in only 27% of the total sample were physicians able to proffer satisfactory scientific theories about causation [21]. Interestingly the distribution of lay theories of causes of epilepsy among Scambler and Hopkins' adults with epilepsy and Tavriger's parents of children with epilepsy were remarkably similar. By far the largest sub-group in each study, 39% in the former and 47% in the latter, identified 'prolonged stress' as the primary cause [18]. This may have been because people could not tolerate the idea of a 'physical' cause; or because they felt that if the seizures were a product of stress there must be hope of a cure; or perhaps because they did not distinguish clearly between factors implicated in the aetiology of the conditions and factors precipitating individual seizures.

Family studies have indicated that parents, wittingly or otherwise, can exercise a considerable long term influence on how well children with epilepsy adjust to their condition and its psychosocial correlates. The damage that overly zealous stigma coaching and protectiveness can do is being documented. Ziegler has argued that epilepsy can severely disrupt a family's sense of autonomy and competence and that physicians must consider how they can best incorporate counselling and support for families into overall treatment plans [22]. If a state of family equilibrium is to be restored, it is important that family members reach a working consensus on what epilepsy is and how it should be accommodated. Such a consensus may or may not be compatible with the scientific perspective of the physicians consulted. It may, for example, involve the construction of what Ferreira terms a 'family myth' – a consensus which unites the family but is quite unrelated or even contrary to scientific rationality [23]. Without a consensus, family disequilibrium and a measure of conflict between members seems assured.

17.3 EPILEPSY AND DISADVANTAGE AT WORK

17.3.1 Disclosing to employers

An individual with epilepsy looking for a job is often advised to disclose his or her condition to potential employers [24]. Those diagnosed whilst in employment are similarly counselled to put their employers in the picture. The chief motivations for defying such advice are, first, a fear of encountering stigmatization, and second, a fear of meeting with 'legitimate' discrimination (e.g. if the job involves driving). A number of studies have shown that non-disclosure is common. It has been estimated that in the US, one-third of all people with epilepsy lie about their conditions on job applications [25]. In Britain, Jones found that only 26% of prospective employees with epilepsy at a steel works admitted their condition at the pre-employment 'medical' [26]. Aston found that only 7% of the men at a motor works who were suffering from epilepsy prior to employment admitted as much before starting work [27].

Scambler and Hopkins found that 53% of those in their community sample who had had two or more full-time jobs after the onset of seizures had never disclosed to an employer [28]. Of those in employment when interviewed, 28% had informed their employers they had epilepsy, 17% had mentioned their attacks but not the diagnosis, and 55% had made no disclosure of any kind. Those who had opted to disclose tended to be having more frequent seizures than those who had not. Presumably they judged that they would almost certainly have a seizure at work sooner or later and that an anticipatory disclosure was the lesser of two evils. Significantly, only 5% actually volunteered a disclosure before starting work and each of these was experiencing daily seizures at the time.

The same authors found that although people who decided not to disclose the diagnosis of epilepsy were not directly vulnerable to stigmatization or 'legitimate' discrimination, they often experienced living with the daily possibility of 'exposure' as highly stressful [10]. Exposure might occur through either 'stigmata' or 'stigma cues'. Stigmata refer to clinical manifestations of people's conditions, usually seizures, which are noticed and lead to exposure; and stigma cues refer to events or happenings like slips of the tongue, witnessed drug-taking or absences from work, any of which might function as cues to others, leading them to suspect the presence of epilepsy.

Scambler and Hopkins found that most of their respondents who *had* disclosed to their employers, and who had no reason therefore to fear exposure through stigmata or stigma cues, remained committed to a policy of 'covering'. Goffman writes: 'It is a fact that persons who are ready to admit possession of a stigma (in many cases because it is known about or immediately apparent) may nonetheless make a great effort to keep the stigma from looming large' [11]. Consider, for example, absences from work. Pasternack has suggested that, given the competitive ethos of economic life in Europe and the US, employers may be reluctant to hire or persevere with employees with epilepsy because they see them as 'less efficient' than others, and therefore as 'poor investments'; and he mentions anticipated high absenteeism as an important factor here [29]. Scambler and Hopkins report that most respondents who had disclosed to their employers felt 'at risk' on occasions, or even 'on trial', and were fully aware that any absence from work could be interpreted as evidence of inefficiency and mistaken investment. As a result they went to great lengths to avoid losing time from work. When an absence was necessary, either because of seizures or their sequelae or because of hospital appointments, they frequently attempted to cover, even if this meant lying outright to their employers. A study of epilepsy in the British Steel Corporation found no difference between employees with epilepsy and other employees for rates of absenteeism for less than twenty days, although longer absences were more common amongst those with epilepsy [30].

17.3.2   Disadvantage in work

Unemployment rates for people with epilepsy are higher than for others both in Europe and in the US. In Britain the unemployment rate has been shown to be particularly high for married women with epilepsy and to be associated with low social class and a high frequency of seizures [28]. Various studies have claimed that between one-quarter and three-quarters of those in the labour market experience employment problems [31]. The authors of most of the relevant studies, however, have used their own distinctive, and sometimes idiosyncratic, definitions of 'employment problems'. Consider, for example, the two studies which generated the highest and the lowest estimates of the prevalence of such problems.

The lowest figure of one-quarter derives from a community survey conducted by the College of General Practitioners [32]. Their figure included the unemployed and all those who fell into a rather vague and heterogeneous category of 'partially employed': 'these were patients whose work had to be modified considerably because of their fits. At home the housewife could only do restricted work; and, outside, sheltered employment was necessary'. The highest figure of three-quarters comes from Jones' study of people with epilepsy who applied for jobs at a steel works [26]. Out of 39 applicants 33 were appointed. However, over half of those who were appointed had subsequently to change their jobs within the steel works in the face of stigmatization or 'legitimate' discrimination: these, together with the six rejected applicants, were defined as having 'employment problems'. It must of course be remembered, on the one hand, that Jones' study omitted those with epilepsy who did not apply for jobs at all; but, on the other hand, that it also omitted those who did not disclose their epilepsy to their employer. Clearly these two studies were conducted with very different populations and utilized very different definitions of employment problems.

Ryan and her colleagues report that 46% of their sample of people with epilepsy suggested they had encountered employment discrimination due to their epilepsy [8]. Twenty-two per cent felt they had been fired from one or more of their last four jobs 'for an epilepsy-related reason'. Scambler and Hopkins found that 42% of those in their sample who had had at least one full-time job since onset thought their careers had been inhibited by either stigmatization or 'legitimate' discrimination [28]. Fourteen per cent complained of a rejected job application, 12% of a loss of responsibility or income, 12% of a reduced chance of promotion, 11% of dismissal, 8% of having to leave a job because of pressure exerted by employers, 3% of being suspended, and 1% of having to settle for sheltered employment. Of the sub-group who had experienced full-time employment after onset 14% felt their careers had been affected by stigmatization.

Consistent with their general analysis of stigma summarized earlier, Scambler and Hopkins maintain that felt stigma (i.e. the fear of stigmatization) causes more anxiety and disquiet in the employment arena than either enacted stigma (i.e. actual stigmatization) or 'legitimate' discrimination. They add that felt stigma can lead to career inhibition in its own right. A number of married women chose not to enter the job market at all because of felt stigma: at the time of interview only 32% of them had full-time jobs, compared with 48% of the married women in the British population as a whole. Furthermore, some of the men and women in employment who had not disclosed their epilepsy had clearly denied themselves opportunities for advancement because they thought promotion would increase the potential personal cost of exposure and hence the stresses associated with future information management.

The work capacity of those who have epilepsy uncomplicated by other problems has been shown to be good [24]. It is evident, however, that many people with epilepsy perceive themselves to be at a disadvantage in relation to employment opportunity. Fearing stigmatization, a policy of concealment is often adopted. This in itself can be extremely stressful. Unemployment rates among those with epilepsy are higher than for the population as a whole; but it must be remembered that epilepsy is sometimes merely one symptom of a condition much more disabling in other ways. Estimates of the prevalence of employment problems vary, and there remains a need for studies of employer discrimination which are independent of the judgments of putative victims. It may also be the case that some individuals with epilepsy consciously decide either not to apply for jobs or to limit their work ambitions because they fear meeting with discriminatory practices.

17.4 DOCTOR AND PATIENT AND THE MANAGEMENT OF EPILEPSY

17.4.1 Patients' perspectives

Early models of the doctor–patient relationship tended to portray the doctor's role as 'active' and the patient's as 'passive'. Haug puts it lucidly: 'The relationship with the physician is asymmetrical; the patient is in a dependent and the physician a superordinate status. It is the "competence gap" between doctor and patient which justifies both the professional's authority and the client's trust, confidence and norm of obedience. Although the objective of care is to return the patient to an active, independent status, he is obligated in the model to become temporarily submissive and to accept the doctor's right to tell him what to do' [33]. Freidson was perhaps the first to challenge this 'bias', insisting that while physicians may expect patients to accept their judgements and recommendations unquestioningly, patients generally 'seek services on their own terms' [34]. He argues that there may well be a 'clash of perspectives', and therefore a potential for conflict. Patients may appear submissive during medical consultations but it does not follow that they are truly acquiescent or 'passive'. Behaviour which seems deferential is not necessarily indicative of agreement or satisfaction or even of a readiness to take medical advice [35].

Scambler and Hopkins argue that, when they are told they have epilepsy, people develop a characteristic 'special view of the world' which turns on the perception of epilepsy as stigmatizing [10]. And they go on to show how this 'special view of the world' can bring people into overt and, more often, covert conflict with their doctors. It was the at times over-riding perception of epilepsy as stigma, for example, which variously prompted patients to reject the diagnosis of epilepsy, or at least to 'negotiate' for a less threatening alternative; to misinterpret normal EEGs as evidence of premature or mistaken diagnosis; and to defy medical advice about the regular taking of anti-convulsants in order to hasten the transition from 'epileptic' to 'normal' status.

The importance of patients' perspectives are clearly demonstrated in relation to the 'problem of non-compliance'. It is known that compliance is poor amongst both adults and children with epilepsy, although it tends to be higher when fewer anticonvulsant drugs are used. Moreover there is some evidence that compliance is *not* improved by special interventions to inform patients of the value of medication [36]. There have been surprisingly few attempts to explore patients' own views on anticonvulsant medication. Stimson had made the point that patients rarely take medication in 'a thoughtless vacuum' [37]. Schneider and Conrad's study in the US has shown that people with epilepsy frequently formulate their own strategies for drug-taking [25]. They found that 'self-regulators' variously altered their prescribed dosages to test their lay theories of seizure control; to avoid becoming dependent; to minimize the risk of drug-taking as a stigma cue or as stigmatizing in its own right; to ensure that seizures did not occur on special occasions; or to enhance their sense of control over their conditions.

Scambler and Hopkins found that patients' sense of stigma also led them to take umbrage at doctors' preoccupation with the diagnosis and treatment of disease. The charge that doctors lacked the inclination or time to show empathy – and hence volunteered little or no information or counsel on coping with the psychosocial correlates of epilepsy – was most often directed at hospital doctors [18]. Most patients preferred treatment by their general practitioners. West has suggested that what doctors lack is a coherent 'stigma ideology' relating to epilepsy: in particular, they have no clear 'set of prescriptions, or "practice theories", to enable the stigmatized themselves to manage their situation as effectively as possible' [14]. One result of this, he believes, is that 'the physician is in danger of legitimating the stigma of epilepsy, not by talking about it, but by *not* talking about it'.

17.4.2 Improving patient care

It needs to be borne in mind that a minority of people with epilepsy are unidentified and have no medical contact: a recent estimate in the US puts the figure at 20–25% [38]. One reason for not seeking medical help, of course, could be the perception of the medical label 'epileptic' as a social liability. Schneider and Conrad write: 'When "blackouts", "headaches" and "spaciness" become "seizures", and when the cause is something called "epilepsy" or a "seizure disorder" certified by a medical expert, one moves to a set of meanings, prescribed courses of conduct, and interaction that alters experience, past, present, and future' [25]. Put bluntly, a doctor's diagnostic utterance 'makes a person into an epileptic' [10].

Some commentators have argued that the diagnosis of epilepsy should be used more sparingly. West has countered that this would almost certainly mean that only the 'worst' seizures would be labelled epileptic; and that this would merely serve to reinforce the negative image of epilepsy held by sections of the public [14]. West himself suggests that more, rather than less, use should be made of the word epilepsy. His argument is that extending the use of the term, by including febrile convulsions for example, should help diminish its associated stigma: the range of people with a history of epilepsy would be increased, and this might lead to a 'broadening of experience and commensurate modification of "negative" stereotypes'. Scambler and Hopkins reject both these contradictory pieces of advice as unrealistic and defeatist [18]. The advice is unrealistic in the assumption that both those who experience seizures and members of the public can be duped by an essentially artificial redefinition of epileptic phenomena. The advice is defeatist in its seeming acceptance of stigmatization against people with epilepsy as a *given* factor in the equations.

Whatever doubts there may be about the optimum criteria for diagnosing epilepsy, it remains the case that physicians need to address the likely effects of labelling on their patients. A precondition of doing so is taking patients' perspectives seriously, even, or especially, when they 'clash' with their own. It has already been implied that patients' perspectives are wide-ranging and touch upon all aspects of health care: the sense of epilepsy as stigma may be central but it does not monopolize patients' thoughts about their illness or its implications. Schneider and Conrad insist that doctors and patients need to be 'coparticipants in treatment' [25]. For doctors, they contend, 'this entails listening carefully to their patients' concerns about seizures, self, the future, the meanings of medications, stigma, relationships of dependence and, perhaps most difficult, about relationships with the doctors themselves'.

Physicians' capacity to help effect a destigmatization of epilepsy is obviously limited, although their collective contribution over the last 100 years has been significant. But they can work to ensure that medical perspectives are purged of myths from the past. Bagley is particularly damning, for example, of post-war medical papers attributing negative and antisocial traits to people with epilepsy; of the then current 'vogue' among some physicians to describe disturbed behaviours as so-called 'epileptic equivalents'; and of the common tendency to postulate causal connections between epilepsy and all kinds of psychiatric disorders [39].

Finally, as many chapters in this volume illustrate in detail, there is room for improvement in the routine management of epilepsy. Hopkins and Scambler have described the current management of epilepsy in Britain as largely ritualistic [21]. In their community study they report unnecessary referral to hospital, unnecessary electroencephalography, inadequate medication and follow-up supervision not related to patient need. Opinion on the potential of the kind of special centres and hospital-based epilepsy units advocated in a number of government sponsored reports to improve routine management is divided. Some commentators believe that epilepsy can generally be managed perfectly adequately in general practice [21]. Others have lamented the fact that specialized epilepsy services have not been made available and maintain that this has put people with epilepsy in Britain at a disadvantage compared with patients in some other countries [40].

Physicians tend not to take time to explore how their patients interpret their epilepsy and its impact on their lives. Evidence is plentiful across a whole range of illnesses that understanding patients' perspectives is an important ingredient of effective medical practice. Arguably, people with epilepsy have as much difficulty adjusting to the diagnostic label 'epilepsy' as they do to the recurring seizures. Both the parents of children with epilepsy and adults with epilepsy need empathy, counsel and support in this process of adjustment. Responsibility for treatment and rehabilitation needs to be shared by doctor and patient. Clinical aspects of the management of epilepsy could clearly be improved, although debates continue about the best ways of organizing care.

REFERENCES

1. Temkin, O. (1945) *The Falling Sickness*, Johns Hopkins Press, Baltimore.
2. Awaritefe, A., Longe, A. and Awaritefe, M. (1985) Epilepsy and psychosis: a comparison of social attitudes. *Epilepsia*, **26**, 1–9.
3. Danesi, M. (1984) Patient perspectives on epilepsy in a developing country. *Epilepsia*, **25**, 184–90.
4. Caveness, W. and Gallup, G. (1980) A survey of public attitudes towards epilepsy in 1979 with an indication of trends over the past thirty years. *Epilepsia*, **21**, 509–18.
5. Caveness, W., Merritt, H. and Gallup, G. (1969) Trends in public attitudes towards epilepsy over the past twenty years in the United States, in *Exploring World Attitudes Towards Epilepsy*, International Bureau for Epilepsy, London. pp. 5–11.
6. Bagley, C. (1972) Social prejudice and the adjustment of people with epilepsy. *Epilepsia*, **13**, 33–45.
7. Albrecht, G., Walker, V. and Levy, J. (1982) Social distance from the stigmatized: a test of two theories. *Soc. Sci. Med.*, **16**, 1319–27.
8. Ryan, R., Kempner, K. and Emlen, A. (1980) The stigma of epilepsy as a self-concept. *Epilepsia*, **21**, 433–44.
9. Blaxter, M. (1976) *The Meaning of Disability: A Sociological Study of Impairment*, Heinemann, London.
10. Scambler, G. and Hopkins, A. (1986) Being epileptic: coming to terms with stigma. *Soc. Health Illness*, **8**, 26–43.
11. Goffman, E. (1968) *Stigma: Notes on the Management of Spoiled Indentity*, Penguin, Harmondsworth.
12. Schneider, J. and Conrad, P. (1981) Medical and sociological typologies: the case of epilepsy. *Soc. Sci. Med.*, **15A**, 211–19.
13. Schneider, J. and Conrad, P. (1980) In the closet with illness: epilepsy, stigma potential and information control. *Soc. Prob.*, **28**, 32–44.
14. West, P. (1979) *An Investigation into the Social Construction and Consequences of the Label 'Epilepsy'*, PhD Thesis, University of Bristol.
15. Lennox, W. (1960) *Epilepsy and Related Disorders*, Vols 1 and 2, Churchill Livingstone, London.
16. Ounsted, C. (1955) The hyperkinetic syndrome in epileptic children. *Lancet*, **2**, 303–11.
17. Lerman, P. (1977) The concept of preventive rehabilitation in childhood epilepsy:

a plea against overprotection and overindulgence, in *Epilepsy: The Eighth International Symposium* (ed. K. Penry), Raven Press, New York, pp. 265–8.

18. Scambler, G. (1983) *'Being Epileptic': Sociology of a Stigmatizing Condition.* PhD Thesis, University of London.
19. Voysey, M. (1975) *A Constant Burden: The Reconstitution of Family Life*, Routledge & Kegan Paul, London.
20. Tavriger, R. (1966) Some parental theories about the causes of epilepsy. *Epilepsia*, **7**, 339–43.
21. Hopkins, A. and Scambler, G. (1977) How doctors deal with epilepsy. *Lancet*, **i**, 183–7
22. Ziegler, R. (1981) Impairments of control and competence in epileptic children and their families. *Epilepsia*, **22**, 339–46.
23. Ferreira, A. (1963) Family myth and homoestasis. *Arch. Gen. Psychiatr.*, **9**, 457–63.
24. Gloag, D. (1985) Epilepsy and employment. *Br. Med. J.*, **291**, 2–3.
25. Schneider, J. and Conrad, P. (1983) *Having Epilepsy: The Experience and Control of Illness*, Temple University Press, Philadelphia.
26. Jones, J. (1965) Employment of epileptics. *Lancet*, **ii**, 486–9.
27. MacIntyre, I. (1976) Epilepsy and employment. *Comm. Health*, **7**, 195–204.
28. Scambler, G. and Hopkins, A. (1980) Social class, epileptic activity and disadvantage at work. *J. Epidemiol. Comm. Health*, **34**, 129–33.
29. Pasternack, J. (1981) An analysis of social perceptions of epilepsy: increasing rationalization as seen through the theses of Comte and Weber. *Soc. Sci. Med.*, **15E**, 223–9.
30. Dasgupta, A., Saunders, M. and Dick, D. (1982) Epilepsy in the British Steel Corporation: an evaluation of sickness, accident and work records. *Br. J. Industr. Med.*, **39**, 145–8.
31. Office of Health Economics (1971) *Epilepsy in Society*, Office of Health Economics, London.
32. College of General Practitioners (1960) A survey of the epilepsies in general practice. *Br. Med. J.*, **2**, 416–22.
33. Haug, M. (1976) Issues in general practitioner authority in the National Health Service, in *The Sociology of the NHS*, (*Sociological Review Monograph 22*) (ed. M. Stacey). University of Keele, Keele. pp. 23–42.
34. Freidson, E. (1961) *Patient Views of Medical Practice*, Russell Sage Foundation, New York.
35. Stimson, G. and Webb, B. (1975) *Going to See the Doctor: The Consultation Process in General Practice*, Routledge & Kegan Paul, London.
36. Pryse-Phillips, W., Jardine, F. and Bursey, F. (1982) Compliance with drug therapy by epileptic patients. *Epilepsia*, **23**, 269–74.
37. Stimson, G. (1974) Obeying doctor's orders: a review from the other side. *Soc. Sci. Med.*, **8**, 97–104.
38. Commissions for the Control of Epilepsy and Its Consequences (1978), in *Plan for Nationwide Action on Epilepsy*, Vols I–IV, US Dept of Health, Education and Welfare, Pub. No. (NIH) 78–276.
39. Bagley, C. (1971) *The Social Psychology of the Child with Epilepsy*, Routledge & Kegan Paul, London.
40. Shorvon, S. (1983) Specialized services for the non-institutionalized patient with epilepsy: developments in the US and the UK. *Health Trends*, **15**, 40–5.

CHAPTER EIGHTEEN

Epilepsy and Psychiatric Disorders

Peter Fenwick

18.1 INTRODUCTION

People with epilepsy have always suffered more from other people's view of them, and of the 'epileptic personality', than from the illness itself. Until the time of Hippocrates, epilepsy was known as the sacred disease. One can understand the fear engendered by seeing a healthy human being suddenly struck down, lying foaming and jerking, and then miraculously restored to life. Aretaeus, in the 2nd Century AD, saw epileptics as 'languid, spiritless, stupid, unsociable . . . slow to learn from torpidity of the understanding and the senses . . .' [1]. The notion of a link between epilepsy and mental illness is longstanding. Galen thought that the lunar cycle was involved, that fits occurred at the full moon, and that epileptics were lunatics. By the mid 19th century, epilepsy and mental illness were included in a unitary view of psychological disturbance. Morel, in 1857, suggested that both were the result of a progressive degenerative strain running from generation to generation, showing itself as moral defects, weakness of character, mental deficiency and epilepsy [2]. The degenerative theory was subscribed to by most of the famous 18th century physicians, including Bleuler, Kraeplin and even Henry Maudsley. Lombroso applied it to the 'born criminal', who was also an epileptic, distinguished by physical degeneration and specific facial features [3]. By the end of the 19th century, bromide had begun to be used in residential epileptic colonies. Epileptics were severely institutionalized and isolated, and bromide toxicity was common. So it was not surprising that support for the idea of an epileptic personality, including violence and aggressive outbursts, slowness, stupidity and inevitable degeneration, grew even stronger.

By the 1930s, with the introduction of phenobarbitone and, more importantly, confirmation by Adrian and Mathews [4] of the discovery of the EEG, a fuller understanding of epilepsy came to be possible. It was realized that seizures arose from epileptic foci within the brain, and that the site of the lesions was as important as the seizure. Lennox and Gibbs in Harvard, Pond, Hill and Murray Falconer at the Maudsley and Penfield and Jasper in Montreal, all contributed to the present understanding of epilepsy and psychiatric illness. The discovery of the temporal lobe focus and thus temporal lobe epilepsy in 1949, with the then current evolving ideas of the limbic system and the Papez circuit, led to the idea of mental illness being linked to epileptic disturbance in specific brain areas, particularly the temporal lobe. And so the modern view of epilepsy and mental illness arose, that people with epilepsy are normal mentally, but it is brain damage and the site of the lesion which leads to an association between epilepsy and mental illness. Dennis Hill [5] provides an excellent review of these concepts.

18.2   PREVALENCE OF PSYCHIATRIC MORBIDITY

Accurate estimates of psychiatric morbidity in epilepsy are hard to find. What estimates there are tend to be biased because of the selection of the populations studied.

   Firstly, there is no one universally used definition of epilepsy. Some studies include only those who have seizures, or who have had seizures, some exclude febrile convulsions and some define their population as including only those on anticonvulsants. Secondly, most studies have relied on self-administered questionnaires rather than more accurate formal interview methods of assessment. Thirdly, the wide use of hospital clinic studies to define prevalence rates will give a falsely high prevalence of psychiatric morbidity. Pond and Bidwell [6], in their study of 14 general practices, showed that twice as many patients with psychological difficulties were referred to hospital compared to those who were not referred. Surveys show that between 4% and 5% of patients living in mental hospitals have epilepsy, 7–8 times the expected rate [7, 8].

   Several helpful community studies include the Icelandic study of Gudmundsson [9], who found that only half the epileptic sample were psychologically normal. Part of this was accounted for by personality disorders (ixoid and ixothyme – terms seldom now used), which makes the true rate of psychiatric illness difficult to disentangle. Comparing his findings to that of Helgason [10] who had studied a general psychiatric survey of the Icelandic population, Gudmundsson found the same rate of neuroticism (10%) for men as Helgason, but a significantly higher rate of 25% for women with epilepsy. Pond and Bidwell give an overall figure of 29% of people with epilepsy with psychological difficulties, which they say may well have been an underestimate. In a survey of all children from the Isle of Wight, the overall rate of psychiatric disorder in children with uncomplicated epilepsy was 28.6%, four times the control rate, rising to 58.3% in those with brain damage [11]. A follow-up study of a sample of children with epilepsy 25 years after they had entered a population survey found that two-thirds of the population 'suffered minimal or no ill-effect' [12, 13]. Morgan *et al.* [14] studying the MRC National Longitudinal Survey of Health and Development of Children born in 1946 in Great Britain, found that by the age of 26 about 35% of the 46 epileptics (mainly those with definite brain damage) in the study were graded as 'complicated', and, both socially and in employment, did not perform as well as the controls, taken from the same street and social class. Those with uncomplicated epilepsy showed no difference in jobs, social class, educational achievement or marriage when compared with controls. Although most of these 'uncomplicated' children had been rated as different by teachers in childhood, no differences could be seen later. Thus, a figure for the prevalence of psychiatric morbidity in people with epilepsy of about one third would seem reasonable. However, it is significant that several studies indicate that childhood psychiatric morbidity does not necessarily lead to psychiatric disturbance in adulthood.

18.3 FACTORS LEADING TO PSYCHIATRIC MORBIDITY

It might be expected that frequently occurring, recurrent bursts of abnormal brain activity resulting in a loss of or altered state of consciousness might lead to a change in brain function and so to the manifestation of psychiatric disorder. Epileptic fits may occur in association with any mental illness, either because the illness itself may give rise to occasional fits, for example the single grand mal fit which sometimes occurs in catatonic schizophrenia, or because drug treatment lowers the seizure threshold, increasing the likelihood of seizure in susceptible individuals. Phenothiazines and tricyclic antidepressants are examples of medications that may precipitate seizures [15–17] (see Chapter 4). Drug withdrawal seizures, especially during withdrawal of barbiturates and alcohol, are common. However, these single fits are not usually considered as epileptic, though they may confound epidemiological studies (Chapter 1).

The patient with epilepsy has recurrent, often widespread, transient disturbances of brain function. Yet despite these, and the accompanying social stigmata caused by the resulting changes in behaviour (see Chapter 17), non-brain damaged patients with epilepsy as a group are relatively normal. A high prevalence of psychiatric morbidity is associated with several different factors, each of which is important, and some of which are cumulative.

18.3.1 Brain damage

An association between brain damage and psychiatric morbidity has been described in many studies. The relationship between epilepsy, brain damage and chronic illness has been shown by Rutter *et al.* [11] in the results of a total survey of the school children on the Isle of Wight. They found an overall rate of psychiatric morbidity of 6.8% for the control sample, and a rate of 11.5% for children with physical handicap not involving the brain. Psychiatric morbidity for uncomplicated epilepsy without brain damage was 28.6% – about four times that of the controls. For those with brain damage only, the rate was higher still at 37.5%. The highest prevalence was found for those with brain damage *and* epilepsy – 58.3%. The association of brain damage with epilepsy is thus an important factor. This study also found that the presence of temporal lobe seizures, emotional instability in the mother and low social class significantly influenced the occurrence of psychiatric morbidity.

Is there, therefore, any evidence that brain damage is widespread in patients with epilepsy, or leads to an intellectual disadvantage? Gastaut [18] has stated that there is associated brain damage, varying from the trivial to the incapacitating, in 95% of all epileptics. Moreover, evidence from CT scanning and MRI studies indicates that small lesions are much commoner than previously reported (see Chapter 8).

Studies of intelligence in patients with epilepsy run into the difficulty that the populations studied may not be representative of the group as a whole. The effects of medication may also influence the results. Residential centres for epilepsy, for example, contain a greater proportion of seriously brain damaged people, and studies carried out on these populations will give lower IQ results than studies conducted in general practices. An old study which tested a random sample of non-institutionalized men with epilepsy of military age found them to have only slightly lower average intelligence scores than non-epileptic men of the same district.

It has been suggested that patients with epilepsy as a group are slower and have longer reaction times than non-epileptics, but that this difference is frequently intensified by anticonvulsant medication. This could reasonably be explained in terms of mild cerebral injury.

Studies by Lennox [19], and Lennox and Lennox [20], showed the importance of brain damage in causing psychiatric morbidity in those with epilepsy. They found that early age of onset of the epilepsy carried a poorer prognosis for mental functioning. In the first study, of 1905 patients with epilepsy, two-thirds were found to be mentally normal. In those whose mental functioning was severely affected there was a higher preponderance of brain damage. In the second study, the IQs were again lower in the brain damaged group than in the controls, suggesting that it was brain damage rather than the seizures that was significant in lowering intelligence. Reitan [21] also showed that the younger the age at which brain damage occurs, the greater will be its effects on the development of the intellect and personality. Personality disorders are found more frequently the earlier the seizures start and the more widespread the convulsions [11, 22].

A more recent study by Betts *et al.* [23] concludes: 'In general terms there is no good evidence in properly matched groups that there is any lowering of intelligence due to epilepsy itself, though of course any causative brain damage may leave an intellectual loss and cognitive impairment.' Scott *et al.* [24] also found no difference in IQ between people with epilepsy and normal controls.

Rutter *et al.* [25], confirmed this finding in school children: 'If epilepsy is uncomplicated, i.e. no obvious brain damage is present, intelligence follows a normal distribution.' A greater incidence of lower IQ was found in people who showed evidence of brain damage.

The level of intellectual performance is also affected by the type of epilepsy and the site of the brain lesion. As would be expected, those epileptics who suffer from idiopathic epilepsy have higher intelligence scores than those whose epilepsy is symptomatic of underlying cerebral damage. Generalized diffuse brain damage tends to produce a global reduction in IQ scores but no specific reduction in sub-test scores, whereas localized lesions may produce focal cognitive deficits. Dominant (L) temporal lesions, for example, generally produce a deterioration in verbal IQ and verbal memory, while non-dominant (R) temporal lesions may show no specific change or, sometimes, impaired verbal memory and reduced verbal IQ. A few studies do, however, show non-verbal memory impairment.

Two authors have described differences for patients with left and right temporal lobe lesions in the expected directions – impaired verbal memory for the left and impaired non-verbal memory for the right [26, 27]. Delaney compared groups with unilateral temporal lobe lesions, frontal lesions and a normal control group, and found that memory impairment was similar in those with right and left temporal lobe lesions, but more severe in those with left temporal lobe lesions for learning word lists. On tests of non-verbal memory, however, those with right temporal lobe lesions showed more impairment than the left temporals and frontals who were the same as normal controls.

Glowinski [28] found rather different results. He compared patients with temporal lobe epilepsy with the then fashionable 'centrencephalic' epilepsy and normal controls, and found that those who had unilateral temporal lobe lesions had greater difficulty in memorizing and integrating verbal material than the other groups. This finding was independent of the side of the lesion, IQ or medication. A study by Milberg *et al.* [29] used the WAIS to construct a special index and compared patients with temporal lobe and generalized epilepsy, and showed similar findings.

The conflict in these studies is more apparent than real. It is not always possible to be certain of the extent of any epileptogenic lesion and many of the patients described may well have had bilateral temporal damage. Epileptic discharges themselves are also known seriously to interfere with cognition [30], and this is an additional variable which cannot be controlled. Thus, focal epileptogenic lesions usually lead to focal cognitive deficits, and those with focal deficits are more at risk from psychiatric illness than those without.

18.3.2 Extent and site of epileptogenic lesions

Diffuse lesions with generalized brain damage lead to intellectual impairment with an increased prevalence of psychiatric morbidity, as described above, and focal lesions may lead to specific cognitive deficits. Of greater importance, however, is the recent finding that temporal lobe lesions have a significant relationship to the genesis of psychiatric morbidity.

The study by Gudmundsson [9] showed that 50% of patients with temporal lobe epilepsy had psychological difficulties compared to 25% of those with other types of attacks. Pond and Bidwell's study [6] showed similar results; nearly 20% of those with temporal lobe epilepsy had been in mental hospitals compared to 7% of the group as a whole.

However, other authors have frequently pointed out that there may be other links with temporal lobe epilepsy which could account for its association with psychiatric morbidity. Stevens [31, 32] has drawn attention to the lack of adequate controls, poor diagnosis and the selected nature of the populations in some studies, and has found no convincing association [32]. Currie [33] found a surprisingly low prevalence rate of psychiatric morbidity. His hospital study of temporal lobe epileptics suffers from all the deficits mentioned above, but in view of the fact already mentioned that patients with temporal lobe epilepsy and psychiatric illness are more frequently referred to hospital, a higher prevalence rate might have been expected. Rodin [34] showed a clear relationship between temporal lobe epilepsy and psychiatric morbidity, but he also showed that patients with temporal lobe epilepsy were more difficult to control, took a greater number of drugs, and frequently had more than one seizure type – all confounding variables. Table 18.1 shows his results.

Table 18.1 Differences between patients with temporal lobe epilepsy and other seizure types, matched for age, sex and IQ (Rodin *et al.* [34])

Temporal lobe seizure patients had:	Student's t	$p<$
Greater number of anticonvulsants used in treatment	3.3	0.01
More commonly more than one seizure type	3.2	0.01
More clusters of major seizures	3.0	0.01
More common history of meningitis	2.7	0.01
Less common hereditary cause for illness only	2.5	0.01
More frequent occurrence of sleep after minor seizures	2.3	0.05
More common bleeding or threatened abortion during pregnancy	2.3	0.05
More random circadian distribution	2.2	0.05
More mixed hereditary and external aetiological factors	2.1	0.05
More frequent major seizures	2.0	0.05
Longer history of major seizures	2.0	0.05
More decreased overall psychomotor activity	2.0	0.05
More impaired peer relations	3.3	0.05
More personality disturbance on psychological tests	2.8	0.01
Poorer performance on information sub-test on WAIS	2.7	0.01
More psychotic tendencies during psychiatric interview	2.4	0.05
Higher elevation on depression scale on MMPI	2.3	0.05
Higher elevation on paranoia scale on MMPI	2.1	0.05
More psychotic tendencies on psychological test results	2.1	0.05
More organic disturbances on psychological test results	2.0	0.05

More recently, Trimble and Perez [35], reviewing those studies which had used questionnaire scoring of psychopathology and type of seizure, showed that there is an association between an increased prevalence of psychiatric morbidity and temporal lobe epilepsy.

An explanation for the discrepancies in these findings may be that within the main diagnostic category of temporal lobe epilepsy, several subgroups can be found. Taylor [36] has consistently emphasized that it is no longer sufficient to lump all patients with temporal lobe epilepsy together. He has shown [37] that in patients undergoing temporal lobectomy 'a number of effects – pathological sinistrality, the balance of cognitive skills, complexity of the aura experience, aggression, extraversion and liability to psychosis – were partially dependent on the time of origin of the temporal lobe lesion, its left or right location, and on the patient's sex'. Taylor also showed [22] that aggressiveness is more often associated with left temporal lobe lesions, and that this behaviour responds well to surgery. Taylor's results are a useful guide if surgery is contemplated.

Comparing children with epilepsy with non-epileptic controls, Stores [38] found that the epileptic children were significantly more socially isolated, inattentive, overactive and anxious. They were also emotionally dependent on their mothers. His most significant finding, however, was that boys with epilepsy were more affected than girls, and children of both sexes who had left temporal epileptic foci rather than right, were more frequently affected. This finding was confirmed in the follow-up study of children with temporal lobe epilepsy by Lindsay *et al.* [39], who again suggested that males with a left temporal focus were particularly at risk.

18.3.3 Family

The family's response to and ability to cope with a disadvantaged child plays an important part in the genesis of psychiatric morbidity. Rutter [11] found that disturbed home backgrounds and broken family relationships were more important causes of psychiatric morbidity for children with and without epilepsy, but that having an epileptic child in the family is a potent source of family stress. One-fifth of the mothers of epileptic children had a nervous breakdown, while those whose children had no fits but had cerebral palsy, had significantly fewer breakdowns.

Sillanpää [40] has also reported increased psychiatric morbidity among parents of epileptic children in Finland, and has shown that parents and guardians of children with epilepsy had higher rates of divorce and family illegitimacy. Mulder and Suurmeijer [41], in a pilot study, looked at the way families of epileptic children behaved in response to the occurrence of epilepsy. Both this study and that of Mattsson [42] found that parents adapted better to their epileptic child when they understood more about the condition and had become more confident in handling their children. These parents were able to develop a warm and accepting relationship with the child, and perhaps most importantly, were able to allow him to become independent. These authors found that school refusal was seldom due to uncontrolled seizures. It was more often due to an interaction between the child and the despairing attitudes of the parents, and of parental lack of control.

It is a general finding that parents of epileptic children are often over-protective [43], (and see Chapter 17), so that the children tend to be emotionally immature and excessively dependent on their families, particularly their mothers. The child's immaturity, lack of social skills and fear of independence may lead to a stormy adolescence and difficulty in breaking free from the family. Often the result is a hostile, dependent adult, who may never succeed in leaving the parental home.

18.3.4   The epileptic personality

The belief in an 'epileptic personality' – described as being 'sticky', 'suspicious', 'quarrelsome', 'aggressive', 'touchy', 'pedantic', 'egocentric', 'circumstantial' and 'religiose' is one of the many reasons for prejudice against people who have epilepsy. Although a few patients – 4% in Pond and Bidwell's study [6] – do undoubtedly show some of these characteristics, these are unlikely to be due to the epilepsy alone. Brain damage, the stigma of epilepsy, difficulties with schooling, employment, and interpersonal relationships all contribute. Personality difficulties may be exacerbated by chronic long term medication and, in a small proportion of patients, institutionalization. Tizard [44] has pointed out that it is impossible to define a specific personality type in patients with epilepsy, because of selection of patients, multiple types of seizure, differing degrees of brain damage, the site and location of the brain lesion, and the confounding effects of medication. The instruments which were used to measure personality in the early studies were inappropriate. Tizard, together with more recent authors, [23, 45, 46] agree that there is no personality disorder associated with epilepsy *per se*.

Gibbs [47], Gastaut [48] and others, have suggested that seizure discharges within the limbic system (temporal lobe epilepsy) lead to a specific temporal lobe syndrome. Waxman and Geschwind [49] and Geschwind [50] suggest that some patients with temporal lobe epilepsy showed altered sexual behaviour and an altered religious view of life, and that they became compulsive writers (hypergraphia). Bear [51] and Bear and Fedio [52] describe a sensory limbic hyperconnection syndrome: 'Our analysis of the psychological changes occurring interictally in temporal lobe epilepsy emphasizes extensive and progressive investment of stimulus complexes with intense affective significance. It was suggested that this phenomenom is produced anatomically by the formation of new, extensive and excessive sensory (or polysensory) limbic bonds.' They suggested that one effect of temporal lobe epilepsy is to add excessive meaning to the patient's world, and that the hyperconnection syndrome was a reverse Kluver and Bucy [53] syndrome. The patients may suffer from hyposexuality, hypermetamorphosis (a tendency to adhere excessively to each thought, feeling and action) and hyperemotionality (irritability and deepened emotion). Bear and Fedio [52], using a questionnaire developed to rate 18 personality traits for patients with epilepsy, found that temporal lobe epileptic patients show a characteristic pattern of traits. They show humourless sobriety, dependence, circumstantiality, obsessionality, undue preoccupation with religious and philosophic concerns, deepened emotion and irritability, when compared to normal controls, and patients with chronic neuromuscular disorder as further controls.

Bear and Fedio [52] also found an association between right temporal lobe foci and displays of excess emotion such as periods of sadness, irritability and elation. Patients who had left temporal lobe foci showed a pattern of internal ideational (verbal) traits. They were philosophically inclined, had a tendency to ruminate on intellectual questions, saw excess meaning in the world, and were excessively religious, with an augmented sense of personal destiny. When views of the patients by external raters were compared to the patients' own views of themselves, it was found that those who had right temporal lesions exaggerated socially acceptable traits and denied undesirable traits (said to be 'polishers') while those with left temporal lobe foci showed a tendency to over-report traits which showed them up in a bad light ('tarnishers').

Current thinking about the epileptic personality has been greatly influenced by these views, but, although persuasive, they are not generally accepted. Several other workers have shown that if those patients with psychiatric illness are removed from the epilepsy group, then most of the differences between patients with temporal lobe epilepsy and other patient groups disappear [54–57]. It is thus likely that the findings of excessive emotion initially reported by Bear and Fedio [52] are related to psychiatric illness rather than specifically to temporal lobe epilepsy. However, there is continuing controversy about whether it is the seizures themselves, or the underlying brain damage, which cause the suggested personality alteration. The most widely accepted view is that of Stevens and Herman [58], who wrote: 'There are a number of factors which increase the risk of psychopathology in patients with temporal lobe epilepsy. The most powerful factors identified are clinical, EEG and radiological evidence of bilateral, deep or diffuse cerebral pathology.'

18.4 CLASSIFICATION OF THE PSYCHIATRIC DISORDERS OF EPILEPSY

The following classification of epilepsy proposed by Desmond Pond in 1957 is still in use today [59].

(1) Psychiatric disorders due to the brain disease which causes the fits.

(2) Psychiatric disorders directly related to the seizures.
(3) Interictal psychiatric disorders – those disorders whose occurrence is unrelated in time to the seizures.

18.4.1 Disorders due to brain disease

This chapter will not review those brain diseases, such as Alzheimer's disease or arteriosclerotic dementia, which result in both epilepsy and psychiatric disorder, which are dealt with elsewhere in this book (Chapter 4). In addition, an excellent review will be found in Lishman [45] or Fenton [60].

18.4.2 Disorders directly related to the seizures

(a) Prodrome

The prodrome is a period of minutes, hours or even days before the onset of the seizure, when psychological changes or changes in behaviour preceding the fit may be apparent to the patients themselves, or to those close to them. These changes vary in intensity and frequently terminate with the start of the fit. They are usually non-specific but include feelings of tension, anxiety, depression, and irritability. As yet, little is known about the mechanism.

(b) Ictus

The form a seizure takes will depend on the precise location of the seizure discharge within the cortex and the extent of its subsequent spread. There may be tingling if the discharge arises from the sensory cortex, movement from the motor cortex, visual patterns from the occipital cortex. Most complex and interesting are the phenomena of seizures arising from the temporal lobe. These may include changes in volition, mood or cognition which may intrude on consciousness, producing distortions in perception, or feelings of anxiety.

Particularly complex hallucinations arise when the discharges invade the association cortices or the temporal lobe. Even though these are often very vivid and real, they are always seen as something independent of the patient, imposed on him – a splitting of the perceptual stream described by Hughlings Jackson as a form of mental diploplia. They are fleeting, occurring only during the aura and tend to be stereotyped, often inappropriate to the situation. They may be accompanied by some clouding of consciousness. (For further details see [61].)

In addition to the complex hallucinations already discussed, complex cognitive, affective and psychomotor symptoms are also seen if the seizure discharge originates in or rapidly invades brain structures involved with the elaboration of higher mental processes.

Cognitive features may include dysmnesic, ideational and other symptoms. Dysmnesic symptoms involve impairment or distortion of memory – particularly the ability to recall some particular thought. Panoramic memories are rarely impaired. Ideational symptoms consist of forced thinking of a particular thought or of several thoughts. Other symptoms include distortions in the perception of time, which seems either speeded up or slowed down, and feelings of unreality [60, 62].

Affective symptoms are very common in people with temporal lobe epilepsy. These experiences are seldom pleasant, but range from the negative to the terrifying, sometimes with fear of imminent death. Gowers [63] studying 505 cases of aura in 1881, found none with positive affect. Lennox [64] found 0.9% of positive auras, but of these only a few were truly pleasant. Cirignotta *et al.* [65] described an ecstatic aura with a non-dominant temporal lobe epileptic seizure [66]. The sudden feelings of familiarity – déjà vu, -entendu, -vécu, (having already seen, heard or experienced) or jamais vu, -entendu, -vécu, a sudden feeling of strangeness, of never having seen, heard or experienced, are seldom classified under affective symptoms, but should be included in this category because they carry either a strong negative or positive affect. Affect is not, however, limited to these experiences, but may be attached to any experience that occurs during an aura. However, anger rarely occurs as an ictal emotion.

Automatisms (psychomotor symptoms) may be defined as 'a state of clouding of consciousness which occurs during or after a seizure, and during which the individual retains the control of posture and muscle tone and performs simple or complex movements without being aware of what is happening.' The time course of an automatism can be divided into three parts. (1) The initial phase, which lasts only seconds and usually consists of staring or simple mouthing and chewing movements. (2) More complex behaviour which is still stereotyped and repetitive, such as fumbling with objects, picking at clothes or standing up and turning. This lasts a further few seconds or minutes. (3) In the final phase behaviour is most complex and may range from the stereotyped to the normal. Complex movements of turning and standing may progress to searching, handling and walking, and then merge imperceptibly into normal behaviour [67].

Memory is always impaired during an automatism, because for the automatism to arise there must have been a bilateral spread of the seizure discharge into both periamygdaloid-hippocampal structures. Jasper [68] has shown that in stimulation experiments at operation, automatisms arise when the bilateral involvement of the amygdaloid-hippocampal structures spreads to the mesial diencephalon and temperoparietal cortex. Automatisms usually arise from temporal lobe lesions, but are also seen in discharging lesions of the frontal lobe and orbitofrontal and parietal regions of the mesial surface of the hemisphere [69, 70]. Consciousness is also interfered with during an automatism, so that actions are poorly directed and executed. The patient behaves as if confused, is dazed and disorientated. Aggressive acts are very rare (see below). Most automatisms are brief. Knox [71] found that 80% last less than 5 min, 12% less than 15 min and the remaining 8% less than an hour.

There is often an interaction between the patient and his environment during such a seizure: the form the automatism takes is at least partly determined by the patient's thought content and surroundings before a seizure begins. Forster and Liske [72] quote the case of an organist who had a seizure while playing a hymn. He stopped during the aura and then played a few bars of jazz before recommencing the hymn again.

(c) Ictal episodes – absence status (petit mal status)

Absence status presents with clouding of consciousness and confusion. The patient is usually unco-ordinated, confused, perseverative and slow, and often appears stuporose and out of contact, motionless and withdrawn. Attacks last from a few minutes to several days, sometimes waxing or ceasing abruptly for several minutes. The onset is rapid. The attack is often terminated by a grand mal seizure. Absence status in younger children may not be so severe; body tone may be preserved and simple motor acts carried out. The most striking feature is the alternation between relative normality and a silly confused state which may mimic hysteria. Occasionally, only cognitive tests may detect subtle mental state changes [73].

The EEG record is dominated by spike and wave activity. This is frequently degraded spike and wave and polyspike activity, and very seldom classical 3 Hz spike and wave.

Absence status is commonest amongst young patients and those who have had previous petit mal attacks. Roger *et al.* [74] found that in 75% of cases, onset is before the age of 20. Dalby [75] found an incidence of 6.2% in patients with primary generalized epilepsy. Lennox [76] first reported its occurrence. Although the term 'absence status' is to be preferred, subsequent authors have suggested alternative names: 'epileptic twilight states' by Zappoli [77], 'spike-wave stupor' by Neidermeyer and Khalifeh [78], 'absence status' by Bruens [79]. However, the fact that the term absence status has also been used for other conditions where it is inappropriate has led to some confusion in the literature. Lugaresi *et al.* [80] have used the term for episodes in young children who have an abnormal EEG, mental dullness and who do not respond to treatment. It has been suggested by Roger *et al.* [74] that, as these form part of the continuum of the Lennox-Gastaut syndrome, they should be classified separately.

Cases of late onset absence status have also been reported [81–83]. These showed a more complex symptomatology ranging from paranoid hallucinatory psychoses, pseudodepressive dementia to depressive psychoses. Metabolic or drug changes, which probably altered cerebral excitability so as to allow the spike-wave and abnormal mental state to arise, were present in most cases.

(d) Temporal lobe status

Continuous temporal lobe ictal activity may lead to a confused or obtunded twilight state. Studies have been described by both Delgado-Escueta *et al.* [84]

and Markand *et al.* [85] in which patients showed continuous and repetitive automatisms, such as picking and chewing movements, while others were withdrawn and obtunded, responding only to insistent stimulation with simple though often co-ordinated behaviour. There may be psychotic features with a paranoid flavour, and paranoid delusion or content may occur. These episodes may end spontaneously with a grand mal seizure or by therapeutic intervention with an intravenous injection of diazepam. They arise in a setting of confusion and disorientation and their organic nature is clearly visible. The EEG frequently shows temporal lobe spiking in an abnormal background of delta and theta rhythms.

(e) Postictal states
The response to a grand mal seizure will depend on the location of the epileptogenic lesion and on any other associated cerebral pathology. Postictal confusional states, lasting from 5–10 min, up to hours or even days and, rarely, as long as one to two weeks commonly follow both grand mal and focal seizures. As the patient regains consciousness after a grand mal seizure, he is confused, disorientated and irritable. He may fall asleep or gradually become less confused until he regains full consciousness. The EEG immediately after the fit is dominated by high voltage delta activity which slowly decreases in amplitude as the normal background rhythms return. If prolonged twilight states or abnormal states follow a seizure, the EEG often shows either focal or generalized delta activity. There may be prolonged effects following a grand mal seizure in some patients. Patients with focal cerebral damage quite commonly show focal cognitive deficits of which they are not always aware for up to two weeks following a seizure. One patient at the Maudsley Epilepsy Unit believed that he had regained his verbal fluency after a grand mal seizure within two days, whereas changes in verbal fluency could be shown for two weeks after the seizure. In elderly patients and patients with significant brain damage there may be deterioration in cognitive state for several days after a grand mal seizure.

Clark and Lesko [86] and Levin [87], who have carried out two of the most important of the few detailed studies on postictal states, found that irritability and confusion are common, although aggression and excitement are also often seen. Visual or auditory hallucinations and delusions are prominent in those who develop a psychosis, and these are usually paranoid in character. Visual hallucinations are often so well structured and persecutory that they may lead to impulsive attempts to escape from the hallucinatory world and occasionally, attempts at suicide. Most of these episodes last up to 72 hours but those with more frankly psychotic features may last up to one week or, more rarely, up to two weeks. They may be terminated by a further grand mal seizure. They are most common between 30 and 40 years, but can arise at any age [87]. They most often arise after a series of grand mal seizures, though they can follow a single grand mal seizure. Treatment is as for any other psychotic episode, preferably by the butyrophenone group of drugs (haloperidol). Anticonvulsant levels should be checked to make sure that further seizures are not likely to occur.

18.4.3 Interictal disorders

The interictal disorders are those states which arise in clear consciousness and are unrelated to seizure activity. They include both psychotic illnesses, consisting predominately of the schizophrenia-like psychoses of epilepsy [88] and the affective psychoses, and the neurotic illnesses, which are predominately affective in character and usually depressive. The degree to which these illnesses are related to the epilepsy is not fully understood, although it is clear that there is a relationship between them. The current view is that either the epilepsy or the psychiatric illness may run a course which is independent of the other.

18.5 PSYCHOSIS AND EPILEPSY

18.5.1 Prevalence

Few studies have attempted to assess the prevalence of psychosis and epilepsy. Community studies cannot give a true picture unless they trace and include those patients with epilepsy who are not in the community but in chronic institutions. Unfortunately, most studies look at selected populations, although there are a few community-based epidemiological studies. A study of 908 patients with epilepsy in northern Norway identified 2% (16 patients) who either were psychotic or had had a history of psychosis [89]. A study of 245 patients with epilepsy in 14 general practices in England found no cases of psychosis [6]. Special populations, such as hospital clinics, tend, not surprisingly, to produce higher prevalence rates, because, as Pond and Bidwell [6] have shown, patients with psychiatric morbidity are sent preferentially to hospital. Neurology clinic studies give rates of 1.4% [90], 2.4% [79], 4.4% [91], and 8% [92]. An earlier study reported a higher prevalence – 9% of 1200 patients with psychomotor epilepsy, compared with fewer than 1% of 5000 patients with grand mal or Jacksonian epilepsy. Currie *et al.* [33] in a study of patients with temporal lobe epilepsy only found a prevalence of 2%, while Stevens [93] found a much higher figure.

Those studies which have used mental hospital populations have, as would be expected, found higher prevalence rates; 4.3% [7], 5.3% [94] and 5.4% [8]. Standage and Fenton [92], in a study in a neurology clinic which is difficult to interpret, found a prevalence of 16%. A long term survey of admissions to four mental hospitals [8], found 72 patients over a six-year period who were diagnosed as having epilepsy, three of whom were thought to have a paranoid psychosis and 12 of whom were endogenously depressed. Specialist populations give even higher rates. Lindsay *et al.* [39] followed children with limbic seizures for a decade and found that 10.3% developed a schizophreniform psychosis. As this population were still young adults at the time of the survey, the eventual rate will probably be even higher. Falconer [95] found a rate of 16% amongst patients with severe epilepsy referred to the Maudsley Hospital neurosurgical unit. Many of these came from mental hospitals, thus still further biasing the sample. The risk of developing psychosis has been shown to be further increased by temporal lobectomy. A study of 14 patients operated on at the University of Oregon found that three out of 11 patients developed a paranoid psychosis two to three years postoperatively [96]. Taylor [22], studying 100 consecutive patients following temporal lobectomy, found that 12 patients were psychotic before surgery whilst 19 were psychotic following surgery. Jensen and Larsen [97] report the postoperative onset of psychosis in nine patients from a group of 74 who underwent temporal lobectomy.

18.5.2 Clinical associations

It seems unlikely that there is a genetic association between epilepsy and psychosis. Slater *et al.*, in the foundation paper, found only three patients with epilepsy and psychosis (two schizophrenic and one paranoid) who had psychotic relatives [88]. These findings were supported by those of Flor-Henry [98]. Several authors have found no specific premorbid personality [88, 97, 99]. The mean age of onset in Slater's [88] study was approximately 15 years after the onset of epilepsy. In the literature age of onset varies widely, from 12–23 years. (For a review, see [100].) It is generally accepted, though not certain, that psychoses start after the onset of the epilepsy and are thus related to the epilepsy rather than to genetic factors [101].

18.5.3 Clinical characteristics

Hill [102] was the first to describe a paranoid hallucinatory psychotic state in association with temporal lobe epilepsy. Pond [59] drew attention to the retention of a warm affect. Slater *et al.* [88] extended these findings and pointed out that although any feature of schizophrenia could be found, some were particularly common. Paranoid, grandiose and mystical delusions with feelings of passivity occurred frequently: auditory hallucinations occurred in a majority of their patients. However, less than half showed any thought disorder. Although disturbances of mood were common, there was little flattening of affect throughout this group. A more objective account, using the Present State Examination (PSE) to quantify precisely the phenomenology of the psychotic states of epilepsy, has been given by Perez and Trimble [103]. They found that affective symptomatology was common and prominent. Toone *et al.* [104] compared both clinically and phenomenologically the psychosis of epilepsy with the functional psychoses. They again found a similarity between the two. In a later paper, Perez *et al.* [105], using the PSE, examined 11 patients with epilepsy and psychosis and nine non-epileptic schizophrenic controls. They found almost identical PSE profiles for the schizophrenics and the epileptic psychoses. The wide range of psychotic features found in their series supported the views of Slater and his colleagues [88] that any of the features of schizophrenia may be present. Although the paranoid hallucinatory psychotic state of epilepsy is widely accepted as an accurate description of the schizophrenia-like epileptic psychoses, it must be stressed that this is a clinical stereotype. In practice any of the features of schizophrenia may be present to a greater or lesser degree. Affect, however, is usually well preserved.

The clinical course is variable. The psychosis remits after one episode in a proportion of patients, but in half it becomes chronic and follows a relapsing episodic course. Several studies have found that patients remained psychotic for up to ten years after the onset of their illness. Where affective psychoses occur, they differ little from those seen in patients without epilepsy. Their clinical characteristics are similar, and they run a similar course. Treatment is considered on p. 529.

18.5.4   Associated factors

The aim of this chapter is not to review in detail the literature relating to the factors which are thought to be important in the precipitation of the psychoses of epilepsy. The central question is whether it is the epilepsy, the underlying brain damage or an interaction of the two which predisposes to the psychosis, and whether the area of the brain involved colours the form the psychosis will take.

It is generally, though not universally, accepted that there is an association between temporal lobe epilepsy and the schizophrenia-like psychoses of epilepsy [106]. Slater *et al.* [88], and Bruens [99], found that psychomotor seizures occurred in the majority of patients with temporal lobe epilepsy. Kristensen and Sindrup [107] and Flor-Henry [98] both described a reduction in psychomotor seizures at the time the patients were psychotic, suggesting a relationship with temporal lobe seizures. Kristensen and Sindrup [107] also found an excess of automatisms, epigastric auras and déjà vu features in their psychotic group. Jensen and Larsen [97] reported an increase in hallucinations and delusions. Hermann and Shabrias [108], using the Minnesota Multiphasic Personality Index (MMPI), showed that those patients who had raised scores on scales of paranoia and schizophrenia were more likely to have auras of ictal fear.

Brain damage has been found to be associated with patients who develop a psychosis. Air encephalography was abnormal in 70% of one psychotic group of patients, [88] and 80% of another [107]. In the latter series, however, there was no significant difference from the control group who had temporal lobe epilepsy but no psychosis. Jensen and Larsen [97] however found an excess of brain damage in their psychotic patients. Flor-Henry [98] found a higher incidence of brain damage in the psychotic group compared to the manic-depressive psychoses, but not compared to his non-psychotic control group. An association between those patients with psychosis and hamartoma ('alien tissue') lesions of their temporal lobe has been shown by Taylor [109]. Gallhofer *et al.* [110] add further evidence for associated brain damage from PET scan studies, which suggest a 'down regulation' of activity in the temporal cortex, frontal cortex, and head of the caudate nucleus. Brain damage is thus clearly a factor, though the extent to which it contributes is still uncertain. An intensive and well-documented study of ten patients with epilepsy and psychosis by Ramani *et al.* [111], failed to demonstrate a unique association between schizophreniform psychosis and complex partial seizures. They conclude that the interictal psychosis in epilepsy is probably a spectrum of disorders determined by a number of different factors.

Which hemisphere is damaged and which temporal lobe contains the focus is now thought to be important in the genesis of the psychoses of epilepsy. Flor-Henry [98] first suggested that the left temporal lobe was involved in patients with schizophreniform psychoses and the right in those with manic-depressive psychosis, a view which has led to considerable subsequent discussion in the literature. It now seems probable that left temporal lobe damage is indeed associated with the schizophreniform psychoses, but that there is a much less clear relationship between a right temporal lobe lesion and manic-depressive psychosis [39, 112–114]. Negative studies also exist [97, 107]. This divergence of opinion in the literature about whether left or right cerebral hemispheres are predominately involved is not surprising. Cerebral dominance is difficult to define in this population, firstly because there is an association with brain damage and secondly as those with psychosis show an excess of left-handedness. The characterization of psychosis using a proper measuring instrument such as the PSE has only been carried out in one or two of the later studies; the early studies leave some doubt as to the exact nature of the psychiatric illnesses involved.

An inverse relationship between psychosis and seizures such that when the patient is psychotic, his seizures are in remission and the EEG tends to be normal, has been suggested by Landolt [114–117]. This is called 'forced normalization'. There is considerable discussion in the literature as to whether or not this relationship truly exists, and the question is not yet resolved. (For reviews see Glaser [118] and Bruens [79].) Ramani *et al.* [111], who carried out intensive long term monitoring on patients with the interictal psychoses of epilepsy, threw considerable doubt onto the concept of forced normalization. The relationship could be demonstrated in only one of their ten patients: they report that in most cases the emergence of the psychosis could not be explained. Non-specific factors may be involved, as during a psychotic episode patients tend to be more aroused; also, because they are in hospital, they are more likely to be taking their anticonvulsants. Both these factors will tend to normalize their EEG.

Whether chronic psychotic illnesses develop in the presence of epilepsy or whether epilepsy is more common in the presence of psychotic illnesses is therefore a question still unresolved. These two views lead to two different theories, an affinity theory, suggesting a relationship between psychosis and epilepsy, and an antagonism theory, which suggests that epilepsy protects against psychosis. Evidence that brain damage and subictal activity are found in association with epilepsy supports the former view, whereas in support of the latter are the biochemical hypotheses which suggest that those chemicals, e.g. dopamine, which are anticonvulsant when present at elevated concentrations are antipsychotic when reduced. This same argument is applied to folate metabolism [119]. For a full review see Toone [100].

18.6 EPILEPSY AND NEUROSIS

18.6.1 Prevalence

The prevalence of psychiatric disorders in people with epilepsy has already been discussed elsewhere in this chapter (p. 524).

18.6.2 Clinical characteristics

A relationship between depression and epilepsy was described by Hippocrates: 'Melancholics ordinarily become epileptics and epileptics melancholics: of these two states, what determines the preference is the direction the malady takes; if it bears upon the body, epilepsy, if upon the intelligence, melancholy' [120, 121].

Few studies have looked specifically at the characteristics of patients with depressive illness and epilepsy, and yet depression is the most commonly described interictal psychiatric illness. Several groups of workers have suggested that depression is common. Betts [8] reported that 31% of their sample were depressed, while Robertson and Trimble [121] suggested that some 40% of their patients had an endogenous pattern of depression, of moderate severity. Mendez *et al.* [122] found that patients with epilepsy attending vocational services for the disabled were significantly more depressed than other disabled controls, and much more likely to have made prior suicide attempts. Depression may be more frequent if the epilepsy is of late onset [123]. It has been suggested by Rodin *et al.* [124] that in those patients with epilepsy, depression scores were higher in patients who had temporal lobe epilepsy, and this was confirmed by Dikman *et al.* [125], who found higher rates in patients suffering from complex partial seizures. This was, however, not found to be so by Robertson [126], possibly because her sample was more severely depressed. She also noted that there was no relationship between the severity and features of the depression, and the site of the focal lesion or the type of epilepsy. Trimble and Perez [35] using the Middlesex Hospital questionnaire, found high anxiety and depression scores in their epileptic population compared to normal controls, but could show no relationship between the depression and the type of epilepsy. Kogeorgos *et al.* [127], in a study of 66 patients with epilepsy attending a neurological outpatient clinic, found that nearly half the sample emerged as probable cases on the General Health Questionnaire and that depression was particularly common. Again, no relationship was found between the type of epilepsy and the characteristics of the depression.

Depressive symptoms range from a depressive reaction to the epilepsy itself or to other life circumstances, to severe endogenous depressive illness. Feelings of sadness, guilt, self-blame and unworthiness are all common. In severely depressed patients vegetative features also occur, and there may be disturbances of sleep, loss of weight and appetite. The depressed patient who threatens suicide has powerful drugs available and should be taken seriously. Suicide is five times more common in patients with epilepsy than in the general population, and 25 times more common in patients with temporal lobe epilepsy [121, 128].

Anxiety states are also said to be associated with epilepsy, but their characteristics do not differ significantly from those of a normal anxiety state [129]. Patients not uncommonly become fearful of their attacks and develop a true phobic state about going out or appearing in public.

18.6.3 Management of psychotic and neurotic illnesses

The fact that a patient has epilepsy does not affect the specific management of neurosis or psychosis. Treatment of both the epilepsy and the psychiatric disorder should be as usual. Acute psychotic symptoms are best treated with phenothiazines or butyrophenones given orally. Maintenance can be by depot preparations such as flupenthixol or fluphenazine given on an outpatient basis. Manic symptoms too are treated by either phenothiazines or butyrophenones, with lithium carbonate as maintenance therapy.

Depressive symptoms are best treated initially by those drugs which are thought to have an anticonvulsant action – the dopamine agonists such as nomifensin [130], (now withdrawn in the UK) or viloxazine, or those antidepressants with least epileptogenic effects such as mianserin. However, caution should be exercised when using these antidepressants, as side-effects have recently been reported for both drugs. If these are not successful, then the monoamine re-uptake inhibiting drugs, or the tricyclic antidepressants, may be used. When using drugs which are liable to cause seizures it is important to make sure that the patient is well 'covered' by anticonvulsant medication.

Behavioural methods for the treatment of neurotic disorders, particularly anxiety states, in epilepsy are becoming more popular (Section 10.5). This subject has been reviewed by Mostofsky and Balaschak [131] and by Fenwick [132]. Reward for seizure-free periods [133] and punishment for having seizures [134], have both been found effective. Ince [135] and Mostofsky [136] report some success with relaxation methods. Behaviour modification has been used by Standage [137] for a patient who was afraid of having seizures in social situations. The patient was asked to rehearse the situations in imagination while relaxed. This lessened the patient's anxiety in the actual provocative situations, with a reduction in fit frequency. Another successful study is reported by Parrino [138]. 'Flooding' has been successfully used in a patient with agoraphobia which was clearly related to her movement epilepsy [139]. She was exposed to the phobic situation for long periods in the presence of the therapist; improvement was reported in both her agoraphobia and her fits.

18.7 DISTURBANCES OF SEXUAL FUNCTION

Several authors have postulated a relationship between sexual dysfunction and sexual deviation with epilepsy. Most of the literature, reviewed by Scott [140] relates to case reports of temporal lobe epilepsy. Sexual dysfunction includes both changes in sexual function which occur in relationship to the seizure, and disorders which arise between seizures.

Partial seizures arising from the medial surface of the hemisphere in the central region can lead to a contralateral genital sensation. Both ictal and postictal epileptic automatisms may simulate crude sexual behaviour. Dressing and undressing automatisms are common, although seldom reported in the literature [33, 141]. Seizures can be triggered during intercourse and occasionally by orgasm [140]. Both fetishism and transvestism have been described in association with temporal lobe epilepsy and temporal lobe lesions. The case of a patient whose safety pin fetish was cured by temporal lobectomy is often quoted [142] but such associations are in fact rare and seldom seen in practice. Sexual deviations are, in any case, extremely common in the general population, although there is some evidence that the left temporal lobe may be involved in a small minority of these.

Most of the evidence suggests that reduced libido and potency are the commonest form of sexual dysfunction among epileptic males. Toone *et al.* [143, 144], Fenwick *et al.* [145] and Dana-Haerai *et al.* [146] have found low serum free testosterone levels in patients taking anticonvulsants. They suggest that this may result from altered metabolism of testosterone and sex-hormone binding globulin due to induction of liver enzymes. Herzog *et al.* [146a] suggest that hyperprolactinaemia may play a part in impaired potency. Anticonvulsants may affect the testes directly [148]. Preliminary work by Daniels *et al.* [147] suggests that testosterone replacement may have a part to play in patients with low free testosterone levels and sexual dysfunction. Little work has been done yet on women with epilepsy, but Herzog [148a] found that

CONTENTS: Preface; Contributors; Definitions and epidemiology of epilepsy; The biology of epilepsy; The different types of epileptic seizures and the international classification of epileptic seizures and of the epilepsies; The causes and precipitation of seizures; The genetic basis of the epilepsy; The first seizure, and the diagnosis of epilepsy; Electro-encephalography and epilepsy; Imaging in the investigation of epilepsy; The treatment of epilepsy by drugs; The management of epilepsy uncontrolled by anticonvulsant drugs - surgery and other treatments; Factors which influence the prognosis of epilepsy; Epilepsy and menstruation; Epilepsy after head injury and intracranial surgery; The management of status epilepticus; Febrile convulsions; Epilepsy in childhood; Sociological aspects of epilepsy; Psychiatric disorders of epilepsy; Epilepsy and the law; Epilepsy and driving; Index.

ORDER FORM

Please return to the Promotion Department, Chapman and Hall, 11 New Fetter Lane, London EC4P 4EE.
All cash orders are sent post & packing free in the UK.
Overseas add postage and packing: £1.75 surface; £5.00 airmail.

Please send me

_____ copy/ies of _____ @ £ _____

_____ copy/ies of _____ @ £ _____

☐ I enclose a cheque/International Money Order payable to Associated Book Publishers (UK) Ltd £ _____

☐ Please invoice me: ☐ Please debit my credit card account

Visa/Access/Diners Club/American Express card account with the sum of £ _____

Account Number _____ Expiry Date _____

Name _____

Address _____

_____

Signature _____ Date _____

If the above address is different from the registered address of your credit card, please give the registered address separately.

Registered Address: Associated Book Publishers (UK) Ltd, 11 New Fetter Lane, London EC4P 4EE.
Reg. No. 937236 England.

EPILEPSY

Edited by Anthony Hopkins, Department of Neurological Sciences, St. Bartholomew's Hospital, London.

There has been renewed interest in the scientific and sociological aspects of epilepsy in the last 15 years, reflected in a large number of meetings and publications. Advances in diagnosis and treatment have stemmed from the use of new imaging modalities and from new drugs, so that the prognosis for sufferers can now be very good indeed.

Epilepsy is a major new text, and its 20 chapters provide a coherent and up-to-date account of the biology, epidemiology, investigation and treatment of epilepsy. It has been written by an international team of authors pre-eminent in their special field, and will become a standard reference for the resident neurologist in training as well as for those who are already established.

1987   Hb 0 412 26520 6   592pp   £45.00

patients with right temporal lobe seizure discharges were particularly likely to lack sexual interest.

Many of the factors previously reported in the literature as being responsible for sexual dysfunction have been shown by Fenwick *et al.* [145] to be of only minor importance. They found no correlation between type and frequency of seizure, type and age of onset of epilepsy, brain damage or institutionalization and sexual dysfunction in patients in an epilepsy centre. What is often overlooked is that many patients with epilepsy are immature, dependent people with poor sexual and social skills and a poor self-image. It is probable that these factors contribute significantly to any sexual problems they encounter.

18.8 AGGRESSIVE BEHAVIOUR IN EPILEPSY

If a connection between epilepsy and aggression does indeed exist, it might be expected that higher prevalence rates of aggressive behaviour would be found in populations of patients with epilepsy. It is, however, difficult to make a comparison between the many studies which have attempted to demonstrate this. First, most lack a precise definition of what constitutes aggressive behaviour. Secondly, higher rates of aggression reported in some populations may be due to the fact that these populations have more intractable epilepsy and therefore higher anticonvulsant medication [32].

A number of different situational, cultural and pathological factors are involved in the genesis of violent behaviour. Socioeconomic factors such as poor housing and education are generally accepted to contribute. A higher proportion of violence is found in social class III and IV than in I and II [149]. Situational violence is determined by specific factors operating at the time it occurs – most murders, for example, are committed within the family, and many acts of violence take place in the context of crime.

18.8.1 Prevalence

Gastaut [150] reports that 50% of a group of patients with temporal lobe epilepsy showed paroxysmal rage – an unusually high prevalence. A much lower rate of aggression – 7% – was reported by Currie and co-workers [33] in a survey at the London Hospital of 666 patients with temporal lobe epilepsy of mixed aetiology and type, and by Rodin [151], who found pathological aggression in only 4.8% of a population of 700 from the Michigan Epilepsy Centre. Rodin reported that the aggressive group were young men of below average intelligence. They had a higher rate of psychiatric problems and more evidence of organic damage in the central nervous system than a control group without aggressive outbursts, matched for age, sex and IQ. A study of 90 patients from both neurological and neurosurgical clinics of a general hospital in Sweden, found aggressive behaviour in 17% of patients with temporal lobe epilepsy [152].

A study of patients with severe epilepsy who were being assessed for temporal lobectomy found that a high proportion showed violent behaviour [95]. Of 50 patients who had a predominately unilateral (mainly left-sided) spike focus, pathological outbursts of aggressive behaviour occurred in 38%; and a further 14%, many of whom were otherwise well adjusted individuals, showed milder or more persistent aggressiveness associated with a paranoid outlook [153, 154].

Because aggressive behaviour commonly leads to imprisonment, it has been argued that prison population should contain a higher proportion of people with epilepsy than the general population. A methodologically comprehensive survey, carried out on the total population of Iceland, found an overall rate of criminal offences which was three times higher in the epileptic population than in the general community [9]. A prevalence rate of epilepsy of 7.2 per thousand was found by Gunn [155], in a survey of prisoners in England and Wales. Britten *et al.* [13] showed an overall prevalence of epilepsy of about 9.5 per thousand in a recent prospective longitudinal study of a national sample of children born one week in March 1946. This study does not support the view that there is a connection between crime and epilepsy. Their sample showed higher prevalence rates in socioeconomic groups III and IV, suggesting that Gunn's figures [155] show a lower, rather than higher prevalence in the prison population. Gunn's survey [155] has been repeated by Channon [156], using a questionnaire sent to prison doctors. Channon found a prevalence rate similar to Gunn's study, of 7.6 people with epilepsy per 1000 prison population. Higher prevalence rates amongst prison populations have been shown in several studies from the States [157–159], but these studies suffer from the disadvantage that the methods used by prison doctors to detect epilepsy (anticonvulsant medication or examination), may be inaccurate. A methodologically sound study by Whitman *et al.* [160] showed a prevalence of epilepsy amongst prisoners some four times higher than that expected for a similar age group. Whitman *et al.* found a surprisingly high number – almost one-half – of the prisoners with epilepsy had a post-traumatic aetiology. They conclude: 'Thus our prison study, along with other studies of more general populations, indicates that epilepsy is directly related to socioeconomic status. These sociologic factors, rather than any intrinsic relationships between the biologic aspects of epilepsy and aggressiveness, largely explain the high prevalence of epilepsy in prisons.'

18.8.2 Relationship of aggressive behaviour to seizure occurrence and seizure type

Aggression has been more frequently reported in patients with temporal lobe seizures. It is convenient to classify aggressive behaviour into that which occurs during the seizure and postictally and that which is interictal, occurring between seizures in a setting of clear consciousness.

(a) Ictal aggression

There is evidence that episodes of violent behaviour are most likely to occur if there are temporal lobe discharges involving the hippocampus, amygdala and hypothalamus [161–164]. These episodes have the characteristics associated with seizure activity – there is a disorder of consciousness, and the aggressive activity is usually disordered, unco-ordinated, and non-directed. Delgado-Escueta *et al.* [165], in probably the most comprehensive study, studied 5400 videotaped seizures collected from different units throughout the world and rated them according to the degree of ictal violence. They found only 13 cases of violent behaviour, of which most were postictal and in a confusional setting. Only three of them involved a physical attack. They concluded that frank ictal violence is very rare. However, it is perhaps not surprising that Delgado-Escueta and co-workers failed to find ictal aggression in the clinical situation of a videotape recording laboratory. The authors have unfortunately failed to recognize that the form an epileptic seizure takes is dependent not only on the spread of the discharge through the brain, but also on the thought content of the patient at the time of the seizure. There are numerous examples in the literature of the way a patient's intended action is modified by the seizure, supporting the view that aggression is likely to occur to a much greater extent in the community than in the 'protected' environment of hospital.

The same point is made in King and Ajmone Marsan's study [166] of 270 epileptic patients with temporal lobe foci. They observed complex partial seizures in 199 of these patients. Although 20 of these had a history of interictal violent behaviour, fighting, striking people and throwing objects, no such episodes occurred in hospital. However, nine of the 199 patients for whom well observed seizures had been recorded showed violent peri-ictal behaviour that was in most cases postictal and confusional in nature. Rodin [151], who recorded 150 patients with seizures in hospital between 1959 and 1964, makes the same point. None of these patients (with one possible exception) ever showed clear evidence of ictal aggression. Rodin and subsequent workers have suggested that this is because ictal violence is rare, but their finding could at least in part be due to the fact that the recordings were made in hospital. Further evidence is needed which could only be obtained by portable recording devices used at home.

However, few cases of ictal aggression have been described in the literature. This is partly because it has not previously been possible to monitor patients continuously in the community [167], and also because it is difficult to be certain that a particular episode is ictal in origin. A systematic study of the relationship between epileptic automatism and violence found aggressive and violent behaviour in only one patient out of a total of 434 epileptic outpatients [71]. A survey of epileptic offenders in prisons and Borstals (places of custody for young offenders) in England and Wales indicated that probably only two persons out of a total of 158 had committed their crimes during or following a seizure. One was a possible postictal automatism and the other occurred in a postictal state [168–170]. A survey of 29 male epileptics at Broadmoor hospital, a special hospital for violent psychiatric offenders, found a definite relationship between crimes and seizures in only two patients; both had behaved violently in a postictal confusional state. Lewis *et al.* [171], studying 78 violent boys in a reform school, found five had committed violent acts during an ictus. They state: 'Clearly, most violence in this group was not caused by epilepsy but neither was the association (with ictal discharge) exceedingly rare' [167]. Thus although some studies provide only doubtful evidence that direct ictal behaviour is the sole cause for aggressive acts, the evidence supports the conclusion that ictal violence does occur. (For a fuller review see Treiman and Delgado-Escueta [172], Fenwick [173], Fenwick and Fenwick [174].)

(b) Interictal aggression

Many of the studies of interictal aggression fail to provide a clear definition of aggression, or to describe the relationship of the aggressive behaviour to the underlying personality. The only relationship found by Mungus [175], using cluster analysis on data derived from 138 neuropsychiatric outpatients who attended the UCLA Neurobehavioural Clinic, was between seizure disorders and a high frequency of impulsive, violent acts. He found no relationship between temporal lobe abnormalities and aggression. He concluded that violent behaviour was not a unitary syndrome and that seizures were not related to all types of violence.

Stevens and Herman [176] have suggested that when the many non-specific factors related to violent behaviour are taken into account, the associations of aggression and violence with epilepsy become weaker. Violent people tend to come from the lower socioeconomic groups where there are higher levels of perinatal mortality, infections and trauma. There is often a family history of violence, and many have shown episodes of violence since youth. They tend to be males under the age of 40; many show 'soft' neurological signs, abnormal EEGs, and cognitive impairment, occasionally with focal cognitive deficits. A high proportion are left handers, and many have a poor attention span. When these factors are taken into account, many of the associations of aggression and violence with epilepsy become weaker.

A positive association between epilepsy and aggression has been shown by several workers. Nuffield [177] developed an aggression score for 322 children with temporal lobe, petit mal and grand mal epilepsy, classified by use of the EEG, and found that children with temporal lobe epilepsy had aggression scores which were nearly four times those of the patients who had petit mal. Kaufman *et al.* [178] have criticized this work on the grounds that EEG abnormalities tend not to be consistent from recording to recording and that mixed forms of abnormality are usually found. Stevens and Herman [176] have made the further criticism that many of the patients with temporal lobe epilepsy also suffered from grand mal seizures, so that the association found by Nuffield could be with grand mal seizures rather than with temporal lobe epilepsy. Currie *et al.* [33], in a retrospective study of 666 patients with temporal lobe epilepsy attending the London Hospital, showed that only 16 of these patients showed rage attacks, while they describe a further five as having 'violent outbursts'. However, it is difficult to know whether or not there is a raised prevalence of aggression without a control formed from other patients in a neurology clinic. Again no indication is given as to what proportion of these patients suffered from grand mal seizures. A 30-year prospective study of a population of 100 epileptic patients by Lindsay and colleagues [39], reports that 36 had rages in childhood. These rages carried a poor adult prognosis in terms of both social and psychiatric outcome. Overt physical violence was more common in the boys than the girls. This study has often been cited to support a relationship of temporal lobe epilepsy to aggression, but, once again, a large proportion of those who showed violent behaviour also had coexisistent brain damage. Only 12 had pure temporal lobe epilepsy without associated brain damage or grand mal seizures, and none of these had significant psychological problems, or a history of rage outbursts. This again supports the view that non-specific factors unrelated to the temporal lobe epilepsy were involved. Whereas 85% of the original group of children had psychological problems in childhood, 75% of those who survived 15 years were then found to be psychologically normal. It therefore seems probable that the psychiatric morbidity noted in childhood was related to an interaction between the epilepsy and those psychosocial factors which lead to a high prevalence of psychiatric morbidity. Psychiatric morbidity was probably not related to the epilepsy itself, but a multifactorial aetiology is most likely.

In conclusion, although much of the evidence makes it clear that a relationship does exist between aggressive behaviour and epilepsy, methodological difficulties and patient selection weaken the correlations found between interictal aggression and temporal lobe epilepsy. This and two recent reviews of the literature conclude that the most significant factor in the relationship is probably the associated brain damage, but that other non-specific factors which are common in both violent populations and patients with epilepsy are also involved. However, when adequate control groups are used, many of the differences which were apparently significant, disappear [176, 179].

(c) Seizure types

It has already been pointed out that methodological flaws exist in nearly all studies which have compared the prevalence rates of different forms of psychopathology associated with different types of seizures. Recognizing this, Herman *et al.* [180] set up a controlled study using the MMPI to determine whether patients with complex partial seizures alone had more psychopathology than those with complex partial seizures and secondary generalized seizures. The 165 adults in the study consisted of one group with complex partial seizures, and one with generalized seizures and complex partial seizures. Matching took into account a number of variables including age, education, age of onset of seizures, duration of seizures, IQ data and a Halstead Impairment Index (test of brain damage). Herman *et al.* found that the group with multiple seizure types scored more highly in the direction of increased psychopathology than the single seizure group on every measure used in the study. It could be argued that a multiplicity of seizure types correlated with higher degrees of brain damage, and that it was the brain damage which led to the increased rates of psychiatric morbidity. It is of interest that one of the scales that showed the greatest difference between the groups was the psychopathic deviance scale of the MMPI, which is known to be associated with poor impulse control. This study can therefore be interpreted as suggesting that aggressive behaviour may be more common in patients with multiple seizure types.

Herman suggests that this study supports the theory put forward by Stevens and Herman [176] that 'there are a number of factors which increase the risk of psychopathology in individuals with temporal lobe epilepsy. The most powerful factors identified are clinical, EEG, and radiological evidence of bilateral, deep, or diffuse cerebral pathology.'

Stevens [181] has argued that the biochemical systems involved in the deveopment of schizophrenia, pathological violence, paranoia and hallucinations respond to drugs which block the catecholamine system. He writes: 'Catecholamine blockade decreases the threshold for epileptic discharge in every model of epilepsy [182, 183]. In contrast, catecholamine precursors and agonists generally increase seizure thresholds. These facts suggest that the catecholamine system may be part of the brain's natural defence against propagation of epileptic discharge.' This theory provides another link between violent behaviour and epilepsy.

18.8.3 Conclusion

Aggressive behaviour in patients with epilepsy is probably caused by a number of factors. Important amongst these are low socioeconomic status, increased perinatal morbidity, brain damage and infections, all of which are found in excess in populations of people with epilepsy. Psychosocial factors, including the stigma of epilepsy, and the increased dependence and poor social skills of many patients are also likely to be significant. Multiple seizure types and specific lesions within the limbic system can undoubtedly lead to poor impulse control and aggressive outbursts. Aggressive outbursts in a setting of clouding of consciousness can also be produced by the spread of seizure discharges into those brain structures involved with the control of aggression.

However, these outbursts usually occur in relation to specific factors in the environment and are thus seldom seen in a hospital setting. It is certainly extremely rare for a sudden aggressive episode to be due entirely to epilepsy, and the notion that most epileptics are aggressive, impulsive people finds little current support in scientific studies. The association that is found is between poor impulse control and brain damage. It seems probable that brain damage and not the epilepsy is the main common factor.

18.9 THE PRECIPITATION OF SEIZURES – PSYCHOGENIC SEIZURES

The term reflex epilepsy has long been used for the precipitation of seizures by specific stimuli [132, 184]. Symonds [186] preferred the term evoked seizures, and this term should be used in preference to the outmoded term reflex epilepsy, particularly for those epilepsies which have a specific external precipitant (see Chapter 4). In this chapter the term 'psychogenic seizure' is used in the correct sense, to describe true epileptic attacks which can be generated by an act of will or by the mind (psyche) without an external stimulus, e.g. seizures which can be triggered by an act of attention, by thinking or calculating, or by a particular emotion. It does not include pseudoseizures, which are non-epileptic phenomena, and are described on p. 539.

18.9.1 Prevalence

Although their true prevalence is not known, and there has as yet been no comprehensive study of their incidence, psychogenic seizures are probably more common than evoked seizures. Symonds [186] reported an incidence of evoked seizures of 6.5%, Servit *et al.* [187] found an incidence of 5.1%. A survey carried out at the Maudsley Hospital, found that in this special population, the prevalence of psychogenic seizures was nearly four times that of evoked seizures. The true prevalence is probably higher still.

18.9.2 Classification

Psychogenic seizures are described as either primary – those seizures which can be precipitated by a direct act of will, or secondary – those which can be precipitated by a specific functioning of the mind without a deliberate intention on the part of the patient to precipitate a seizure and without a clear evoking peripheral stimulus, [132]. The thinking epilepsies of Ingram and Ryman [188] fall into the latter category.

(a) Primary psychogenic seizures

Primary psychogenic seizures are true epileptic attacks deliberately precipitated by the patient by a direct act of will. The mechanism used by the patient to induce a seizure seems to be the raising of excitability in the area of the epileptogenic focus, so that he enhances the physical sensations or emotional states which experience has taught him can often precipitate an attack. Motor seizures, for example, can be triggered by attending to the motor aura and mimicking precisely the body movements which occur at the beginning of the seizure. Patients with temporal lobe epilepsy and damage to the limbic system will often induce a seizure by enhancing emotions which tend to precipitate an attack. A patient in our clinic, for example, learnt to induce seizures by intensifying feelings of sadness and self-pity. Patients with generalized seizures and no focal discharge may learn to manipulate their attention to precipitate seizures. One patient, who had had generalized epilepsy from early childhood, found that he could precipitate a generalized seizure by lying on his bed and making his mind a blank. Another discovered that he could induce petit mal attacks at will by suddenly swinging his attention to the periphery of his attentional field – a technique he found particularly useful when being scolded by his mother! [132]

(b)   Secondary psychogenic seizures

Secondary psychogenic seizures are not deliberately produced by the patient, but occur because a particular mental process has precipitated epileptic discharge in a specific, damaged, cortical area. Cases have been described of seizures precipitated by simple calculation [188] and by mental arithmetic and other psychological tasks requiring parietal lobe functioning [189]. Other authors have reported seizures specifically related to mental activity [186, 190–195].

18.9.3   Mechanism

The mechanism postulated for the evoked epilepsies is that sensory inputs initiate activity in those areas which are epileptogenic, and so trigger seizure discharge. An extension of this hypothesis has been put forward to explain the mechanism of both primary and secondary psychogenic seizures. It is suggested that specific forms of voluntary or involuntary mental activity are associated with the activation of specific neural circuits. If these circuits are epileptogenic, seizures will be precipitated. If the damaged areas are well localized, very specific activities are required to trigger a seizure [185].

   Wilkins *et al.* [196] has recently extended his proposed mechanism for photogenic seizures to the thinking epilepsies. He suggests a two stage model 'when normal physiological excitations exceed some (slightly variable) limit, paroxysmal disturbance is triggered. When the disturbance exceeds some topographic limit, complete generalization occurs.' This model implies that in the case of both primary and secondary psychogenic seizures, areas of cortex are damaged and so epileptogenic. Mental activity in these areas will evoke abnormal activity and then, if the threshold is exceeded, generalize to a seizure.

18.9.4 Stress as a precipitant of seizures

Many patients with epilepsy report an association between their seizure frequency and various life-events, such as their menstrual cycle (p. 374), and stressful situations. It is not uncommon for patients to report that, when under stress, their seizures increase, and when the stress is removed (for example, when they are on holiday) that their seizure frequency is reduced. It is widely accepted that patients who may be fitting frequently outside hospital, often have a seizure-free honeymoon of two weeks on admission to the hospital. This may be partly due to increased drug compliance, but it cannot be entirely attributed to it. An as yet unpublished study at the Maudsley Hospital of the families of epileptics looked at the relationship between expressed emotion and seizure frequency in families with epileptic members. High expressed emotion (frequent use of emotionally charged words) was found to correlate with higher seizure frequency.

18.10 PSEUDOSEIZURES

A problem often facing those treating epilepsy is the patient whose behaviour might be due to epilepsy, but which is atypical. If a diagnosis of epilepsy is finally excluded in these patients, their behaviour has been variously described as hysteroepilepsy, pseudoseizures, psychogenic seizures and non-epileptic convulsions. The terms hysteroepilepsy, psychogenic seizures and non-epileptic convulsions are ambiguous and so best avoided. Pseudoseizures is the term to be preferred because it is entirely descriptive and does not imply an aetiology or a mechanism.

Pseudoseizures do not usually occur in people who have no experience of epileptic attacks or other disorders of consciousness on which they can model the seizure. It is also usual for patients who have pseudoseizures or other hysterical symptoms to have accompanying disease of the nervous system.

18.10.1 Clinical description

A pseudoseizure can range from apparent minor transient impairments of consciousness to status epilepticus with apparent unconsciousness lasting for several hours. Behaviour during the seizure is usually atypical and non-physiological in some important respect. The sequence of tonic-clonic convulsions during a grand mal pseudoseizure for example is usually either too long, or contains movements which are clearly not epileptic in nature. The patients may move about the floor during the fit, bumping into the furniture in a provocative way. Examination is often resisted, and if examination of the pupils is attempted the patients may screw up their eyes. Although after the pseudoseizure the patients may feel tired and go to sleep, close questioning may show that, even while apparently unconscious, they were aware of what was going on around them. Pseudoseizures tend to respond more to the needs of the moment than to the dictates of physiology. There is often a clear psychological reason as to why a pseudoseizure should occur at a particular time; patients often feel tense and anxious before an attack begins. Some report that they feel much better after an attack, as though it has cleared the air. Seizures seldom occur if the patient is alone, and patients rarely hurt themselves by falling during an attack.

It can be difficult to distinguish small transient pseudoimpairments of consciousness, in their most complex form, from genuine complex partial seizures. Points of distinction are the psychological nature of the prodrome, which is usually related to an increase in tension and anxiety, and the fact that a pseudoseizure usually lasts longer than the few seconds of a genuine partial seizure. Consciousness may be maintained during the seizure and patients often feel tired once the episode is over. The patient's subjective experience can be complex and difficult to differentiate from that of a genuine seizure; tongue biting, urinary or faecal incontinence all occur in pseudoseizures as well as genuine seizures. Pseudoseizures may occur only occasionally or may happen several times a day; their frequency is not modified by drug therapy. Pseudoseizures should be suspected in patients who have frequent seizures which do not respond to medication and who have a normal EEG.

Several different sub-types of pseudoseizures have been described by Gumnit [197].

(1) Misinterpretation of normal physiological stimuli. Here the patient misinterprets a normal physiological event such as palpitations, dizziness, depersonalization, etc. as a seizure episode.
(2) A true aura or seizure is followed by a pseudoseizure.
(3) Manipulation. This refers to overt, conscious manipulation of the environment for unconscious use of seizures as a manipulative technique without major psychopathology.
(4) Outright malingering.
(5) Neurotic conflicts. This is often the group with typical pseudoseizures.
(6) Psychosis. Here the pseudoseizures are a manifestation of a major psychopathology.

18.10.2 Prevalence

There have been few studies of the prevalence of pseudoseizures, but they probably occur relatively frequently. Ljungberg [198] found pseudoseizures in approximately one-third in his sample of patients with hysterical conversion symptoms. Trimble [199] in a study of patients who had the diagnosis of hysteria at the National Hospital in London, reported a frequency of just over

19%. A study of hysteria in Athens suggested that the commonest presenting symptom was pseudoseizures [200].

18.10.3 Differential diagnosis

A detailed history directed towards the minutiae of the behaviour during the 'seizures', together with associated psychiatric symptomatology, will usually distinguish between pseudoseizures and genuine convulsions. Special attention should be paid to the first 'convulsion', as this frequently sets the pattern for subsequent attacks. It is often possible to see the direct effect of psychological factors more easily in the first 'convulsion'. Roy [201, 202], in a study of 22 patients with pseudoseizures and a control group of patients with epilepsy, found five factors which helped distinguish the two groups. They were a family history and past history of psychiatric disorder, sexual maladjustment, attempted suicide and a current affective illness. Conversely Vanderzant *et al.* [202a] found no difference in MMPI scores between those with pseudoseizures and those with generalized seizures.

The most difficult cases should be treated within a unit where trained nursing staff can observe the seizures. Videotape recording with split screen EEG presentation together with 24 hour EEG monitoring, can be helpful, Telemetry and video monitoring were used by Rowan *et al.* [203] who were able to distinguish between epilepsy and pseudoseizures in just over half of their 52 cases. Pseudoseizures and true seizures often exist together [204]. In a group of 52 patients, 42% showed pure pseudoseizures, 30% probable mixed seizures and 28% definitely mixed seizures. Lesser *et al.* [205] report that only five of their 50 patients had both pseudoseizures and true seizures, but this is probably due to different patient selection. Riley and Berndt [206] describe an interesting approach to distinguishing between true and pseudoseizures. They were able to produce pseudoseizures in the EEG recording laboratory by asking the EEG technician to comment on the likelihood of their arising.

Trimble [207] confirmed the previous work done on ECT convulsions and showed a rise in serum prolactin after a spontaneous grand mal seizure, which he found was absent in patients with pseudo grand mal seizures. Trimble therefore suggested that a prolactin level should be taken 20 min after a fit, work which has since been extended using ambulatory monitoring [208, 209]. A rise in prolactin also occurs in complex partial seizures and in simple partial seizures if the seizure discharge spreads to mesial limbic structures [210]. Prolactin rises after both types of seizures are very large and levels below 800 μU/ml are not significant.

18.10.4 Management

A full psychiatric history should first be taken, and pathological factors in the patient's family and life situation detected, so that treatment for any affective disorders or other psychiatric conditions can begin. Anticonvulsant medication should be withdrawn slowly, to avoid withdrawal seizures which might complicate the picture. Tranquillizers or relaxation methods may be helpful if the patient's attacks occur in special situations or in response to anxiety.

The outcome can be good providing support can be given and the patient's life situation modified. However, prolonged psychiatric intervention is necessary in the more severely disturbed cases. Usually the pattern is for the patient to have recurrent admissions to different hospitals with further prescriptions of anticonvulsant medication. It is certainly worthwhile making sure that there is a good liaison between hospitals and general practitioners so that these patients can be protected from themselves. When they appear in hospital casualty departments, or in yet another family doctor's surgery, information should then be available and unnecessary treatment avoided.

18.11 CONCLUSION

This chapter illustrates the difficulty in disentangling those factors which are responsible for the increased psychiatric morbidity in patients with epilepsy. Whether seizures by themselves are a cause of psychiatric pathology is still debatable. The nature and extent of the relationship between psychiatric morbidity and epilepsy has yet to be precisely determined. Brain damage is clearly responsible for many of the changes seen, but also involved are nonspecific factors such as the social stigma of epilepsy, the habitual overprotection by the parents of the child, the increased prevalence of epilepsy in lower socio-economic groups (p. 11) and the cognitive deficits from which patients with epilepsy frequently suffer.

REFERENCES

1. Guerrant, J., Anderson, W. W., Fischer, A. *et al.* (1962) *Personality in Epilepsy*, Charles C. Thomas, Springfield, Ill.
2. Morel, B. A. (1857) *Traite des Degenerescences Physiques, Intellectuelles et Morales de l'Espece Humaine et des Causes qui Produisent ses Varietes Maladaptives*, Vol. 1, Balliere, Paris.
3. Hibbert, C. (1963) *The Roots of Evil*, Weidenfeld and Nicholson, London.
4. Adrian, E. D. and Mathews, B. H. C. (1934) The Berger rhythm: potential changes from the occipital lobes in man. *Brain*, **57**, 355–85.
5. Hill, D. (1981) Historical review, in *Epilepsy and Psychiatry* (eds E. Reynolds and M. Trimble), Churchill Livingstone, Edinburgh, pp. 1–11.
6. Pond, D. and Bidwell, B. (1960) A survey of epilepsy in 14 general practices. II Social and psychological aspects. *Epilepsia*, **1**, 285–99.
7. Liddell, D. W. (1953) Observations on epileptic automatisms in a mental hospital population. *J. Ment. Sci.*, **99**, 732–48.
8. Betts, T. A. (1974) A follow up study of a cohort of patients with epilepsy admitted to psychiatric care in an English city, in *Epilepsy: Proceeding of the Hans*

Berger Centenary Symposium (eds P. Harris and C. Mawdsley), Churchill Livingstone, Edinburgh, p. 326.

9. Gudmundsson, G. (1966) Epilepsy in Iceland: a clinical and epidemiological investigation. *Acta Neurol. Scand.*, **23** (Suppl. 25), 100–14.

10. Helgason, T. (1964) Epidemiology of mental disorders in Iceland. *Acta Psychiatr. Scand.*, **40** (173), 1.

11. Rutter, M., Graham, P. and Yule, W. (1970) A neuropsychiatric study in childhood, in *Clinics in Developmental Medicine*, Nos 35 and 36, Heinemann and Spastics International Medical Publications, London.

12. Harrison, R. M. and Taylor, D. C. (1976) Childhood seizures: a 25-year follow-up. *Lancet*, **i**, 948–51.

13. Britten, N., Wadsworth, M. and Fenwick, P. (1984) Stigma in patients with early epilepsy: a national longitudinal study. *J. Epidemiol. Comm. Health*, **38**, 291–5.

14. Britten, N., Morgan, K., Fenwick, P. and Britten, H. (1986) Epilepsy and handicap from birth to age 36. *Devl Med. Child Neurol.*, **28**, 719–28.

15. Dallos, V. and Heathfield, K. (1969) Iatrogenic epilepsy due to antidepressant drugs. *Br. Med. J.*, **4**, 80–2.

16. Toone, B. K. and Fenton, G. W. (1977) Epileptic seizures induced by psychotropic drugs. *Psychol. Med.*, **7**, 265–70.

17. Edwards, G. (1979) Antidepressants and convulsions. *Lancet*, **ii**, 1368–9.

18. Gastaut, H. (1976) Conclusions: computerised transverse axial tomography in epilepsy. *Epilepsia*, **17**, 325–35.

19. Lennox, W. (1942) Brain injury, drugs and environment as causes of mental decay in epilepsy. *Am. J. Psychiatr.*, **99**, 174–80.

20. Lennox, W. and Lennox, M. (1960) *Epilepsy and Related Disorders*, Vols 1 and 2, Little Brown and Co., Boston.

21. Reitan, R. M. (1974) Psychological testing of epileptic patients, in *The Epilepsies (Handbook of Clinical Neurology Vol. 15)* (eds P. Vinken and G. Bruyn), North Holland Publishing Co., Amsterdam, pp. 559–75.

22. Taylor, D. C. (1972) Mental state and temporal lobe epilepsy. *Epilepsia*, **13**, 727–65.

23. Betts, T. A., Merskey, H. and Pond, D. A. (1976) Psychiatry, in *A Textbook of Epilepsy* 1st Edition (eds J. Laidlaw and A. Richens), Churchill Livingstone, Edinburgh, pp. 145–184.

24. Scott, D., Moffat, A., Mathews, A. and Ettlinger, G. (1967) The effect of the epileptic discharges on learning and memory in patients. *Epilepsia*, **8**, 188–94.

25. Rutter, M., Tizard, J., Yule, W. *et al.* (1976) Research Reports IOW Studies, 1964–1974. *Psychol. Med.*, **6(2)**, 313–32.

26. Fedio, P. and Mirsky, A. F. (1969) Selective intellectual defects in children with temporal lobe or centrencephalic epilepsy. *Neuropsychologia*, **7**, 287–300.

27. Delaney, R., Rosen, A., Mattson, R. and Novelly, R. (1980) Memory function in focal epilepsy: a comparison of non-surgical, unilateral temporal lobe and frontal lobe sample. *Cortex*, **16(1)**, 103–17.

28. Glowinski, H. (1973) Cognitive deficits in temporal lobe epilepsy. An investigation of memory functioning. *J. Nerv. Ment. Dis.*, **157**, 129–37.

29. Milberg, W., Greiffenstein, M., Lewis, R. and Rourke, D. (1980) Differentiation of temporal lobe and generalised seizure patients with the WAIS. *J. Consult. Clin. Psychol.*, **48(1)**, 39–42.

30. Fenwick, P. (1981) EEG studies, in *Epilepsy and Psychiatry* (eds E. Reynolds and M. Trimble), Churchill Livingstone, Edinburgh, Chap. 18.
31. Stevens, J. R. (1966) Psychiatric implications of psychomotor epilepsy. *Arch. Gen. Psychiatr.*, **14**, 461–71.
32. Stevens, J. R. (1975) Interictal clinical manifestations of complex partial seizures. *Adv. Neurol.*, **11**, 85–107.
33. Currie, S., Heathfield, W., Henson, R. and Scott, D. (1971) Clinical course and prognosis of temporal lobe epilepsy: a survey of 666 patients. *Brain*, **94**, 173–90.
34. Rodin, E. A., Katz, M. and Lennox, K. (1976) Differences between patients with temporal lobe seizures and those with other forms of epileptic attacks. *Epilepsia*, **17**, 313–20.
35. Trimble, M. and Perez, M. (1980) The phenomenology of the chronic psychoses of epilepsy. *Adv. Biol. Psychiatr.*, **8**, 98–105.
36. Taylor, D. (1981) Brain lesions, surgery, seizures, and mental symptoms, in *Epilepsy and Psychiatry* (eds E. Reynolds and M. Trimble), Churchill Livingstone, Edinburgh, pp. 227–41.
37. Taylor, D. C. (1985) Psychological aspects of chronic sickness, in *Child and Adolescent Psychiatry: Modern Approaches* (eds M. Rutter and L. Hersov), Blackwell Scientific Publications, Oxford, Chap. 38, pp. 614–24.
38. Stores, G. (1978) Schoolchildren with epilepsy at risk for learning and behaviour problems. *Devl Med. Child Neurol.*, **20**, 502–8.
39. Lindsay, J., Ounsted, C. and Richards, P. (1979) Long-term outcome in children with temporal lobe seizures. (3) Psychiatric aspects in childhood and adult life. *Devl Med. Child Neurol.*, **21**, 630–6.
40. Sillanpää, M. (1973) Medico-social prognosis of children with epilepsy. *Acta Paediatr. Scand.*, (Suppl. 237), 3–104.
41. Mulder, H. C. and Suurmeijer, T. P. B. M. (1977) Families with a child with epilepsy: a sociological contribution. *J. Biosoc. Sci.*, **9**, 13–24.
42. Mattsson, A. (1972) Long-term physical illness in childhood: a challenge to psychosocial adaptation. *Paediatrics*, **50**, 801–11.
43. Hartledge, L. C. and Green, J. B. (1972) The relationship of parental attitudes to academic and social achievement in epileptic children. *Epilepsia*, **13**, 21–6.
44. Tizzard, B. (1962) The personality of epileptics: a discussion of the evidence. *Psychol. Bull.*, **59**, 196–210.
45. Lishman, W. A. (1978) *Organic Psychiatry*, Blackwell Scientific Publications, London.
46. Scott, D. (1978) Psychiatric aspects of epilepsy. *Br. J. Psychiatr.*, **132**, 417–30.
47. Gibbs, F. A. (1951) Ictal and non-ictal psychiatric disorders in temporal lobe epilepsy. *J. Nerv. Ment. Dis.*, **113**, 522–8.
48. Gastaut, H. and Collomb, H. (1954) Etude du comportement sexuel chez les epileptiques psychomoteurs. *Ann. Medico-Psychol.*, **2**, 657–96.
49. Waxman, S. G. and Geschwind, N. (1975) The interictal behaviour syndrome of temporal lobe epilepsy. *Arch. Gen. Psychiatr.*, **32**, 1580–6.
50. Geschwind, N. (1979) Behavioural changes in temporal lobe epilepsy. *Psychol. Med.*, **9**, 217–19.
51. Bear, D. (1979) Temporal lobe epilepsy – a syndrome of sensory limbic hypoconnection. *Cortex*, **15**, 357–84.

52. Bear, D. and Fedio, P. (1977) Quantitative analysis of inter-ictal behaviour in temporal lobe epilepsy. *Arch. Neurol.*, **34**, 454–67.
53. Kluver, H. and Bucy, P. (1939) Preliminary analysis of functions of the temporal lobe in man. *Arch. Neurol. Psychiatr.*, **42**, 979–1000.
54. Herman, B. P. and Riel, P. (1981) Interictal personality and behavioural traits in temporal lobe and generalised epilepsy. *Cortex*, **17**, 125–8.
55. Mungus, D. (1982) Interictal behaviour abnormality in temporal lobe epilepsy. *Arch. Gen. Psychiatr.*, **39**, 108–11.
56. Bear, D., Levin, K., Bloomer, D. *et al.* (1982) Interictal behaviour in hospitalised temporal lobe epileptics: relationship to idiopathic psychiatric syndromes. *J. Neurol. Neurosurg. Psychiatr.*, **45**, 481–8.
57. Sensky, T. and Fenwick, P. (1982) Religiosity, mystical experience and epilepsy, in *Progress in Epilepsy* (ed. F. C. Rose), Pitman, London, pp. 214–20.
58. Stevens, J. R. and Herman, B. P. (1981) Temporal lobe epilepsy. Psychopathology and violence: the state of the evidence. *Neurology* (NY), **31**, 1127–32.
59. Pond, D. A. (1957) Psychiatric aspects of epilepsy. *J. Ind. Med. Prof.*, **3**, 1441–51.
60. Fenton, G. W. (1981) Psychiatric disorder of epilepsy: classification and phenomenology, in *Epilepsy and Psychiatry* (eds E. H. Reynolds and M. R. Trimble), Churchill Livingstone, Edinburgh, Chap. 2.
61. Gastaut, H. (1964) Proposed international classification of epileptic seizures. *Epilepsia*, **5**, 297–306.
62. Gastaut, H. (1973) *Dictionary of Epilepsy*, World Health Organisation, Geneva.
63. Gowers, W. R. (1881) *Epilepsy and Other Chronic Convulsive Disorders*, Churchill, London.
64. Lennox, W. (1960) *Epilepsy and Related Disorders*, Vols 1 and 2, Churchill, London.
65. Cirignotta, F., Todesco, C. and Lugaresi, E. (1980) Dostoievskian epilepsy. *Epilepsia*, **21**, 705–10.
66. Fenwick, P. (1983) Some aspects of the physiology of the mystical experience, in *Psychology Survey*, No. 4 (eds J. Nicholson and V. Foss), British Psychological Society, Leicester, Chap. 8.
67. Fenton, G. W. (1972) Epilepsy and automatism. *Br. J. Hosp. Med.*, **7**, 57–64.
68. Jasper, H. (1964) Some physiological mechanisms involved in epileptic automatism. *Epilepsia*, **5**, 1–20.
69. Geier, S., Bancaud, J., Talairach, J. *et al.* (1976) Automatisms during frontal lobe epileptic seizures. *Brain*, **99**, 447–58.
70. Geier, S., Bancaud, J., Talairach, J. *et al.* (1977) The seizures of frontal lobe epilepsy. *Neurology*, **27**, 951–8.
71. Knox, S. (1968) Epileptic automatisms and violence. *Med. Sci. Law*, **8**, 96–104.
72. Forster, P. M. and Liske, E. (1963) Role of environmental clues in temporal lobe epilepsy. *Neurology (Minneap.)*, **13**, 301–5.
73. Rennick, M., Perez-Borja, C. and Rodin, E. A. (1969) Transient mental deficits associated with current prolonged epileptic clouded state. *Epilepsia*, **10**, 397–405.
74. Roger, J., Lob, H. and Tassinari, C. A. (1974) *Status Epilepticus* (*Handbook of Clinical Neurology*, Vol. 15) (eds P. J. Vinken and G. W. Bruyn), North Holland Publishing Co., Amsterdam and Elsevier Publishing Co., New York.
75. Dalby, M. A. (1969) Epilepsy and three per second spike and wave rhythms. A

clinical electroencephalographic and prognostic analysis of 346 patients *Acta Neurol. Scand.*, (Suppl. 40), **45**, 1–183.

76. Lennox, W. (1945) The treatment of epilepsy. *Med. Clin. N. Am.*, **29**, 1114–28.
77. Zappoli, R. (1955) Two cases of prolonged epileptic twilight state with almost continuous 'wave-spikes'. *Electroenceph. Clin. Neurophysiol.*, **7**, 421–3.
78. Neidermeyer, E. and Khalifeh, R. (1965) Petit mal status ('spike-wave stupor'): An electro-clinical appraisal. *Epilepsia*, **6**, 250–62.
79. Bruens, J. H. (1974) Psychosis in epilepsy, in *The Epilepsies* (*Handbook of Clinical Neurology*, Vol. 15) (eds P. J. Vinken and G. W. Bruyn), North Holland Publishing Co., Amsterdam and Elsevier Publishing Co., New York.
80. Lugaresi, E., Pazzaglia, P. and Tassinari, C. A. (1971) Differentiation of 'absence status' and 'temporal lobe status'. *Epilepsia*, **12**, 77–87.
81. Schwartz, M. S. and Scott, D. (1971) Isolated petit mal status presenting de novo in middle age. *Lancet*, **ii**, 1399–401.
82. Wells, C. E. (1975) Transient ictal psychosis. *Arch. Gen. Psychiatr.*, **32**, 1201–3.
83. Ellis, J. M. and Lee, S. I. (1978) Acute prolonged confusion in later life as an ictal state. *Epilepsia*, **19**, 119–28.
84. Delgado-Escueta, A. V., Boxley, J., Stubbs, N. *et al.* (1974) Prolonged twilight state and automatisms. A case report. *Neurology*, **24**, 331–9.
85. Markand, O. N., Wheeler, G. and Pollak, S. (1978) Complex partial status epilepticus (psychomotor status). *Neurology*, **28**, 189–96.
86. Clark, R. A. and Lesko, J. M. (1939) Psychoses associated with epilepsy. *Am. J. Psychiatr.*, **96**, 595–607.
87. Levin, S. (1952) Epileptic clouded states. *J. Nerv. Ment. Dis.*, **116**, 214–25.
88. Slater, E., Beard, A. W. and Clithero, E. (1963) The schizophrenia-like psychoses of epilepsy. *Br. J. Psychiatr.*, **109**, 95–150.
89. Krohn, W. (1960) Study of epilepsy in Northern Norway: its frequency and character. *Acta Psychiatr. Neurol. Scand.*, **Suppl. 150**, 215–25.
90. Alving, J. (1978) Classification of the epilepsies. An investigation of 1508 consecutive adult patients. *Acta Neurol. Scand.*, **58**, 205–12.
91. Small, J. G. and Small, I. F. (1967) A controlled study of mental disorders associated with epilepsy. *Rec. Adv. Biol. Psychiatr.*, **9**, 171–81.
92. Standage, K. F. and Fenton, G. W. (1975) Psychiatric symptom profiles of patients with epilepsy. A controlled investigation. *Psychol. Med.*, **5**, 152–60.
93. Stevens, J. R. (1983) Prevalence of psychosis in temporal lobe epilepsy. *Arch. Neurol.* (Chicago), **4**, 773.
94. Mann, S. and Cree, W. (1976) 'New' long-stay psychiatric patients: a national sample survey of 15 mental hospitals in England and Wales. 1972/73. *Psychol. Med.*, **6**, 603–16.
95. Falconer, M. (1973) Reversibility by temporal lobe resection of the behavioural abnormalities of temporal lobe epilepsy. *N. Engl. J. Med.*, **289**, 451–5.
96. Stevens, J. R. (1980) Biological background of psychoses in epilepsy, in *Advances in Epileptology*, XIth Epilepsy International Symposium (eds R. Canger, F. Angeleri and J. K. Penry), Raven Press, New York, pp. 167–72.
97. Jenssen, I. and Larsen, J. K. (1979) Mental aspects of temporal lobe epilepsy. *J. Neurol. Neurosurg. Psychiatr.*, **42**, 256–65.
98. Flor-Henry, P. (1969) Psychosis and temporal lobe epilepsy. *Epilepsia*, **10**, 363–95.

99. Bruens, J. H. (1971) Psychosis in epilepsy. *Psychiatr. Neurol. Neurochirurg.*, **74**, 174–92.

100. Toone, B. K. (1981) Psychoses of epilepsy, in *Epilepsy and Psychiatry* (eds E. H. Reynolds and M. R. Trimble), Churchill Livingstone, Edinburgh, Chap. 10, pp. 113–37.

101. Slater, E. and Moran, P. (1969) The schizophrenia-like psychoses of epilepsy: relation between ages of onset. *Br. J. Psychiatr.*, **115**, 599–600.

102. Hill, D. (1953) Psychiatric disorders of epilepsy. *Med. Press*, **229**, 473–5.

103. Perez, M. and Trimble, M. (1980) Epileptic psychosis – diagnostic comparison with process schizophrenia. *Br. J. Psychiatr.*, **137**, 245–9.

104. Toone, B., Garralda, M. and Ron, M. (1982) The psychosis of epilepsy and the functional psychoses. A clinical and phenomenological comparison. *Br. J. Psychiatr.*, **141**, 256–61.

105. Perez, M., Trimble, M., Murray, M. and Reider, I. (1985) Epileptic psychosis: an evaluation of PSE profiles. *Br. J. Psychiatr.*, **146**, 155–63.

106. Small, J. G., Milstein, V. and Stevens, J. R. (1962) Are psychomotor epileptics different? *Arch. Neurol.*, **7**, 187–94.

107. Kristensen, O. and Sindrup, E. H. (1978) Psychomotor epilepsy and psychosis. 1. Physical aspects. *Acta Neurol. Scand.*, **57**, 361–9.

108. Herman, B. P. and Shabrias, S. (1982) Interictal psychopathology in patients with ictal fear: a quantitative investigation. *Neurology*, **32**, 7–11.

109. Taylor, D. C. (1975) Factors influencing the occurrence of schizophrenia-like psychoses in patients with temporal lobe epilepsy. *Psychol. Med.*, **5**, 249–54.

110. Gallhofer, B., Trimble, M., Frackowiak, R. *et al.* (1985) A study of cerebral blood flow and metabolism in epileptic psychosis using positron emission tomography and oxygen. *J. Neurol. Neurosurg. Psychiatr.*, **48**, 201–96.

111. Ramani, V. and Gumnit, R. (1982) Intensive monitoring of interictal psychoses in epilepsy. *Arch. Neurol.*, **11**, 613–22.

112. Sherwin, I. (1977) Clinical and EEG aspects of temporal lobe epilepsy with behaviour disorder. The role of cerebral dominance, in *McLean Hospital Journal, Special Issue* (eds D. Blumer and K. Levin), p. 40.

113. Toone, B. K. and Driver, M. V. (1980) Psychosis and epilepsy. *Res. Clin. Forum. 2*, **2**, 121–7.

114. Landolt, H. (1953) Some clinical electroencephalographical correlates in epileptic psychoses (twilight states) *Proc. Electroenceph. Clin. Neurophysiol.*, **5**, 121.

115. Landolt, H. (1955) Uber verstimmungen dammerzostande und schizophrene zustanbidder bie epilepsie. *Schweiz Arch. Neurol. Psychiatr.*, **76**, 313.

116. Landolt, H. (1956) L'electroencephalographie dans les psychoses epileptiques et les episodes schizophrenique. *Rev. Neurol.* **95**, 597–9.

117. Landolt, H. (1958) Serial EEG investigations during psychotic episodes in epileptic patients during schizophrenic attacks, in *Lectures on Epilepsy* (ed. A. M. Lorentz de Haas), Elsevier, Amsterdam, pp. 91–133.

118. Glaser, G. H. (1964) The problem of psychosis in psychomotor temporal lobe epileptics. *Epilepsia*, **5**, 271–8.

119. Reynolds, E. (1981) Biological factors in psychological disorders associated with epilepsy, in *Epilepsy and Psychiatry* (eds E. Reynolds and M. Trimble), Churchill Livingstone, Edinburgh, pp. 264–90.

120. Lewis, A. (1934) Melancholia: a historical review. *J. Ment. Sci.*, **80**, 1–42.

121. Robertson, M. and Trimble, M. (1983) Depressive illness in patients with epilepsy: a review. *Epilepsia*, **24**, 5109–16.
122. Mendez, M. F., Cummings, J. L. and Benson, F. (1986) Depression in epilepsy. *Arch. Neurol.*, **43**, 766–70.
123. Mignone, R., Donnelly, E. and Sadowsky, D. (1970) Psychological and neurological comparisons of psychomotor and non psychomotor epileptic patients. *Epilepsia*, **11**, 345–59.
124. Rodin, E., Rhodes, R. and Velarde, N. (1965) The prognosis for patients with epilepsy. *J. Occupat. Med.*, **7**, 560–3.
125. Dickman, S., Herman, B., Wilensky, A. and Rainwater, G. (1983) Validity of the Minnesota Multiphasic Personality Inventory (MMPI) to psychopathology in patients with epilepsy. *J. Nerv. Ment. Dis.*, **171**, 114–22.
126. Robertson, M. (1986) *Ictal and Inter-ictal Depression in Patients with Epilepsy*, Author's address, National Hospital, Queen Square, London, (in preparation).
127. Kogeorgos, J., Fonagy, P. and Scott, D. F. (1982) Psychiatric symptom patterns of chronic epileptics attending a neurological clinic: a controlled investigation. *Br. J. Psychiatr.*, **140**, 236–43.
128. Barraclough, B. (1981) Suicide and epilepsy, in *Epilepsy and Psychiatry* (eds E. H. Reynolds and M. R. Trimble), Churchill Livingstone, Edinburgh, Chap. 7, pp. 72–76.
129. Betts, T. A. (1981) Psychiatry and epilepsy, in *A Textbook of Psychiatry*, 2nd edn, (eds J. Laidlaw and A. Richens), Churchill Livingstone, Edinburgh, Chap. 6, pp. 227–81.
130. Robertson, M. and Trimble, M. (1985) Treatment of depression in patients with epilepsy. A double-blind trial. *J. Affect. Dis.*, **9**, 127–36.
131. Mostofsky, D. I. and Balaschak, B. A. (1977) Psychobiological control of seizures. *Psychol. Bull.*, **84(4)**, 723–59.
132. Fenwick, P. (1981) Precipitation and inhibition of seizures, in *Epilepsy and Psychiatry* (eds E. Reynolds and M. Trimble), Churchill Livingstone, Edinburgh, Chap. 22.
133. Gardner, J. (1967) Behaviour therapy treatment approach to a psychogenic seizure case. *J. Consult. Psychol.*, **31**, 209–12.
134. Wright, L. (1973) Aversive conditioning of self-induced seizures. *Behav. Ther.*, **4**, 712–13.
135. Ince, L. P. (1976) The use of relaxation training and a conditioned stimulus in the illumination of epileptic seizures in a child: a case study. *J. Behav. Ther. Expl Psychiatr.*, **7**, 39–42.
136. Mostofsky, D. I. (1975) Teaching the nervous system. *NY Univ. Educ. Quart.*, **Spring**, 8–13.
137. Standage, K. F. (1972) Treatment of epilepsy by reciprocal inhibition of anxiety. *Guy's Hosp. Rep.*, **121**, 217–19.
138. Parrino, J. (1971) Reduction of seizures by desensitization. *J. Behav. Ther. Expl Psychiatr.*, **2**, 215–18.
139. Pinto, R. (1972) A case of movement epilepsy with agaraphobia treated successfully by flooding. *Br. J. Psychiatr.*, **121**, 287–8.
140. Scott, D. (1978) Psychiatric aspects of sexual medicine, in *Epilepsy '78*, British Epilepsy Association, Wokingham, England, pp. 89–97.

141. Hooshmand, J. and Brawley, B. (1969) Temporal lobe seizures and exhibitionism. *Neurology*, **19**, 1119–24.

142. Mitchell, W., Faulkner, M. A. and Hill, D. (1954) Epilepsy with fetishism relieved by temporal lobectomy. *Lancet*, **ii**, 626–30.

143. Toone, B. K., Wheeler, M. and Fenwick, P. (1980) Sex hormone changes in male epileptics. *Clin. Endocrinol.*, **12**, 391–5.

144. Toone, B., Fenwick, P., Ededeh, J. *et al.* (1983) Sex hormones, sexual activity and plasma anticonvulsant levels in male epileptics. *J. Neurol. Neurosurg. Psychiatr.*, **46**, 824–6.

145. Fenwick, P., Mercer, S., Grant, R. *et al.* (1985) The relationship of nocturnal penile tumescence and serum testosterone levels in patients with epilepsy. *Arch. Sex. Behav.*, **15**, 13–21.

146. Dana-Haerai, J., Oxley, J. and Richens, A. (1982) Reduction of free testosterone by anti-epileptic drugs. *Br. Med. J.*, **284**, 85–6.

146a. Herzog, A. G., Seibel, M. M., Schomer, D. L. *et al.* (1986) Reproductive endocrine disorders in men with partial seizures of temporal lobe origin. *Arch. Neurol.*, **43**, 347–50.

147. Daniels, O., Fenwick, P., Lelliott, P. *et al.* (1984) Sex hormone replacement therapy in male epileptics, in *Advances in Epileptology: XVth Epilepsy International Symposium* (eds R. J. Porter and A. A. Ward), Raven Press, New York, pp. 291–96.

148. Christiansen, P., Deigaard, J. and Lund, M. (1975) Potens, Fertilitet, og Kønhormonudskillelse hos yngre mandlige epilepsilidonde. *Ugeskr. Laeger.*, **137**(41), 2402–5. (Eng. Abstr.).

148a. Herzog, A. G., Seibel, M. M., Schomer, D. L. *et al.* (1986) Reproductive endocrine disorders in women with partial seizures of temporal lobe origin. *Arch. Neurol.*, **43**, 341–46.

149. Whitman, S., Colman, T., Borg, B. *et al.* (1980) Epidemiological insights into the socioeconomic correlates of epilepsy, in *A Multidisciplinary Handbook of Epilepsy* (ed. B. Herman), Charles C. Thomas, Springfield, Ill., pp. 243–71.

150. Gastaut, H., Morrin, G. and Lesevre, N. (1955) Etudes du comportement des epileptiques psychomoteur dans l'interval de leurs crises. *Ann. Med. Psychol.*, **113**, 1–29.

151. Rodin, E. (1973) Psychomotor epilepsy and aggressive behaviour. *Arch. Gen. Psychiatr.*, **28**, 210–13.

152. Bingley, T. (1958) Mental symptoms in temporal lobe epilepsy and temporal lobe gliomas with special reference to laterality of lesion and the relationship between handedness and brainedness. *Acta Psychiatr. Scand.*, **33** (Suppl. 120), 1–151.

153. Serafetidines, E. (1965) Aggressiveness and temporal lobe epilepsy and its relationship to cerebral dysfunction and environmental factors. *Epilepsia*, **6**, 33–7.

154. Taylor, D. (1969) Aggression and epilepsy. *J. Psychosomat. Res.*, **13**, 229–36.

155. Gunn, J. (1977) *Epileptics in Prison*, Academic Press, London.

156. Channon, S. (1982) The resettlement of epileptic offenders, in *Abnormal Offenders, Delinquency, and the Criminal Justice System*, Vol. 1 (eds J. Gunn and D. P. Farrington) (*Current Research in Forensic Psychiatry and Psychology*), John Wiley and Sons, Chichester, pp. 339–73.

157. King, D. and Young, Q. (1978) Increased prevalence of seizure disorders among prisoners. *JAMA*, **239**, 2674–5.

158. Derro, R. (1978) Admission health evaluation of a city-county workhouse. *Minnesot. Med.*, **61**, 333–7.
159. Norvik, L., Dellapenna, R., Schwartz, M. *et al.* (1977) Health status of the New York city prison population. *Med. Care*, **15**, 205–17.
160. Whitman, S., Coleman, T. E., Patman, C. *et al.* (1984) Epilepsy in prison: elevated prevalence and no relationship to violence. *Neurology (NY)*, **34**, 775–82.
161. Heath, R. (1963) Electrical self-stimulation of the brain in man. *Am. J. Psychiatr.*, **120**, 571–7.
162. Heath, R. and Mickle, W. (1960) Evaluation of seven years' experience with depth electrode studies in human patients, in *Electrical Studies of the Unanaesthetised Brain* (eds E. Ramey and D. O'Doherty), Paul B. Hober, New York, pp. 214–47.
163. Mark, V. and Ervin, F. (1970) *Violence and the Brain*, Harper and Row, New York.
164. Wieser, H. (1983) Depth recorded limbic seizures in psychopathology. *Neurosci. Behav. Rev.*, **7(3)**, 427–40.
165. Delgado-Escueta, A., Mattson, R. and King, L. (1981) The nature of aggression during epileptic seizures. *N. Engl. J. Med.* **305**, 711–16.
166. King, D. and Ajmone Marsan, C. (1977) Clinical features and ictal patterns in epileptic patients with EEG temporal lobe foci. *Ann. Neurol.*, **2**, 138–47.
167. Lewis, D. and Pincus, J. (1983) Psychomotor epilepsy and violence. *Am. J. Psychiatr.*, **140**, 646–8.
168. Gunn, J. (1979) Forensic psychiatry, in *Recent Advances in Clinical Psychiatry* (ed. K. Granville-Grossman), Churchill Livingstone, Edinburgh, pp. 271–95.
169. Gunn, J. and Fenton, G. (1969) Epilepsy in prisons. A diagnostic survey. *Br. Med. J.*, **4**, 326–8.
170. Gunn, J. and Fenton, G. (1971) Epilepsy, automatism and crime. *Lancet*, **i**, 1173–6.
171. Lewis, D., Pincus, J., Shanok, S. and Glaser, G. (1982) Psychomotor epilepsy and violence in a group of incarcerated adolescent boys. *Am. J. Psychiatr.*, **139**, 882–7.
172. Treiman, D. and Delgado-Escueta, A. (1983) Violence and epilepsy: a critical review, in *Recent Advances in Epilepsy, Vol. 1* (eds T. Pedley and B. Meldrum), Churchill Livingstone, Edinburgh, pp. 179–210.
173. Fenwick, P. (1986) Epilepsy and aggression, in *Psychiatric Disorders of Epilepsy* (eds T. Bolwig and M. Trimble), John Wiley, Chichester, pp. 31–60.
174. Fenwick, P. and Fenwick, E. (eds) (1985) *Epilepsy and the Law – A Medical Symposium on the Current Law (International Congress and Symposium Series*, No. 81) The Royal Society of Medicine, London.
175. Mungus, D. (1983) An empirical analysis of specific syndromes of violent behaviour. *J. Nerv. Ment. Dis.*, **171**, 354–61.
176. Stevens, J. R. and Herman, B. (1981) Temporal lobe epilepsy, psychopathology and violence: the state of the evidence. *Neurology (NY)*, **31**, 1127–32.
177. Nuffield, E. (1961) Neurophysiology and behaviour disorders in epileptic children. *J. Ment. Sci.*, **107**, 438–58.
178. Kaufman, K., Harris, R. and Shaffer, D. (1980) Problems in the categorization of child and adolescent EEGs. *J. Child Psychol. Psychiatr.*, **21**, 333–42.
179. Kligman, D. and Goldberg, D. T. (1975) Temporal lobe epilepsy and aggression. *J. Nerv. Ment. Dis.*, **160**, 324–41.
180. Herman, B. P., Dikmen, S., Schwartz, M. S. and Karnes, W. E. (1982) Interictal

psychopathology in patients with ictal fear: a quantitative investigation. *Neurology*, **32**, 7–11.

181. Stevens, J. R. (1977) All that spikes is not fits, in *Psychopathology and Brain Dysfunction* (eds C. Shagass, S. Gershon and A. Friedhoff), Raven Press, New York, pp. 183–98.

182. Corcoran, M., Fibiger, H., McCoughran, J. *et al.* (1974) Potentiation of amygdaloid kindling and metrazol induced seizures by 6-hydroxydopamine. *Expl Neurol.*, **45**, 118–33.

183. Browning, R. and Symondton, R. (1978) Antagonism of the anticonvulsant action of phenytoin, phenobarbital and acetazolamide by 6-hydroxydopamine. *Life Sci.*, **22**, 10.

184. Merlis, J. K. (1974) Reflex epilepsy, in *The Epilepsies (Handbook of Clinical Neurology, Vol. 15)* (eds P. Vinker and G. Bruyn), North–Holland Publishing Co., Amsterdam, pp. 440–56.

186. Symonds, C. (1959) Excitation and inhibition in epilepsy. *Brain* **82(2)**, 133–46.

187. Servit, Z., Macher, J., Stercova, A. *et al.* (1962) Reflex influences in the pathogenesis of epilepsy in the light of clinical statistics. *Epilepsia*, **3**, 315–22.

188. Ingram, A. and Ryman, H. (1962) Epilepsia arithmetica. *Neurology (Minneapol.)*, **12**, 282–7.

189. Wilkins, A., Zifkin, B., Anderman, F. and McGovern (1981) Seizures induced by thinking. *Ann. Neurol.* **11**, 608–12.

190. Bingel, A. (1957) Reading epilepsy. *Neurology*, **7**, 752–6.

191. Gomez, G. and Delgado-Escueta, A. V. (1977) In *Reflex Epilepsy, Behavioural Therapy and Conditional Reflexes* (ed. F. Forster), Charles C. Thomas, Springfield, Ill.

192. Ch'en, H., Ch'in, C. and Ch'u, C. (1965) Chess epilepsy and card epilepsy. *Chin. Med. J.*, **84**, 470–4.

193. Forster, F. M., Richards, J. F., Panitch, H. S. *et al.* (1975) Reflex epilepsy evoked by decision making. *Arch. Neurol.*, **32**, 54–6.

194. Forster, F. (ed.) (1977) In *Reflex Epilepsy, Behavioural Therapy and Conditional Reflexes*, Charles C. Thomas, Springfield, Ill., p. 318.

195. Cirignotta, F., Cicogna, P. and Lugaresi, E. (1980) Epileptic seizures during card games and drafts. *Epilepsia*, **21**, 137–40.

196. Wilkins, A. J., Binnie, C. D. and Darby, C. E. (1980) Visually induced seizures, *Prog. Neurobiol.*, **15**, 85–117.

197. Gumnit, R. (1985) Behaviour disorders related to epilepsy, in Long Term Monitoring and Epilepsy. *Electroenceph. Clin. Neurophysiol.*, **Suppl. 37**, 313–23.

198. Ljungberg, L. (1957) Hysteria: a clinical, prognostic and genetic study. *Acta Psychiatr. Scand.*, (Suppl. 112), pp. 1–162.

199. Trimble, M. (1981) Antidepressant drugs at the seizure threshold, in *Advances in Epileptology: XIIth Epilepsy International Symposium* (eds M. Dam, L. Gram and J. K. Penry), Raven Press, New York, pp. 51–7.

200. Stephanis, C., Markidis, M. and Christodoulou, G. (1976) Observations on the evolution of a hysterical symptomatology. *Br. J. Psychiatr.*, **128**, 269–75.

201. Roy, A. (1977) Hysterical fits previously diagnosed as epilepsy. *Psychol. Med.*, **7**, 271–3.

202. Roy, A. (1979) Hysterical seizures. *Arch. Neurol.* **36**, 447.

202a. Vanderzant, C. W., Giordani, B., Bereut, S. *et al.* (1986) Personality of patients with pseudoseizures. *Neurology*, **36**, 664–68.

203. Rowan, A., Binnie, C., Overweg, J. *et al.* (1980) The value of prolonged EEG/video monitoring as a routine diagnostic procedure in epilepsy, in *Advances in Epileptology: XIth Epilepsy International Symposium* (eds R. Canger, F. Angeleri and J. K. Penry), Raven Press, New York, pp. 139–42.

204. Gates, J., Ramani, V. and Whalen, S. (1982) *Ictal Characteristics of Pseudoseizures*, Abstracts, American Epilepsy Society Meeting, Phoenix, Az.

205. Lesser, R., Lueders, H. and Dinner, D. (1983) Evidence for epilepsy is rare in patients with psychogenic seizures. *Neurology (Minneap.)*, **33**, 502–4.

206. Riley, T. and Berndt, T. (1980) The role of the EEG technologist in delineating pseudo-seizures. *Am. J. EEG Technol.*, **20**, 89–96.

207. Trimble, M. (1978) Non-monoamine oxidase inhibitor antidepressants and epilepsy: a review. *Epilepsia*, **19**, 241–50.

208. Oxley, J., Roberts, M., Danahaeri, J. and Trimble, M. (1980) Evaluation of prolonged four channel EEG taped recordings and serum prolactin levels in the diagnosis of epileptic and non-epileptic fits, in *Advances in Epileptology: XIIth Epilepsy International Symposium* (eds M. Dam, L. Cram and J. K. Penry), Raven Press, New York, pp. 343–55.

209. Trimble, M. and Perez, M. (1982) The phenomenology of the chronic psychoses of epilepsy, in *Temporal Lobe Epilepsy, Mania, Schizophrenia and the Limbic System* (eds W. Koella and M. Trimble), Karger, Basel, pp. 98–105.

210. Sperling, M. R., Pritchard, P. B., Engel, J. *et al.* (1986) Prolactin in partial epilepsy: an indicator of limbic seizures. *Ann. Neurol.*, **20**, 716–22.

CHAPTER NINETEEN

Epilepsy and the Law

Peter Fenwick

Epilepsy, throughout its history, has inspired fear and derision in those witnessing an attack. Ignorance, superstition and misunderstanding have not only been present in the common people, but also in the patricians and law-makers. For epileptics, the law has always been restrictive. Temkin quotes the Babylonian code of Hammurabi, in approximately 2000 BC, as protecting the interests of slave buyers against the possibility of a slave developing epilepsy within a month of purchase. The vendor was required to give a money-back guarantee in the case of a slave developing bennu (epilepsy) within a month of purchase [1].

Gunn, in his introduction to an article on the medicolegal aspects of epilepsy, gives a historical background to legal discrimination against people with epilepsy [2]. He records that Sweden, in 1757, was probably the first country in modern times to legislate against marriage for those with epilepsy, and some US States still have laws making such marriages illegal, void or voidable on their statute books, though they are not enforced. Sterilization of epileptics, either voluntary or by court order, has also been practised in the past in many States. Even today, some countries, for example Australia, refuse immigration visas to people with epilepsy. However, attitudes towards epilepsy are probably changing, as was evident from surveys repeated in 1969 and 1979 [3]. In 1969, only 57% of people thought people with epilepsy 'should be employed like other people', whereas this had increased to 78% in 1979. In 1969, 68% would not object to having their 'children associate with people who had fits'. This had increased to 88% by 1979. This change in attitude hopefully reflects the growing understanding and knowledge that the general public now has about epilepsy. However, the disadvantage of such surveys is that responses may only reflect the attitude that the respondent believes he ought to have, and may not reflect his actions in real-life situations (p. 498).

This chapter considers only English law, not because of any chauvinistic ideas about its worth, but because a number of recent cases concerning epilepsy and automatism and aggressive acts have been appealed, and analysed in some detail. Furthermore, the author has no first hand knowledge of the legal systems and case law in different states and countries. It is hoped, however, that the arguments used in English courts may be useful to doctors preparing evidence in such cases in other countries.

Epilepsy. Edited by Anthony Hopkins.
Published in 1987 by Chapman and Hall Ltd, 11 New Fetter Lane, London EC4P 4EE.

19.1 EPILEPSY AND THE CRIMINAL LAW

Everyone who has reached the age of discretion is, unless the contrary is proved, presumed by law to be sane, and to be accountable for his/her actions. This is the doctrine of *mens rea*. 'Actus non facit reum nisi mems sit rea' – the deed does not make a man guilty unless his mind is guilty. This is the fundamental basis of the English law. To make a man liable to imprisonment for an offence that he does not know he is committing and is unable to prevent, is against the spirit of justice.

Unless the offence is a statutory one which carries an absolute liability (e.g. in the UK, driving with a blood alcohol level above 80 mg/100 ml), the doctrine of *mens rea*, or the presence of a guilty mind, can only be negated by three major considerations. Firstly, that the mind is not guilty because it is innocent, secondly, because the mind is diseased, and thirdly, because at the time of the act there was an absence of mind.

The defence of innocence is seldom used and is applied sometimes to mental subnormality, but is of little relevance to epilepsy. A defence of disease of the mind rests in England on the McNaghten Rules, which arose as a consequence of the case of Daniel McNaghten, tried in 1843. The House of Lords established that for a defence on the grounds of insanity to be successful, it must be clearly proved that *at the time of committing the act the party accused was labouring under such a defect of reason, from disease of the mind, as not to know the nature and quality of the act he was doing, or, if he did know it, that he did not know he was doing what was wrong.* This defence can only be used by patients with epilepsy who, at the time they commit an offence, have an associated mental illness. It might thus be used in people with epilepsy, who have for example, either a postictal or an interictal paranoid psychosis, and who at the time they commit their crime are suffering from an insane delusion. In these circumstances, epilepsy is very little different from any other functional psychotic illness. The rules applying to people with epilepsy in this instance are no different from those applying to the mentally ill population as a whole.

The law relating to epilepsy is, however, distinct, when we consider the third category of defence – that no mind was present at the time of the act. For it can be claimed that during an epileptic seizure the mind is absent, and so any action carried out is automatic. An act carried out in the absence of mind is known legally as an automatic act, and the defendant may wish to establish the defence of automatism. The legal definition of automatism and the medical definition of automatism are quite different, and must not be confused. This may be more clearly understood if it is recognized that the law has to deal with the protection of the public, as well as with the rights of the individual. The law is not overly concerned with the brain and its mechanisms. Medicine is concerned primarily with brain mechanisms, their disorder and cure, and is not unduly concerned with the rights of society and the protection of one individual from another. Thus although both the law and medicine use the same word – automatism – they mean different things.

19.1.1 Automatism

An epileptic automatism is defined medically as:

'A state of clouding of consciousness which occurs during or immediately after a seizure, during which the individual retains control of posture and muscle tone, but performs simple or complex movements without being aware of what is happening. The impairment of awareness varies. A variety of initial phenomena before the interruption of consciousness and the onset of automatic behaviour may occur' [4].

By that definition, automatisms are really very common, and can be divided into two groups: ictal automatisms, which occur during a fit, and postictal automatisms, which occur after a fit.

The accepted legal definition of automatism as given by Viscount Kilmuir LC [5] in the House of Lords Appeal in the case of Bratty v. Attorney General for Northern Ireland is as follows:

'The state of a person who, though capable of action, is not conscious of what he is doing . . . it means unconscious, involuntary action and it is a defence because the mind does not go with what is being done.' Viscount Kilmuir continued: 'This is very like the words of the learned President of the Court of Appeal of New Zealand (P. Gresson) in Reg. v. Cottle where he said: "With respect, I would myself prefer to explain automatism simply as action without any knowledge of acting, or action with no consciousness of doing what was being done".'

This definition is very close to the medical definition, and it would thus seem that the doctors and the lawyers are in agreement about what constitutes an automatism. This is, however, not so, because the law, unlike medicine, defines two types of automatisms: sane (*automatism simpliciter*), for example, sleepwalking, and insane (*automatism due to disease of the mind*), for example, resulting from arteriosclerosis. Either kind of automatism can be put forward as a defence and if accepted by the Court, will enable the defendent to plead not guilty. However, the consequences of a successful defence are quite different in the two cases. In the case of a sane automatism, the defendent will walk free from the Court. But in the case of an insane automatism the defendent does not go free, but must be compulsorily committed to a mental hospital for an indefinite period at the discretion of the Home Secretary.

19.1.2 Sane and insane automatism

The distinction between insane and sane automatism is arbitrary, and makes little medical sense. A review of several legal cases which have attempted to clarify this distinction, and tried to categorize epileptic automatisms, shows the extent of the confusion.

(a) Epilepsy is automatism simpliciter: Reg. v. Charlson

In the case of Reg. v. Charlson in 1955, epilepsy was defined as a non-insane automatism. At the trial of Charlson, the following facts were admitted: 'The accused, who was a shopkeeper, lived in a house, the backroom windows of which overlooked a river two feet deep. The accused called his 10-year-old son Peter into the back room, telling him that there was a rat to be seen standing on a stone in the river. When the boy came to the window, the accused picked up a wooden mallet from the floor, and struck the boy twice on the head, breaking the skin of the scalp and causing blood to flow . . . The accused thereupon picked the boy up and threw him out of the window.' In his summing up, Mr Justice Barry said: 'If he struck his son with the mallet, knowing what he was doing, and by those blows caused the injuries, then he is guilty . . . . If he did not know what he was doing, if his actions were purely automatic, and his mind had no control over the movement of his limbs, if he was *in the same position as a person in an epileptic fit* (my italics), then no responsibility rests upon him at all, and the proper verdict is, not guilty.' [6]

There was thus no doubt at that time that epilepsy was a sane automatism, requiring an acquittal and the defendant going free.

(b) Automatism due to disease of the brain is insane automatism: Reg. v. Kemp

In the case of Reg. v. Kemp, in 1956, held before Mr Justice Devlin, it was held that an automatic act could be a disease of the mind. Mr Kemp was accused of causing grievous bodily harm to his wife. 'During one night he made an entirely motiveless and irrational attack upon his wife, striking her with a hammer with such violence as to cause a grievous wound. The accused suffered from a physical disease, namely arteriosclerosis, or hardening of the arteries . . . It is a well recognized consequence of arteriosclerosis that it may lead to a congestion of blood in the brain due to a sudden rise of blood pressure. As a result of such a congestion, the accused suffered a temporary lapse of consciousness, so that he was not conscious when he picked up the hammer or that he was striking his wife with it. In that mental condition he was not responsible for his actions.' [7]

In his further discussion of the case Mr Justice Devlin continued: 'The broad submission that was made to me on behalf of the accused was that this is a physical disease and not a mental disease; arteriosclerosis is a physical condition primarily and not a mental condition. But that argument does not go so far as to suggest that, for the purpose of the law, diseases that affect the mind can be divided into those that are physical in origin and those that are mental in origin. There is such a distinction medically . . . The distinction between the two categories is quite irrelevant for the purposes of the law, which is not concerned with the origin of the disease, or the cause of it, but simply with the mental condition which has brought about the act. It does not matter for the purpose of the law, whether the defect of reason is due to degeneration of the brain or to some other form of mental derangement. That may be a matter of importance medically, but it is of no importance to the law, which merely has to consider the state of mind in which the accused is, not how he got there . . . Hardening of the arteries is a disease which is shown on the evidence to be capable of affecting the mind in such a way as to cause a defect, *temporarily* or permanently, of its reasoning, understanding and so on, and so is in my judgment a disease of the mind which comes within the meaning of the Rules' [7].

(c) Epileptic automatism is disease of the mind: Bratty v. Attorney General

Thus a malfunction of the brain leading to an automatic act was seen to be a disease of the mind even if it was temporary. So it was not surprising that when epilepsy was put forward as automatism simpliciter (sane automatism) in the case of Bratty v. The Attorney General of Northern Ireland, this was disallowed. In 1961, Bratty was charged with killing a girl whom he had taken for a ride in his car. He maintained that a 'blackness' came over him at the time of the killing, and that he did not know what he was doing. The medical evidence suggested that he might be suffering from psychomotor epilepsy, although a close reading of the medical history cannot possibly support this. The defence asked the jury to acquit the accused on a plea of automatism, or to find him guilty of manslaughter, or to find him not guilty by reason of insanity. The trial judge discounted the plea of automatism for lack of evidence, and Bratty was convicted of murder. The case on appeal reached the House of Lords on the question of whether or not the trial judge was correct in dismissing the plea of automatism. It is of interest that it was in this case that medical expert witnesses themselves suggested that epilepsy was a disease of the mind.

Lord Denning, in his opinion said: 'This brings me to the root of the question in the present case: was a proper foundation laid here for the defence of automatism, apart from the plea of insanity? There was the evidence of George Bratty himself, that he could not remember anything because "this blackness was over me". He said, "I did not realize exactly what I was doing," and added afterwards, "I didn't know what I was doing. I didn't realize anything." He said he had four or five times previously had "feelings of blackness", and frequent headaches. There was evidence, too, of his odd behaviour at times, his mental backwardness and his religious leanings. Added to this there was the medical evidence. Dr Sax, who was called on his behalf, said there was a possibility that he was suffering from psychomotor epilepsy. It was, he said, practically the only possibility that occurred to him. Dr Walker, his general practitioner, said you could not leave the possibility out of account. Dr Robinson, a specialist, who gave evidence on behalf of the Crown, said he thought it was extremely unlikely that it was an epileptic attack, but one could not rule it out. *All the doctors agreed that psychomotor epilepsy, if it exists, is a defect of reason due to disease of the mind* (my italics) and the judge accepted this view. No other cause was canvassed.'

Lord Denning said 'In the circumstances, I am clearly of the opinion that, if the act of George Bratty was an involuntary act, as the defence suggested, the evidence attributed solely to disease of the mind and the only defence open was the defence of insanity. There was no evidence of automatism apart from insanity' [8].

Lord Denning also discussed Mr Justice Barry's statement that epilepsy was automatism simpliciter (sane automatism) and not a disease of the mind (insane automatism). He says: 'that in Charlson's case, Barry J. seems to have assumed that other diseases such as epilepsy or cerebral tumour are not diseases of the mind, even when they are such as to manifest themselves in violence. I do not agree with this. It seems to me that any mental disorder which has manifested itself in violence and is prone to recur, is a disease of the mind. At any rate, it is the sort of disease for which a person should be detained in hospital rather than being given an unqualified acquittal' [8].

This case can be seen to state, both from the medical point of view and from the legal point of view, that an epileptic seizure should be considered a disease of the mind, and that crimes committed during an epileptic seizure could not use the defence of automatism simpliciter (sane automatism).

The case of Bratty v. The Attorney General for Northern Ireland was unsatisfactory from the medical point of view as a foundation case on which to base the concept that a violent act occurring during an epileptic seizure was an insane automatism; the accounts of the offence provide very little medical evidence that the act was committed during an epileptic seizure. Indeed, the defence recognized this by running simultaneously the defence of automatism, insanity or manslaughter. From the legal point of view, it was also unsatisfactory, as there were additional legal points which were being tested besides that of automatism alone. It was thus in the case of Regina v. Sullivan that the argument about whether an epileptic automatism was a sane or an insane automatism was first put to the test.

(d)　Appeal – epileptic automatism as disease of the mind: Reg. v. Sullivan

Sullivan, a man of previous good character, was an epileptic who suffered complex partial seizures with occasional secondary generalization from the age of eight. He had had two severe head injuries resulting in widespread brain damage, and some degree of change in personality. His major attacks ceased in 1979, and only the complex partial seizures remained. These seizures spread rapidly and bilaterally into both amygdala and hippocampal structures, so that Sullivan had no memory for the seizure or events immediately after the seizure [9].

During a partial complex seizure, Sullivan attacked and seriously injured an elderly neighbour. The seizures and the attack were witnessed, so that there was no medical doubt that the assault took place during an epileptic automa-tism, and this was accepted by both the prosecution and the defence. Sullivan wished to establish the defence of sane automatism (automatism simpliciter), and pleaded not guilty. The trial judge, His Honour Judge Lymbery, ruled that this plea was not available to the defence, and that if Mr Sullivan carried out the act during an epileptic fit, then he must plead not guilty because of automatism due to disease of the mind. If Mr Sullivan had pleaded 'insane automatism' and his plea had succeeded, as it undoubtedly would, it would have meant that the court would have had to send him to hospital, possibly a special hospital. Mr Sullivan's defence lawyers were not willing to risk this possibility, and so Mr Sullivan was persuaded to plead guilty to an act which he could not remember committing and over which he had no control. Because of the difficulty in which Mr Sullivan was placed by not being allowed the plea of sane automatism, the case went to the Court of Appeal, and finally to the House of Lords. The Appeal was rejected, thus confirming that in legal terms epilepsy is a disease of the mind, and that a criminal act perpetrated during an epileptic seizure is an insane automatism [9].

Commenting on the verdict of the House of Lords, Mr Lionel Swift who presented the Appeal, said: 'From the point of view of the administration of the law and justice to epileptics and others, the reasoning of the House of Lords is, with respect, impeccable . . . It matters not whether the impairment (of mind) is organic, as in epilepsy, or functional. It matters not whether the impairment is permanent or transient, or capable of control by drugs. Provided that (impairment) is his condition at the material times, he comes within the definition of being temporarily insane. At the time he committed the act, Sullivan was completely unaware of what he was doing and, therefore, he was insane at the time' [9].

(e) Present definition of sane and insane automatism: Reg. v. Quick

The definition of automatism simpliciter (sane automatism) was extended in the case of Reg. v. Quick, 1972. Quick, a nurse at a mental hospital, was charged with assaulting a patient while hypoglycaemic due to the effects of insulin. Quick was a diabetic, and on the morning of the assault he had taken his insulin as prescribed, drunk a quantity of spirits, but had eaten little food. He had no recollection of the assault. The trial judge, quite logically in view of Lord Denning's judgment in the Bratty case, felt that the defence of automa-tism simpliciter (sane automatism) was not available to Quick but that he must plead automatism due to a disease of the mind. This was, however, reversed in the Court of Appeal. The Court of Appeal cited Lord Denning's discussion in the case of Bratty and went on to record: 'If that opinion is right, and there are no restricting qualifications which ought to be applied to it, Quick was setting up a defence of insanity. He may have been, at the material time, in a condition of mental disorder manifesting itself in violence. Such manifestations had occurred before and might recur. The difficulty arises as soon as the question is asked, whether he should be detained in a mental hospital. No mental hospital would admit a diabetic merely because he had a low blood sugar reaction; and common sense is affronted by the prospect of a diabetic being sent to such a hospital, when in most cases the disordered mental condition can be rectified quickly by pushing a lump of sugar, or a teaspoonful of glucose, into the patient's mouth' [10]. Thus, the Appeal Court countered Lord Denning's argument that a disordered mind leading to an automatic act which was prone to recur must be a disease of the mind.

The Appeal Court also dealt with Justice Devlin's comments in the case of Kemp, [7], where he stressed the importance of the accused's state of mind at the time of the act, and not the underlying physiological mechanisms. 'Applied without qualification of any kind, Devlin J.'s statement of the law would have some surprising consequences. Take the not uncommon case of the rugby player who gets a kick on the head early in the game and plays on to the end in a state of automatism. If, while he was in that state, he assaulted the referee, it is difficult to envisage any court adjudging that he was not guilty by reason of insanity. Another type of case that could occur is that of the dental patient who kicks out while coming round from an anaesthetic. The law would be in a defective state if a patient accused of assaulting a dental nurse by kicking her while regaining consciousness could only excuse himself by raising the defence of insanity' [10]. They concluded . . . 'In this case Quick's alleged mental condition, if it ever existed, was not caused by his diabetes but by his use of the insulin prescribed by his doctor. Such malfunctioning of his mind as there was, was caused by an external factor and not by a bodily disorder in the nature of a disease which disturbed the working of his mind.' Thus the defence of automatism simpliciter, sane automatism, should have been allowed to Quick.

This case defines in English law the present standing of the difference between sane and insane automatism. Automatism simpliciter (sane automatism) occurs when the mind is disordered by an external factor such as an injection of insulin, a blow on the head, or the injection of an anaesthetic. An insane automatism occurs when the mind is disordered due to an intrinsic factor which leads to a situation that is prone to recur and may result in violence. Thus any organic condition of the brain or the body resulting in a disorder of the mind, even if temporary, is an insane automatism. This clearly leads to differences which appear to be nonsensical. For a violent act committed while the mind is disordered due to an excess of insulin is automatism if the insulin is injected, while it is an insane automatism simpliciter if the insulin comes from an insulinoma of the pancreas. It is this author's opinion that the distinction between sane and insane automatism is a meaningless one.

19.2 EPILEPSY AND CRIMINALITY

Not infrequently, hospital psychiatrists are called upon to decide whether or not a crime has been committed during an epileptic seizure, and whether or not the defence of automatism is one that can be substantiated by the medical facts of the case. Usually the offence is fairly trivial, for example shoplifting during either a postictal confusional state or during the automatism of a partial complex seizure. Occasionally, however, defendents may claim the defence of epileptic automatism when there is little evidence to support this. The psychiatrist should satisfy himself on the following six points before going to court to substantiate the diagnosis of epileptic automatism.

(1) The patient should be a known epileptic. It is clearly unlikely that a crime will be committed during a first seizure. Thus, unless there is overwhelming evidence, the diagnosis of epilepsy should be rejected if the act is said to have occurred during a first seizure. The case of epilepsy is strengthened if there is evidence that the patient is either subject to ictal or postictal automatisms (Chapter 18, p. 521), and that the behaviour described during the crime is consistent with behaviour that has been previously described during such an automatism.

(2) The act should be out of character for the individual and inappropriate for the circumstances. Clearly, if the defendent is habitually aggressive and commits a violent and aggressive crime, it is much more difficult to substantiate the diagnosis of epileptic automatism than if the act occurred in a patient who was mild mannered and tolerant. It is also important that the act should be inappropriate in the circumstances in which it occurred. A violent act of automatism during a fight, although it may occur, is less likely to persuade the court than one which occurs during a Sunday stroll.

(3) There must be no evidence of premedication or concealment. An epileptic automatism must arise *de novo* from ongoing behaviour. If there is any suggestion that there was preplanning for the act, then it is not possible to substantiate a diagnosis of automatism. Concealment is also unlikely after an automatism. On regaining consciousness, a patient emerges from a state of confusion or amnesia, and thus he is unlikely to register the full meaning of the events which have occurred. His natural response to such a situation is immediately to seek help, and not to conceal the evidence of any crime.

(4) If a witness is available, they should report a disorder of consciousness at the time of the act. Unfortunately, witnesses are not always available, but when they are, detailed questioning about the defendent's behaviour to establish a disorder of consciousness is essential. Features to seek are those of automatism; staring eyes, stereotyped movements, confusion, and evidence that the person was out of touch with his surroundings.

(5) Because the act occurs during an automatism or a postictal confusional state, a disorder of memory is the rule. It is unlikely that an epileptic automatism can occur in the setting of clear consciousness. Thus, memory for the act should be impaired.

(6) The diagnosis of automatism is a clinical diagnosis. Although weight will clearly be given to abnormal investigations, such as a focal lesion on the

CT scan or evidence of focal neuropsychological deficit or of generalized or focal EEG epileptiform discharges, none of these make the diagnosis of epilepsy. Epilepsy is a clinical diagnosis. Any physician who enters court unable to substantiate the diagnosis on clinical grounds alone is likely to find himself in trouble [9].

This chapter deals with the legal aspects of epilepsy relevant to the UK. Information regarding North American practice can be found in the publication *Legal Rights of Persons with Epilepsy*, 6th edn (1987). It is published by the Epilepsy Foundation of America, at 4351 Garden City Drive, Landover, MD 20785, USA.

REFERENCES

1. Temkin, O. (1945) *The Falling Sickness*, Johns Hopkins Press, Baltimore.
2. Gunn, J. (1981) Medico-legal aspects of epilepsy, in *Epilepsy and Psychiatry* (eds F. H. Reynolds and M. R. Trimble), Churchill Livingstone, Edinburgh, Chapter 13.
3. Caveness, W. and Gallup, G. (1980) A survey of public attitudes towards epilepsy in 1979, with an indication of trends over the past thirty years. *Epilepsia*, **21**, 509–18.
4. Frenton, G. (1972) Epilepsy and automatism. *Br. J. Hosp. Med.*, **7**, 57–64.
5. In *Bratty*, (1961) 46 Criminal Appeal Reports **1** at pp. 7–8 [1963] A.C. at p. 401.
6. The Weekly Law Reports. March 29th 1955. pp. 317–25.
7. The Law Reports. 1Q.B. Queen's Bench Division. (1957) *R. v Kemp*, pp. 339–408.
8. *Bratty* v. *Att. Gen.* for Northern Ireland. (1961) Northern Ireland Law Reports 1961. pp. 78–110.
9. Fenwick, P. and Fenwick, E. (eds) (1985) *Epilepsy and the Law – A Medical Symposium on the Current Law. Royal Society of Medicine International Congress and Symposium Series, No. 81*. The Royal Society of Medicine, London.
10. *R. v. Quick* [1973] 3 Weekly Law Reports p. 26.

CHAPTER TWENTY

Epilepsy and Driving

Anthony Hopkins and Peter K. P. Harvey

One of the problems that looms largest in the life of someone newly diagnosed as epileptic is their eligibility to hold a driving licence. Indeed much time during the first few consultations are, in our experience, taken up with discussion of this point. Although laws and regulations vary between different countries and political systems, virtually all developed countries do impose some restrictions in order to prevent injury to other road users caused by a driver's impairment of consciousness during a seizure. This chapter reviews (1) the evidence that the risk of an accident is increased if a driver has epilepsy; (2) the types of road traffic accident arising during seizures; (3) some of the different regulations in existence (basing this section largely on the UK Regulations); (4) the efficacy of such regulations; (5) the advice given by neurologists; and (6) certain special situations.

20.1 IS THE RISK OF HAVING AN ACCIDENT ACTUALLY INCREASED IF A DRIVER HAS EPILEPSY?

There are certainly good grounds for preventing some people with epilepsy from driving. Hierons [1] recounted some case histories of accidents caused by seizures. Millingen [2] estimated that 0.3% of all road traffic accidents in Tasmania between 1967 and 1975 were caused by an epileptic seizure. Waller [3] reviewed the experience of those *licensed* drivers with epilepsy in California – subjects who might reasonably have been expected to drive in reasonable safety. Table 20.1 is derived from Table 6 of Waller's paper. The observed accident rate was approximately twice the expected accident rate based upon

Table 20.1 Three-year accident and traffic violation rates for Californian drivers with *known* epilepsy compared to age-adjusted control drivers – per million miles

Accidents		Violations	
Expected	Observed	Expected	Observed
8.2	16.2	34	47

From Waller [3].

the experience of a group of Californian drivers not known to have epilepsy. The rate of traffic violations was, moreover, rather more amongst epileptic drivers. An earlier, less sophisticated study from Finland had also shown an excessive number of accidents by epileptic drivers [4].

Taylor, who is the Chief Medical Officer to the Department of Transport in the UK, reports on the medical background to 1605 accidents reported by the police in which the driver collapsed at the wheel, survived, and who was injured only to the extent that he could resume driving subsequently [5]. No less than 38% of such accidents were due to a witnessed generalized seizure. 'Blackouts' of an unspecified nature (but not clearly due to vascular disease or insulin-treated diabetes) accounted for a further 23%. Taylor estimated that about half of these 'blackouts' were epileptic in nature, making epilepsy responsible over all for 50% of such events. There must of course, as Taylor points out, be other cases in which subjects are severely injured or killed, and it is impossible to determine at autopsy whether a seizure occurred immediately before impact. Parsons [5a] reported that, of 92 patients who attended his clinic having lost consciousness or had a fit at the wheel, epilepsy was the cause in 42%.

All this evidence makes it clear that accidents not infrequently result from seizures, and make the imposition of some sort of restriction justifiable.

20.2 IF A DRIVER WITH EPILEPSY HAS AN ACCIDENT, IS THE TYPE OF ACCIDENT DIFFERENT FROM THAT EXPERIENCED BY OTHER DRIVERS?

As might be expected from Taylor's figures [5], a detailed analysis of accidents caused by epileptic seizures shows that single vehicle accidents – the car leaving the road, or colliding with a stationary object – are much more likely to occur to epileptic than control drivers. Figures from the Netherlands [6] are shown in Table 20.2.

Table 20.2 The features of 155 traffic accidents caused by epileptic seizures in the Netherlands, 1959–1968

	Drivers with epilepsy		Controls	
	No.	%	No.	%
Driver's car+immovable object	92	59	39 000	22
Driver's car only, i.e. 'off the road'	32	21	5 000	2.8
Involving other vehicles	30	19	134 000	75
Unknown	1	0.6	1 000	0.5

From van der Lugt [6].

20.3 WHAT RESTRICTIONS ARE PLACED ON DRIVERS WITH EPILEPSY?

Restrictions vary so much from country to country that all we can do here is to give some indication of the situation in the UK, as a model, and touch upon variations in other legal systems.

The current UK Regulations came into operation in April 1982 in *The Motor Vehicles (Driving Licences) (Amendment) (No. 3) Regulations 1982*:

'Epilepsy is prescribed for the purposes of section 87 (3) (*b*) of the Act of 1972 and an applicant for a licence suffering from epilepsy shall satisfy the conditions that—

(a) he shall have been free from any epileptic attack during the period of two years immediately preceding the date when the licence is to come into effect; or

(b) in the case of an applicant who has had such attacks whilst asleep during that period, he shall have had such attacks only whilst asleep during a period of at least three years immediately preceding the date when the licence is to have effect; and

(c) the driving of a vehicle by him in pursuance of the licence is not likely to be a source of danger to the public.'

Summarized, this means that a patient with epilepsy will be allowed to drive after demonstrating that for two years he/she has had complete freedom from epileptic events. If the attacks occur only while the patients are asleep then they may drive after three years during which time they have had only such seizures. This particular ruling leads to more misunderstanding than any others, and is often interpreted as meaning that a patient who has had a sleep seizure may ignore it as far as his driving is concerned. Nobody may hold a licence entitling them to drive heavy goods vehicles (HGV licence) or public service vehicles (PSV licence) such as buses, if they have had any epileptic event of any type, isolated or multiple, after the age of five. This is a recent concession to allow people who have had febrile convulsions to hold PSV and HGV licences. This Regulation recognizes the mileage covered by such drivers, the chances of further seizure activity occurring while they are at the wheel, and, in the case of public service vehicles, the chances of many people being involved in any accident caused by epilepsy. However, no such regulations apply to people such as commercial travellers who may spend a large proportion of their waking hours driving.

Patients in the UK presenting after a single seizure will lose their licence for one year, unless there is a predictable continuing liability to seizures, in which case they will not regain it until they have had no seizures for two years. This requirement is not specifically mentioned in the Regulations, but under (c) above is applied at the discretion of the Secretary of State for the Environment on the advice of his advisers in the Driving and Vehicles Licencing Centre

(DVLC). It is to the DVLC that patients in the UK who have had either one seizure, or who have developed epilepsy, are obliged to report themselves. Their driving licence is rescinded until they have been free for one year, two years, or three years. After this time, they may apply for the restoration of their driving licence. They will never again receive a driving licence current until age 70, as do the rest of the population. The licence will at first be subjected to annual review, and thereafter every three years.

Patients who are unhappy about the revocation of their licence have the right of appeal to an advisory panel of neurologists and neurosurgeons who advise the DVLC, and they have also the right of appeal through the local Magistrate's Court. In our experience, such appeals are often precipitated by inaccurate and conflicting advice given by doctors at the time of the diagnosis of epilepsy.

In the US the regulations vary from State to State, as little as three months freedom from seizures being required by a few, the majority requiring a year, and others two years. In Canada the two year rule applies.

Europe, Belgium, Denmark, Eire, Finland, France, Holland, Hungary, Luxembourg, Norway, Sweden, Switzerland and West Germany require two years of freedom from seizures, while Austria, Bulgaria, Czechoslovakia, Greece, Italy, Spain, Turkey and Yugoslavia do not allow 'people with seizures' to drive.

In the UK, subjects with epilepsy themselves have the responsibility of informing the licencing authorities. Seven states in the USA (California, Connecticut, Delaware, Indiana, Nevada, New Jersey and Oregon) require the doctor treating a patient with epilepsy to report that patient to the Licencing Authorities, by law. Furthermore, in Connecticut, any doctor knowing that a patient represents a hazard on the road is obliged to report that patient, irrespective of who is treating the patient. Although doctors in both systems of health care have long been accustomed to mandatory reporting of certain illnesses such as tuberculosis, the idea of mandatory reporting of epilepsy to legal authorities responsible for the issue of driving licences seems repugnant to many. It could be argued that patients, knowing that they are likely to be reported, may not seek medical help for conditions that might jeopardize their ability to drive. It has been argued that the breaking of confidentiality between doctor and patient leads to mistrust on the part of the patient, to the detriment of the standard of care that he/she will receive. There are other arguments: a doctor reporting his patient could, in theory, be sued for breach of confidentiality, but this has been protected by granting the doctor privilege in such circumstances in the US. In the UK both the major malpractice insurance organizations will defend such doctors vigorously. Indeed it is the advice of the Medical Defence Union that it is a doctor's duty to report a patient who he knows to be driving when medically unfit to do so, for the 'greater good'. A doctor failing to report a patient with epilepsy who is driving and who is involved in an accident could be responsible for claims by an injured party. This has happened in the US: in a state where it was mandatory for doctors to report patients with epilepsy, one had failed to do so, his patient was involved in a crash, and other injured parties sued the doctor. In two recent forums of British neurologists it was the overwhelming consensus that neurologists should not report patients, despite the advice of the British Medical Association Ethical Committee that it was their responsibility to do so.

The arguments that can be used with a patient in an attempt to convince him that he should not drive are many. Subjects may be asked to anticipate their response if one of their children were to be killed by another driver, or by themselves as a result of an epileptic attack. The more cold blooded assurance that involvement in any accident, whatever the cause, will render the driver's insurance null and void if they are driving illegally is often similarly effective.

20.4 HOW EFFECTIVE ARE SUCH RESTRICTIONS?

Table 20.3 reviews Millingen's experience from Tasmania [2]. Eight out of the 43 accidents (19%) due to a seizure resulted, at least allegedly, from a first ever seizure. In Taylor's series [5] 11% were due to a first seizure. Clearly these attacks cannot be prevented. However, the vast majority of accidents resulting from seizures occur as a result of epilepsy not previously admitted (77% of the Tasmanian series and 82% of the UK series). Clearly no regulation will prevent accidents due to epilepsy if the epilepsy is undeclared.

The worth of sensible assessment and restriction of drivers with known epilepsy can also be judged from the Tasmanian experience (Table 20.4). Using criteria similar to the UK criteria (p. 565), no patient initially approved to drive had a subsequent seizure or accident. Even amongst those about whom there were some reservations, only five of 50 had a subsequent seizure, in two cases resulting in an accident [2].

There is good evidence that many currently ineligible people with epilepsy are driving. There is a shortfall of people declaring epilepsy when applying for a licence compared to the expected figures derived from known figures of incidence and prevalence [3, 5]. There is a mismatch between referrals to an

Table 20.3 Accidents due to epileptic seizures in Tasmania, 1967–1975

	No.
Accidents resulting from epileptic seizure (0.3% of total number of accidents in that period)	43
Accidents as a result of epilepsy not previously admitted	33
Accidents as a result of first seizure	8
Accidents as a result of a seizure in licensed driver with epilepsy	2

From Millingen [2].

Table 20.4 Worth of sensible assessment of drivers with known epilepsy in Tasmania, 1967–1975

Drivers with epilepsy		Subsequent seizure
Initially approved to drive	122	0
Initially unacceptable	83	
Ultimately approved	50	5*

*In two cases resulting in an accident.
From Millingen [2].

EEG department for definite epilepsy, and the numbers of these patients subsequently found from licensing authority records to hold a driving licence. From such a study by Maxwell and Leyshon [7] it was estimated that nine out of ten people with epilepsy applying for a licence concealed their epilepsy. There is a difference between information given in different social situations. On examination for military service in the Netherlands in 1966 and 1967, 1268 men claimed to have epilepsy. Five years later, 699 held a driver's licence, of whom only 65 (19%) had admitted epilepsy in answer to a direct question on the application form [8]. Finally, when enquiry about driving, with promised confidence, is made of people with epilepsy, driving is often admitted. In one community survey [9] nineteen of 62 subjects (31%) currently ineligible to hold a licence under British Regulations, admitted that they were driving.

Mandatory reporting does not necessarily improve the situation. In California, only a quarter of people with epilepsy who were driving had been reported by their physicians [10].

20.5 WHAT ADVICE IS GIVEN BY NEUROLOGISTS TO DRIVERS WITH EPILEPSY?

It might be thought that those countries or States with regulations or restrictions on epilepsy and driving would have defined the conditions in such a way that physicians and people with epilepsy could be in no doubt as to what is intended. However, a survey by these authors in 1983 showed areas of gross confusion [11, 12]. These authors submitted clinical vignettes of patients with seizure problems to all members of the Association of British Neurologists, inviting their views as to whether the subjects of the vignettes should drive. For example:

'An engineer of 40 had ten grand mal seizures between the ages of 10 and 22, when his medication was changed to phenytoin 400 mg daily, and he had no more seizures. He holds a current driving licence. He is admitted to hospital for a minor surgical procedure, and the house surgeon orders his serum phenytoin to be estimated. This is 100 μmol/l. Despite there being no evidence of clinical toxicity, he reduces the dosage to 200 mg daily. Ten days later the engineer has a grand mal seizure while awake. He immediately goes back to taking 400 mg of phenytoin a day and consults you a few weeks later having had no further seizures. When may he drive?'

Faced with this credible clinical vignette, 20% of responding British neurologists wrote that the engineer could drive at once, 4% after three months, 22% after six months, 11% after one year and 39% after three years. Similar marked variations in the understanding of the Regulations, and in the advice given, was encountered in the response to other vignettes. Faced with this confusion amongst experienced neurologists, it is not surprising that many primary care physicians and their patients with epilepsy are also confused. Indeed, many patients with epilepsy probably use such professional confusion to negotiate a situation in which they can believe that they have been told that they can drive.

20.6 CERTAIN SPECIAL SITUATIONS

In our experience, confusion between people with epilepsy, their physicians and neurologists and legal regulations arise in the following areas:

(1) A surprising number of patients say that they 'have never had an attack while driving'. This statement, of course, logically offers no prediction about future events.

(2) 'I always know when I am going to have an attack.' This often may be true, but there is good evidence that cognition may be impaired during the initial symptoms (auras) of partial seizures (p. 2). Furthermore, seizures may become secondarily generalized with a latency that varies in the same subject.

(3) 'I only have minor attacks.' The same arguments apply as in (2) above.

(4) 'I must drive for my work/to get the children to school, etc.' Personal inconvenience does not overrule the Regulations, or safety.

(5) 'The only attacks I've had were brought on by stress, and I'm much more relaxed now.' This statement is possibly true but irrelevant to the Regulations; the effect of stress in precipitating seizures in any event is probably overrated (pp. 131–33).

Other problems which confront neurologists are:

(6) The lack of definition of 'epilepsy' in most statutory regulations, which encourages confusion about what to advise after the first seizure, which some consider insufficient to make a diagnosis of epilepsy (see Chapter 1).

(7) The special case of seizures occurring only during sleep. There is good evidence that, of those who initially have attacks only during sleep, a substantial proportion eventually have attacks whilst awake [13]. In spite of

this, some regulations allow concessions to those whose seizures have hitherto occurred only during sleep.

(8) Seizures occurring as a result of an acute neurological illness, or following the ingestion of certain drugs such as amitriptyline which are known to precipitate seizures. If the precipitating drug is withdrawn, the 'epileptic' status of the patient, and the legitimacy of his driving, is unclear. The problem of seizures recurring after cessation of, or a reduction in, medication has already been mentioned in the vignette on p. 568.

(9) Finally, there remains those patients at risk from seizures. Examples include patients after a craniotomy for a middle cerebral artery aneurysm that has bled, or after a head injury into a depressed fracture and dural tear. As Chapter 13 demonstrates, such patients may have a substantial risk of later epilepsy, and their first seizures may possibly occur while driving. Not every set of Regulations includes such subjects; in Britain a driving licence contains the statement 'You are required by law to inform Drivers and Vehicle Licencing Centre, Swansea, at once if you have any disability which is *or may become* likely to affect your fitness as a driver'. If the medical advisers consider that the risk of seizures following trauma or craniotomy is significant, then the licence may be revoked, even if no seizures have occurred.

Finally, there is the problem of the results of investigations, such as electroencephalography, which do not reliably provide information about the probability of relapse, and which few, if any, statutory regulations take into consideration. However, our experience is that, after a first seizure, the Department of Transport in the UK often makes enquiry about the results of such investigations, and various quasi-official publications suggest that such results are relevant.

REFERENCES

1. Hierons, R. (1956) The epileptic driver. *Lancet*, **i**, 206–7.
2. Millingen, K. S. (1976) Epilepsy and driving. *Proc. Aust. Assoc. Neurol.*, **13**, 67–72.
3. Waller, J. A. (1967) Chronic medical conditions and traffic safety. *N. Engl. J. Med.*, **273**, 1413–20.
4. Hormio, A. (1961) Does epilepsy mean higher susceptibility to road traffic accidents? *Acta Psychiatr. Scand.*, **150** (Suppl.), 210–12.
5. Taylor, J. F. (1983) Epilepsy and other causes of collapse at the wheel, in *Driving and Epilepsy – And Other Causes of Impaired Consciousness (Royal Society of Medicine, International Congress and Symposium Series, Vol. 60)* (eds R. B. Godwin-Austen and M. L. E. Espir), Royal Society of Medicine, London, pp. 5–7.
5a. Parsons, M. (1986) Fits and other causes of loss of consciousness while driving. *Qtly. J. Med.*, **58**, 295–304.
6. Van der Lugt, P. J. M. (1975) Traffic accidents caused by epilepsy. *Epilepsia*, **16**, 747–51.
7. Maxwell, R. D. H. and Leyshon, G. E. (1971) Epilepsy and driving. *Br. Med. J.*, **3**, 12–15.

8. Van der Lugt, P. J. M. (1975) Is an application form useful to select patients with epilepsy who may drive? *Epilepsia*, **16**, 743–6.

9. Hopkins, A. P. and Scambler, G. (1977) How doctors deal with epilepsy. *Lancet*, **i**, 183–6.

10. Quaglieri, C. E. (1977) The epileptics' compliance with motor vehicle laws. *J. Legal Med.*, **5**, 8AA–8BB; reported in Masland, R. L. (1985) in *The Epilepsies* (eds R. J. Porter and P. L. Morselli), Butterworths, London, pp. 356–75.

11. Harvey, P. and Hopkins, A. (1983) Views of British neurologists on epilepsy, driving and the law. *Lancet*, **i**, 401–4.

12. Harvey, P. and Hopkins, A. (1983) Neurologists, epilepsy and driving, in *Driving and Epilepsy – And Other Causes of Impaired Consciousness (Royal Society of Medicine, International Congress and Symposium Series, Vol. 60)* (eds R. B. Godwin-Austen and M. L. E. Espir), Royal Society of Medicine, London, pp. 9–15.

13. Gibberd, F. B., Bateson, R. C. (1974) Sleep epilepsy: its pattern and prognosis. *Br. Med. J.*, **2**, 403–5.

Index

Page numbers in italics refer to illustrations